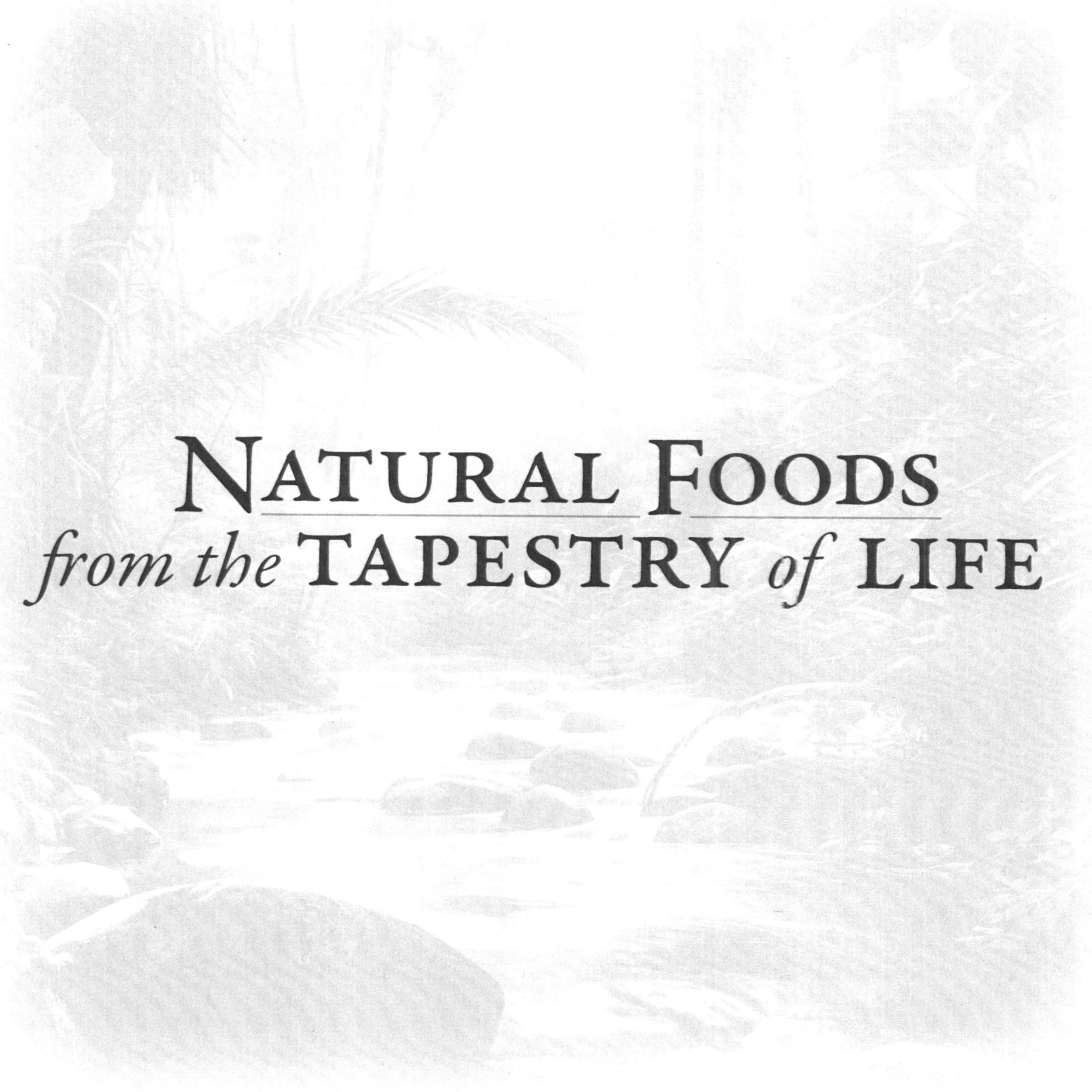

NATURAL FOODS *from the* TAPESTRY *of* LIFE

Natural Foods *from the* Tapestry *of* Life is intended solely for informational and educational purposes, and not as medical advise. Please consult a medical or health professional if you have questions about your health.

First Printing 2025.
Second Printing 2026.

Printed in the United States of America
ISBN: 979-8-9985183-0-0
Library of Congress Control Number: 2025907839

Published by Nutrition in a Nutshell, LLC, Amy J. Wing, Founder and Owner
Book Design: Eagle Lady Design Studio, Sandra L. Jones
Cover Illustration: Rima Al Turk, ©Dreamstime.com
Published in Prescott, Arizona, United States of America

Nutrition in a Nutshell, LLC

NutritioninaNutshell.com
Visit our website to find:

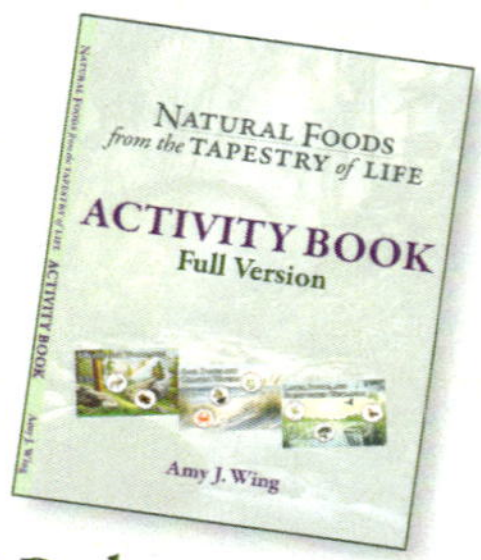

- **Natural Foods *from the* Tapestry *of* Life and companion ACTIVITY BOOK–Full Version**

  Nutrition Charts and Natural Foods Sticker Gift Package

  These exquisite and detailed educational materials are designed for educators and anyone studying nature and holistic health

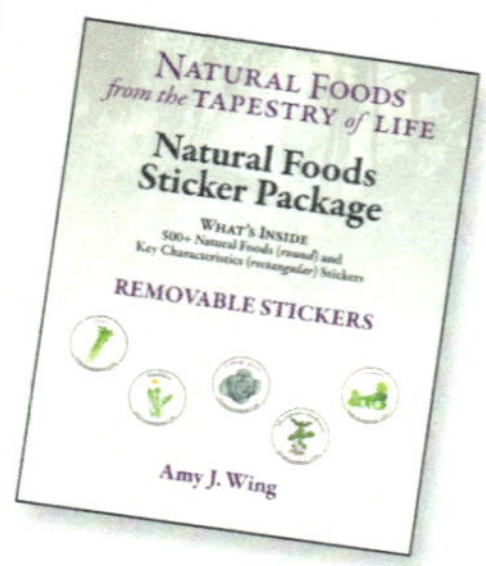

- **Organic, regenerative farm store links to traditional, artisan-prepared natural foods**

DEDICATION

The *Tapestry* books are dedicated to individuals and families who seek the benefits of natural health. Furnishing a compendium of resources, these books describe the high-quality nourishment that can be obtained from traditionally-prepared foods and offer a unique opportunity to study the breadth of natural foods' health-giving properties.

Author Amy J. Wing

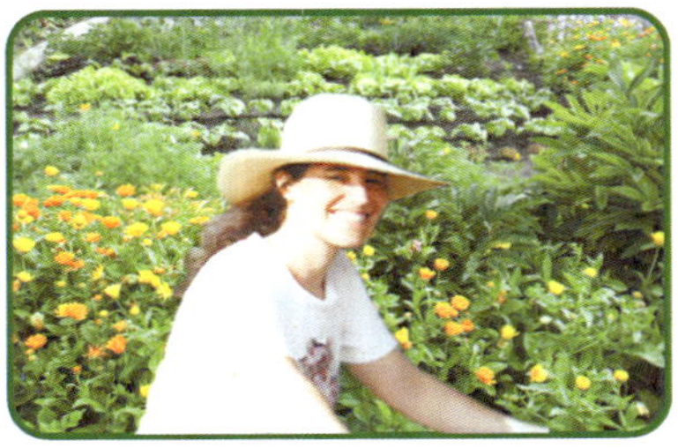

Amy is the founder of Nutrition in a Nutshell, LLC. She has a Master of Science in Health and Nutrition Education degree from Hawthorn University, California, and a Master of Arts in Interdisciplinary Studies degree–with an emphasis in biodiversity conservation–from George Mason University, Virginia. Amy has 30 years of experience as an ecologist, National Wildlife Refuge System planner, and trainer working for the U. S. Fish and Wildlife Service. Throughout her career, she worked on family farms in Arizona, Kansas, Maine, Ohio, Scandinavia, Washington, and West Virginia. Amy has studied how the field of natural health has taken shape over the last century and draws on the sound principles of natural healing in writing about natural foods.

Designer and Illustrator Sandra L. Jones

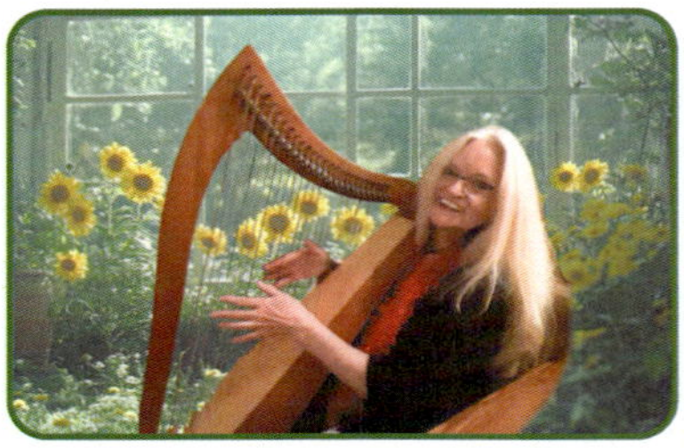

Sandy is an award winning graphic designer. She has successfully designed for authors and businesses for more than four decades, as the designer, illustrator, and owner of Eagle Lady Design Studio. With positivity and confidence, Sandy brings creativity and 'madskillz' to her work for all of her clients. She has an MBA in Marketing, a BA in Graphic Design, and an AA in Fine Art. Additionally, she has completed the UCLA Extension Certificate Program, majoring in Graphic Design, Computer Graphics, and Multimedia. Sandy's vision is for all her clients' designs to unfold as innovative and compelling. She focuses on launching clients' businesses and books from a winning vantage point.

FOREWORD

"As a physician deeply committed to integrative and naturopathic medicine, it's a true honor to write the foreword for this inspiring work. This book is a heartfelt blend of wisdom and science—one that empowers readers to take charge of their health using nature's pharmacy. Amy's passion for holistic wellness shines through every page, offering practical, evidence-informed insights on vitamins, herbs, and healing traditions. It's more than a guide—it's an invitation to reconnect with the body's innate ability to heal."

Your natural partner in health,
Dr. Linda Khoshaba, NMD, FABNE

Specialized Relationships in Richly Diverse Tropical Rainforests

Brazil nuts are a nourishing forest food. They are the seeds of the Brazil nut tree and grow in clusters high up in the canopy. Towering above other trees in tropical rainforests, Brazil nut trees have adapted essential and intricate relationships with several species in their natural habitat, illustrated below.

(Read about these symbiotic relationships on page 78)

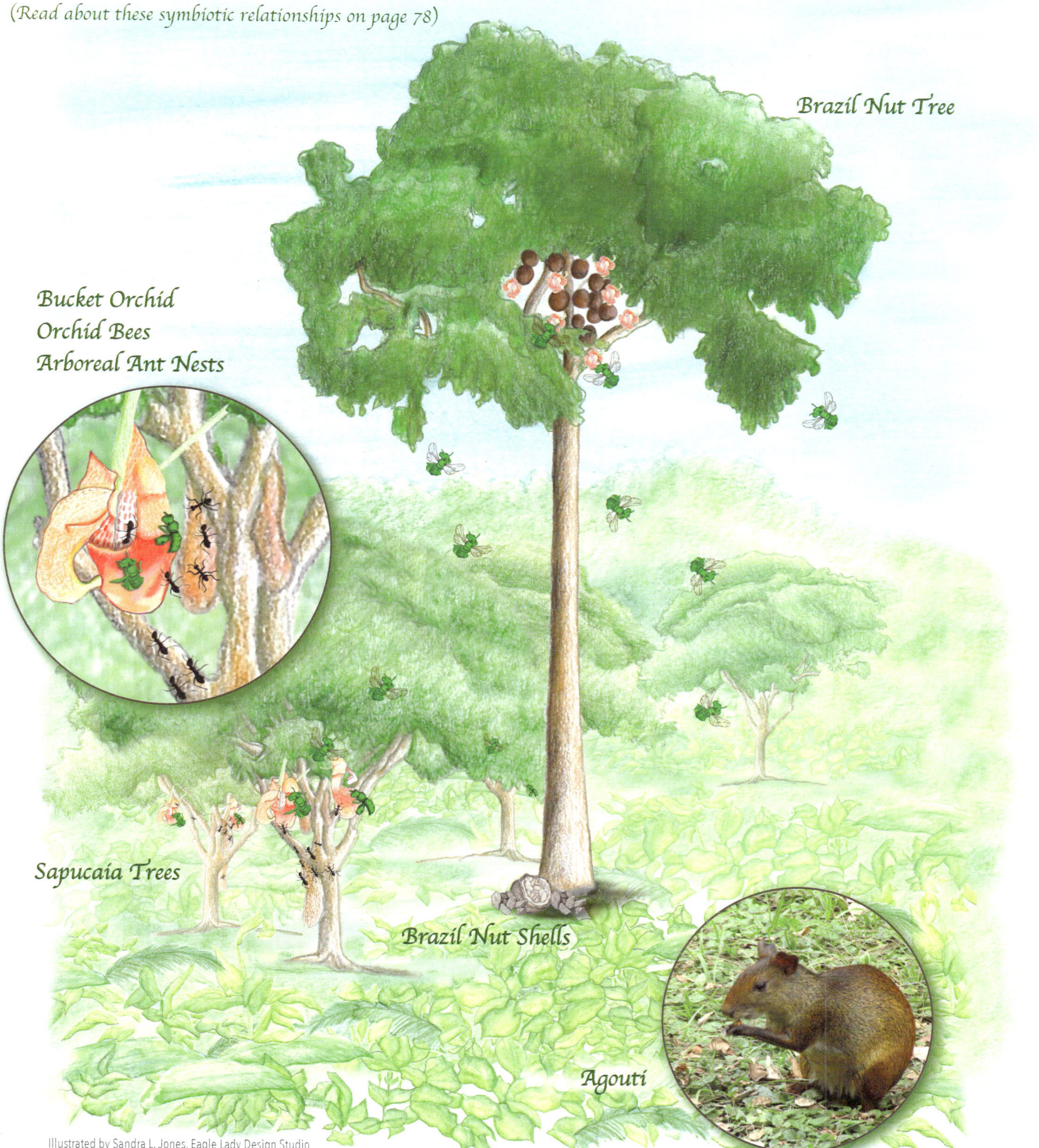

Illustrated by Sandra L. Jones, Eagle Lady Design Studio
Photography by Cleverson Felix, © Dreamstime.com, ants illustrated by Andjelka Simic, © Dreamstime.com

CONTENTS

PART I
Introduction **3**
Nourishing Traditional Foods **5**

PART II
Foods *from* Nature **17**

PART III
The Tapestry *of* Life **57**

PART IV
Nutrient Library **111**

PART V
Study Of **169**

PART VI
Natural Foods Support *the* 11 Systems *of the* Body **179**

PART VII
Human Health *and* Homeostasis **205**

PART VIII
Natural Living **213**

PART IX
Planning Nourishing Meals **243**

PART X
Inspiration **281**

282 Appendix: Federal Natural Resources Conservation Statutes

291 Special Thank You and Acknowledgements

295 Reference for Companion **ACTIVITY BOOK**

Living Vibrantly

Sunshine, fresh air, clean water, nutrition, sound sleep, physical activity, and a nurturing community opens doors to our best health and enjoying what we love most in life.

PART I

INTRODUCTION

Our Long Relationship with Natural Foods

NOURISHING TRADITIONAL FOODS

A Lasting Foundation for Our Health

The Journey & Findings of Dr. Weston A. Price, D.D.S.

INTRODUCTION

Our Long Relationship with Natural Foods

As humans, we have depended on natural foods from the land and sea for ~300,000 years. Over that time, our species (*Homo sapiens*) adapted to the foods our ancestors hunted, pastured, fished, foraged, and cultivated. During a pivotal window of time, Weston A. Price, D.D.S. studied ancestral food practices in great depth. For over a decade, he traveled to diverse bioregions of the world and documented the traditional diets of indigenous people and their high immunity to disease.

Dr. Price's research began in 1931. At this time, airplanes became accessible for public transportation,[1] enabling him to cross continents to carry out his research. Advances were also made around this time in 35-millimeter (lightweight) cameras making it possible for him to efficiently document his work with photographs and film.[2,3] In conducting his investigations, Dr. Price observed that the ". . . displacing foods of modern civilization. . ."[4] were substantially undermining peoples' health. In his research findings and landmark book, *Nutrition and Physical Degeneration*, he shares what he learned from indigenous people about their time-honored selection and preparation of natural foods. Therein, Dr. Price informs us on the nourishment that nature provides and the remarkable potential for human health.

References

[1]Road Warrior Voices. (2016), January 10. *This is what it was like to fly in the 1930s*. USA Today. https://www.usatoday.com/story/travel/roadwarriorvoices/2016/01/10/this-is-what-it-was-like-to-fly-in-the-1930s/83283086.

[2]Lenshunters. (2021, August 23). *The birth of 35mm photography — Leica and Contax*. Lenshunters. https://lenshunters.com/history/35mm-photography-leica-contax.

[3,4]Price, W.A. (2019). *Nutrition and Physical Degeneration* (8th ed., p. xv, 1). Lemon Grove, CA: Price Pottenger.

NOURISHING TRADITIONAL FOODS

A Lasting Foundation for Our Health

The Journey & Findings of Dr. Weston A. Price, D.D.S.

NOURISHING TRADITIONAL FOODS
A Lasting Foundation For Our Health
The Journey & Findings of Dr. Weston A. Price, D.D.S.

I. INTRODUCTION

During the 1930's, Weston A. Price, D.D.S. (1870-1948) conducted a comprehensive study that revealed the types of food needed to build human health. For over a decade, he traveled with his wife and kindred soul, Florence, to some of the most remote places on Earth where they learned from different groups of indigenous people about their traditional diets that sustained them for thousands of years. In 1939, Dr. Price published his book, *Nutrition and Physical Degeneration*. Eighty years later in the 2019, David J. Getoff, Traditional Naturopath, Board Certified Clinical Nutritionist, and Fellow of the American Association of Integrative Medicine, stated, "*Nutrition and Physical Degeneration* remains the single most important treatise on human nutrition and dietary health ever written."[1]

Dr. Price's story begins in the backwoods of southern Ontario, Canada, where he and his eleven siblings grew up on their 200-acre family farm, homesteaded in the wilderness by their great grandparents. In 1893, he received his degree in dentistry at the University of Michigan in Ann Arbor, Michigan. While practicing at his clinic in Grand Forks, North Dakota, he became very ill with typhoid fever and nearly died. His eldest brother brought him back to the family farm and helped him recover his health. While home, his uncle took him camping and fishing, which included time at Lake Massanoga (now called Lake Mazinaw). Later, Dr. Price's grand-nephew, Donald Delmage Fawcett, wrote, "The fresh air, sunshine, good water, the salmon, trout, huckleberries, wild raspberries and probably small game, did Weston a world of good."[2] This experience instilled in Dr. Price a deep appreciation for nature.

Once Dr. Price recuperated, he opened a dental practice in Cleveland, Ohio. Here he began to see a decline in his patients' health, and it was not long before he noticed their decline coincided with the advent of modernization and the mass production of processed food. At the time, big agribusinesses were out competing and taking over small farms across the country. Small farms were replaced with vast fields of monocrops, mainly wheat, soybeans, and corn, and sprayed heavily with chemical fertilizers, pesticides, and herbicides. Factories were established to make processed food products distributed throughout the country in chain grocery stores. This included refined white flour, sugar, and salt and industrialized oils (such as cottonseed, canola, safflower, soybean, and corn) extracted at high temperatures and with hexane gas.[3]

Lake Mazinaw
Ontario, Canada

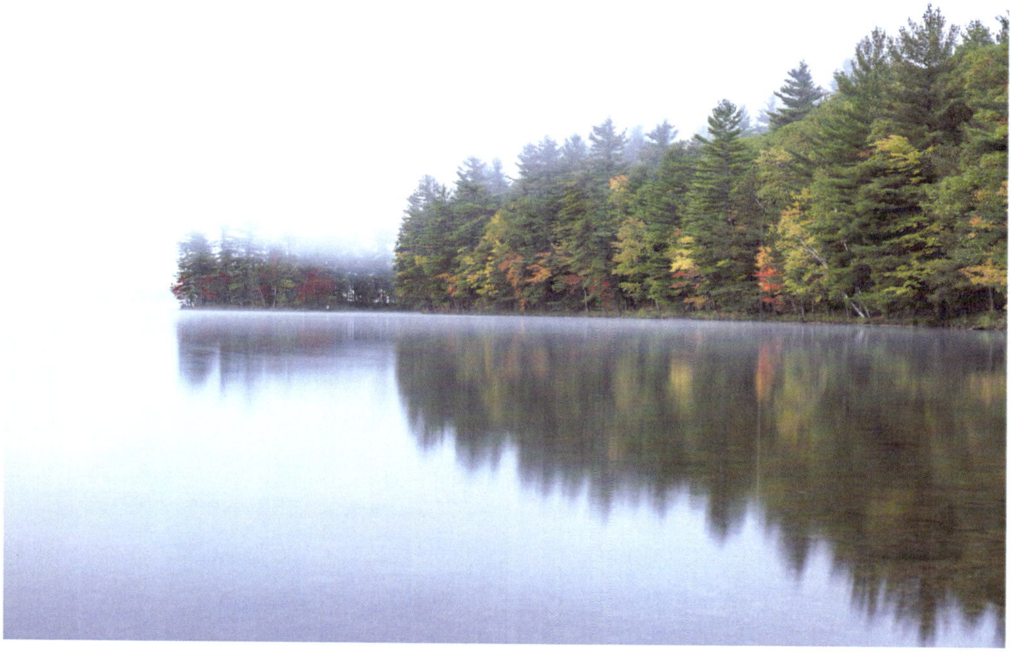

While investigating the cause of the degeneration in his patients, Dr. Price noticed that the results strongly indicated there was an "absence of some essential factors . . ."[4] He decided to take a positive approach and study first-hand the traditional diets of indigenous people who were known in the scientific literature to have high immunity to disease and degeneration.[5]

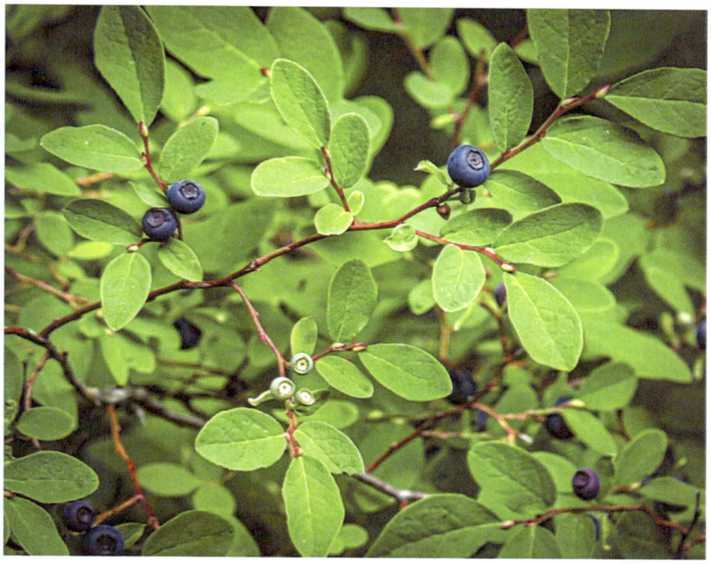

Wild Huckleberries

II. THE PRICES' JOURNEY

In 1931, financed by income from his dental practice, Dr. Price and his wife Florence dedicated themselves to the quest of studying traditional diets.[6] They made their way by airplane, steamship, railway, small river boat, truck, and on foot to meet with nomadic tribes and villagers who inhabited wilderness, untouched by modern society. Often traveling with interpreters, Dr. Price and Florence earned the trust of indigenous people everywhere they went. Receiving their consent, he conducted dental examinations of the individuals and was advised on what they ate and how they prepared their food. Dr. Price shared with them the results of his studies, relaying the wisdom he saw in their selection of foods for their health. He cautioned them about the degenerative consequences of the modern diet, evident in his research. Dr. Price's investigation included narrative reports and "some fifteen thousand photographs, four thousand slides, and many filmstrips."[7]

III. BIOREGIONS & INDIGENOUS TRADITIONAL DIETS

Dr. Price documented the condition of each individual in the indigenous groups. He consistently found that they had sturdy bone structure and ample room for straight teeth. In his comparative analysis of members of the indigenous groups who left their isolated communities and adopted the ". . . displacing foods of modern civilization. . ." Dr. Price discovered deformities, including narrowed skulls and dental arches, crooked teeth, and dental decay.[8] He wrote a summary of the traditional diets he studied, condensed below:[9]

- Switzerland Alpine Valley Swiss – exceptionally high-vitamin [raw] dairy products and sour dough rye bread; meat about once a week; vegetables as available, chiefly in the summer
- Outer Hebrides Islands off the Coast of Scotland Gaelics – sea foods; oat cake and oat porridge; limited vegetables in season; marine plants
- Alaskan and the Far North Eskimos and Indians – sea and land animals, including organs; limited vegetables; greens in season; very limited seeds
- Polynesian, Melanesian, and Micronesian South Sea Islanders – sea animal foods, marine and land plants, limited seeds, lily roots or taro
- African Cattle Tribes – [raw] milk, blood and meat, supplemented by plant foods
- African Agricultural Tribes – domestic animals, including their organs; fresh water animal life; insects; and a variety of plants
- Australian Aborigines – large and small wild animal life; wild plants; and, where available, fresh water or marine sea life, large and small
- New Zealand Maori – sea animal life; marine plants; marine birds, and their eggs; land birds; seeds of trees and plants; and vegetables, particularly fern root
- North and South American Plains Indians – organs and tissues of wild animal life, a large variety of plant foods, and fresh and salt water animal life
- North and South American Coastal Tribes – sea animal and plant life
- Amazon Jungle Indians – fresh water animal life, small land animals, birds, wild plants, and seeds

Of the fourteen indigenous groups Dr. Price researched, three of them from the following locations are described in detail on the next four pages: 1) Lötschental Valley in Switzerland, 2) Northern British Columbia and Yukon Territory of Canada, and 3) Amazon Jungle at the foothills of Peruvian Andes.

Alpine Village in the Lötschental Valley

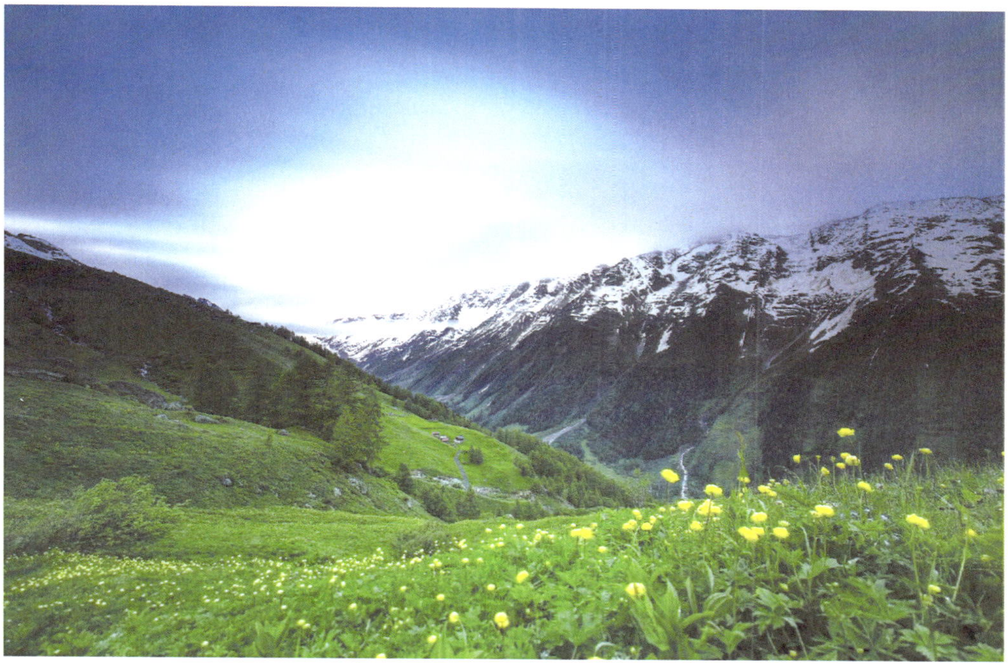

Lötschental Valley

Almost completely enclosed by three high snow-capped mountain ranges, the alpine Lötschental Valley in Switzerland was isolated for centuries. Shortly before Dr. Price and Florence arrived, an eleven-mile tunnel had been built which gave them access; and, a footpath took them the rest of the way. The villagers' foods were still produced locally except for a few items including sea salt.[10] Their traditional diet consisted of raw cow and goat milk, butter, cheese, and cream; rye sourdough bread; greens in the brief summer months; and meat once per week. In the summer, the cows followed the retreating glacial snowmelt, leaving the lower valley to be harvested for hay and rye. Cultured rye sourdough bread was a staple, eaten with raw cheese and milk. The superior quality of the first butter that was made after the cows reached their glacial pastures in June was a celebrated occasion every year in the villages of Lötschental Valley.[11]

In examining each of the individuals in the villages, Dr. Price found that these isolated communities, dependent on locally-produced natural foods, had nearly complete immunity to dental caries (cavities). He wrote that "Of all the children in the valley still using the primitive diet of whole rye bread and dairy products the average number of cavities per person was 0.3 percent."[12] Dr. Price found that the substitution of modern diets for these foods destroyed this immunity, whether in elevated areas or the fertile plains. He stated that the individuals in the modernized districts were found to have widespread tooth decay ranging from 85 to 100 percent.[13] Many had marked irregularity of the teeth with narrowing of the dental arch.[14] These conditions were associated with the use of refined white flour and a high intake of sweets, canned vegetables goods, sweetened fruits and chocolate, and greatly reduced use of dairy products.[15]

In 1931, the villages of Lötschental Valley were the first destination in Dr. Price's decade-long quest to study indigenous people living in remote locations that were untouched by modern civilization.

Moose in Yukon Territory

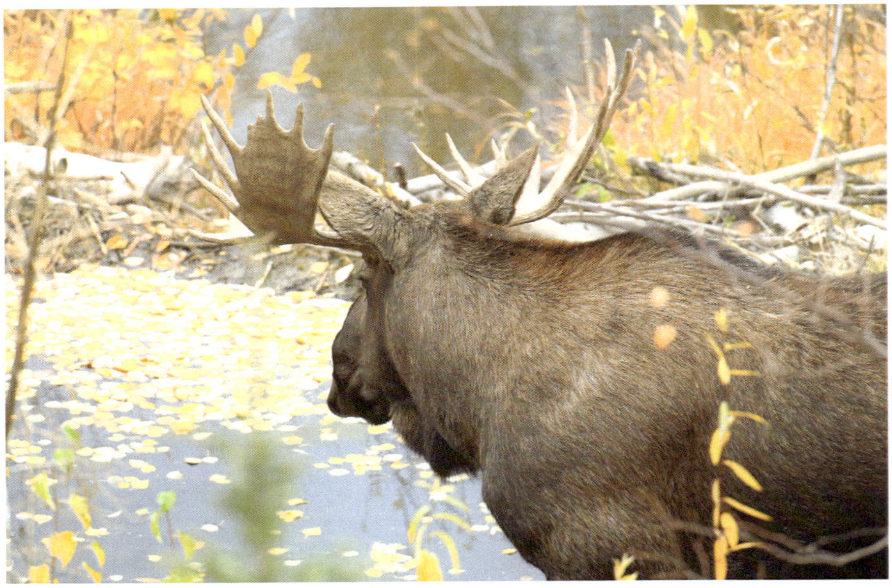

Northern British Columbia and Yukon Territory of Canada

One of the Prices' expeditions was to Northern British Columbia and Yukon Territory, beyond the Rocky Mountain Divide where the rivers flowed north to the Arctic. Once he and Florence arrived, they met with some of the nomadic tribes that followed the seasonal migrations of the moose and caribou. Dr. Price noticed that no animal life was accessible from the sea and farming was infeasible because of the extreme cold. The tribes' diets consisted almost entirely of wild animals, including the organs and tissues and particularly the walls of the second stomach and adrenal glands. Dr. Price noted that the adrenal glands in their diet contained more vitamin C than any other known plant or animal source.[16] In examining all the individuals of these northern tribes, Dr. Price found that each person was in superb health. He wrote, "Indeed, in several groups examined not a single tooth was found that had ever been attacked by tooth decay." In total, he found only 0.16 percent dental caries in these nomadic tribes.[17] In contrast, Dr. Price described their return, stating "As we came down the Stikine River to the Alaskan frontier towns, the dental caries problem increased to 40 percent of all teeth."[18]

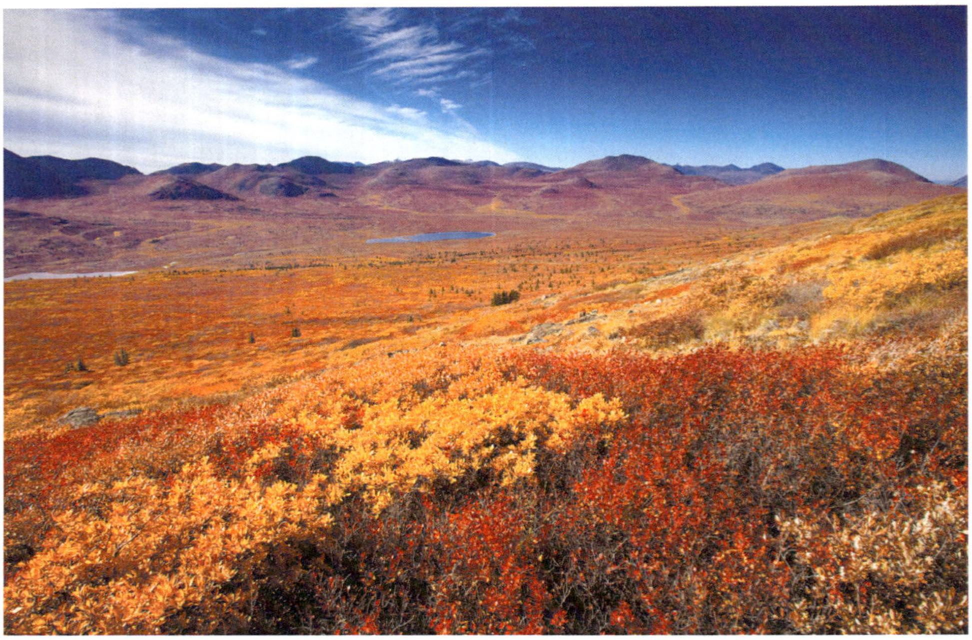

Yukon Territory
Autumn Tundra

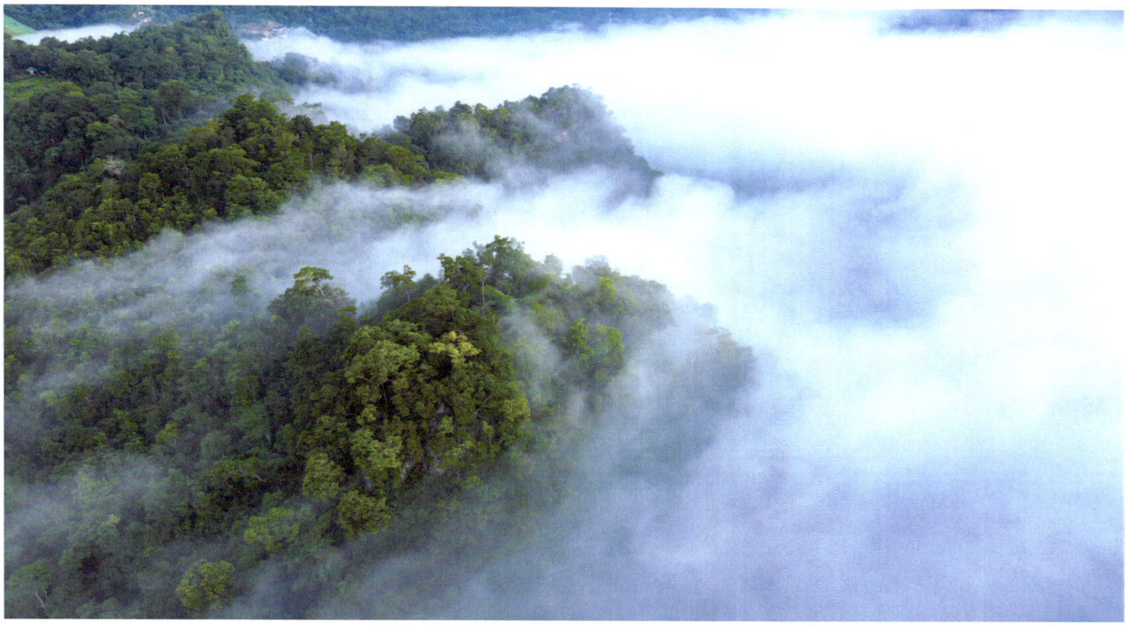

Morning Mist in the Amazon Jungle

Amazon Jungle

The Amazon Jungle on the eastern slopes of the Peruvian Andes was another destination for Dr. Price and Florence. Upon arriving, he described the area, "The abundance of rain, the fertility of the soil, and the warm climate make plant growth most luxuriant on the eastern slopes of the Andes."[19] Initially, they met with a tribe of thirty members from an isolated area of the jungle. Their diet consisted of abundant fish from the Amazon River and its branches; animal life from the forest and thickets; bird life, including many water fowl and their eggs; and plants and fruits. Andean yucca was commonly eaten.[20] In this tribe, Dr. Price did not find a single tooth that had been attacked by dental caries. However, in another related tribe whose members had converted to a modern diet, Dr. Price found rampant tooth decay and extensive loss of teeth.[21]

IV. TRADITIONAL DIETS CONFERRED HIGH IMMUNITY

Dr. Price found that the indigenous people who exclusively ate their traditional foods had high immunity to disease and degeneration. Their immunity not only protected their teeth but their health overall. Like the Northern British Columbia and Yukon Territory and Amazon Jungle tribes, the Lötschental Valley Swiss villagers had nearly complete immunity to dental caries; and whereas tuberculosis was absent from the Lötschental Valley villages, it was the most prevalent disease in the rest of Switzerland.[22]

Conducting a biochemical analysis of the food, soil, and saliva samples in his lab, Dr. Price identified the nutrients that were bringing these groups robust health and high immunity to disease, throughout all stages of life and from generation to generation. His research demonstrated that while the foods differed greatly among the indigenous groups, their diets were very similar when reduced to the mineral and vitamin content.[23] In a broader context, he stated, "We humans have the same rigid restrictions regarding food selection as the simpler forms of life when foods are evaluated from their chemical basis."[24]

Dr. Price documented how malnutrition was the cause of the degeneration in his patients and the indigenous groups he studied elsewhere in the world who had adopted industrially-processed food products. He stated, "Modern commerce has deliberately robbed some of nature's foods of much of their body-building material. . . For example, in the production of refined white flour approximately eighty percent or four-fifths of the phosphorus and calcium content are usually removed, together with the vitamins and minerals provided in the embryo or germ."[25]

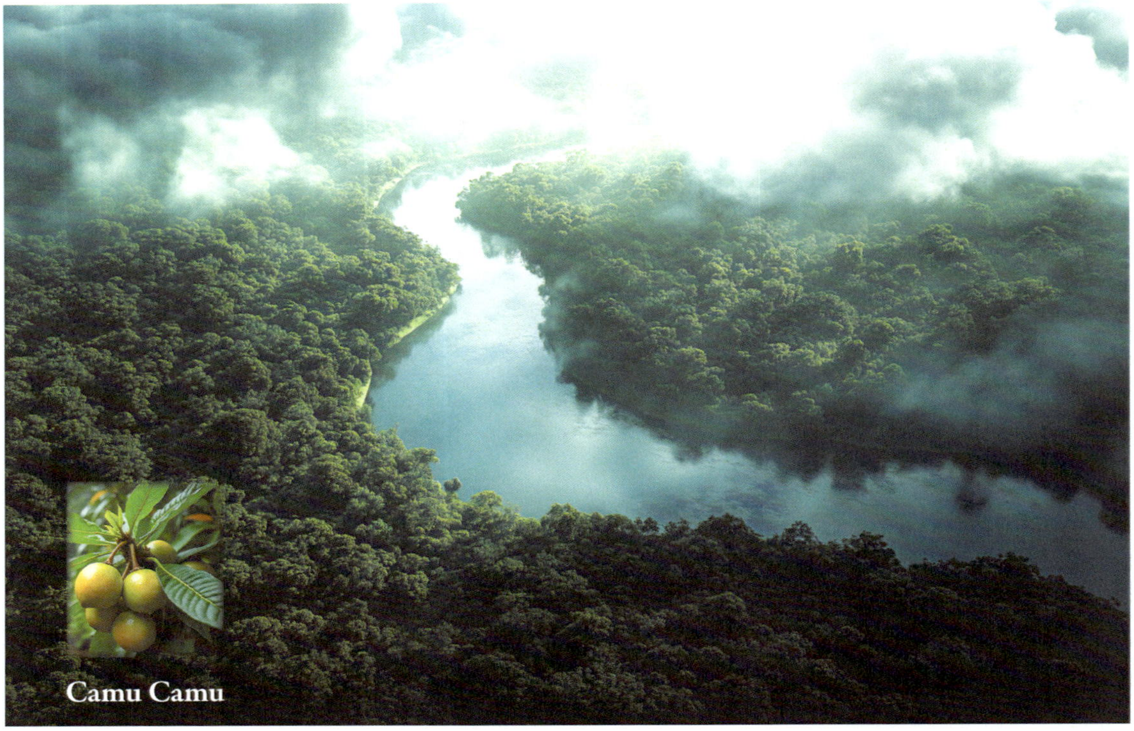

Amazon River Winding through the Rainforest

Based on what he learned, Dr. Price designed a program to restore health with traditional foods that he discovered built superb health and high immunity to disease.

V. NUTRITION PROGRAM TO RESTORE HEALTH

Dr. Price developed a nutrition program to restore teeth with incipient dental decay, concentrating on improving the chemistry of the saliva so that harmful acids and pathogenic bacteria no longer dissolved the tooth enamel. Eliminating the industrially-processed foods of the modern diet was imperative to improving the saliva chemistry. Once corrected, the saliva nourished the teeth rather than damaged them. Dr. Price's restorative diet encompassed high-vitamin butter from cows that pastured on early summer grasses and high-vitamin cod liver oil, seafood, the organs and bone marrow of animal foods, vegetables, and raw milk.[26] Based on all the traditional diets he studied, Dr. Price placed particular emphasis on the importance of the fat-soluble vitamins (A, D, E, and K), especially vitamin K_2 MK-4 which he called 'activator X.'[27]

VI. CHARACTERISTICS OF TRADITIONAL DIETS

In 1999, Sally Fallon Morell and Mary G. Enig, Ph.D. established the Weston A. Price Foundation (WAPF) to carry on the work of Dr. Price with an emphasis on research and education. The WAPF has local chapters around the world and advocates for small, organic, regenerative farms. Drawing on Dr. Price's research, the WAPF describes the Characteristics of Traditional Diets, condensed below:[28]

- Animal food, such as fish and other seafoods; land and water fowl; land and sea mammals; eggs; [raw] milk and milk products; reptiles; and insects. "The whole animal is consumed–muscle meat, organs, bones and fat, with the organ meats and fats preferred."[28]
- At least four times the minerals and water-soluble vitamins, and TEN times the fat-soluble vitamins found in animal fats (vitamin A; vitamin D; and Activator X, now thought to be vitamin K_2) compared to the average American diet
- Cooked animal foods and a portion of their animal foods raw
- High content of food enzymes and beneficial bacteria from lacto-fermented vegetables, fruits, beverages, [raw] dairy products, meats and condiments
- Seeds, grains and nuts are soaked, sprouted, fermented or naturally leavened to neutralize naturally occurring anti-nutrients such as enzyme inhibitors, tannins and phytic acid
- Total fat content varied from 30 percent to 80 percent of calories but only about 4 percent of calories come from polyunsaturated oils naturally occurring in grains, legumes, nuts, fish, animal fats and vegetables. The balance of fat calories is in the form of saturated and monounsaturated fatty acids.
- Nearly equal amounts of omega-6 and omega-3 essential fatty acids
- Natural sea salt
- Animal bones, usually in the form of gelatin-rich bone broths
- Special nutrient-rich animal foods for parents-to-be, pregnant women and growing children; proper spacing of children; and teaching the principles of right diet to the young

Dr. Price's findings about one hundred years ago are profoundly relevant today. Through his research, he identified the common characteristics of traditional diets that conferred excellent health and high immunity to disease. Traditionally-prepared, organic natural foods from the land and sea can be the bedrock for tailoring a nourishing diet for ourselves and our families. For example, traditionally-fermented natural foods contain probiotic bacteria and micro-fungi that make the nutrients more bioavailable and supply digestive, metabolic, and synthesizing enzymes that support the body's innate ability to achieve optimal health.

References

[1, 2, 4, 5, 6, 9, 10, 11, 12, 13, 14, 15, 16, 17, 18, 19, 20, 21, 22, 23, 24, 25, 26]Price, W.A. (2019). *Nutrition and Physical Degeneration*. (8th ed., pp. xxxv, xxxi – xxxii, 1, 1, xxxiii, 433, 22, 25, 25, 35, 36, 40, 69, 69, 71, 223, 228, 225, 39, 432, 424, 255, 392). Lemon Grove, CA: Price-Pottenger.

[3]WAPF. (2017). *The dangers of industrial fats & oils* [Brochure]. Washington, D.C.: The Weston A. Price Foundation.

[7]Price-Pottenger Nutrition Foundation. (1948). The classic studies of Weston A. Price, D.D.S. devitalized foods and physical degeneration, *Dental Items of Interest*, 70, 426.

[8]Fallon Morell, S. (2008). *Nourishing Traditional Diets: The Key to Vibrant Health* [Film]. Washington, D.C.: New Trends Publishing and More Productions.

[27]Schlinsog, D. & Schlinsog, E. (2023, December 7). *Vitamin K_2 MK-4 Dr. Price's activator X and its transformational potential.* Washington, D.C.: The Weston A. Price Foundation. https://www.westonaprice.org/health-topics/ vitamin-k_2-mk-4-dr-prices-activator-x-and-its-transformational-potential/#gsc.tab=0.

[28]Nienhiser, J. (2000, January 1). *Characteristics of traditional diets*. Washington, D.C.: The Weston A. Price Foundation. https://www.westonaprice.org/health-topics/abcs-of-nutrition/characteristics-of-traditional-diets/#gsc.tab=0.

Building and Maintaining Human Health with Nourishing Traditional Foods

Weston A. Price Foundation Dietary Guidelines:[1]

Characteristics of Traditional Diets (page 13)

and

Timeless Principles of Healthy Traditional Diets (page 253)

Tailor the diet, as needed, to remedy an illness or an allergy. For healing the digestive system and related ailments, reference the GAPS Diet (pages 231-233).

References

[1]Nienhiser, J. (2000, January 1). *Weston A. Price Foundation Dietary Guidelines*. Washington, D.C.: The Weston A. Price Foundation. https://www.westonaprice.org/health-topics/abcs-of-nutrition/dietary-guidelines/#gsc.tab=0.

PART II

Foods from Nature

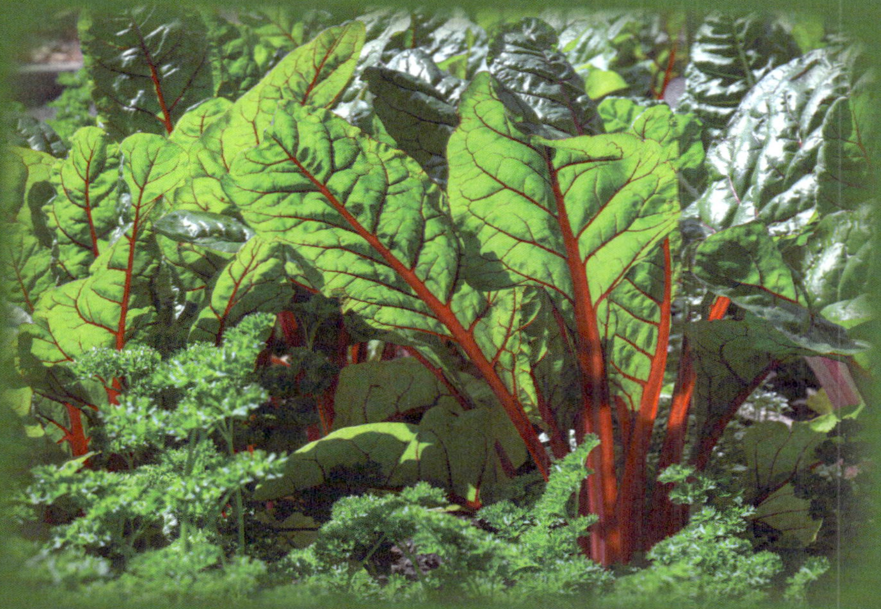

Animal

Animalia Kingdom

Plant

Plantae Kingdom

Mushroom

Fungi Kingdom

Algae

Plantae and Chromista Kingdoms

Probiotic

Bacillati (*Bacteria* Domain) and *Fungi* Kingdoms

Foods from Nature

Animal Foods - Seafoods

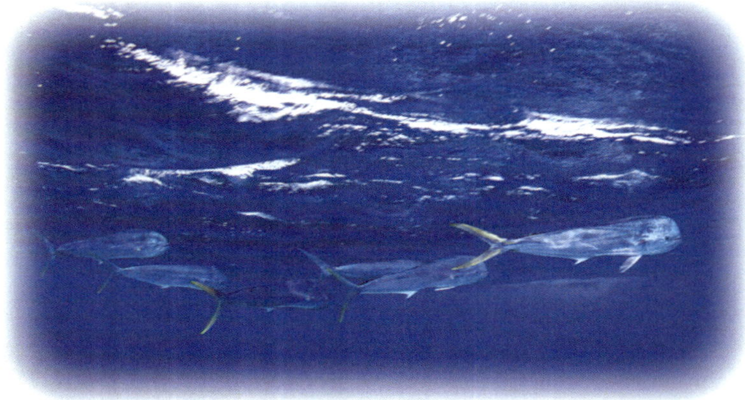

Kingdom: *Animalia*
Phylum: *Chordata*
Class: *Actinopterygii* (ray-finned fish)
Order: *Carangiformes*
Family: *Coryphaenidae*
Genus and species: *Coryphaena hippurus*
Common name: Mahi Mahi

Mahi Mahi are ray-finned fish that live near the ocean surface in temperate, tropical, and subtropical waters worldwide. They school together, feeding on mackerel; flying fish; squid; crabs, and other crustaceans. As part of the marine food web, they are hunted by seals, sea lions, tuna, marlin, swordfish, sharks, and toothed whales.

Kingdom: *Animalia*
Phylum: *Chordata*
Class: *Actinopterygii* (ray-finned fish)
Order: *Clupeiformes*
Family: *Engraulidae* (anchovies)
Genus and species: many genera and species
Common name: Anchovy

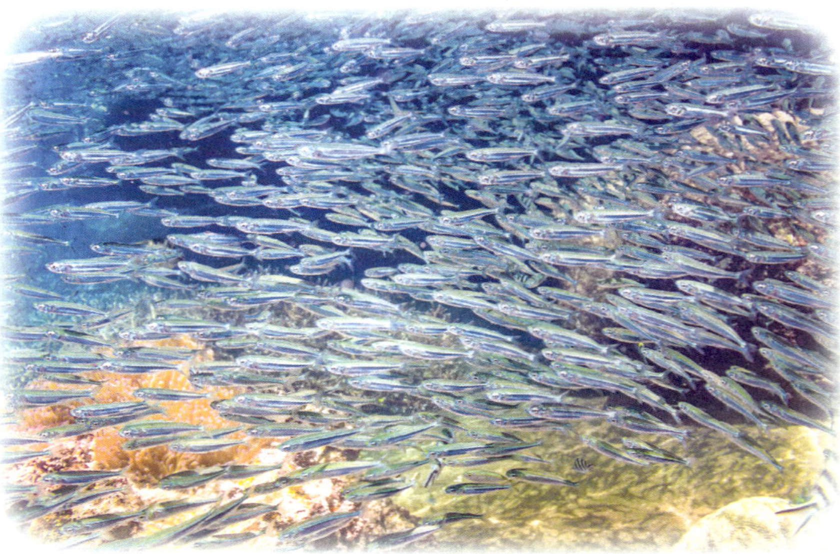

The anchovy family of small fish species inhabit shallow temperate and tropical waters. They are abundant in the open ocean, estuaries, and bays; additionally, a few species live in freshwater. Moving in schools, they forage for plankton, zooplankton, *copepoda* eggs and larvae.

continued...

Foods from Nature

Animal Foods - Seafoods

Kingdom: *Animalia*
Phylum: *Chordata*
Class: *Actinopterygii*
(ray-finned fish)
Order: *Clupeiformes*
Family: *Clupeidae*
Genus and species:
many genera and species
Common name:
Herring and Sardines

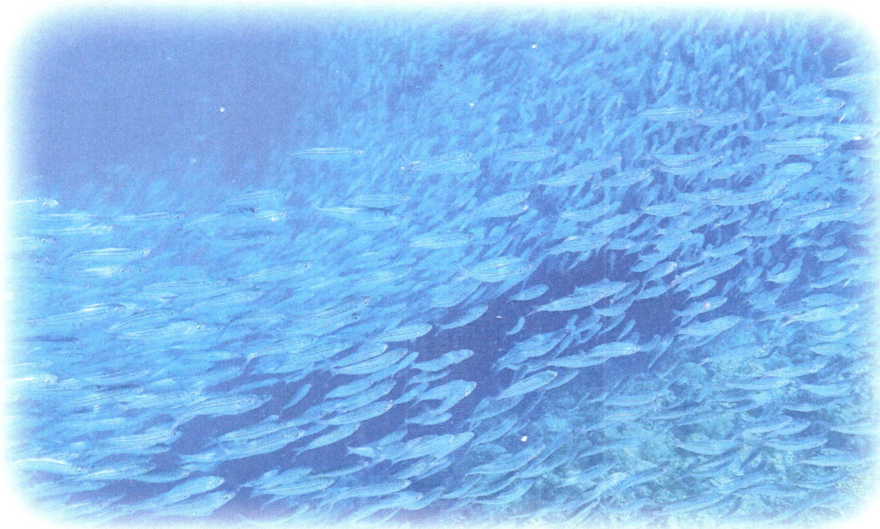

Sardines and herring are widely distributed throughout temperate, subarctic, and occasionally arctic oceans of the Northern Hemisphere. Both migrate to their natal waters. Like salmon, river herring are anadromous and return to spawn in the freshwater habitats where they were born. Coming inland via these rivers to spawn, the river herring bring life-sustaining nutrients into these freshwater ecosystems.

Kingdom: *Animalia*
Phylum: *Chordata*
Class: *Actinopterygii*
(ray-finned fish)
Order: *Gadiformes* (Cod)
Family: *Gadidae*
Genus and species: *Gadus*
(with a few species of cod,
including haddock:
Melanogrammus aeglefinus)
Common name: **Cod and Haddock**

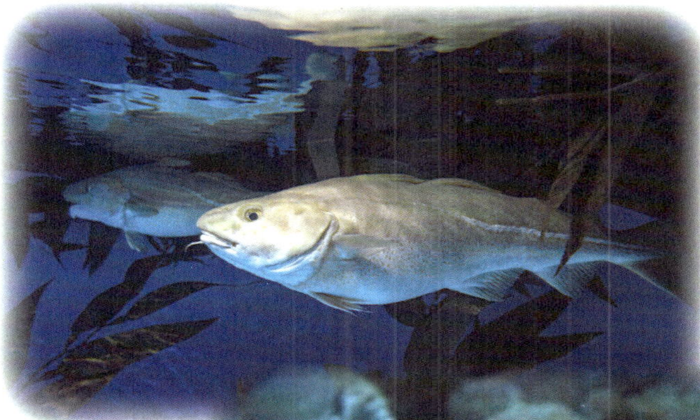

Cod

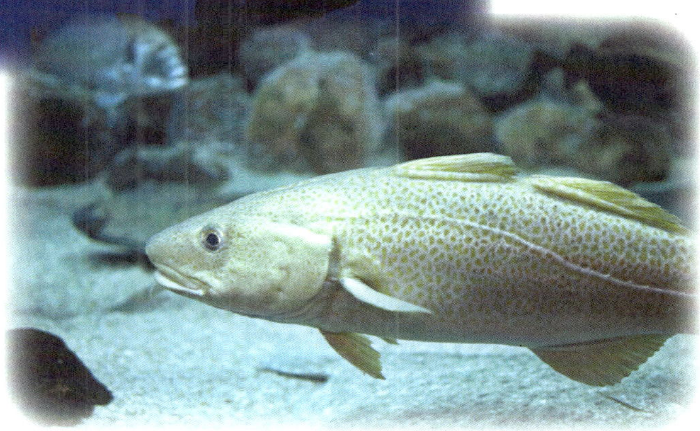

Haddock

Cod, including haddock are cold-water, ray-finned fish that live deep in the ocean. They live in temperate to sub-polar latitudes. Along the ocean floor, cod feed on clams, worms, shrimp, and small fish. They are also found along underwater rocky slopes and ledges. The females come to the edge of the continental shelf (submerged portion of a continent) to spawn.

continued...

Foods from Nature

Animal Foods - Seafoods

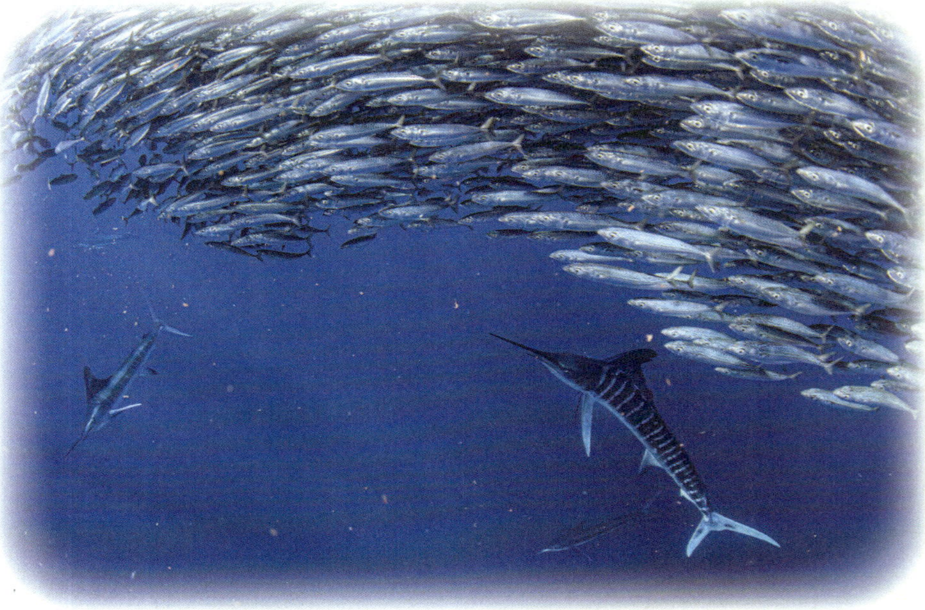

Kingdom: *Animalia*
Phylum: *Chordata*
Class: *Actinopterygii* (ray-finned fish)
Order: *Istiophoriformes*
Family: *Xiphiidae*
Genus and species: *Xiphias gladius*
Common name:

Swordfish

Swordfish, known for their long bill, are one of the largest and fastest predators in the ocean, with the ability to travel fifty miles per hour. They live in the open ocean (pelagic zone), feeding at great depths; and they migrate widely, covering thousands of miles.

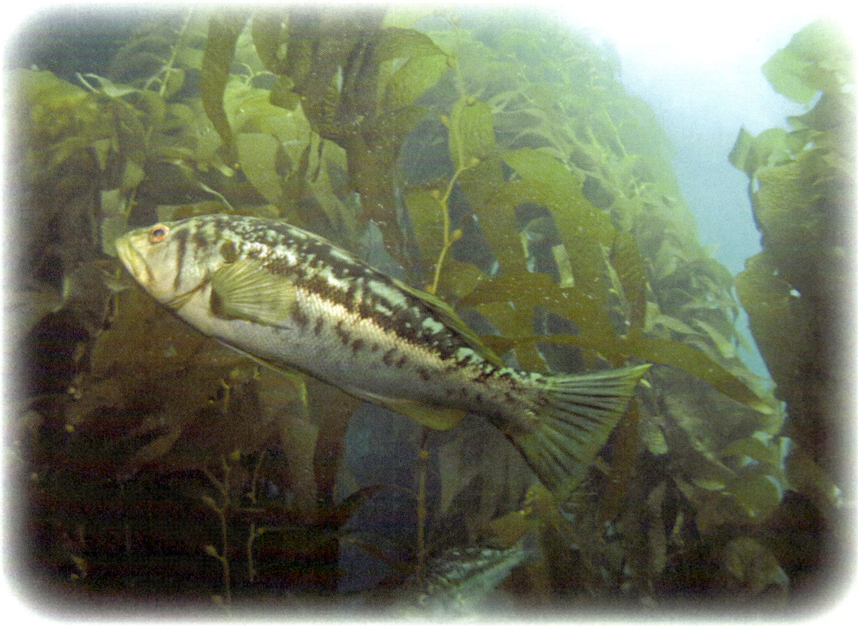

Kingdom: *Animalia*
Phylum: *Chordata*
Class: *Actinopterygii* (ray-finned fish)
Order: *Perciformes*
Family: *Centrarchidae*
Genus and species: several genera and species
Common name:

Bass

Bass mainly inhabit freshwater lakes, ponds, and slow-moving rivers and streams; some bass species are adapted to the brackish waters of estuaries (with moderate salinity). During the day, they may rest under lily pads or algae in the shade. In the evening, they become more active. Their varied diet includes: crawfish, minnows, worms, insects, frogs, salamanders, snakes, lizards, and birds.

continued...

Foods from Nature

Animal Foods - Seafoods

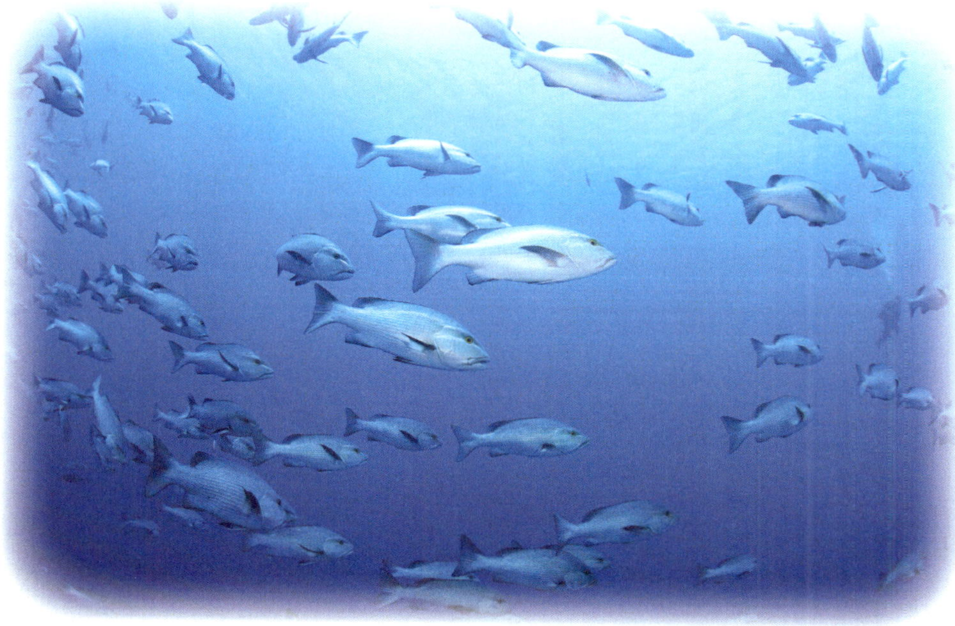

Kingdom: *Animalia*
Phylum: *Chordata*
Class: *Actinopterygii* (ray-finned fish)
Order: *Istiophoriformes*
Family: *Lutjanidae*
Genus and species: *Lutjanus campechanus*
Common name: **Red Snapper**

Red snapper reside in temperate and tropical waters. Their larva swim freely in open water. When they become juveniles, they move to shallow water over sandy or muddy sediment. As adults, they live on the continental shelf (with a hard substrate) where they feed on fish, octopus, squid, crustaceans, and plankton. Red snapper may be preyed on by groupers, sharks, barracudas, and morays, turtles, and marine mammals.

Kingdom: *Animalia*
Phylum: *Chordata*
Class: *Actinopterygii* (ray-finned fish)
Order: *Istiophoriformes*
Family: *Serranidae*
Genus and species: several genera and species
Common name: **Grouper**

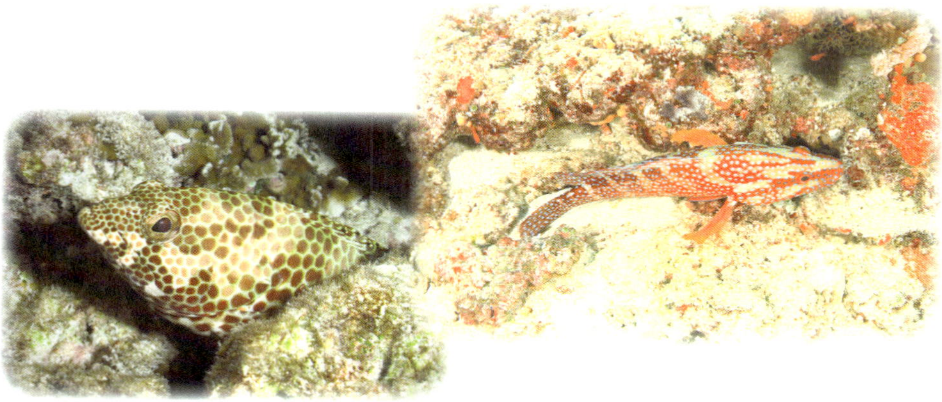

Groupers are tropical reef fishes. They camouflage themselves to evade detection from predators. Their larvae begin life in the open ocean and then come inshore to nursery grounds where they grow into juveniles. When they mature, they move offshore to join adult populations. As groupers move from one habitat to another at each life stage, their diet changes from plankton to bottom-dwelling crustaceans to fish.

continued...

Foods from Nature

Animal Foods - Seafoods

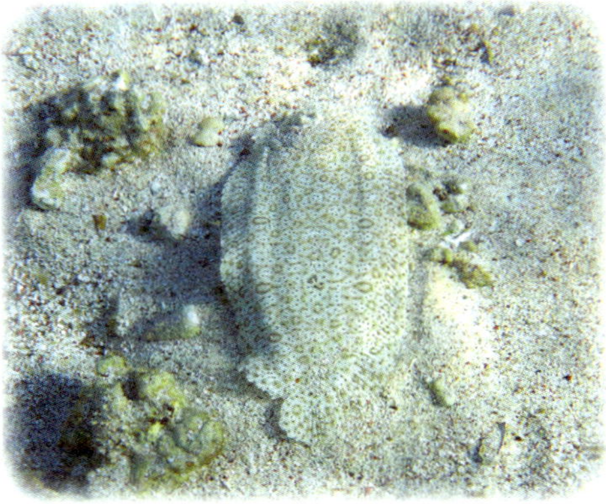

Flounder and Pacific halibut are flatfish. Like some other fishes, amphibians, and insects, they undergo metamorphosis (major structural and physiological change) during their lifetime. Metamorphosis occurs for flounder from the larval stage to the juvenile stage. This entails one eye migrating to the same side of the body as the other eye. This way, they can use both eyes while lying flat on the ocean, stream, or lake floor where, as adults, they spend most of their lives burrowed in the sand. Camouflaged, they hide from predators and wait to ambush prey.

Kingdom: *Animalia*
Phylum: *Chordata*
Class: *Actinopterygii* (ray-finned fish)
Order: *Pleuronectiformes*
Family: *Pleuronectoidei* (flatfish)
Genus and species: several genera and species
Common name: **Flounder** (including Pacific halibut)

Kingdom: *Animalia*
Phylum: *Chordata*
Class: *Actinopterygii* (ray-finned fish)
Order: *Salmoniformes*
Family: *Salmonidae*
Genus and species:
several genera and species
Common name:
Salmon and Sea Trout

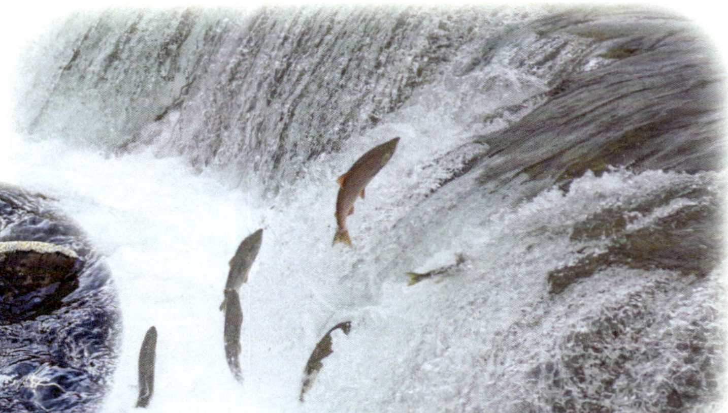

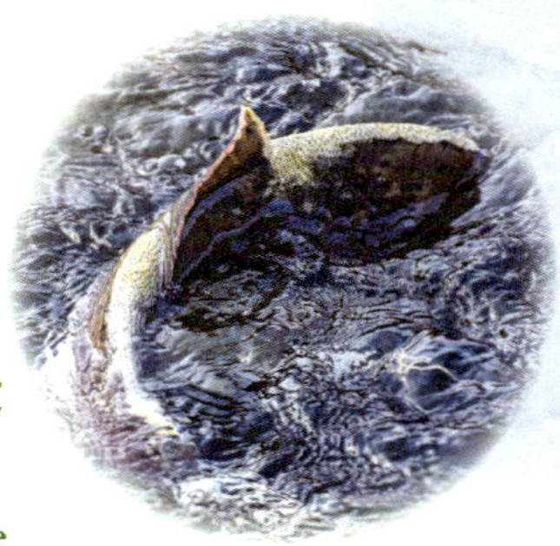

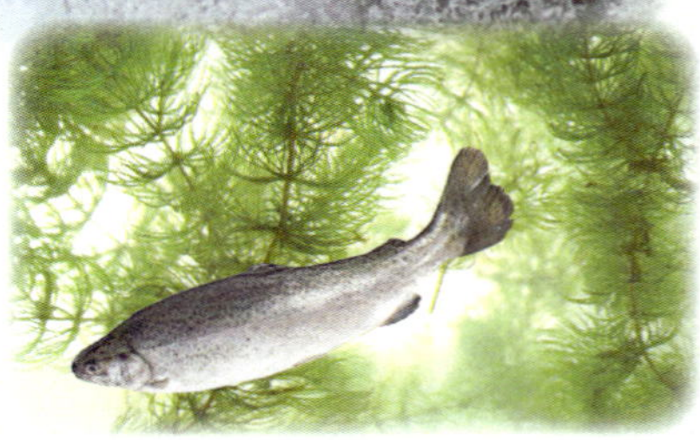

Salmon and sea trout increase the productivity of terrestrial and aquatic ecosystems. They are a major food source of orca, sea lions, seals, sea and river otters, bears, mink, eagles, osprey, common murre (guillemot), king fishers, and many other species. When they move up rivers to spawn and die, they bring nutrients from the ocean into the forest. Their carcasses enrich the streams, and their nutrients are carried further into forest by floods and wildlife. Songbirds benefit from an abundance of insects and larvae on decaying salmon carcasses along rivers and streams.[1] Salmon and trout juveniles find suitable habitat in estuaries where freshwater flows into deltas and inlets, where they can hide from predators, grow, and mature before heading out to the ocean.

References

[1]Lovette, I. (2008, July 15). *How salmon help songbirds*. Cornell Lab of Ornithology: All About Birds. https://www.allaboutbirds.org/news/how-salmon-help-songbirds/#.

continued...

Foods from Nature

Animal Foods - Seafoods

Kingdom: *Animalia*
Phylum: *Chordata*
Class: *Actinopterygii* (ray-finned fish)
Order: *Scombriformes*
Family: *Scombridae* (mackerel family most of the families in this order are in this family)
Genus and species: several genera and species
Common name: **Mackerel**

Mackerel are schooling pelagic (open ocean) fish. Some species migrate vertically, staying in deeper water during the day and rising to the surface to feed at night. Mackerel larvae and juveniles migrate in the opposite direction. Like tuna, mackerel are swift and agile swimmers. They have a cylindrical shape and can become more streamlined by retracting their fins into grooves on their bodies.

Kingdom: *Animalia*
Phylum: *Chordata*
Class: *Actinopterygii* (ray-finned fish)
Order: *Scombriformes*
Tribe (subgroup): *Thunnini* (tuna)
Genus and species: five genera (15 species)
Common name: **Tuna**

Tuna are among the most active and fast swimming predators in the world. They expend high amounts of energy searching the open ocean for food. Environmental conditions, such as layers of different temperature, delineate habitat niches among the various species of tuna. For example, the cold tolerance of bluefin tuna allows them a deeper niche in the ocean than yellowfin tuna.

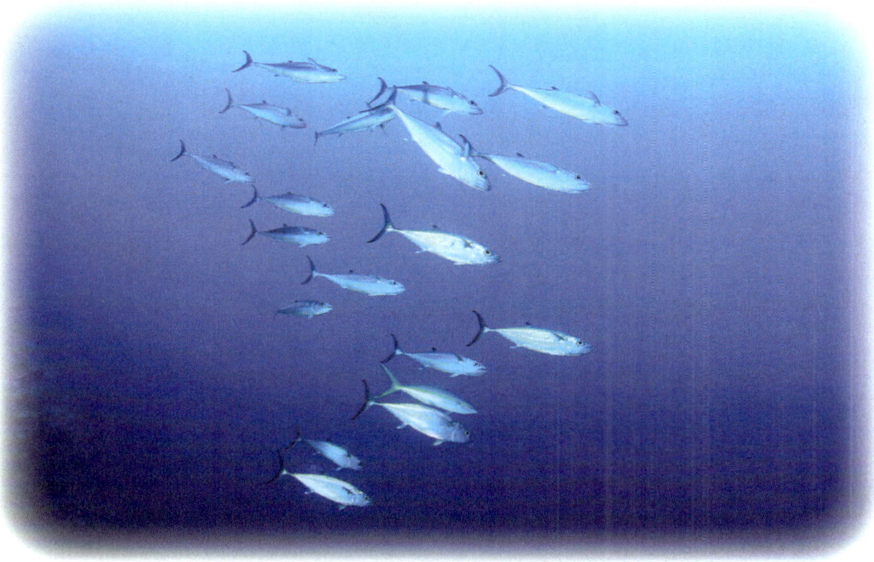

continued...

Foods from Nature

Animal Foods - Seafoods

Kingdom: *Animalia*
Phylum: *Arthropoda*
Subphylum: *Crustacea*
(a form of shellfish)
Class: *Malacostraca*
Order: *Decapoda*
Suborder: *Pleocyemata*
Family, genus, and species:
90+ families, 25 genera,
7,000 species
Common name: **Crab**

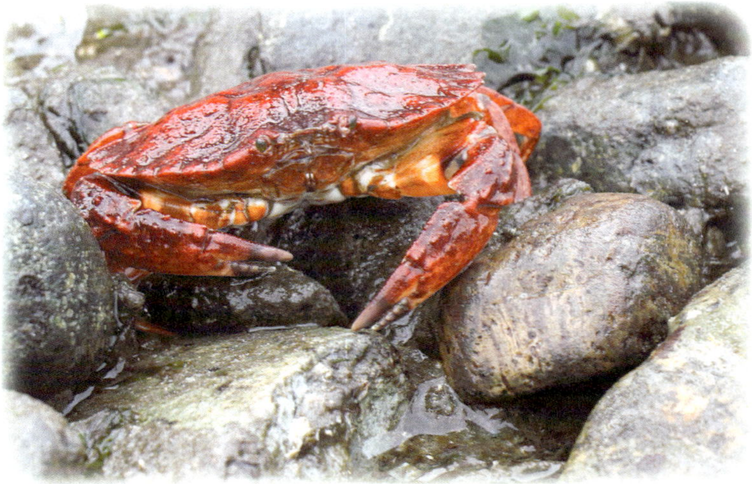

Most species of crabs live in the ocean; although, some species reside in freshwater. Others live on land, even several miles from bodies of water. Crabs often burrow in the sand or mud for shelter and protection. Some crabs make their home in the abandoned shells of snails, oysters, mussels, or other shellfish. Algae beds provide nursery areas for juvenile crabs.

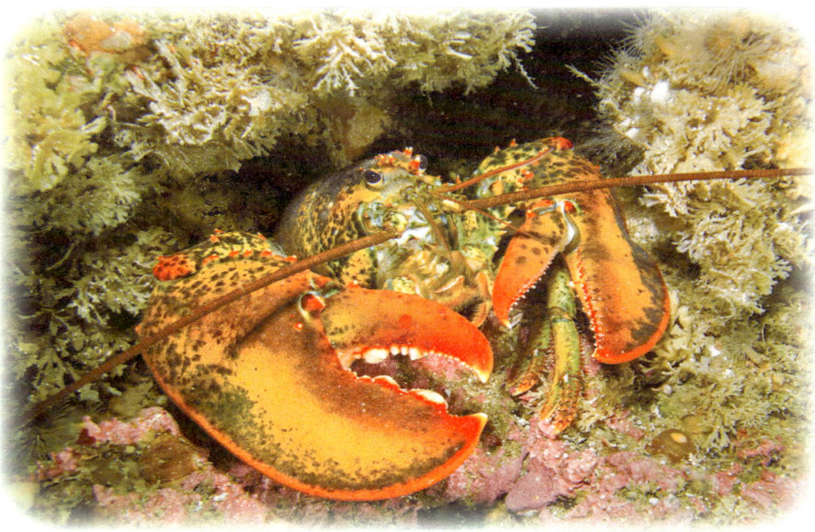

Kingdom: *Animalia*
Phylum: *Arthropoda*
Subphylum: *Crustacea*
(a form of shellfish)
Class: *Malacostraca*
Order: *Decapoda*
Suborder: *Pleocyemata*
Family: *Nephropidae*
Genus and species:
20 genera and many species
Common name: **Lobster**

Lobsters are benthic organisms, residing on rocky, sandy, or muddy substrates along the shoreline, and beyond to the edge of the continental shelf. They are non-migratory, remaining within a home range of a few square kilometers/yards. Juveniles frequently settle into crevices or burrow under rocks while adults walk slowly across the sea floor exploring deeper water.

continued...

Foods from Nature

Animal Foods - Seafoods

Kingdom: *Animalia*
Phylum: *Arthropoda*
Subphylum: *Crustacea* (a form of shellfish)
Class: *Malacostraca*
Order: *Decapoda*
Genus and species: many genera and thousands of species
Common name: Shrimp

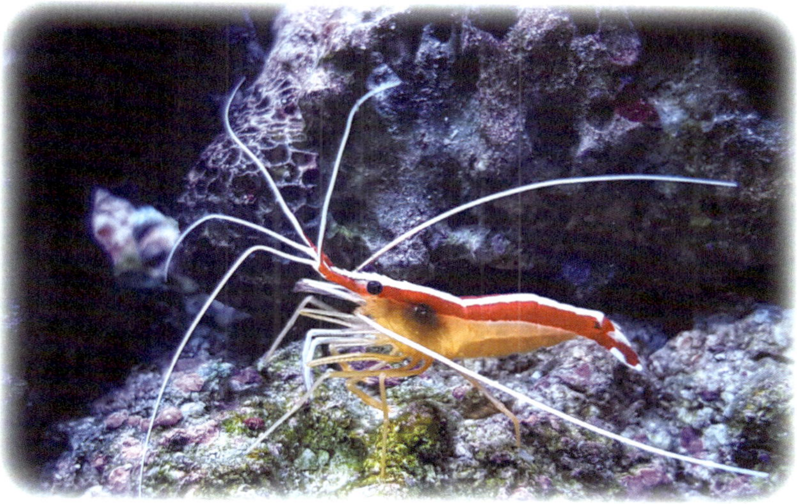

Shrimp are abundant in a variety of habitats from tropical to polar waters. They live near the ocean floor along most coasts and estuaries; and they are also found in rivers and lakes. Their pleopods (appendages) are adapted for swimming. As needed, shrimp slip into the sediment to evade predators. While mostly solitary, shrimp travel in schools during spawning season. In reciprocity, 'cleaner shrimp' (*Lysmata amboinensis*) remain in place where they are visited by fish that depend on them to remove parasites and clean up wounds. In return, the cleaner shrimp benefit by consuming the parasites as food; plus they are protected by the host fish.

Kingdom: *Animalia*
Phylum: *Mollusca*
Class: *Bivalvia* (bivalves)
Orders: many orders
Family, genus, and species: many families and genera, thousands of species
Common name: Mussels

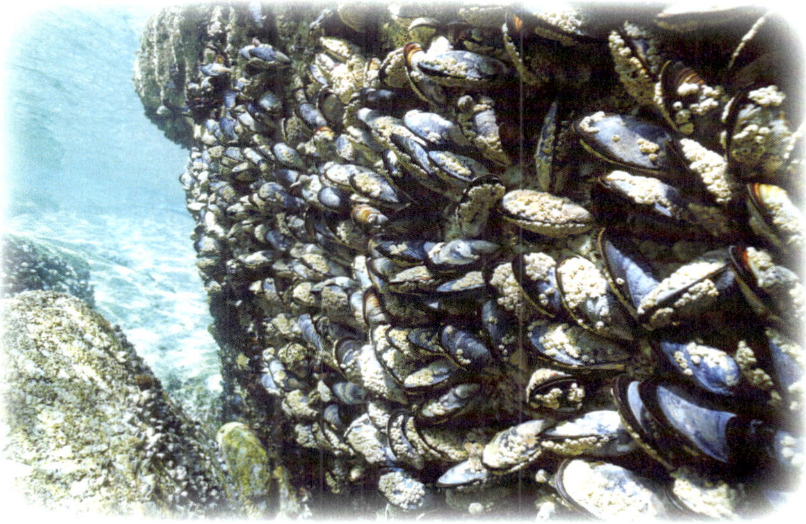

Mussels live in marine, estuarine, and freshwater environments. They are a major food source for sea and river otters, raccoons, birds, and other wildlife. To survive, mussel larvae, released into open water, must find a host fish to attach to for completing their development. When they are ready after several weeks of maturing, the mussels drop from their host fish into the water column and settle into the sediment. As adults, mussels are sessile, attaching themselves to a rock or shell substrate; only rarely do they move along the ocean or river bottom. Mussels filter voluminous amounts of water through their gills for oxygen and food (mostly plankton). Through this filtering process, they significantly improve the water quality in aquatic ecosystems worldwide.

continued...

Foods from Nature

Animal Foods - Seafoods

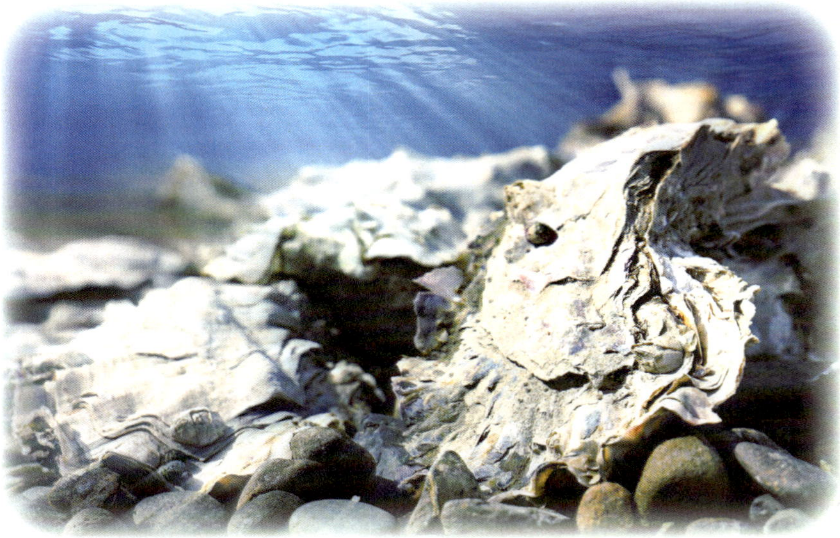

Kingdom: *Animalia*
Phylum: *Mollusca*
Class: *Bivalvia* (bivalves)
Order: *Ostreida*
Family: *Ostreidae*
Genus and species:
several genera and species
Common name: Oyster

In shallow coastal and estuarine waters, oysters start out as free-floating larvae, then attach to rocks or shells. When they mature, they form their own shells. Over time, the oyster shells pile up on one another and turn into a reef that serves as a barrier to storms and tides, prevents erosion, and provides shelter for sea life. Like coral reefs; oyster reefs support hundreds of species. Mussels, barnacles, and sea anemones settle on the oyster reefs. Additionally, algae beds get established and fish come to forage for invertebrates and other shellfish. The oyster reef ecosystem also becomes a nursery for many species.

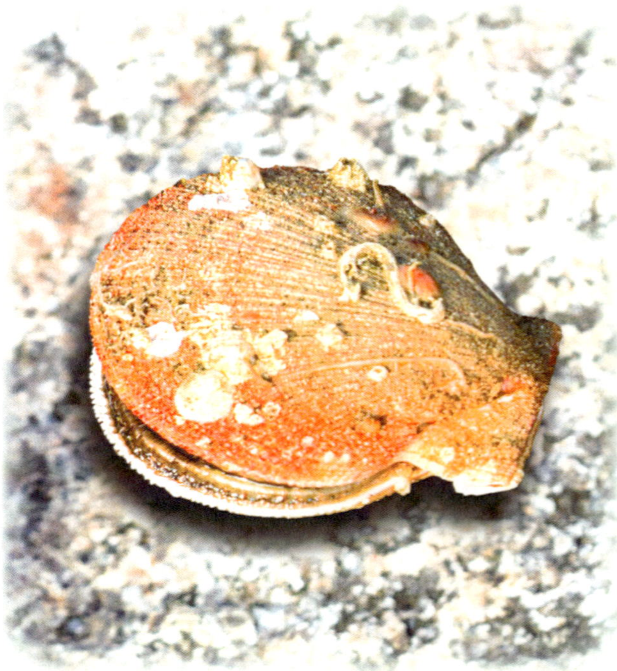

Kingdom: *Animalia*
Phylum: *Mollusca*
Class: *Bivalvia* (bivalves)
Order: *Pectinida*
Family: *Pectinidae*
Genus and species:
several genera and species
Common name: Scallop

Most scallop species are active swimmers, propelling themselves through the water by clapping (opening and closing their shells). This causes a rapid intake and expulsion of water. Other scallop species attach themselves to rock on the ocean floor with byssal threads (silky fibers) that extend from their muscular foot. Sometimes scallops carry symbiotic epibionts on their shells. For example, sponges protect the scallops by attaching onto them; this interferes with the adhesion of predatory sea-stars and the settling of harmful barnacles on the scallop's shells.

Foods from Nature

Animal Foods

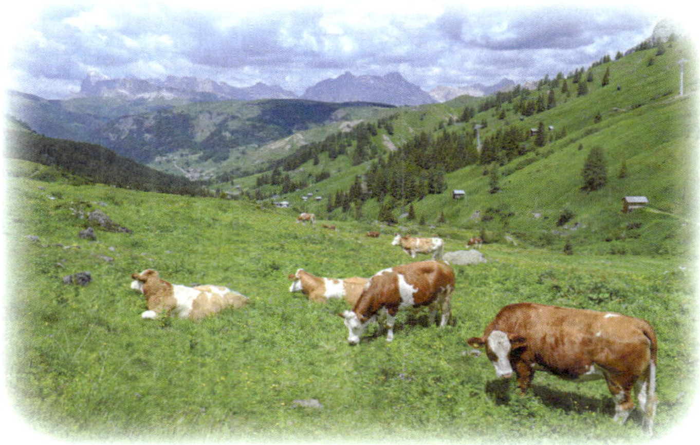

Kingdom: *Animalia*
Phylum: *Chordata*
Class: *Mammalia*
Order: *Artiodactyla*
Family: *Bovidae* (ruminants)
Genus and species:
several genera and species
Common name: Cow

Heritage cows are breeds that have been grazing on natural pasturelands for centuries, such as: guernsey from the Isle of Guernsey and Jersey from the Isle of Jersey, in the British Channel Islands, and ancient white park from England, Scotland, and Wales. Aurochs (*Bos primigenius*), believed to be the ancestor of all cows, once inhabited Northern Africa, Asia, and Europe. Nomadic, indigenous people in different regions of the world accompanied, hunted, and drew milk from migrating ruminant, grazing mammals on pastureland for thousands of years. On contemporary regenerative farms, cows, goats, and sheep graze pastureland, improving soil quality, supporting intact plant root systems, and enhancing biodiversity.

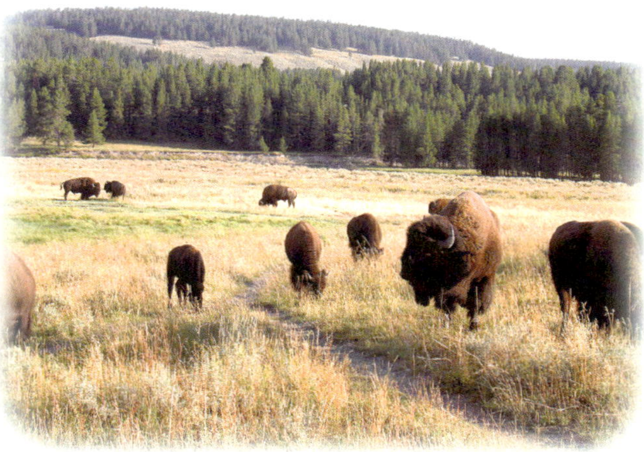

Kingdom: *Animalia*
Phylum: *Chordata*
Class: *Mammalia*
Order: *Artiodactyla*
Family: *Bovidae* (ruminants)
Genus and species: *Bison bison*
Common name: Bison

For millennia, bison have been keystone species in the North American tall, mixed, and short-grass prairies. Grazing across the prairies, their manure is integrated into the topsoil, facilitating nitrogen availability and plant productivity. Bison roll around on the earth, creating wallows. After rainfall, the wallows become temporary pools that support a variety of prairie species. In the warmer months, while bison roam as they graze, their hooves aerate the soil, dispersing seeds and promoting plant growth.

continued...

Foods from Nature

Animal Foods

Kingdom: *Animalia*
Phylum: *Chordata*
Class: *Mammalia*
Order: *Artiodactyla*
Family: *Bovidae* (ruminants)
Genus and species:
Capra hircus and Ovis aries
Common name: Goat and Sheep

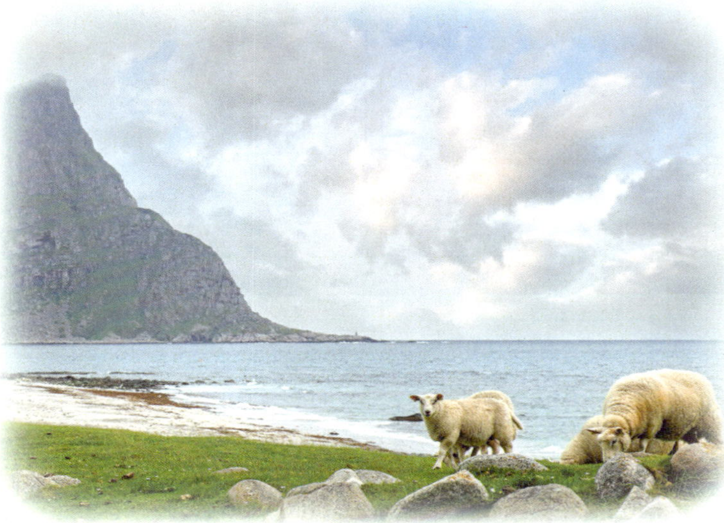

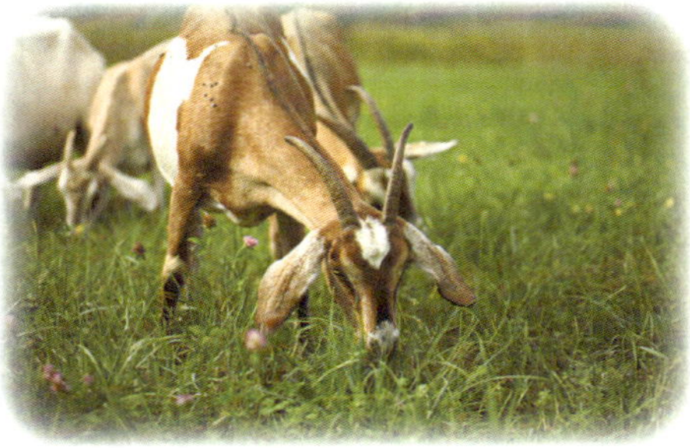

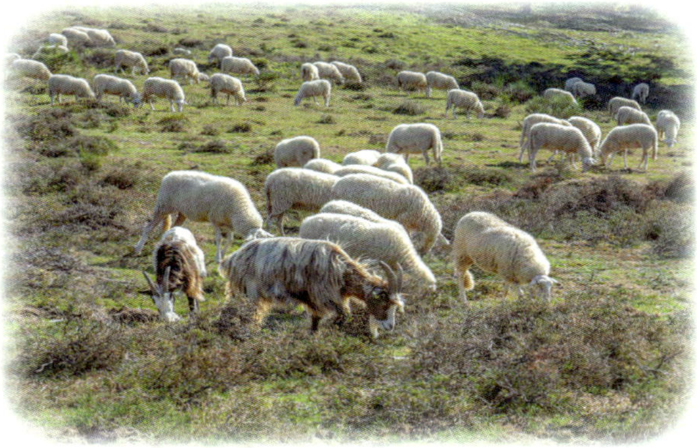

Goats and sheep primarily graze and occasionally browse a wide variety of vegetation. As small ruminant species, they thrive on shrublands, savannahs (grasslands with a few trees), woodlands, forests, and regenerative farm pasture lands. These natural and regeneratively cultivated areas, even where semi-arid, provide ample green grasses, herbs, and forbs for goats and sheep. Ideally for them, these landscapes include a mix of evergreen and deciduous plants throughout the year.

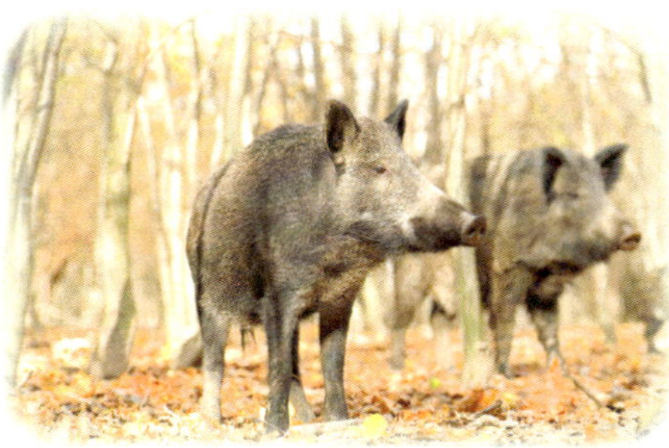

Kingdom: *Animalia*
Phylum: *Chordata*
Class: *Mammalia*
Order: *Artiodactyla*
Family: *Suidae*
Genus and species:
many genera and species
Common name: Pig

Heritage pigs are forest-dwelling. They rest and sleep on the cool forest floor. Heritage pigs forage for leaves, fruits, and flowers and hunt for fish in creeks and streams. Pigs have a scent-sensitive and strong snout that helps them find and dig up roots and tubers to eat. Since they lack sweat glands, pigs lay in the loose soil they dig up to cool themselves. Native seeds and plants benefit from this freshly aerated soil.

continued...

Foods from Nature

Animal Foods

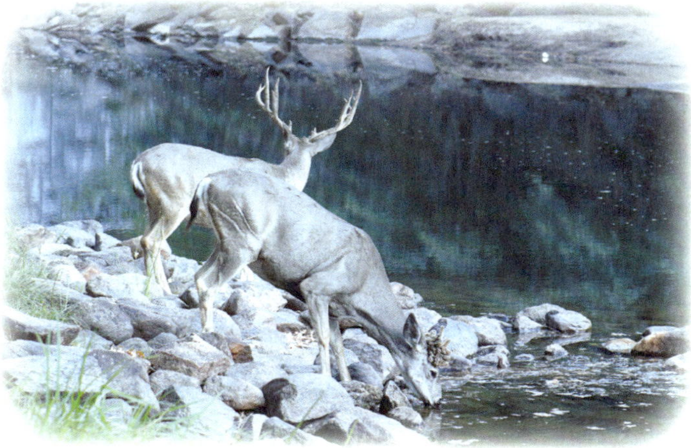

Kingdom: *Animalia*
Phylum: *Chordata*
Class: *Mammalia*
Order: *Artiodactyla*
Family: *Cervidae*
Genus and species:
many genera and species
Common name: Deer

Deer browse in forests, meadows, and woodlands that provide them with food, bedding, and cover. They forage around and drink from lakes and streams. Deer are folivores, consuming foliage, including: the soft shoots, buds, and tender twigs on shrubs and trees; herbs and forbs; acorns and other nuts; fruits, such as berries and apples; mushrooms; and lichens. In natural ecosystems, deer browsing invigorates the regrowth of plants.

Kingdom: *Animalia*
Phylum: *Chordata*
Class: *Mammalia*
Order: *Artiodactyla*
Family: *Cervidae*
Genus and species:
many genera and species
Common name: Elk

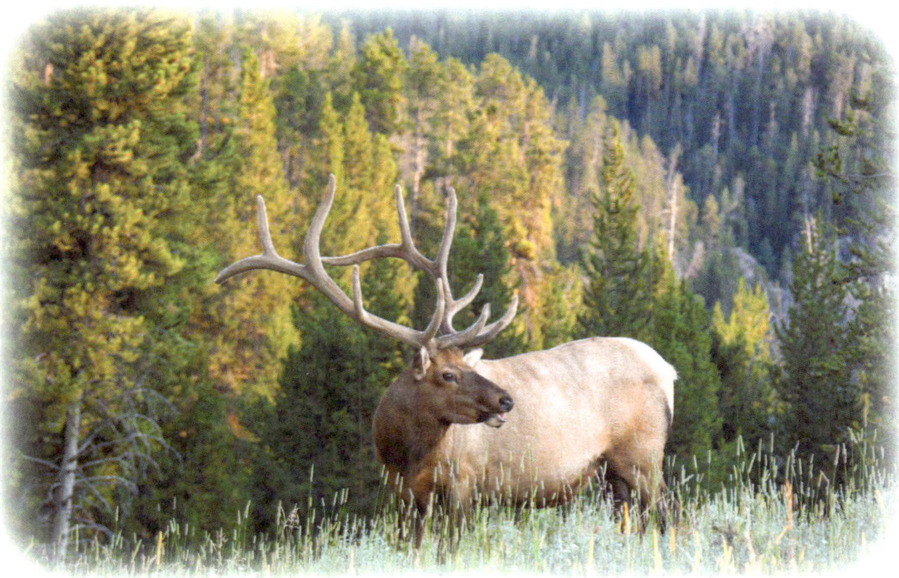

Elk herds migrate through forests, alpine meadows, sagebrush steppe, prairie, and wetlands in North America and Central and East Asia. In the spring and summer, they consume grasses, sedges, and other herbaceous plants. During autumn and winter, they feed on lichens, conifer needles, softwood bark, and green shoots. As a grazing herbivore, elk maintain grassland ecosystems, promoting plant diversity, building rich topsoil, and contributing to nutrient cycling. Elk are important to the diet of cougars, grizzly bears, wolves, and mountain lions; and their carcasses are food for carrion-eating birds and small mammals.

continued...

Foods from Nature

Animal Foods

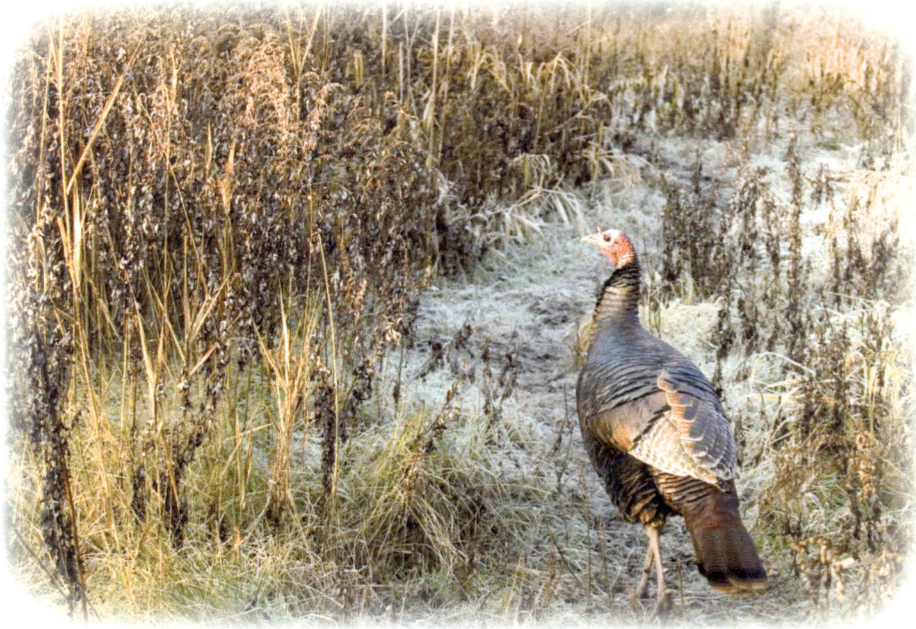

Kingdom: *Animalia*
Phylum: *Chordata*
Class: *Aves* (birds)
Order: *Galliformes*
Family: *Phasianidae*
Genus and species:
Meleagris gallopavo
Common name: Turkey

Turkeys reside in hardwood and mixed conifer-hardwood forests and woodlands, interspersed with pastures and wetlands. During daylight, they tend to stay close to the ground, foraging for acorns and hazel, chestnut, hickory, and pinyon pine nuts as well as seeds, berries, buds, leaves, fern fronds, roots, and insects. Occasionally, they consume salamanders, lizards, and small snakes. At twilight, turkeys fly up to roost overnight in the trees.

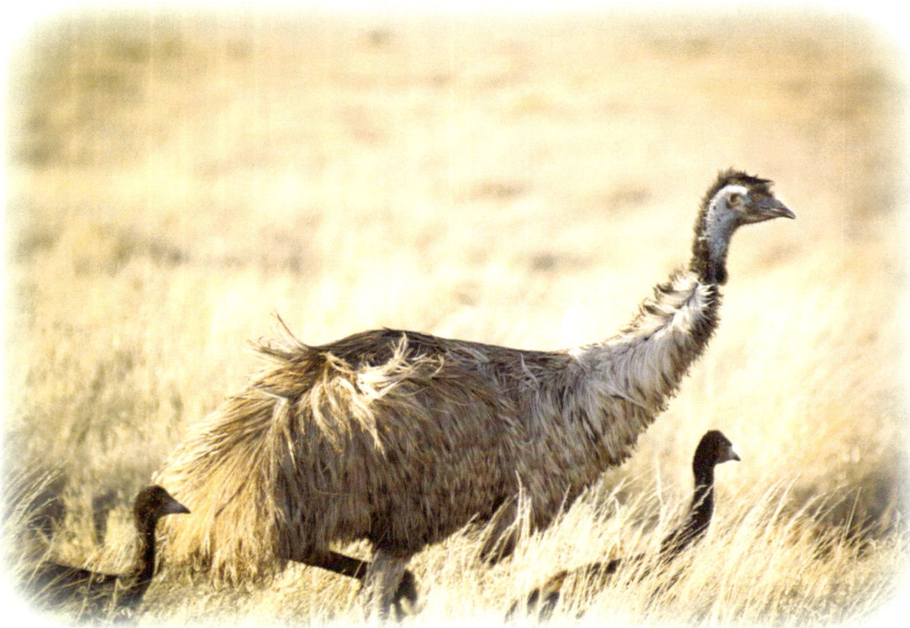

Kingdom: *Animalia*
Phylum: *Chordata*
Class: *Aves* (birds)
Order: *Galliformes*
Family: *Casuariidae*
Genus and species:
Dromaius novaehollandiae
Common name: Emu

Emus are tall land birds endemic to Australia. They are nomadic and often follow rainclouds in search of food that emerges after the rain. Emu have been found in Australia's eucalyptus forests, woodlands, savannah, grasslands, and desert shrub. They eat young shoots, herbs, seeds, fruits, insects, reptiles, and small mammals. Traveling long distances, they disperse plant seeds widely.

continued...

Foods from Nature

Animal Foods

Kingdom: ***Animalia***
Phylum: ***Chordata***
Class: ***Aves*** **(birds)**
Order: ***Galliformes***
Family: ***Phasianidae***
Genus and species:
Gallus **(many species)**
Common name: Chicken

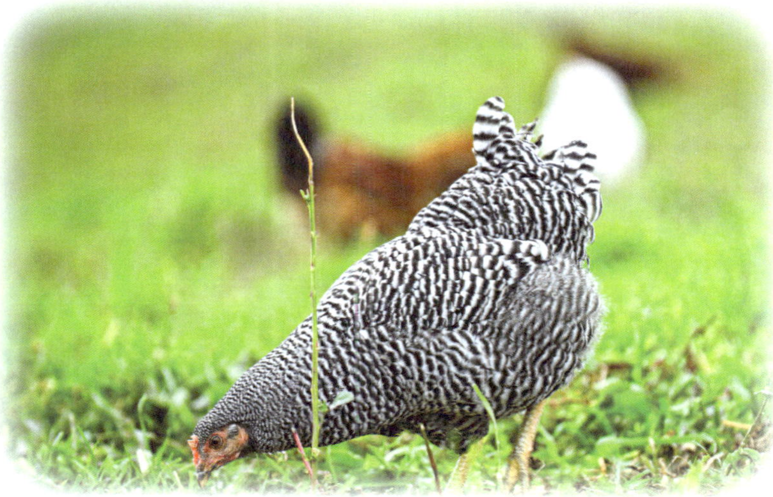

Contemporary chickens are believed to be descended from junglefowl in Asia.[1] The main habitat of their indigenous ancestors, red (*Gallus gallus*) and grey (*Gallus sonneratii*) junglefowl, was likely tropical and subtropical moist broadleaf forests.[1] On regenerative farms that simulate this historic habitat, the chickens may, for example, live under canopies of trees with clearings of open meadow. The trees and woody perennials help protect chickens from inclement weather, including direct sun, and predators. The chickens forage for herbs, seeds, worms, and insects, naturally fertilizing the area with their manure.

References

[1]Pitt, J. C. (2017, March). *The ecology of chickens: An examination of the introduction of the domestic chicken across Europe after the Bronze Age*. Poole, Dorset, United Kingdom: Bournemouth University.

Kingdom: ***Animalia***
Phylum: ***Chordata***
Class: ***Aves*** **(birds)**
Order: ***Galliformes***
Family: ***Phasianidae***
Genus and species:
many genera and species
Common name: Quail

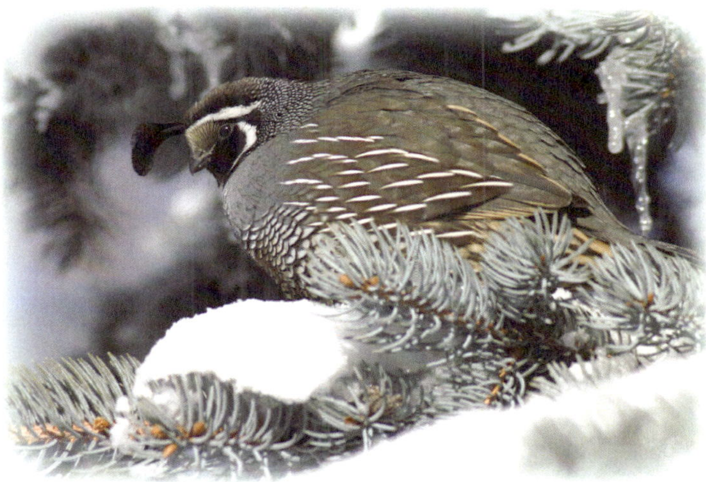

Quail move together in small flocks called 'coveys' until late spring and early summer when they form pair bonds for the breeding season. Their newly hatched chicks are covered in down, weigh about one-quarter of an ounce, and are not much larger than bumblebees.[1] Quail inhabit prairies, with early successional plant communities, maintained by periodic wildfires. They forage for insects, seeds, leaves, and berries.

References

[1]Pierce, R. A. & Gallagher, E. (2022, December). *Ecology of northern bobwhite quail in Missouri*. University of Missouri Extension. https://extension.missouri.edu/publications/g9431.

continued...

Foods from Nature

Animal Foods

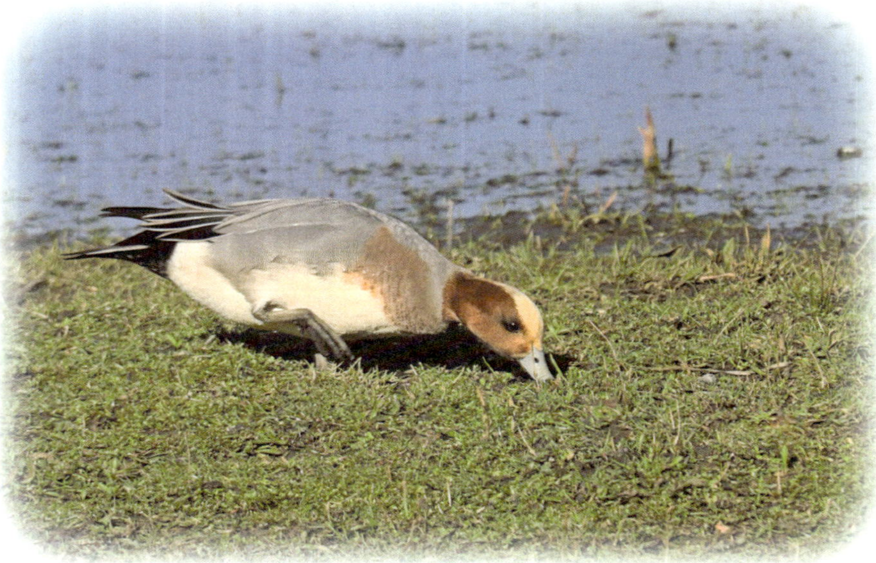

Kingdom: ***Animalia***
Phylum: ***Chordata***
Class: ***Aves*** **(birds)**
Order: ***Anseriformes***
Family: ***Anatidae***
(ducks, geese, and swans)
Genus and species:
many genera and species
Common name: Duck

Ducks, like geese and swans, are in the *Anatidae* (water bird) family. They are adapted for swimming, diving to forage for food, and floating while resting on the surface of the water.[1] More than one hundred species of ducks annually migrate, including: bufflehead, cinnamon teal, eider, gadwall, green-winged teal, harlequin, mallard, merganser, northern pintail, and wood duck. They frequent wetlands, such as marshes and swamps, associated with lakes, ponds, rivers, streams, bays, and oceans. Though they are water birds, they need upland habitat for shelter and nesting. Their food sources include: algae and aquatic plants, insects, fish, worms, small mollusks, and amphibians.

References

[1]All About Birds. (2024). *Ducks*. Ithica, NY: Cornell Lab of Ornithology, Cornell University. https://www.allaboutbirds.org/news.

Kingdom: ***Animalia***
Phylum: ***Mollusca***
Class: ***Gastropoda***
Order: ***Stylommatophora***
Family: ***Helicidae***
Genus and species: ***Helix pomatia***
Common name: Snail (escargot)

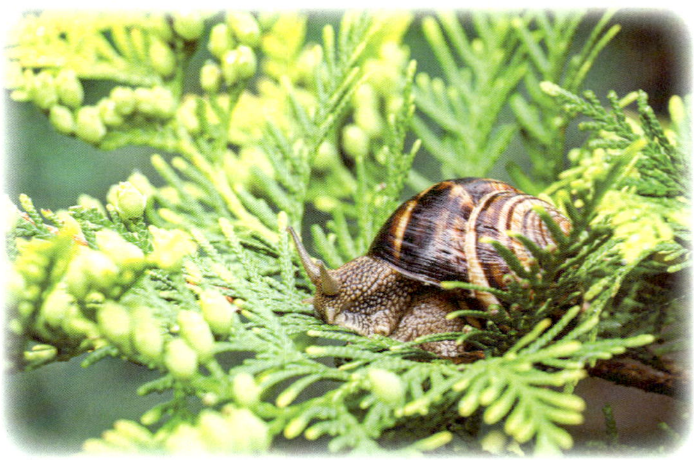

Escargot (*Helix pomatia*) land snails are indigenous to Central and Southeast Europe. They live in grasslands and savannahs, and depend on humid and mild temperatures. As terrestrial snails, they are nocturnal, becoming active in the cooler temperatures at night, consuming leaves, tender green shoots and stems, flowers, fruit, sap, and other plant substances. When foraging, land snails produce a slime trail to reduce water loss and protect themselves from rough or slick surfaces. In winter, land snails hibernate.

Foods from Nature

Plant Foods

FRUITS

Kingdom: *Plantae*
Phylum: *Tracheophytes*
Class: *Magnoliopsida*
Order: *Malpighiales*
Family: *Malpighiaceae*
(tropical and subtropical flowering plants)
Genus and species:
Malpighia emarginata
Common name: Acerola

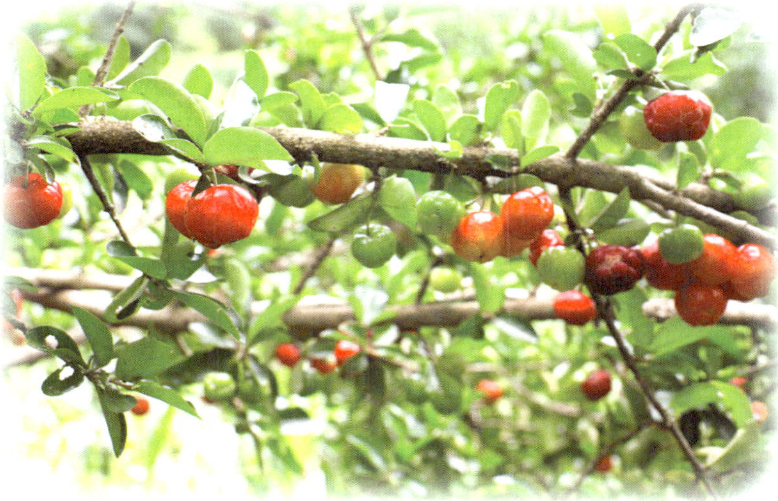

In warm climates, the acerola cherry/West Indian cherry, a drupe (stone) fruit, grows on the acerola evergreen shrub or small tree. The flowers are pollinated by insects, such as honey bees of the *Centris* and *Epicharis* genera. The bees land on the firmest petal of acerola's five-petaled flower and use it as a platform to gather oils and pollen from the flowers; the flowers are then pollenated as the bees travel from one flower to another. When the bees return with the floral oil and pollen to their nests, they feed it to the young bee larvae.

Kingdom: *Plantae*
Phylum: *Tracheophytes*
Class: *Magnoliopsida*
Order: *Malpighiales*
Family: *Phyllanthaceae*
(tropical and subtropical flowering plants)
Genus and species:
Phyllanthus emblica
Common name: Amla Berry/ Indian Gooseberry

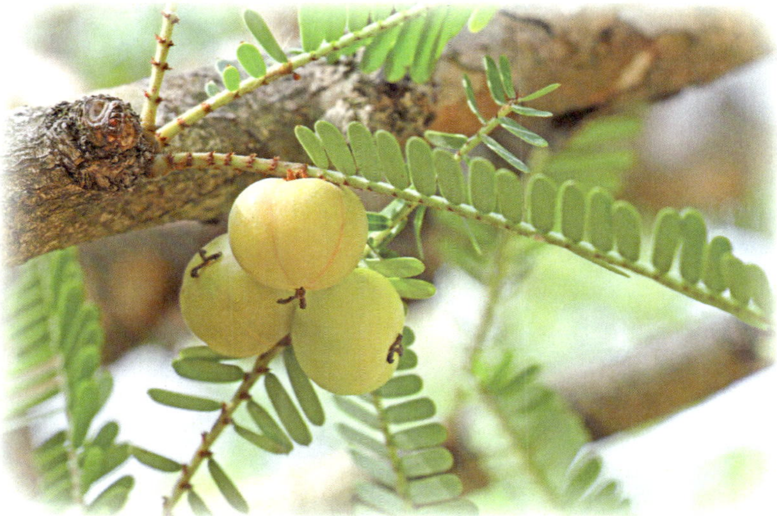

The small deciduous amla tree is indigenous to semi-arid tropical, subtropical, and tropical forests of South Asia. It is a mountainous, hardy, and drought-resistant tree. The length of daylight initiates the development of floral buds on the amla tree.[1]

References

[1]Pushpokumara, D. K. N. G. & Heenkenda, H. M. S. Chapter 6: Nelli (Amla) *Phyllanthus emblica* L. (p. 199). Sri Lanka: University of Peradeniya. https://apps.worldagroforestry.org/downloads/Publications/PDFS/BC07317.pdf.

continued...

Foods from Nature

Plant Foods

GRAINS

Kingdom: ***Plantae***
Phylum: ***Tracheophytes***
Class: ***Liliopsida***
Order: ***Poales***
Family: ***Poaceae***
(grass family)
Genus and species:
Hordeum vulgare
Common name: Barley

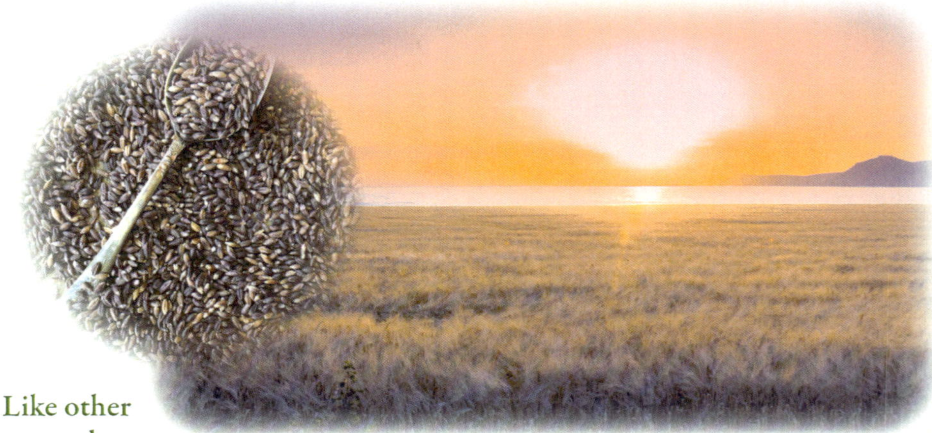

Purple barley is an ancient grain. Like other barley varieties, it is a cool-season annual grass. Herbivores, such as cows, goats, sheep, deer, and elk, graze on the young grasses before the seeds (grain) develop. Later, the grain provides food for many birds and small mammals. Regenerative farmers plant barley as ground cover, which captures moisture and retains it in the soil; replaces nutrients lost in earlier harvests; increases organic matter, adding to the topsoil; maintains the soil structure and microbiome; and reduces erosion.

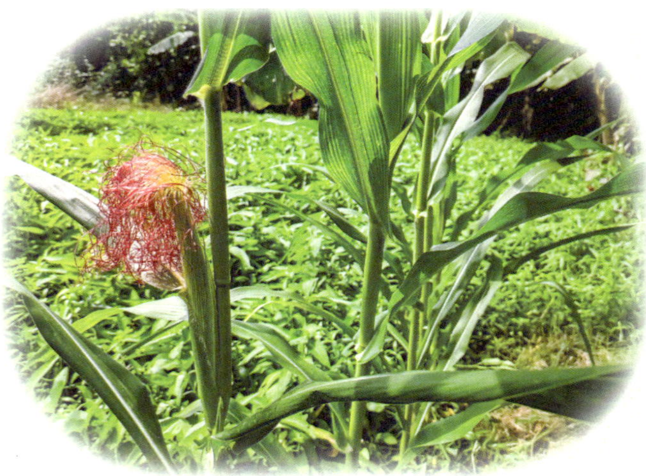

Kingdom: ***Plantae***
Phylum: ***Tracheophytes***
Class: ***Liliopsida***
Order: ***Poales***
Family: ***Poaceae*** **(grass family)**
Genus and species: ***Zea mays***
Common name: Corn/Maize

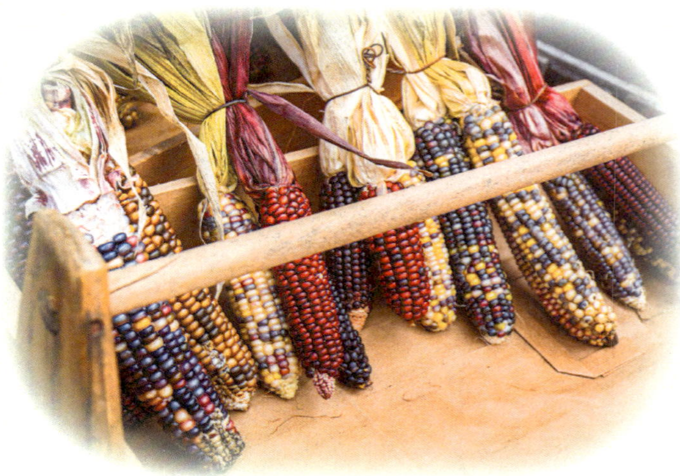

Over thousands of years, indigenous farmers in Mexico and Central America selectively bred corn for the characteristics they favored, generating a wide variety of colors and traits in the corn/maize. Syncing with pollination by wind and insects, indigenous farmers continue to plant teosinte, the wild ancestor of corn/maize, near their farm fields. This way, wild teosinte naturally breeds with the maize they planted, making the plants hardier.

continued...

Foods from Nature

Plant Foods

LEGUMES

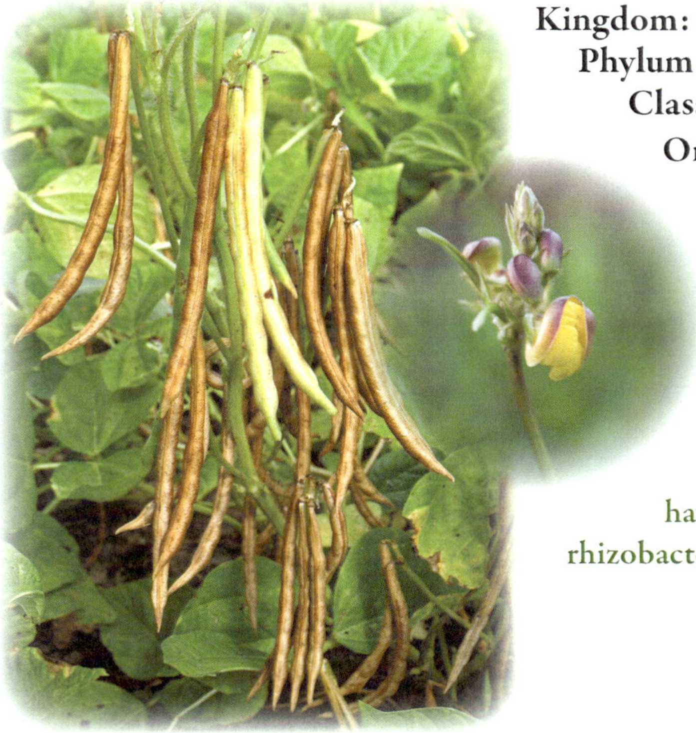

Kingdom: ***Plantae***
Phylum: ***Tracheophytes***
Class: ***Magnoliopsida***
Order: ***Fabales***
Family: ***Fabaceae*** **(legume family)**
Genus and species: ***Vigna angularis***
Common name: Adzuki Bean

Adzuki is an annual vine adapted to a temperate climate and cultivated throughout East Asia. As a member of the legume (*Fabaceae*) family, adzuki plants have symbiotic relationships with nitrogen-fixing rhizobacteria that inhabit nodules in their roots.

Kingdom: ***Plantae***
Phylum: ***Tracheophytes***
Class: ***Magnoliopsida***
Order: ***Fabales***
Family: ***Fabaceae*** **(legume family)**
Genus and species: ***Phaseolus vulgaris***
Common name: Black Bean

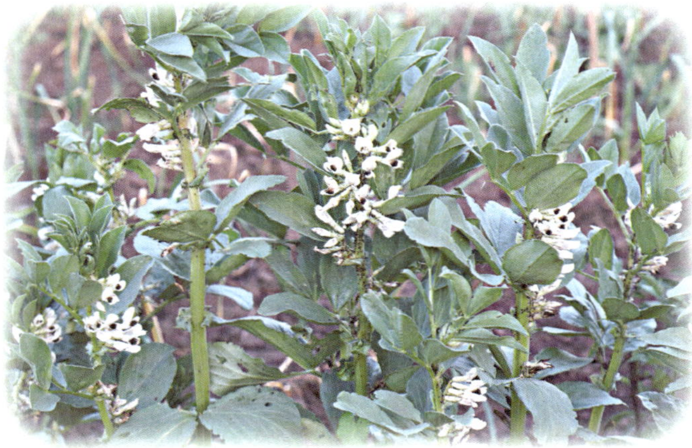

Black beans are part of the 'Three Sisters' tradition of companion planting started by the Haudenosaunee (Ho-deh-no-shaw-nee) people (Iroquois). Haudenosaunee live around the Great Lakes in the Northeastern United States and Canada. They plant corn, bean, and squash seeds together in a mound, which aids with drainage to avoid water logging the plant roots given the abundant rainfall in the summer. "The corn provides a sturdy structure for the bean vines to climb, preventing them from competing with sprawling squash vines. The beans, in turn, enrich the soil with nitrogen and help stabilize the corn. The squash's broad leaves provide shade, preserving soil moisture and inhibiting weed growth."[1]

References

[1]Marinaro, L. (2016, May 27). *How to grow a Three Sisters Garden*. Tucson, Arizona: Native Seed/SEARCH. https://www.nativeseeds.org/blogs/blog-news/how-to-grow-a-three-sisters-garden.

continued...

Foods from Nature

Plant Foods

TREE NUTS

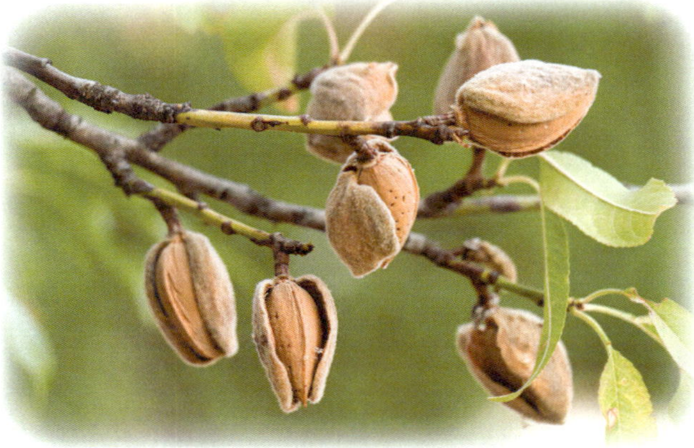

Kingdom: ***Plantae***
Phylum: ***Tracheophytes***
Class: ***Magnoliopsida***
Order: ***Fabales***
Family: ***Rosaceae*** **(rose family)**
Genus and species: ***Prunus amygdalus***
Common name: Almond

Almond trees are native to the Middle East and thrive in the mild climates including the Mediterranean. They require a certain amount of cold weather in the winter to prepare for new growth in the spring. Regenerative farmers plant other edible plant foods between the almond trees to enhance water infiltration and groundwater recharge. This also reduces run-off and evaporation, and increases the amount of organic matter in the soil so it can hold more water in the future. Flowering plants, shrubs, and hedgerows around almond trees provides habitat for pollinators.

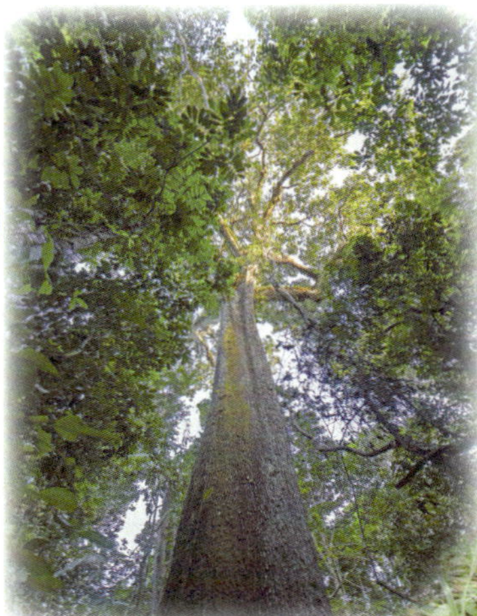

Kingdom: ***Plantae***
Phylum: ***Tracheophytes***
Class: ***Magnoliopsida***
Order: ***Ericales***
Family: ***Lecythidaceae*** **(tropical woody plants)**
Genus and species: ***Bertholletia excelsa***
Common name: Brazil Nut

The Brazil nut is only harvested in the wild where it is interdependent with several species in its habitat. The nuts are harvested from the forest floor where they fall when ripe. Brazil nut trees tower above the Amazon rainforest, reaching heights of 49 metres (160 feet) with canopies spanning 30 metres (100 feet).[1] *Euglossine* bees "... use other plants as a stepladder to reach the Brazil nut flowers. Without the forest complexity of trees with diverse heights leading a path to the Brazil nut flowers, the bees will stick to flowers they don't have to fly so high to reach. The male bees also need access to wild orchids to perfume themselves to attract mates. These Brazil nut tree pollinators require intact rainforest to reproduce and pollinate Brazil nut trees."[2]

Agouti's use sharp, chisel-like teeth to crack open the shells to eat the Brazil nuts inside.[1] They also bury some nuts to eat later. Some of the stored nuts sprout and grow into mature Brazil nut trees, thereby, continuing the cycle of life for these interconnected species.

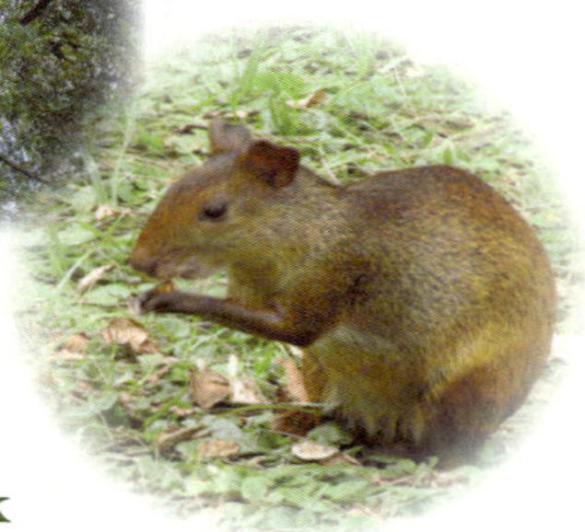

References

[1]Rainforest Alliance. (2023, September 14). *Brazil nut tree: Bertholletia excelsa*. Species Profiles. https://www.rainforest-alliance.org/species/brazil-nut-tree.

[2]Sevigny, C. (2021, May 3). *Postcard from the field: Brazil nuts and rainforest biodiversity*. Water Production Connections. https://www.waterproductionconnections.hs.umt.edu/post/postcard-from-the-field-brazil-nuts-and-rainforest-biodiversity. *continued...*

Foods from Nature

Plant Foods

SEEDS

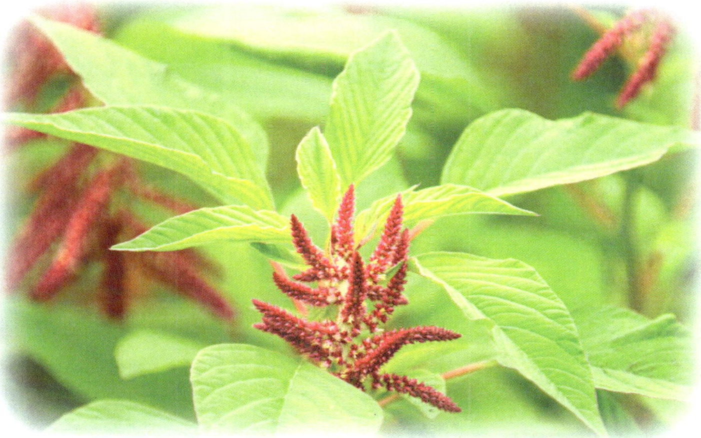

Kingdom: ***Plantae***
Phylum: ***Tracheophytes***
Class: ***Magnoliopsida***
Order: ***Caryophyllales***
Family: ***Amaranthaceae***
(amaranth family)
Genus and species: ***Amaranthus***
(with more than 60 species)
Common name: Amaranth

Amaranth is an ancient plant from South America with tiny edible seeds. The young leaves and shoots are edible too. Amaranth's cascading tassels of flowers bloom in vibrant magenta, red, orange, and yellow. Overall, the *Amaranthaceae* family is ". . . quite a unique plant family, because many species have evolved adaptations to grow in stressful environments such as those characterized by high soil salinity and/or extreme drought."[1]

References

[1]Vandelook, F., Newton, R. J., Bobon, N., Bohley, K., & Kadereit, G. (2021, May 7). Evolution and ecology of seed internal morphology in relation to germination characteristics in *Amaranthaceae, Annals of Botany. 127*(6) 799 – 811. https://doi.org/10.1093/aob/mcab012.

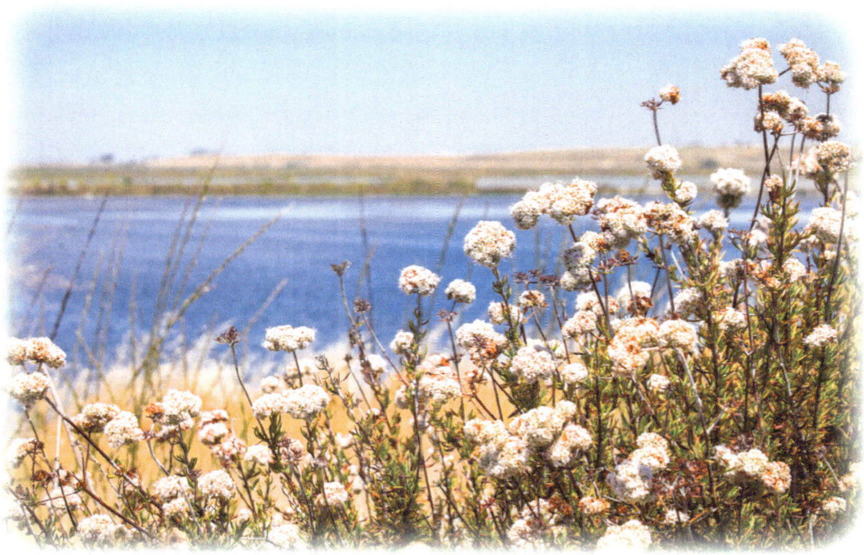

Kingdom: ***Plantae***
Phylum: ***Tracheophytes***
Class: ***Magnoliopsida***
Order: ***Caryophyllales***
Family: ***Polygonaceae***
(buckwheat family)
Genus and species:
Fagopyrum esculentum
Common name:
Buckwheat/Kasha

Common throughout Asia, Russia, and the Americas, buckwheat is a cool climate annual plant. It flourishes in grasslands, woodlands, and forests from near sea level to alpine habitats. Fast growing and robust, buckwheat provides excellent ground cover for regenerative gardens and farms. The edible buckwheat groat is a small, dry, triangle-shaped fruit. Botanically, buckwheat groats are 'achenes' (small nutlets) encased in a hull (protective shell).

continued...

Foods from Nature

Plant Foods

SEASONINGS

Kingdom: *Plantae*
Phylum: *Tracheophytes*
Class: *Magnoliopsida*
Order: *Myrtales*
Family: *Myrtaceae*
Genus and species:
Pimenta dioica (myrtle family)
Common name: Allspice

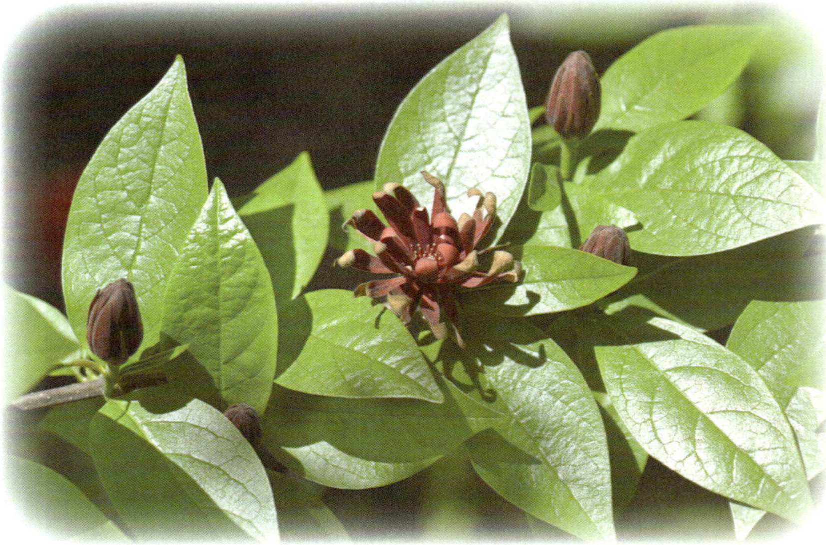

Allspice is a tropical evergreen tree. The unripe, dried allspice berry is a spice, resembling the combined flavors of cloves, cinnamon nutmeg, and black pepper. Without being closely related, allspice shares common compounds with these other species. Specifically, the biochemical compound eugenol is a constituent of cloves, nutmeg, cinnamon, and allspice. Additionally, the biochemical compound piperine, which is prominent in black pepper, is also present in allspice.

Kingdom: *Plantae*
Phylum: *Tracheophytes*
Class: *Magnoliopsida*
Order: *Apiales*
Family: *Apiaceae* (mint family)
Genus and species:
Pimpinella anisum
Common name: Anise

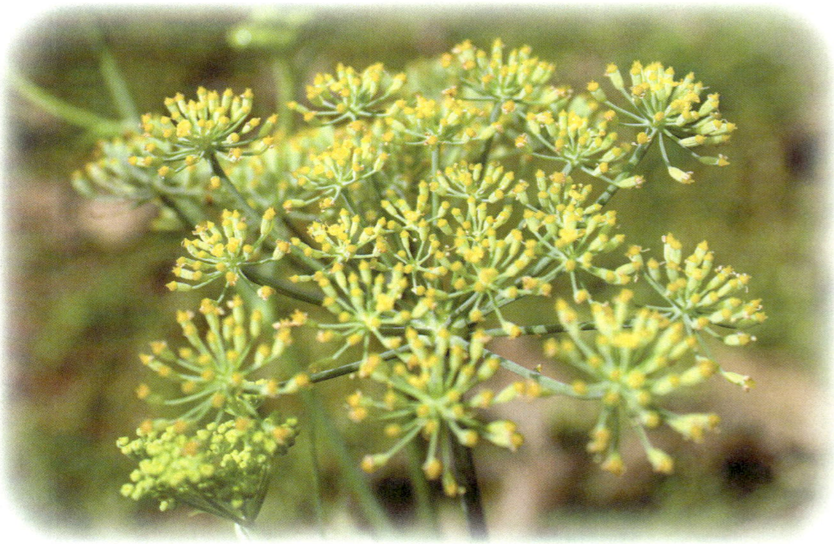

Many wildlife species depend on the anise plant. Pollinating honey and bumble bees, beetles, butterflies, moths, and hummingbirds feed on the nectar. Then, when the flowers go to seed, they are food for songbirds and small mammals. Although in different families, anise seed (*Apiaceae*) and licorice root (*Fabaceae*) have similar flavors and aromas because they both contain the biochemical compound anethole.

continued...

Foods from Nature

Plant Foods

LEAFY GREENS

Kingdom: *Plantae*
Phylum: *Tracheophytes*
Class: *Magnoliopsida*
Order: *Brassicales*
Family: *Brassicaceae*
(cruciferous/mustard/cabbage family)
Genus and species: *Eruca vesicaria*
Common name: Arugula

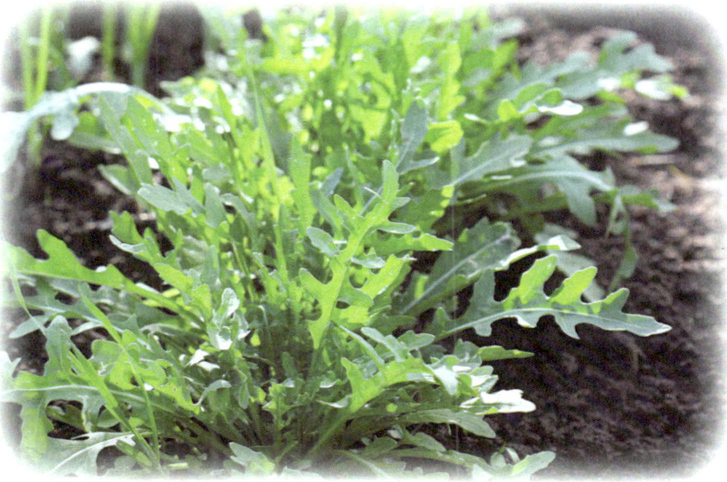

Native to the Mediterranean, arugula is a cold-season, leafy green plant. It is commonly grown in organic gardens. Arugula has a shallow root system and flourishes in moist, fertile soil with plenty of sunshine (dappled with shade in hot climates). Companion planting with strong-scented plants, such as chives, radishes, thyme, or nasturtiums, may discourage pest insects. Edible arugula leaves can be harvested throughout the growing season.

Kingdom: *Plantae*
Phylum: *Tracheophytes*
Class: *Magnoliopsida*
Order: *Caryophyllales*
Family: *Amaranthaceae*
(amaranth family)
Genus and species: *Beta vulgaris*
Common name: Beet Greens

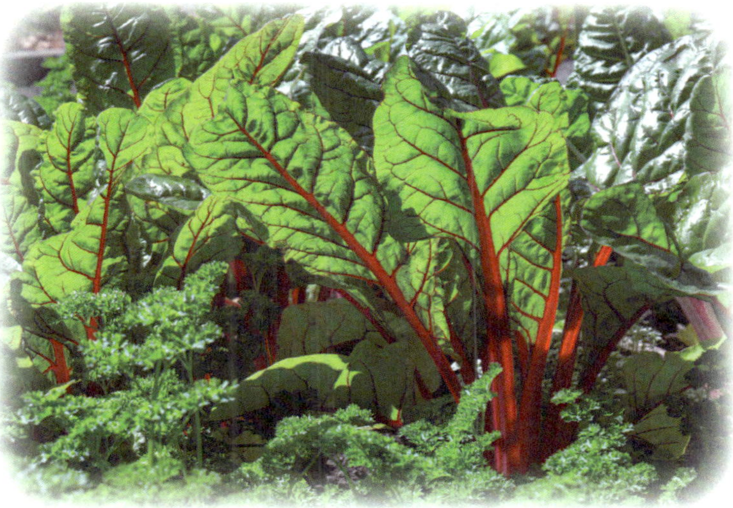

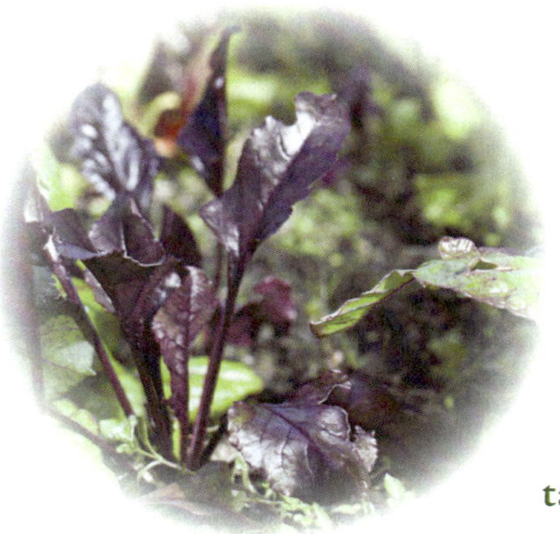

Beets are cool-season, biennial plants. They have green or red-veined leaves (and a purple variety) with a deep red, golden, or Chioggia (alternating red and white) taproot. Through their first spring, summer, and autumn, beet plants grow leaves and taproots. Protected from the cold underground, the taproot stores nutrients and energy for the plant to use over winter and to grow flowers and seeds in the spring of the second year. Once the flowers are pollinated, the plant dies, and the seeds carry on the next generation of beet plants.

continued...

Foods from Nature

Plant Foods

VEGETABLES

Kingdom: *Plantae*
Phylum: *Tracheophytes*
Class: *Magnoliopsida*
Order: *Caryophyllales*
Family: *Asterales*
(aster family)
Genus and species:
Cynara cardunculus
Common name: Artichoke

Artichoke plants put on a large floral display to attract pollinators. Their (edible) buds bloom as a composite of thousands of purple florets. Like their aster family relative, sunflowers, after pollination, a cone-shaped arrangement forms of the seeds as they grow and replace the florets.

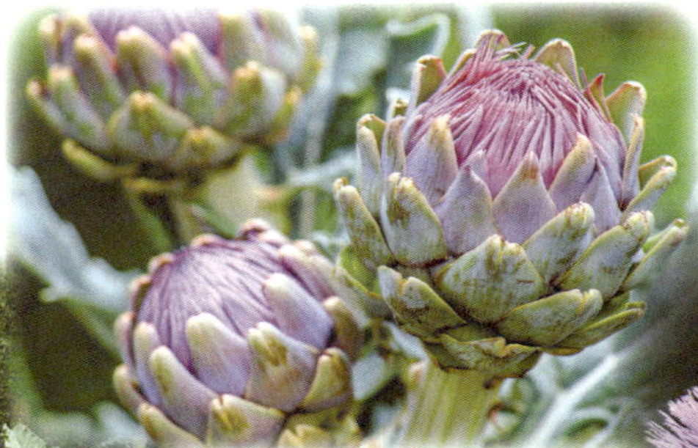

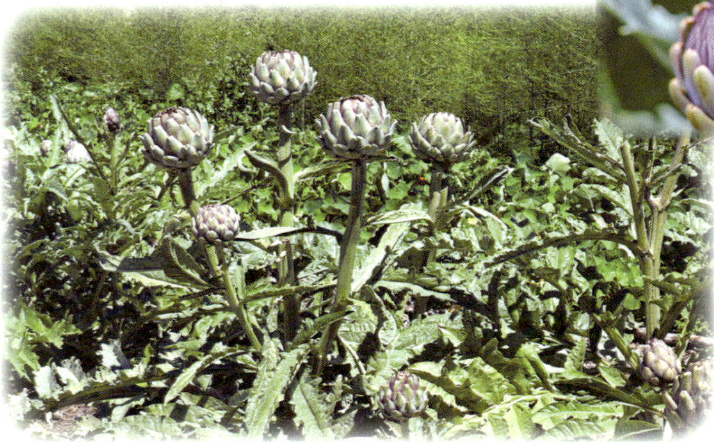

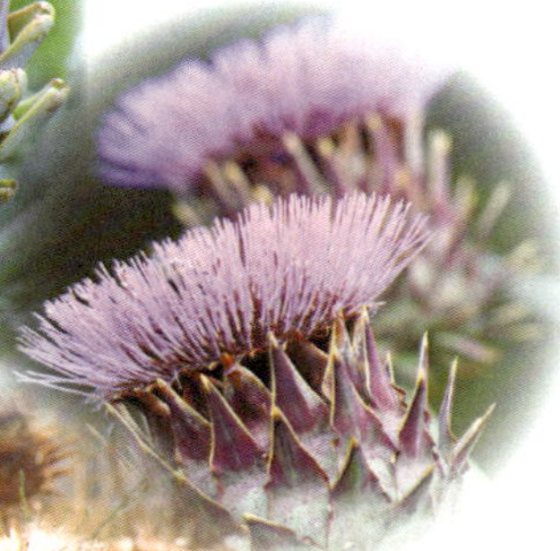

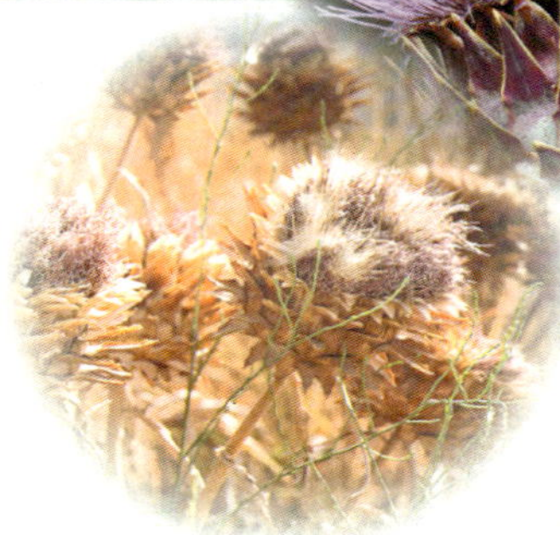

Kingdom: *Plantae*
Phylum: *Tracheophytes*
Class: *Liliopsida*
Order: *Asparagales*
Family: *Asparagaceae*
(asparagus family)
Genus and species: *Asparagus*
(several species)
Common name: Asparagus

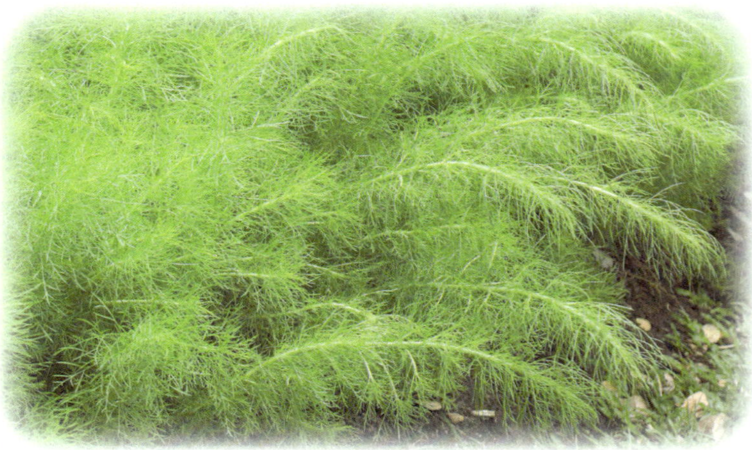

Asparagus species are native to maritime habitats, including coastal dunes and shrubland. They are hardy, evergreen plants that live for fifteen to twenty years. Each individual asparagus plant produces unique blends of volatile oils that comprise their floral scents to attract specific pollinator species.[1] Several wild asparagus species are threatened with extinction in their natural habitats.

References

[1]Llorens L., Tomàs J., Ferriol P., García, M. T., & Gil, L. (2023, September 10). Floral aroma and pollinator relationships in two sympatric late-summer-flowering Mediterranean asparagus species. *Journal of Plants*. Basel, Switzerland. *12*(18):3219. https://www.ncbi.nlm.nih.gov/pmc/articles/PMC10537274.

Foods from Nature

Mushrooms

CAUTION **Edible and Poisonous Mushroom Look-Alikes**
As an adaptation, there are many edible mushrooms that look like poisonous mushrooms; therefore, it is very important to accurately identify them before consuming them. Poisonous mushrooms are still poisonous when cooked.

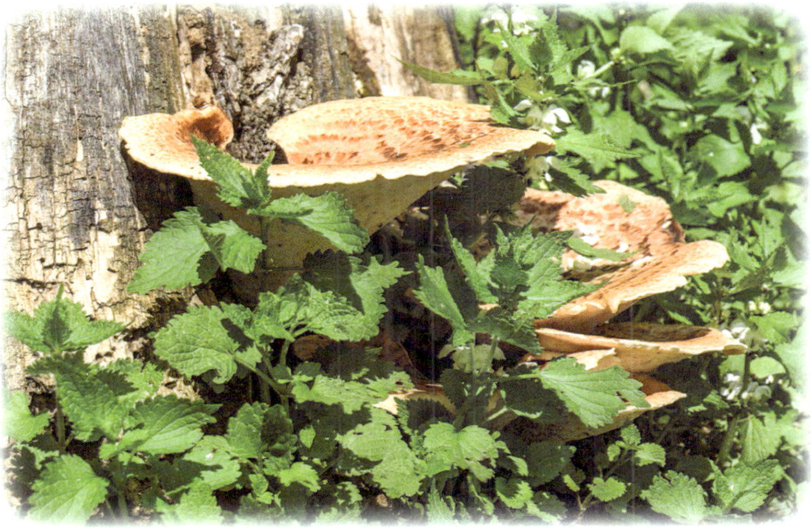

Kingdom: *Fungi*
Phylum: *Basidiomycota*
Class: *Agaricomycetes*
Order: *Hymenochaetaceae*
Family: *Hymenochaetaceae*
Genus species:
Inonotus obliquus
Common name: Chaga

Chaga is a slow-growing parasitic fungus that primarily grows on birch trees and occasionally other deciduous hardwoods. It is adapted to the cold climate of boreal forests in the northern hemisphere. Since chaga is not the fruiting body of mycelium it is, therefore, not a mushroom; instead, chaga is a dense mass of decayed tree tissue with mycelium incorporated into it. When the host tree dies, chaga produces spores to complete its life cycle, which are dispersed by wind and insects.

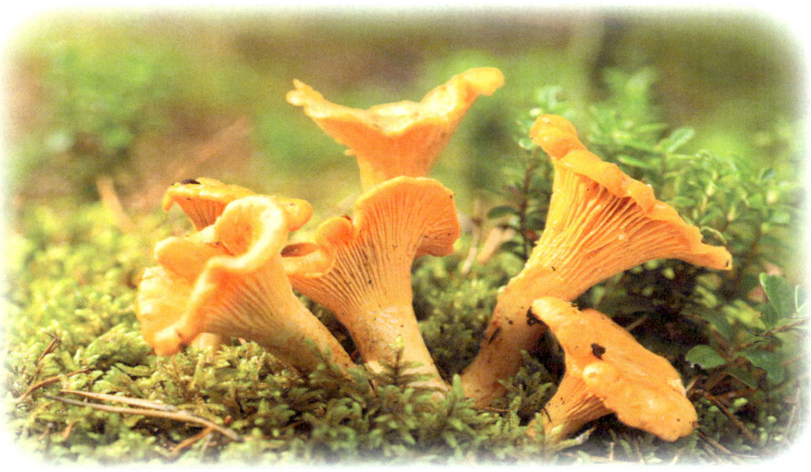

Kingdom: *Fungi*
Phylum: *Basidiomycota*
Class: *Agaricomycetes*
Order: *Cantharellales*
Family: *Cantharellaceae*
Genus: *Cantharellus, Craterellus, Gomphus, Polyozellus*
(~70 species total in these genera)
Common name: Chanterelle

Chanterelle mushrooms are found on every continent. They grow in clusters on the forest floor, including mossy clearings. Abundant in coastal forests, they live near Sitka spruce trees. They are also common in mid-seral stage Douglas fir and western hemlock forests.

continued...

Foods from Nature

Mushrooms

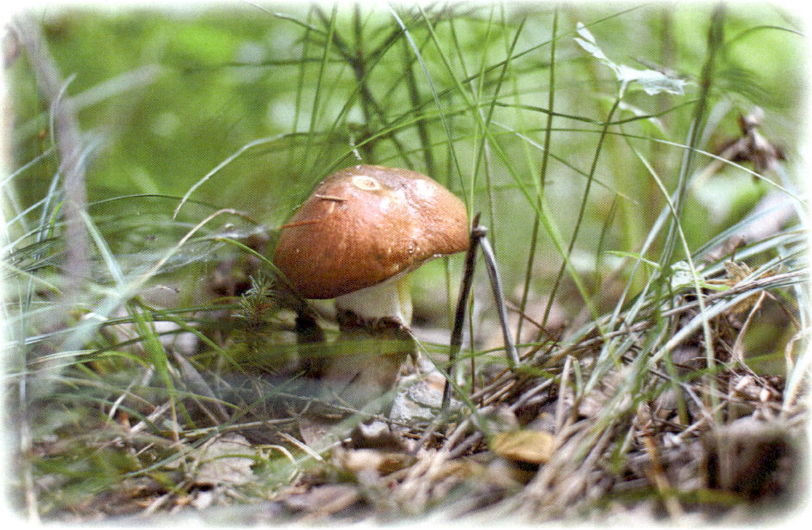

Kingdom: *Fungi*
Phylum: *Basidiomycota*
Class: *Agaricomycetes*
Order: *Agaricales*
Family: *Agaricaceae*
Genus and species:
Agaricus bisporus
Common name: Cremini

Cremini mushrooms, known as 'meadow mushrooms,' are native to grasslands in Eurasia and North America. On grassland landscapes and pasturelands they are frequently found growing in the dung of large grazing herbivores.

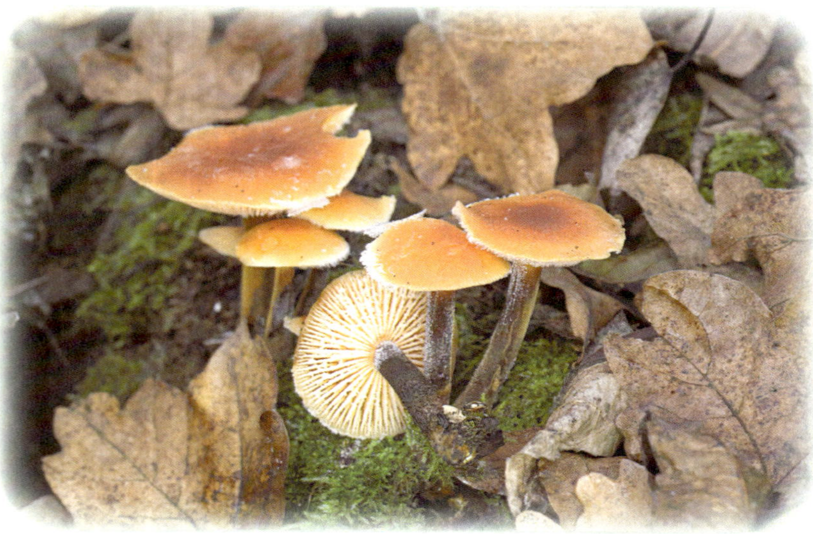

Kingdom: *Fungi*
Phylum: *Basidiomycota*
Class: *Agaricomycetes*
Order: *Cantharellales*
Family: *Physalacriaceae*
Genusand species:
Flammulina velutipes
Common name: Enoki

Enoki (velvet foot) are gilled mushrooms. The gills are located under the cap of the mushroom and used for dispersing spores. Enoki reside in clusters on decaying standing or fallen trees, where they can receive full sunlight. They often grow in the vicinity of similar looking poisonous mushrooms, particularly the deadly galerina (*Galerina marginata*).

continued...

Foods from Nature

Mushrooms

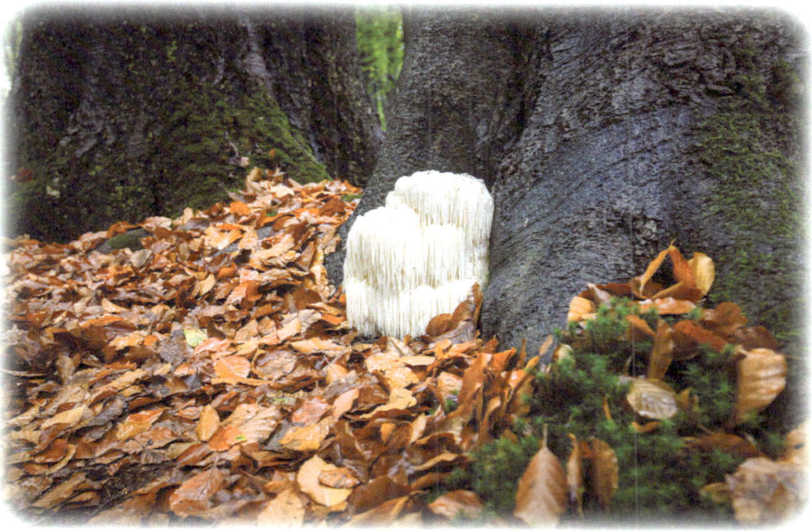

Kingdom: *Fungi*
Phylum: *Basidiomycota*
Class: *Agaricomycetes*
Order: *Russulales*
Family: *Hericiaceae*
Genus and species:
Hericium erinaceus
Common name:
Lion's Mane

Lions mane mushrooms are found throughout the northern hemisphere. Solitary, they are found by themselves on the trunks or at the base of decaying oak, walnut, beech, maple, sycamore, and other broad-leaf trees. They also thrive on fallen decaying trees.

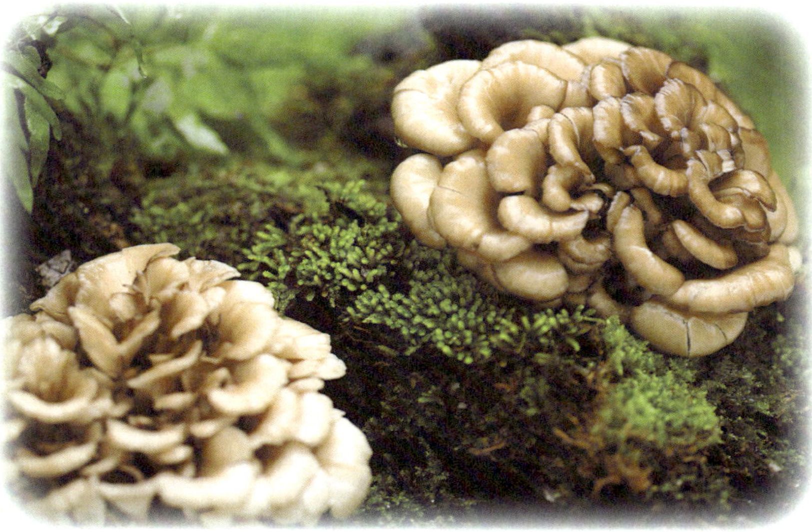

Kingdom: *Fungi*
Phylum: *Basidiomycota*
Class: *Agaricomycetes*
Order: *Polyporales*
Family: *Meripilaceae*
Genus and species:
Brifola frondose
Common name: **Maitake**

Maitake mushrooms grow in a circular cluster at the base of trees or on fallen trees, particularly old growth oaks or maples. They are common in hardwood forests on mature and aging trees, particularly in moist woodlands and along rivers.

continued...

Foods from Nature

Mushrooms

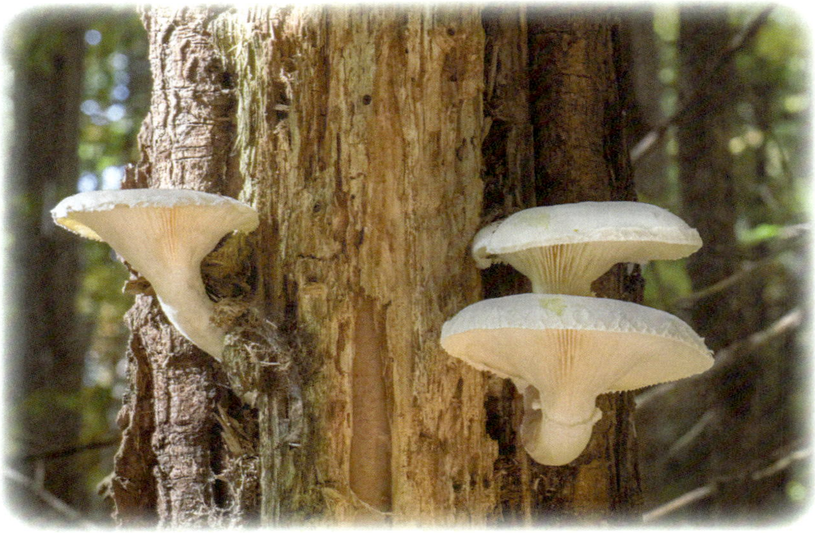

Kingdom: ***Fungi***
Phylum: ***Basidiomycota***
Class: ***Agaricomycetes***
Order: ***Agaricales***
Family: ***Hericiaceae***
Genus and species:
Pleurotus ostreatus
Common name: Oyster

Oyster mushrooms grow together in tiers on decaying standing or fallen trees, especially beech trees. They are present year-round, especially after a cold snap which can trigger the fungus into fruiting. Oyster mushrooms are carnivorous; as a source of nitrogen, they secrete a toxin and then consume nematodes that pass by them in the trees.

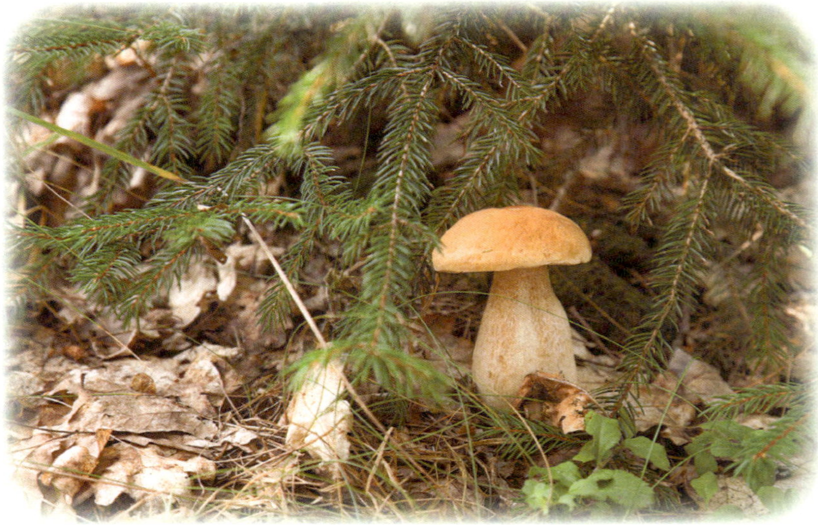

Kingdom: ***Fungi***
Phylum: ***Basidiomycota***
Class: ***Agaricomycetes***
Order: ***Boletales***
Family: ***Meripilaceae***
Genus and species:
Boletus edulis
Common name: Porcini

Porcini fungi and their mushrooms encompass an exceptional diversity of species with a wide distribution across tropical, temperate, and subalpine environments worldwide.[1] Closely adapted to the specific ecological conditions of small forest patches, porcini possess a high degree of genetic distinctiveness associated with their local niche.[2,3]

References

[1]Hosen, M. I., Feng, B., Xu, J., Wu, G., Zeng, N.-K., Li, Y-C., et al. (2012, August 13). DNA sequence analyses reveal abundant diversity, endemism and evidence for Asian origin of the porcini mushrooms. *Journal of PLoS ONE*. 7(8): https://doi.org/10.1371/annotation/e918501c-a3a9-4c14-9ea6-bcc6cf53062e.

[2]Tremble, K., Hoffman, J. I., & Dentinger, T. M. (2022, October 5). Contrasting continental patterns of adaptive population divergence in the holarctic ectomycorrhizal fungus Boletus edulis. *New Phytologist*. https://nph.onlinelibrary.wiley.com/doi/10.1111/nph.18521.

[3]Lewis, E. (2022, December 7). *Unusual discoveries made in the evolutionary patterns of porcini mushrooms*. Utah Public Radio. https://www.upr.org/utah-news/2022-12-07/unusual-discoveries-made-in-the-evolutionary-patterns-of-porcini-mushrooms.

continued...

Foods from Nature

Mushrooms

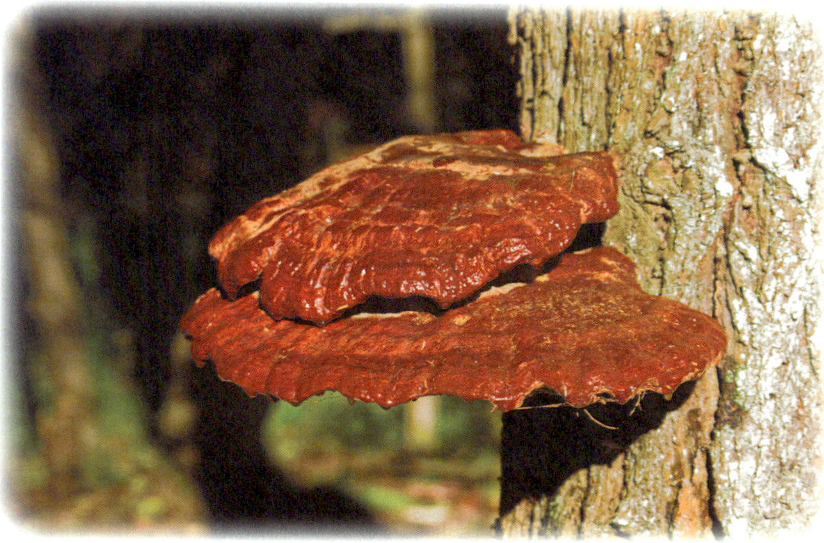

Kingdom: *Fungi*
Phylum: *Basidiomycota*
Class: *Agaricomycetes*
Order: *Polyporales*
Family: *Ganodermataceae*
Genus and species:
Ganoderma lucidum
Common name: Reishi

Reishi mushrooms grow on, or at the base of, living or decaying deciduous hardwood trees. They are particularly common on hemlock trees, and found on oak, elm, black gum, beech, maple, and larch trees as well. Reishi prefer wooded areas with high humidity and plenty of shade.

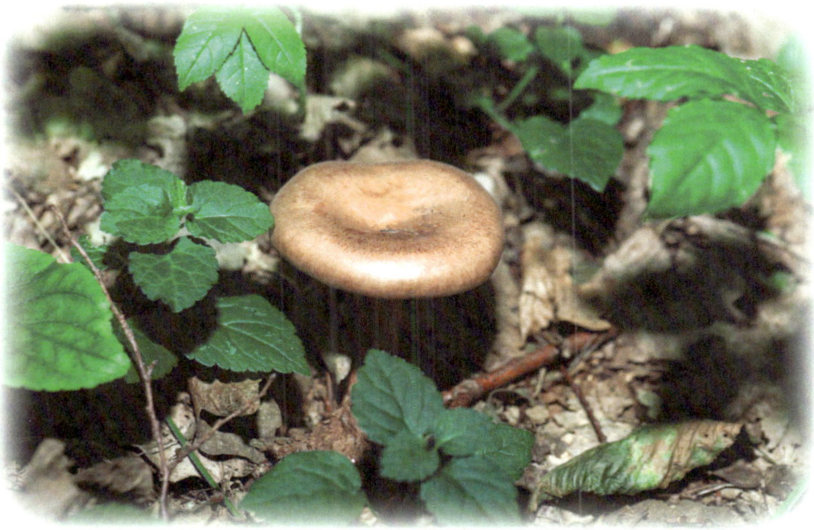

Kingdom: *Fungi*
Phylum: *Basidiomycota*
Class: *Agaricomycetes*
Order: *Agaricales*
Family: *Omphalotaceae*
Genus and species:
Lentinula edodes
Common name: Shiitake

Shiitake mushrooms are native to warm, moist mountainous climates in southeast Asia. They grow in clusters on the decaying wood of deciduous trees, particularly the shii tree, *Castanopsis cuspidata*, which is native to southern Japan and Korea. They also grow on chestnut, chinquapin (dwarf chestnut), oak, maple, beech, sweetgum, poplar, ironwood, and mulberry trees.

continued...

Foods from Nature

Mushrooms

Kingdom: *Fungi*
Phylum: *Basidiomycota*
Class: *Agaricomycetes*
Order: *Polyporales*
Family: *Polyporaceae* (polypore family)
Genus and species: *Trametes versicolor*
Common name: **Turkey Tail**

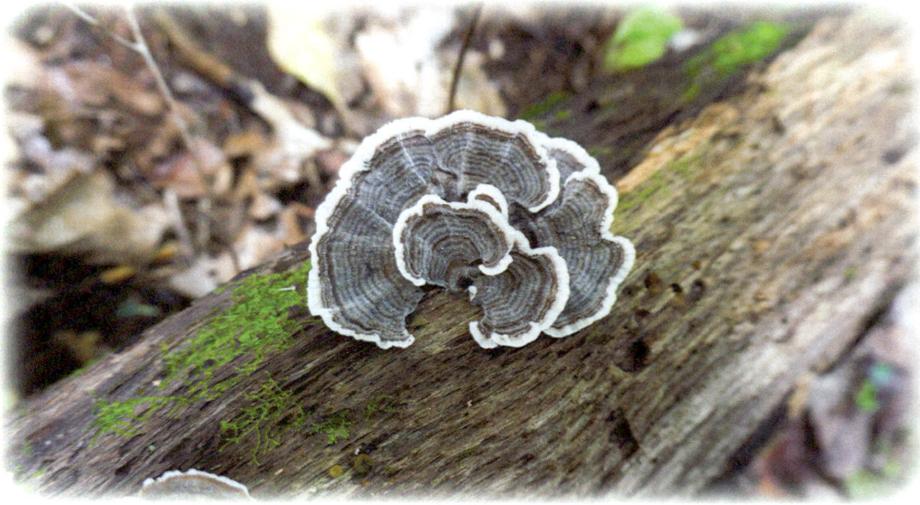

Turkey tail mushrooms grow in tiered layers with multicolored stripes. Being in the polypore family, they have small pore structures on their underside that hold their reproductive spores (rather than gills, which many other mushrooms have). Turkey tail are most often found on decaying fallen trees.

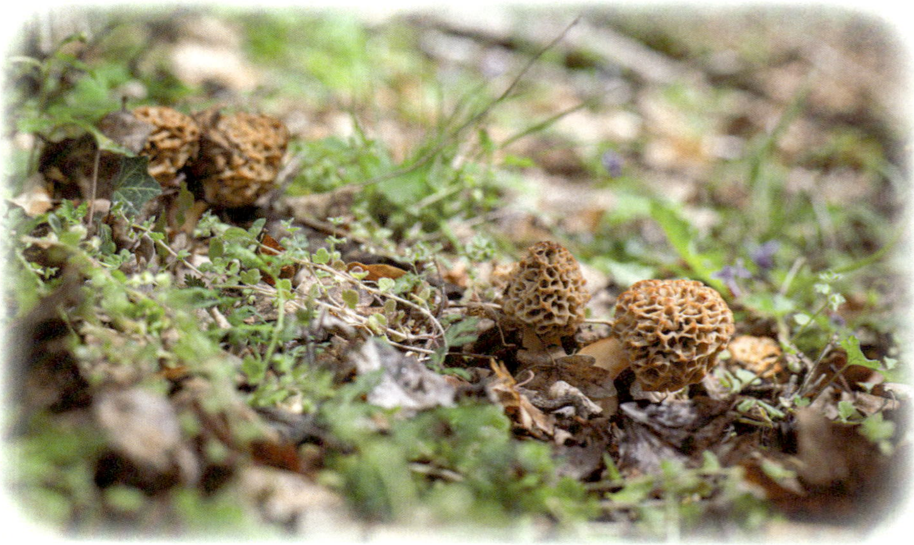

Kingdom: *Fungi*
Phylum: *Ascomycota*
Class: *Pezizomycetes*
Order: *Pezizales*
Family: *Morchellaceae*
Genus and species: many genera and species
Common name: **Morel**

Morel mushrooms flourish in grasslands, woodlands, and forests where there is high humidity, including nearby evaporating bodies of water. Morels prefer living in soil that is rich in organic matter with neutral to slightly acidic pH.

continued...

Foods from Nature

Mushrooms

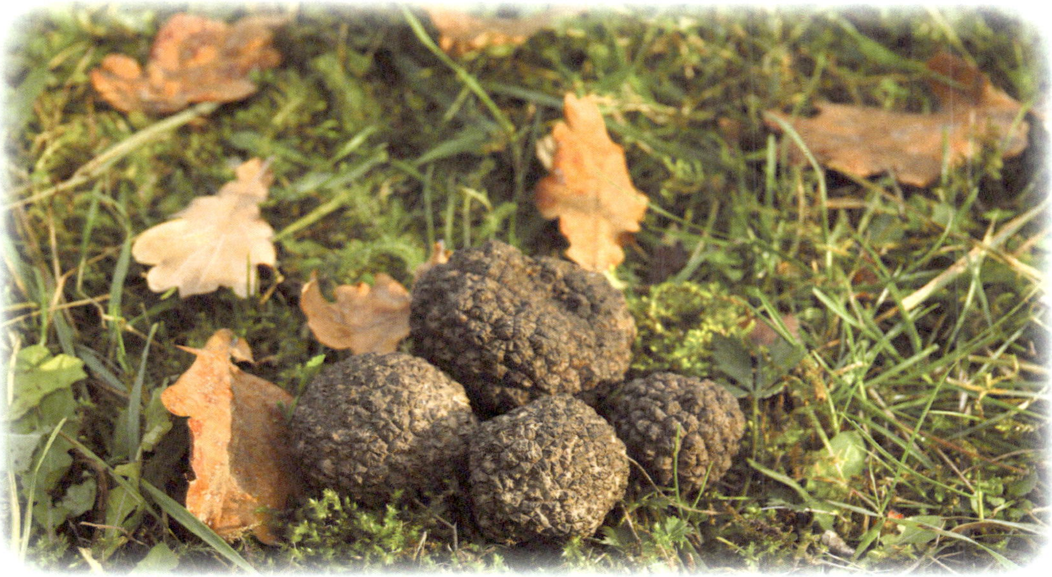

Kingdom: *Fungi*
Phylum: *Basidiomycota*
Class: *Agaricomycetes*
Order: *Polyporales*
Family: *Tuberaceae* (mycorrhizal fungi that first appeared in the Jurassic period (140–180 million years ago)
Genus and species: 55 different truffle genera and more than 350 truffle species
Common name: Truffle

Truffles are subterraneous. Living underground is an adaptation that insulates them from the cold climates they inhabit. Fairly easy to find, truffles are generally found near the surface of the topsoil, beneath the leaf litter. They are a major food source for hundreds of forest-dwelling animals that dig them up, consume them, and, through their excrement, disperse truffle spores throughout the forest. Truffles give off an aroma that attracts these symbiotic truffle-eating animals.

Foods from Nature

Algae

GREEN

Kingdom: ***Plantae***
Phylum: ***Chlorophyta***
Class: ***Trebouxiophyceae***
Order: ***Chlorellales***
Family: ***Chlorellales***
Genus: ***Chlorella*** **(13 species)**
Common name: Chlorella

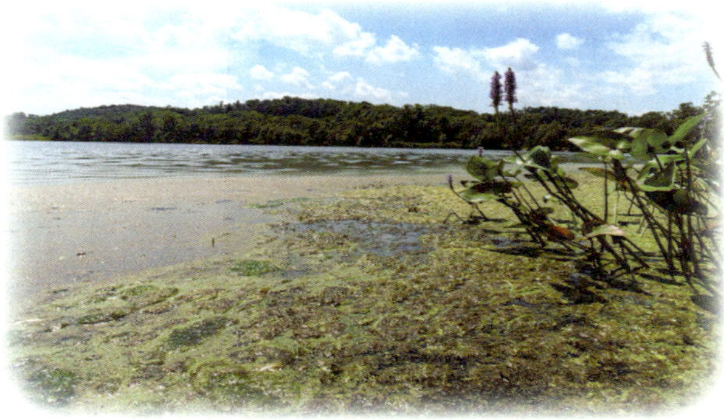

Chlorella are tiny spherical-shaped, single-celled algae. In their chloroplasts, they have photosynthetic pigments (chlorophyll-a and -b) that enable chlorella to grow when they receive sunlight, carbon dioxide, water, and nutrients. Most chlorella species live in freshwater but some have been found in saltwater. As part of the *Chlorellaceae* family, chlorella are adapted to extreme temperatures, atmospheric pressures, and desiccating winds. They self-shade and guard against harsh conditions by forming cell aggregates and excreting mucilage to create an insulating matrix.[1]

References

[1]Darienko, T., Rad-Menéndez, C., Campbell, C., & Pröschold, T. (2019, December 23). Are there any true marine Chlorella species? Molecular phylogenetic assessment and ecology of marine Chlorella-like organisms, including a description of *Droopiella gen. nov. Systematics and Biodiversity. 17*(8), 811 – 829. https://www.tandfonline.com/doi/full/10.1080/14772000.2019.1690597.

Kingdom: ***Plantae***
Phylum: ***Chlorophyta***
Class: ***Ulvophyceae***
Order: ***Bryopsidales***
Family: ***Caulerpaceae***
Genus and species: ***Caulerpa***
(~200 species, including *lentillifera*)
Common name: Sea Grape

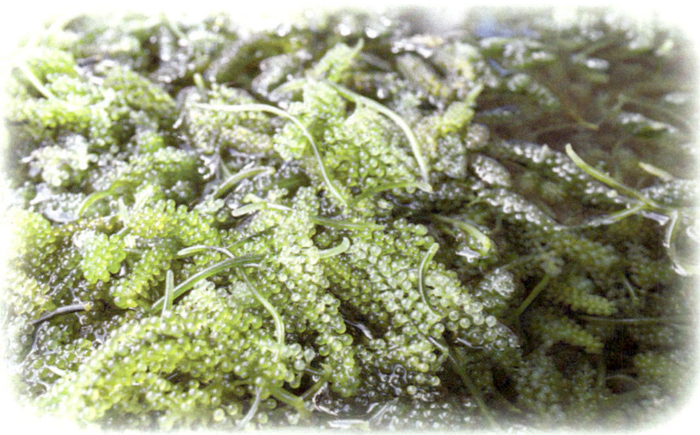

Sea grapes inhabit sandy substrates and rock pools in shallow tropical and temperate waters of the coastal Asia-Pacific region. Vesicle-rudiments give sea grapes their succulent texture. As an algal organism, sea grapes are composed of a single cell with multiple nuclei (one continuous multinucleate cell) that can reach several meters long. Therein, sea grapes are likely the largest single-celled organisms on Earth.[1]

References

[1]Arimoto, A., Nishitsuji, K., Narisoko, H., Shoguchi, E., & Satoh, N. (2019, November 11). Differential gene expression in fronds and stolons of the siphonous alga, *Caulerpa lentillifera,* development. *Journal of Growth, and Differentiation*. https://doi.org/10.1111/dgd.12634Citations: 8.

continued...

Foods from Nature

Algae

GREEN

Kingdom: *Plantae*
Phylum: *Chlorophyta*
Class: *Ulvophyceae*
Order: *Ulvales*
Family: *Ulvaceae*
Genus and species: *Ulva*
(4,300 known species, including *lactuca***)**
Common name: Sea Lettuce

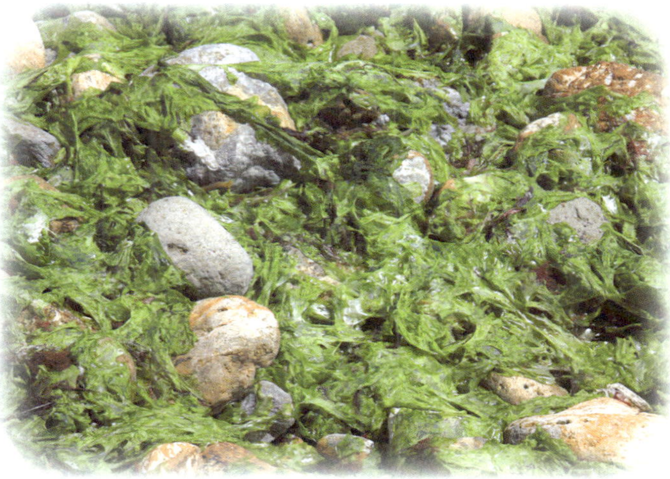

Sea lettuce grows in semi-protected intertidal and shallow subtidal areas. With its small, disk-like holdfast, it attaches to a substrate, such as rocks, shells, or seagrass. Sometimes, sea lettuce can be found free-floating. While its fronds are thin and sheet-like, it has a tough gelatinous, protective sheath. As a perennial, sea lettuce dies back in the winter and regrows in the spring. Its reproductive cycle entails alternating between spore-producing and gamete-producing generations.

BROWN

Kingdom: *Chromista*
Phylum: *Phaeophyta*
Class: *Phaeophyceae*
Order: *Laminariales*
Family: *Lessoniaceae*
Genus and species: *Eisenia bicyclis*
Common name: Arame

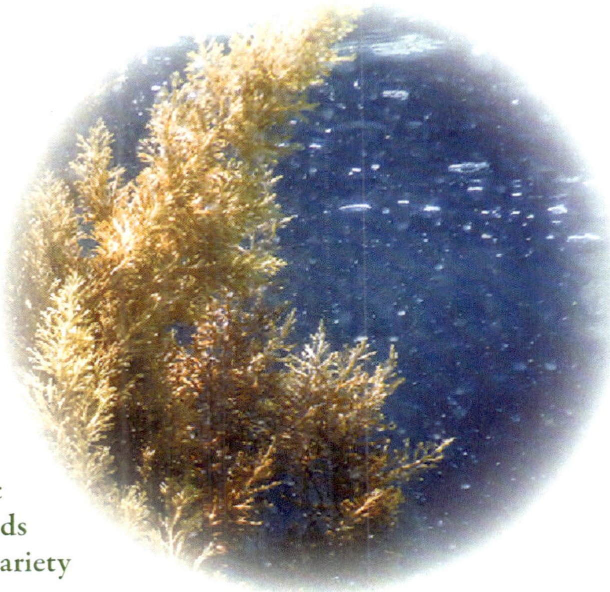

Arama/sea oak has a feathery nature, fanning out from two fronds at the top of its stipe (stem-like structure) which grows to about meter (3.3 feet) high. The fronds are shed and new ones are formed each year. Arame lives in the low intertidal and subtidal zones of the Pacific Ocean. In a temperate climate, arame grows in dense stands on rocky shores and reefs where it provides habitat for a variety of sea life, such as clams, abalone, and fish.

continued...

Foods from Nature

Algae

BROWN

Kingdom: ***Chromista***
Phylum: ***Phaeophyta***
Class: ***Phaeophyceae***
Order: ***Laminariales***
Family, genus, and species:
several families, genera, and species
Common name: Kelp

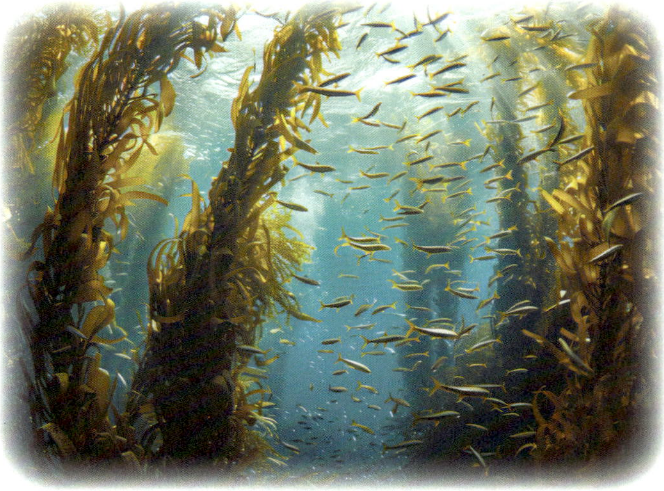

Dense, underwater kelp forests support a wide array of marine life in subtropical, temperate, and sub-Antarctic oceans of the Southern Hemisphere and northeast Pacific Ocean. The giant kelp attach themselves to the seafloor with their holdfasts, and grow to the water's surface where they can receive needed sunlight for photosynthesis. They may reach heights of 45 meters (150 feet). Kelp forests provide a home to hundreds of thousands of species, including invertebrates, fishes, and marine mammals, furnishing shelter from predators and storms. Many species congregate and spawn in kelp forests and use them as nursery habitats. Sea otters are a keystone species. They maintain kelp forest ecosystems by consuming sea urchins that would otherwise overharvest the kelp.

Kingdom: ***Chromista***
Phylum: ***Phaeophyta***
Class: ***Phaeophyceae***
Order: ***Fucales***
Family: ***Sargassaceae***
Genus and species:
Sargassum fusiforme
Common name: Hijiki

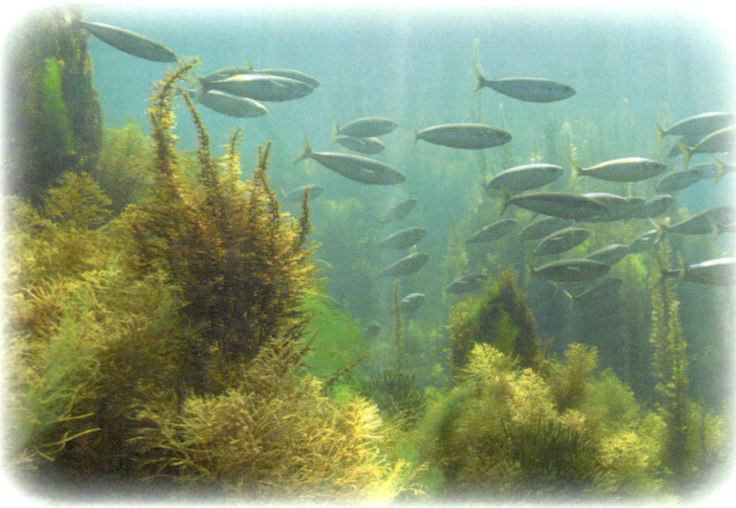

Hijiki grows wild on the rocky coasts of East Asia. Maintaining their traditional practices of harvesting hijiki off the shores of Japan, villagers cut hijiki at low tide with hand-held sickles (a knife with a curved blade).
The villagers synchronize with hijiki's natural life cycle to foster future harvests; they leave plenty of the algae intact above the base to regenerate.
The hijiki is washed in freshwater and laid on racks to dry in the sun.

continued...

Foods from Nature

Algae

BROWN

The Shiretoko Peninsula 'Kombu Garden' Supports a Diverse Trophic Organization (Food Chain)

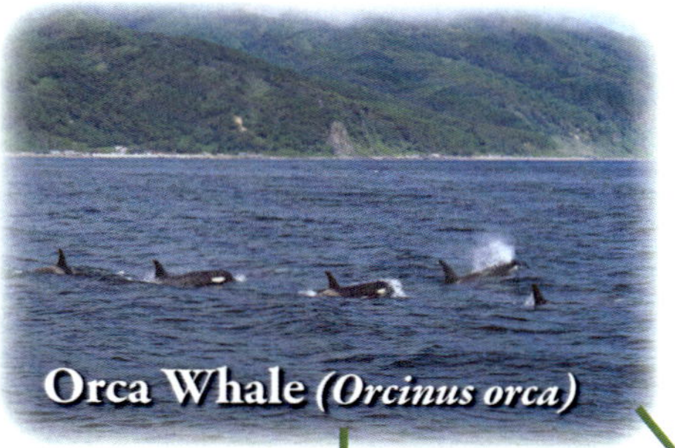
Orca Whale *(Orcinus orca)*

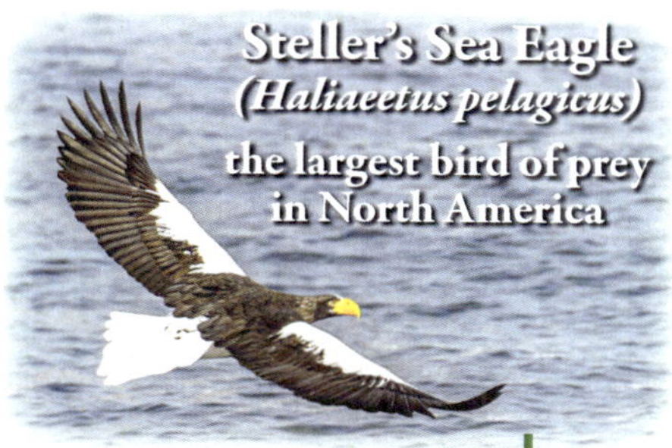
Steller's Sea Eagle *(Haliaeetus pelagicus)* the largest bird of prey in North America

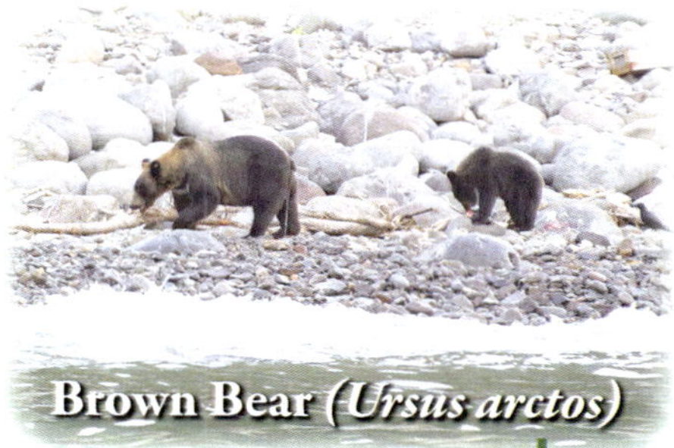
Brown Bear *(Ursus arctos)*

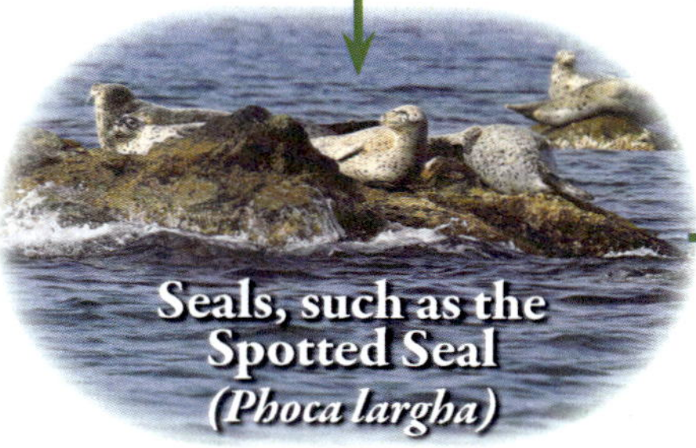
Seals, such as the Spotted Seal *(Phoca largha)*

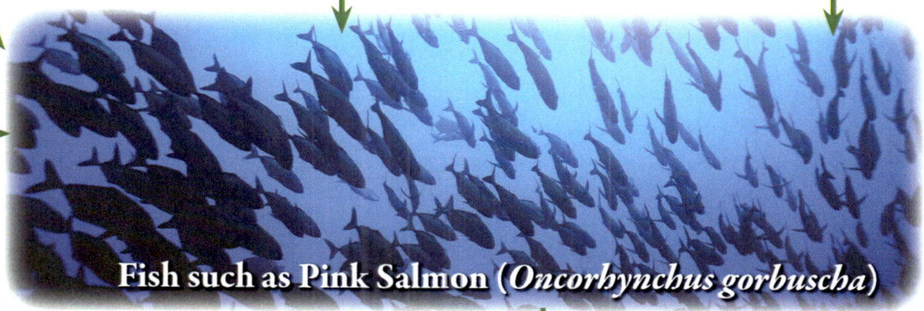
Fish such as Pink Salmon (*Oncorhynchus gorbuscha*)

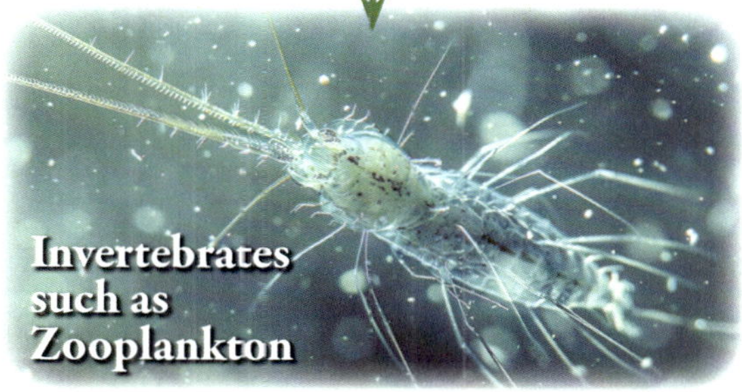
Invertebrates such as Zooplankton

Kingdom: *Chromista*
Phylum: *Phaeophyta*
Class: *Phaeophyceae*
Order: *Fucales*
Family: *Sargassaceae*
Genus and species: *Laminaria digitata*
Common name: Kombu

The Shiretoko Peninsula is a World Natural Heritage Site, recognized for its rich biodiversity and interaction between marine and terrestrial ecosystems[1]

Kombu grows in lower intertidal and shallow subtidal waters along the coasts of the northwest Pacific Ocean. The shores of East Hokkaido, Japan, are known as the 'kombu garden of the world.' Each year, mineral-rich sea ice is carried in the Amur River, by currents and wind from Siberia, to the coast of East Hokkaido's Shiretoko Peninsula. As the ice melts, the mineral-rich sea water nourishes the kombu garden.

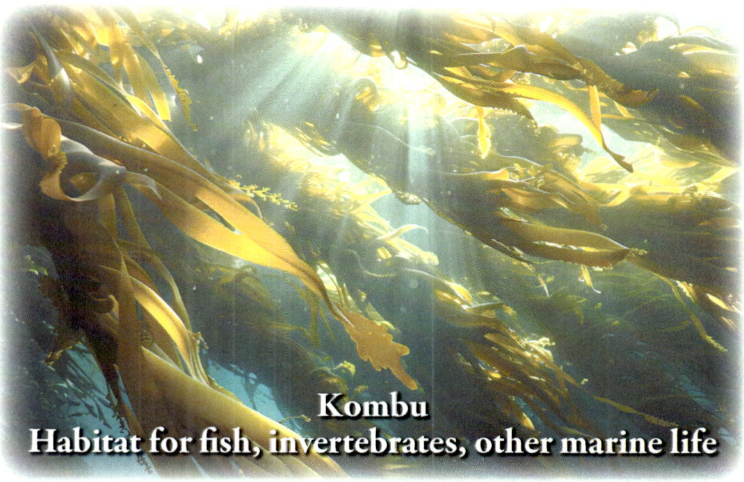
Kombu
Habitat for fish, invertebrates, other marine life

References

[1]World Heritage Convention. (2024). *Shiretoko*. UNESCO. https://whc.unesco.org/en/list/1193.

continued...

Foods from Nature

Algae

BROWN

Kingdom: *Chromista*
Phylum: *Phaeophyta*
Class: *Phaeophyceae*
Order: *Fucales*
Family: *Alariaceae*
Genus and species:
Undaria pinnatifida
Common name: Wakame

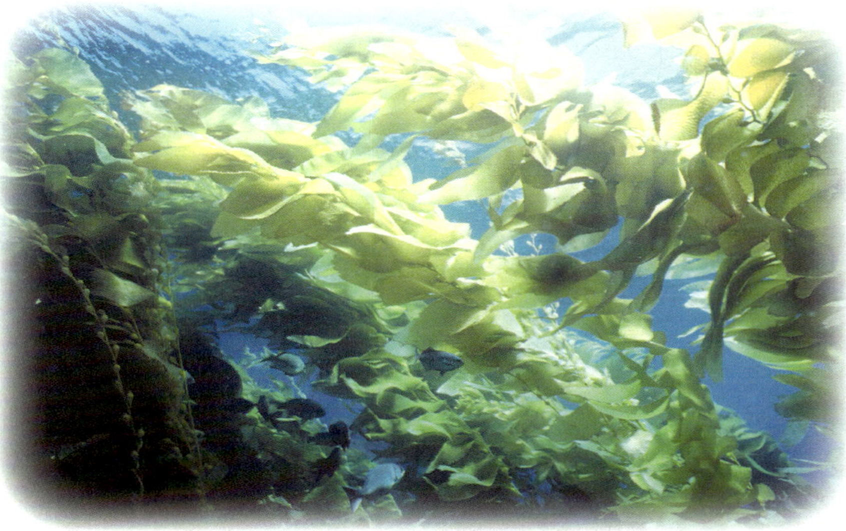

Wakame, like kombu, is native to the cold waters on rocky shores of the northwest Pacific Ocean. Well-adapted to strong wave action, wakame lives mostly in lower intertidal and shallow subtidal areas. It can also tolerate a wide range of salinity, persisting in marine and estuarine environments. Growing in thick stands, wakame provides a buffer against storm surges which protects sea life and reduces coastal erosion by preventing sediment from being swept away from the beaches.

RED

Kingdom: *Plantae*
Phylum: *Rhodophyta*
Class: *Florideophyceae*
Order: *Palmariales*
Family: *Palmariaceae*
Genus and species:
Palmaria palmata
Common name: Dulse

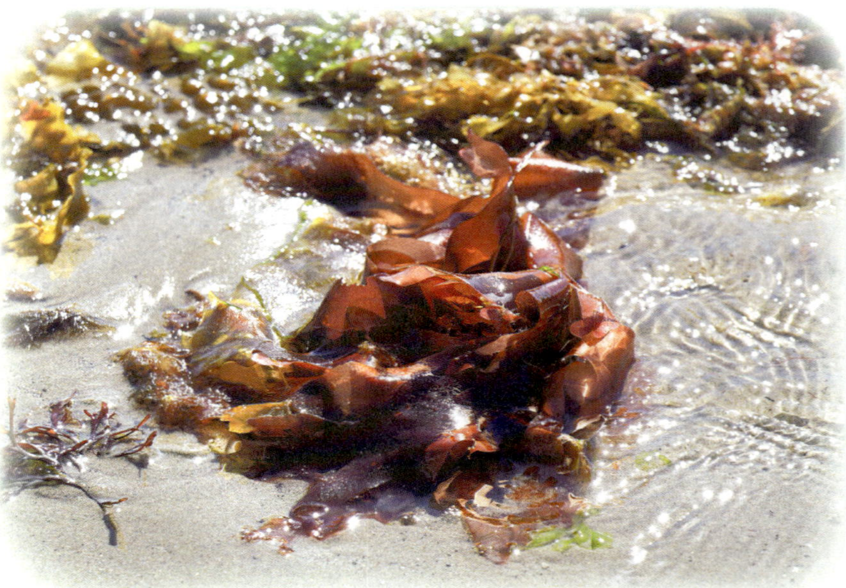

Dulse has a broad temperature tolerance. It grows in the cold and freezing waters of the Arctic Sea as well off the coast of South America. It grows predominantly in the upper sub-tidal zone, where it anchors its holdfasts to rocks and shells. Dulse may also exist as an epiphyte, attaching to other macroalgae, usually on the stipes of large species of kelp. Dulse is a perennial, regrowing new fronds every year. It is often covered with bryozoans, filter-feeding invertebrates.

continued...

Foods from Nature

Algae

RED

Kingdom: *Plantae*
Phylum: *Rhodophyta*
Class: *Florideophyceae*
Order: *Gigartinales*
Family: *Gigartinaceae*
Genus and species: *Chondrus cristus*
Common name: **Sea/Irish Moss**

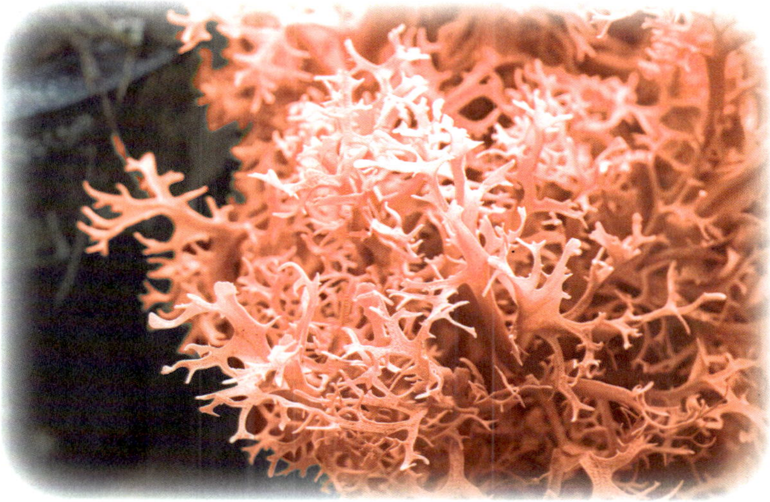

Sea/Irish moss grows in the mid to subtidal zone on rocks and boulders along the Atlantic coast of Europe and North America. It thrives in cold water; although, it can tolerate warmer temperatures. Sea/Irish moss attaches to rocks with its holdfasts or exists in free-floating mats. It is a relatively small algae, only 7 to 8 inches (~20 cm) in length. In light of its small size, sea moss furnishes food and provides refuge for crustaceans, snails, juvenile mussels, crabs, star fish, and other small sea life.

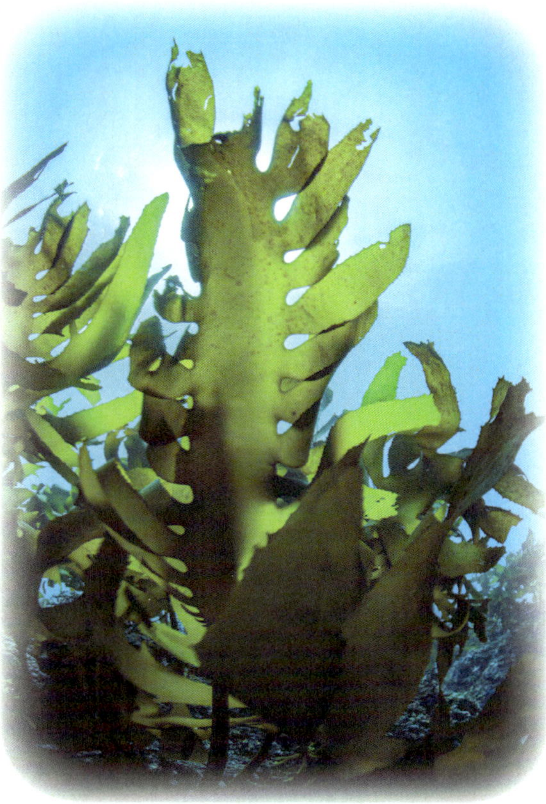

Kingdom: *Plantae*
Phylum: *Rhodophyta*
Class: *Bangiophyceae*
Order: *Bangiales*
Family: *Bangiaceae*
Genus and species: *Pyropia* (about 130 species, including *yezoensis and tenera)*
Common name: **Nori**

Nori occurs in tropical, subtropical, temperate, and northern boreal waters. It has a very thin, sheet-like frond emerging from its holdfast, with no stipe. Nori is an exceptionally hardy algae, growing along exposed coastlines where there are temperature extremes and strong waves. It flourishes in the upper tidal zones where other seaweed species cannot survive. Limpets and other sea snails feed on nori, scraping off layers of the algae with their radula (ribbon-like structure with rows of chitinous toothlets). Some limpets are territorial and actively protect their patch of nori.

Foods from Nature

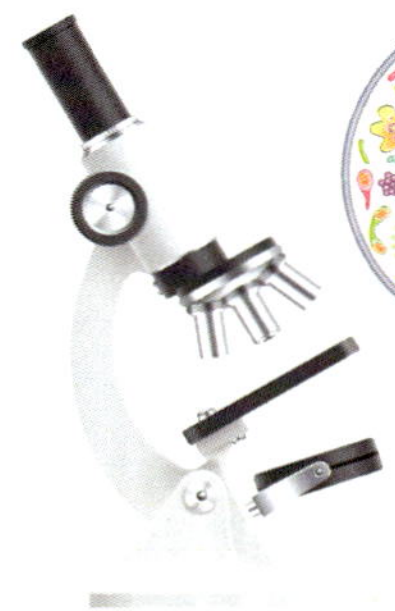

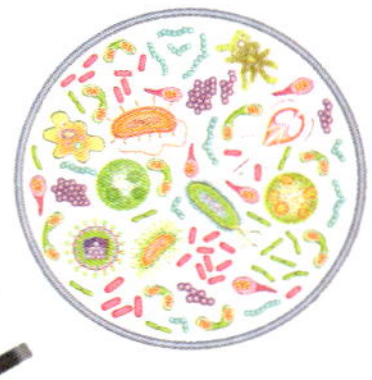

Bacteria and Micro-Fungi Probiotics

BACTERIA in milk ferments, such as yogurt and kefir

Kingdom: ***Bacillati*** **(*Bacteria* Domain)**
Phylum: ***Bacillota***
Class: ***Bacilli***
Order: ***Lactobacillales***
Family: ***Lactobacillaceae***
Genus and species:
Lactobacillus acidophilus

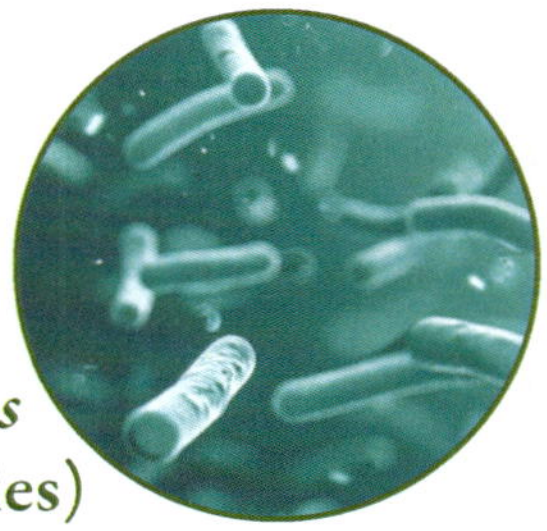

Lactobacillus
(many species)

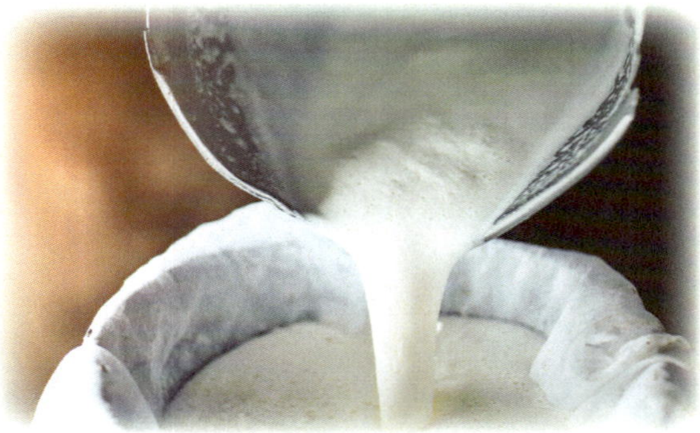

Raw Milk
Habitat for *Lactobacillus* and *Bifidobacterium*

Kingdom: ***Bacillati*** **(*Bacteria* Domain)**
Phylum: ***Actinomycetota***
Class: ***Actinomycetes***
Order: ***Bifidobacteriales***
Family: ***Bifidobacteriaceae***
Genus: ***Bifidobacterium***
Species: ***Bifidobacterium bifidum***

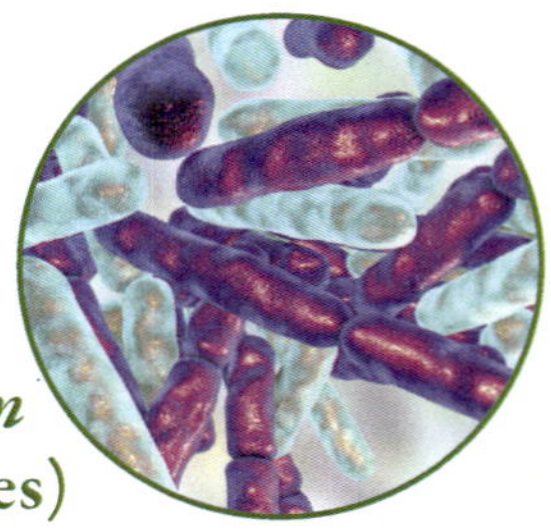

Bifidobacterium
(many species)

BACTERIA in natto soybean ferment

Kingdom: ***Bacillati*** **(*Bacteria* Domain)**
Phylum: ***Bacillota***
Class: ***Bacilli***
Order: ***Caryophanales***
Family: ***Bacillaceae***
Genus and species:
Bacillus subtilis

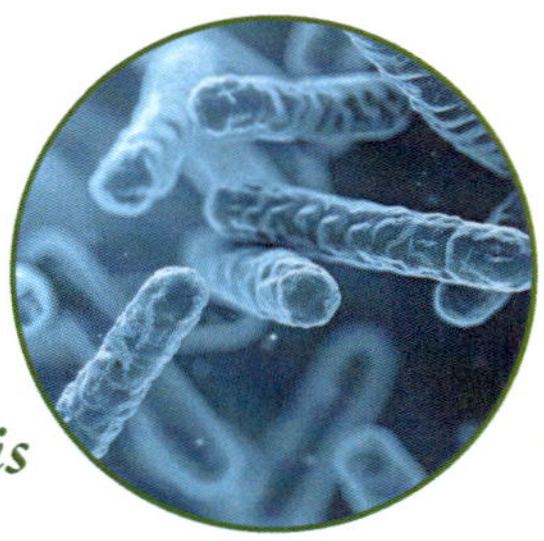

Bacillus subtilis

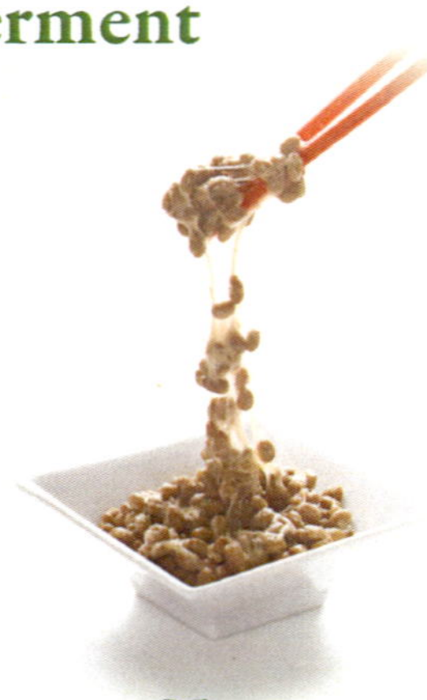

Natto
Habitat for *Bacillus subtilis*

continued...

Foods from Nature

Bacteria and Micro-Fungi Probiotics

BACTERIA and *FUNGI* – starter culture for kefir and kombucha

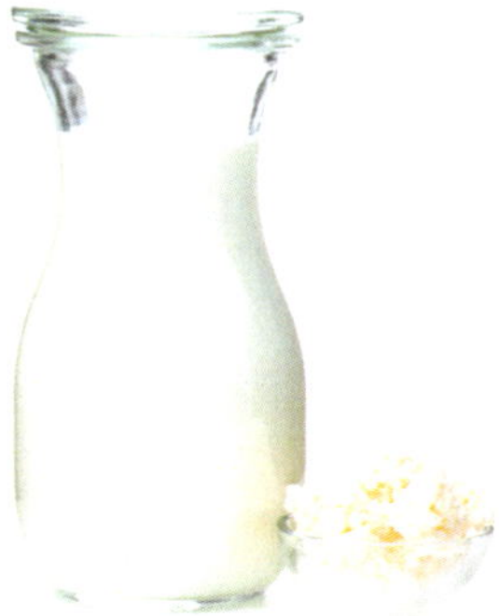

Kefir and kefir grains
Habitat for *Lactobacillus*
and *Saccharomyces cerevisiae*

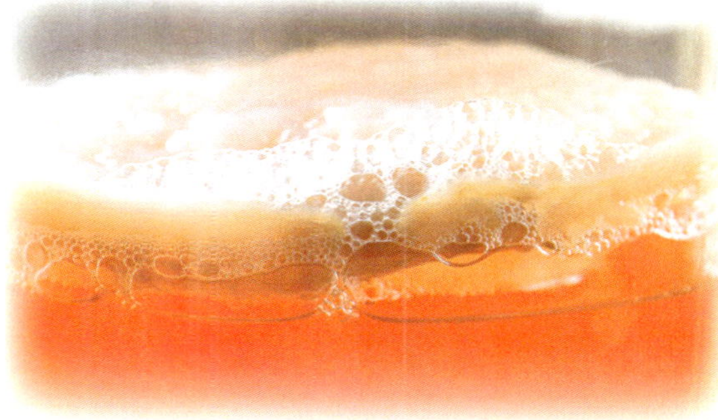

Kombucha
Habitat for *Saccharomyces cerevisiae*

Kingdom: *Fungi*
Phylum: *Ascomycota*
Class: *Saccharomycetes*
Order: *Saccharomycetales*
Family: *Saccharomycetaceae*
Genus and species: *Saccharomyces cerevisiae*

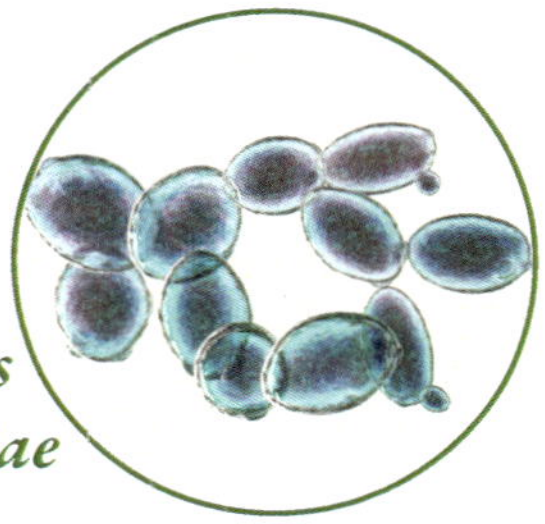

Saccharomyces cerevisiae

FUNGI – starter culture for miso and tamari soybean ferment

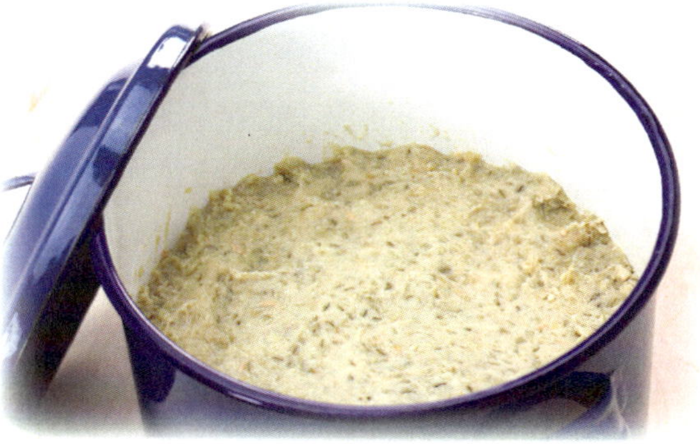

Miso
Habitat for *Aspergillus oryzae*

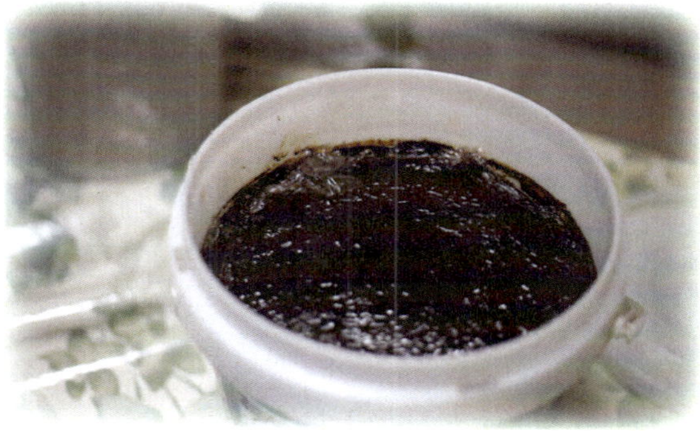

Tamari
Habitat for *Aspergillus oryzae*

Kingdom: *Fungi*
Phylum: *Ascomycota*
Class: *Eurotiomycetes*
Order: *Eurotiales*
Family: *Aspergillaceae*
Genus and species: *Aspergillus oryzae*

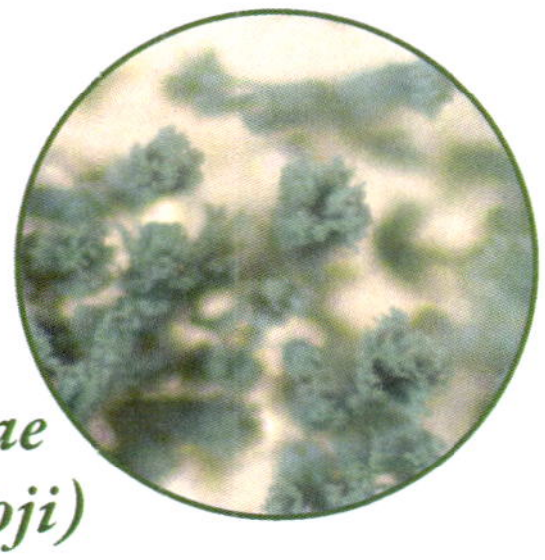

Aspergillus oryzae (Koji)

PART III

The Tapestry of Life

The Tapestry of Life

Ecosystems have non-living (abiotic/inorganic) and living (biotic/organic) constituents that adhere to the laws of physics. Living organisms and, over geologic time, species are self-organizing, self-regulating (maintaining homeostasis), and self-repairing. In carrying out their life cycles, organisms alter their environment. Beaver families, for example, build dams that flood forests, creating habitat for themselves and other aquatic species. *Throughout the world, the activities of organisms generate feedback loops with cumulative effects that influence ecosystems, bioregions, and the biosphere–emerging as a coherent system of life.*[1]

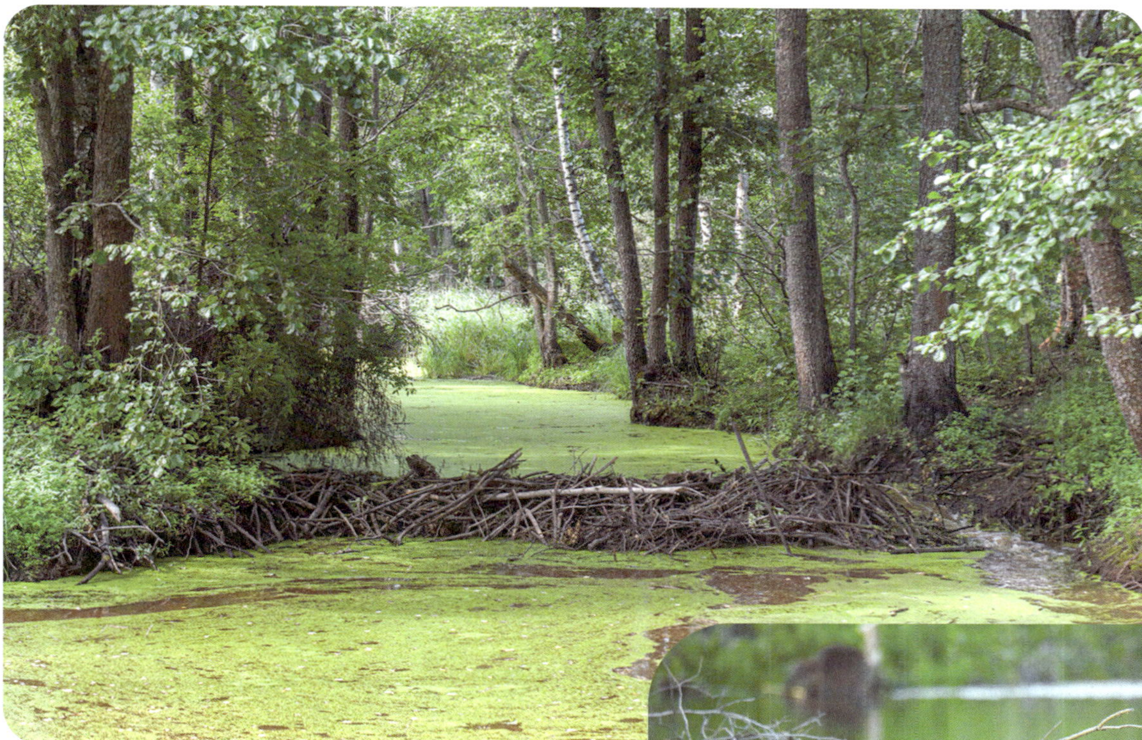

Photographer Denis Kostroma, Dreamstime

Flooded forest caused by the beaver dam

Beaver parents build dams, backing up streams that develop into lakes; and the beaver kits assist with repairs as needed.

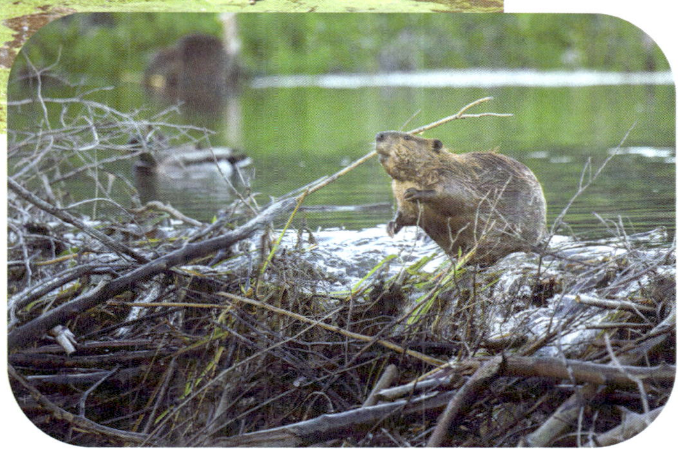

Photographer Chase Dekker, Dreamstime

Beaver building a dam

I. Interfacing Abiotic and Biotic Phenomena

Minerals – Cornerstone to Life Since the Beginning

Micro Level

Minerals (abiotic/non-living/inorganic) from disintegrated rock, along with molecules from the air and water, are integral to the existence of life. "The first living entity emerged from interactions of air, water, and rock–the same raw materials that sustain life today," Robert Hazen, astrobiologist and mineralogist, explains in his book, *Genesis: The Scientific Quest for Life's Origins.*[2] Hazen points out that minerals must have played ". . . a sequence of crucial roles, beginning with the synthesis of biomolecules and during their subsequent assembly into growing and evolving structures."[3] He states that "Many of the molecules that enable today's living cells to process energy have, at their core, a mineral-like cluster of iron or nickel and sulfur atoms."[4] In addition to minerals having been cornerstone to the origin of life, all organisms to this day have a saline (mineral) solution in their bodies, mirroring the primeval seas where life began. In his book, *The Body Is the Hero*, Ronald J. Glasser, M.D. describes how "The concentration of salts, of sodium, potassium and chloride in our bloodstream, the cobalt, magnesium and zinc in our tissues, are the same as those that existed in the earliest seas."[5]

Elements – Earth, Fire, Air, and Water – Set the Stage for Life

Macro Level

Elements–including the minerals in rocks and abiotic/inorganic components of fire, air, and water–and their geologic, climatic, and hydrologic processes make life possible on Earth. Magnetism (gravitational force) from the Earth's fiery core holds ~80% of the atmospheric gases within ten miles of the Earth's surface, delineating the upper boundary of the biosphere. Beyond the atmosphere, the gases thin as they transition into outer space. The ozone layer in the lower stratosphere shields life from extreme temperatures, harmful ultraviolet radiation, and deflects meteorites. The oceans and other water bodies are also held to the Earth's surface. Gravitation pull from the Moon, and to an extent the Sun, drive the ocean tides.

Naturalist and Explorer
Alexander von Humboldt (1769 – 1859)
Broadly investigating nature (including inter-relationships of abiotic and biotic phenomena at multiple scales), Alexander von Humboldt laid the foundation for the study of earth systems and biogeography.

Watersheds and Wetlands

Fine water droplets evaporate from oceans, lakes, and ponds and transpire from plant leaves, forming clouds. When the water in clouds is heavy enough, it falls as rain, hail, snow, and sleet. Most precipitation returns to the water bodies and rainforests where it came from, and wind carries some precipitation to other seascapes and landscapes. When dropping onto land, water divides into 'watersheds;' seeps into the soil; recharges groundwater and aquifers; emerges as springs; and forms tributaries that converge into streams and rivers. The movement of streams and rivers–in waterfalls, eddies, and ripples flowing through grasslands, woodlands, forests, and deserts–oxygenates, energizes, and structures water[6] making it more suitable for life. Moving through wetlands on these landscapes, such as marshes and swamps, water is slowed by water-adapted plants (hydrophytic vegetation) that filter and improve the water quality, hold the soil in place, and support an abundance of aquatic and terrestrial wildlife.

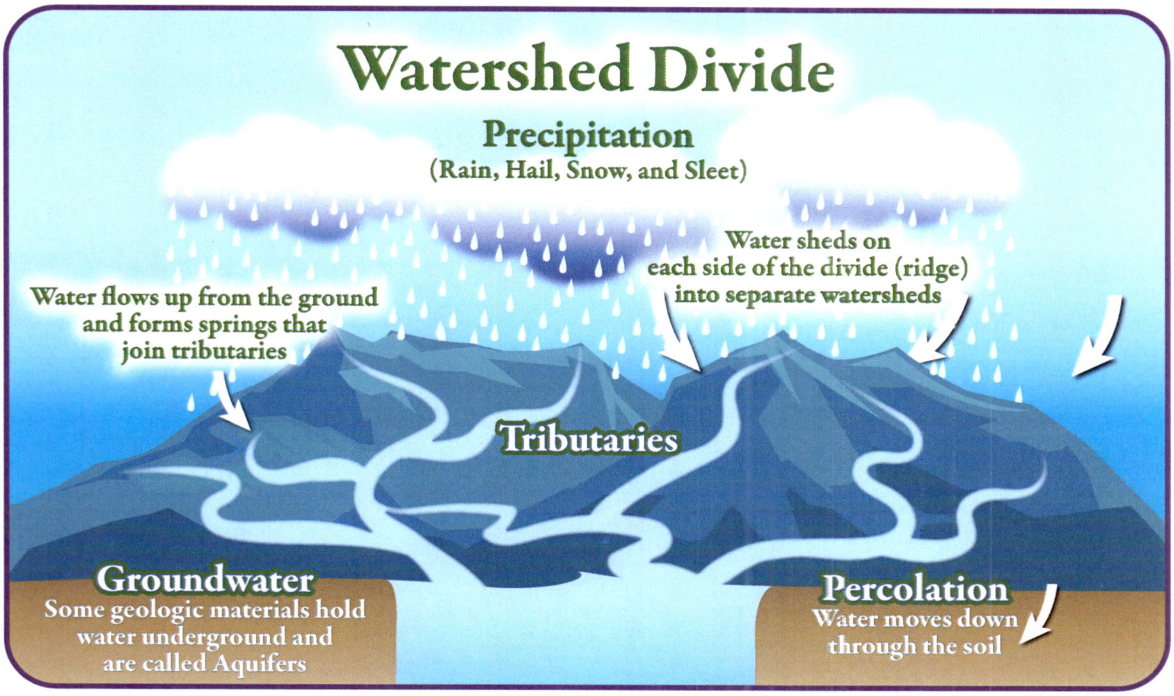

Illustration and Composition by Sandra L. Jones with Dreamstime images- credited in Acknowledgements

Abiotic Disturbance Regimes

- **Geologic, climatic, and hydrologic**

Coastal dunes example: rocks and shells are broken down into sand by regular ocean wave action. Then, carried ashore, wind erosion and the accretion of sand forms dune ecosystems. Algae along the coast stabilizes the ever-shifting sand, develops hummocks (mounds), and enables plants to take root and harbor sand-dwelling invertebrates, a source of food for shorebirds.

Windblown Sand from Nearby Canyons Maintains a Desert Dune Ecosystem

Desert Sand Dunes Example:

Over millennia, monsoons eroded small canyons in the Indio Hills of California; and winds carried the sand across the Coachella Valley, depositing it on the valley floor. This geologic process, including the ceaseless valley winds, created the 200 square-mile Coachella Valley dune ecosystem. The last remaining dunes support a diverse assemblage of dune-adapted species, including the federally-listed threatened Coachella Valley fringe-toed (CVFTL).[7] Collaborative management of the Coachella Valley Preserve System, including the Coachella Valley National Wildlife Refuge, protects the dune habitat in perpetuity. However, the corridor of wind-blown sand from the Indio Hills, replenishing the dunes, is vulnerable to urban development.

The endemic, found nowhere else, and highly specialized CVFTL runs across the dunes at high speeds and then dives into the sand.[8] The fringed scales on their toes make it easy for them to 'swim beneath the sand' to escape predators and the desert heat which can reach 160° F (71.11° Celsius). Gliding into the sand, the CVFTLs' shovel-shaped snout spreads the sand apart and their fringed eyelids seal shut, keeping sand out of their eyes.[9]

Coachella Valley Sand Dune Ecosystem

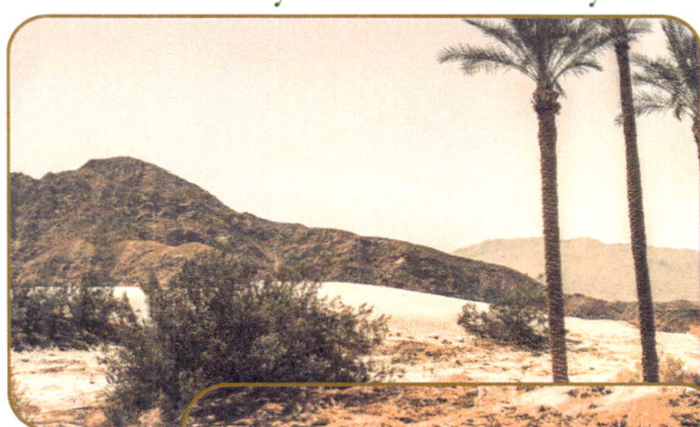

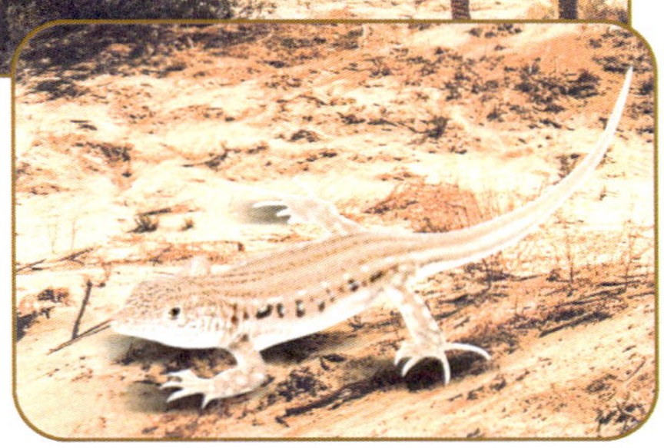

Coachella Valley Fringe-Toed Lizard (*Uma inornata*)

Desert Scene - Photographer Welcomia, Dreamstime
Lizard - Photographer Farinoza, Dreamstime

• Climatic (fires–storms, including lightning)

Coniferous (cone-bearing) forest example: In certain-dry-climate conifer forests, lightning historically ignited wildfires every three to five years. As an adaptation, ponderosa pine trees grow thick bark and drop their lower branches to protect themselves from fire. Some fire-dependent trees and shrubs require fire to melt the seed coat resin before they can germinate.

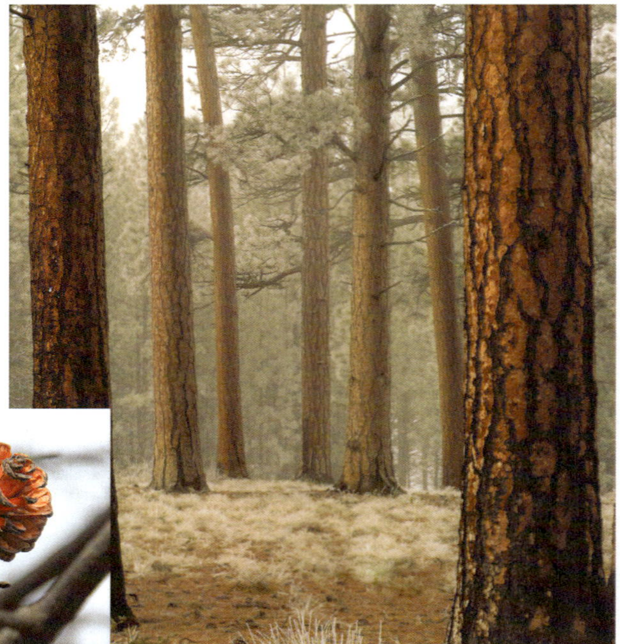

Photographer Kannan Sundaram, Dreamstime

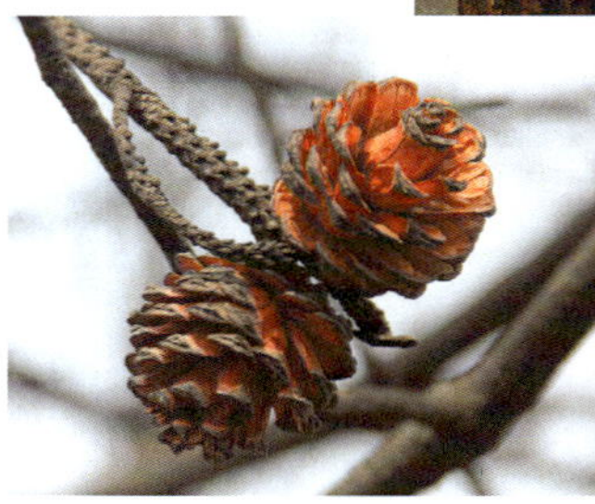

Cones with Resin-Covered Seeds

Ponderosa Pine (*Pinus ponderosa*), Lodgepole Pine (*Pinus contorta*), and Grey Pine (*Pinus banksiana*)

Photographer Lehmanphotos, Dreamstime

• Hydrologic (flooding)

Tropical rainforest example: During the rainy season in the Amazon basin when flood waters are high, jaguars, although agile swimmers, may spend several months living in the tree canopy where the felines hunt and raise their cubs. Their rosette pattern of spots camouflages them in the sunlit forest.

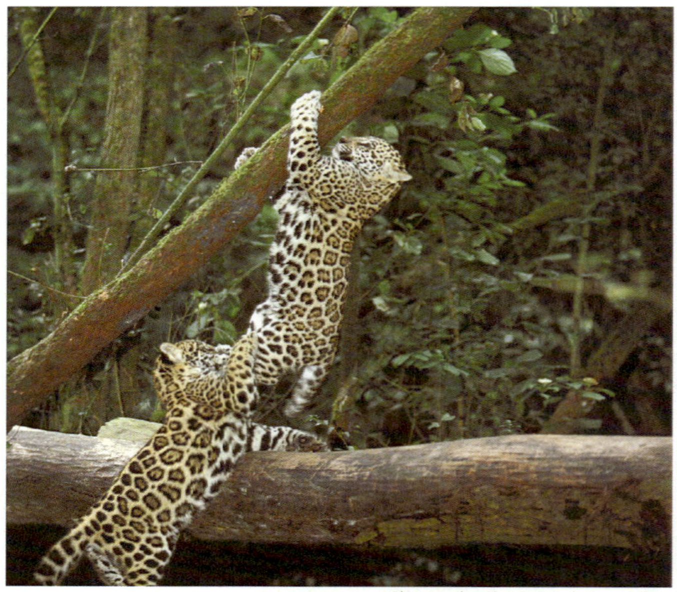

Jaguar (*Panthera onca*) Cubs

Photographer Slowmotiongli, Dreamstime

Abiotic Disturbance Regimes–Fire and Water–Sustain Resilient Forest Ecosystems

Naturally-Occuring Wildfires and Prescribed Burns Interact with the Hydrological Cycle, Supporting a Wide Variety of Forest and Freshwater Habitats and Species

Frequent, Low-Intensity, Slow-Burning Fires:

- reduce the fuel (dry plant matter); therein, future fires will be less likely to burn too hot
- open the forest to more sunlight
- re-mineralize the soil
- stimulate new plant growth
- create a mosiac of habitats across the landscape
- increase snowpack persistance (gradually releasing water as the snow melts during warmer months), the abundance of springs, streamflow, and groundwater storage

River and Wetland Fire Breaks
River corridors and their wetlands act as fire breaks, providing refuge for wildlife and people.

Biotic Disturbance Regimes

- **Biotic disturbance regimes – animal activities cause significant plant and soil disturbance**

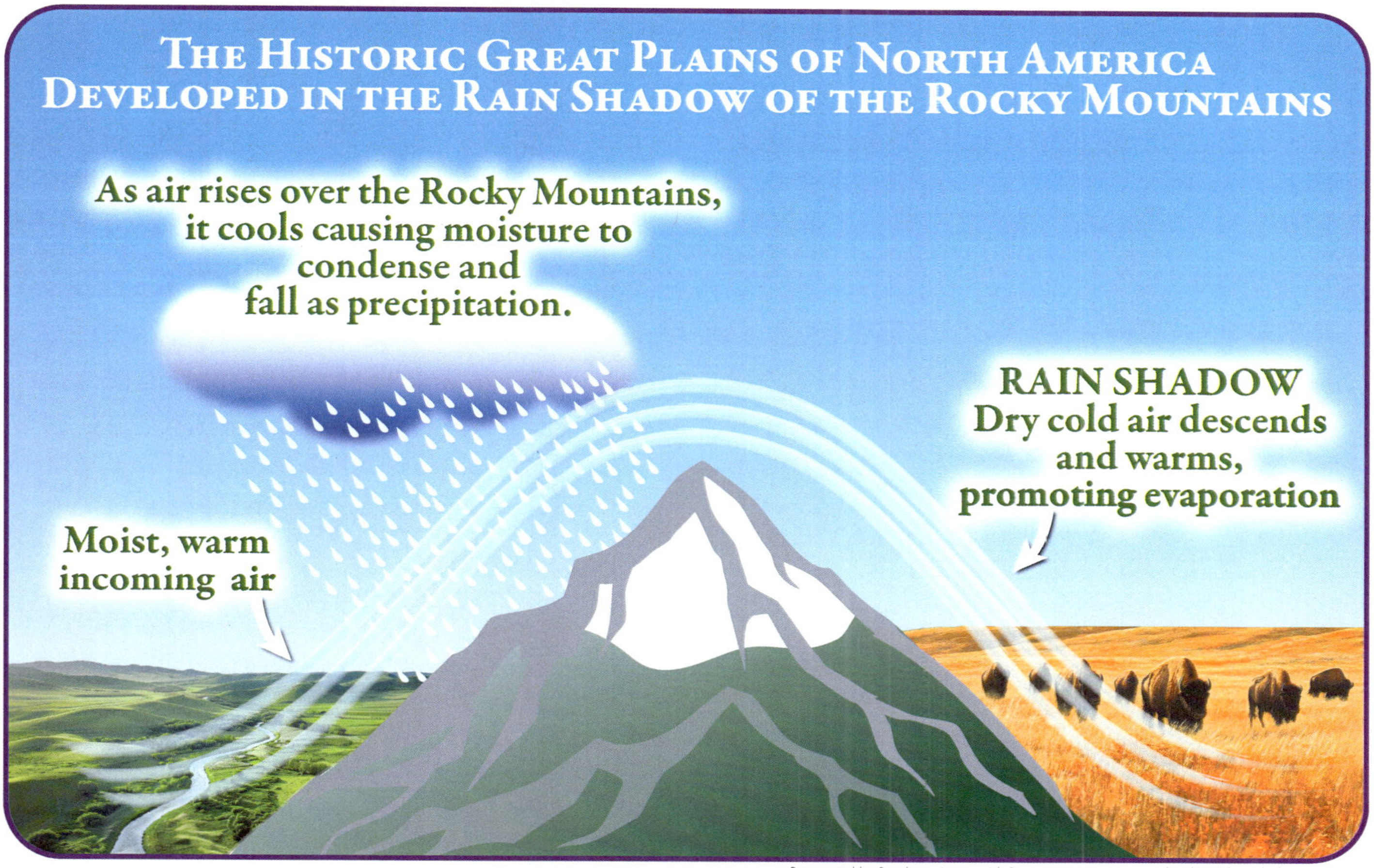

Composed by Sandra L. Jones with Dreamstime images- credited in Acknowledgements

Prairie species example: The Great Plains developed in the 'rain shadow' created by the geologic uplift of the Rocky Mountains. In this semi-arid climate of gently rolling hills and wide river valleys, there were tall, mixed, and short-grass prairie ecosystems. Hundreds of species of grasses; forbs, such as goldenrod; and lichens flourished on the vast prairies, supporting a diversity of insects, neotropical migratory songbirds, reptiles, and mammals. In addition to wildfires that were ignited by lightning and Native American tribes, a variety of biological disturbance regimes maintained the prairies. This included the grazing of bison and elk; mound-building by gophers and ants; and hole-digging by badgers and prairie dogs. These disturbances, though especially wildfires, kept the prairies at early seral stages of succession, preventing trees from establishing; woodlands were limited to isolated buttes and riparian areas. Bison wallows became ephemeral (temporary) wetlands, such as fens (mineral-rich peatlands), sedge meadows, marshes, and ponds that supported amphibians, such as frogs and salamanders. Historically, wide-ranging mountain lions, wolves, bears, and birds of prey hunted in the prairie ecosystems, maintaining balance among species' populations.

The composition of plants across the Great Plains was once greatly influenced by the activities of bison

"Across the Great Plains, it is estimated that there may have once been five or more very small to very large bison wallows per acre. With a historic extent of 500,000 square miles, the Great Plains could have once been marked with over 1.5 billion bison wallows. Today, very old wallows can still be seen, especially from an airplane. This is because the different types of grasses and other plants that still grow in the ancient wallows often have different colors and textures that make the old wallow distinctly noticeable from the surrounding landscape."[10]

Up until the late 1880s, ". . . large herds of bison, elk, deer, and pronghorn moved across the plains. Through grazing, browsing, trampling, wallowing, and defecating, these large herbivores altered the vegetation composition, habitat structure, soils, nutrient cycling, and fire regimes, creating heterogeneous landscapes that included suites of grassland species that associate with open and intensely grazed habitat."[11]

• Traditional Practices Cultivated Biodiversity and Productivity

Indigenous people of North America influenced ecological succession across the landscape. Subsisting on the wildlife inhabiting wetlands, grasslands, forests, deserts, and tundra, they made these ecosystems more diverse and productive. Ethnoecologist Kat Anderson, in her article, "Tending the Wilderness," describes how indigenous people guided the composition of plant communities by: burning, pruning, coppicing (activating new shoots by cutting plants to the ground level), dispersing seeds, transplanting, weeding, and irrigating.[12] They burned prairies extensively to clear brush and encroaching trees, inhibit disease, and re-mineralize soil, encouraging new plant growth. Omer C. Stewart, in his book, *Forgotten Fires*, explains how Native Americans used fire: to warm hearths, heighten the palatability of meats and vegetables, aid in nighttime fishing, hollow out tree trunks for making dugout canoes, construct earth lodges, and keep predators at bay.[13] Anderson illustrates how Native Americans gathered plant materials for dyes, medicines, basketry, musical instruments, tools, firewood, thatching, and clothing. In conclusion she states, ". . . nature and culture were profoundly united through the harvesting of plants and the hunting of animals."[14] Present-day Native American tribes continue traditional practices that cultivate biodiversity and ecosystem productivity (ref. pages 92-94).

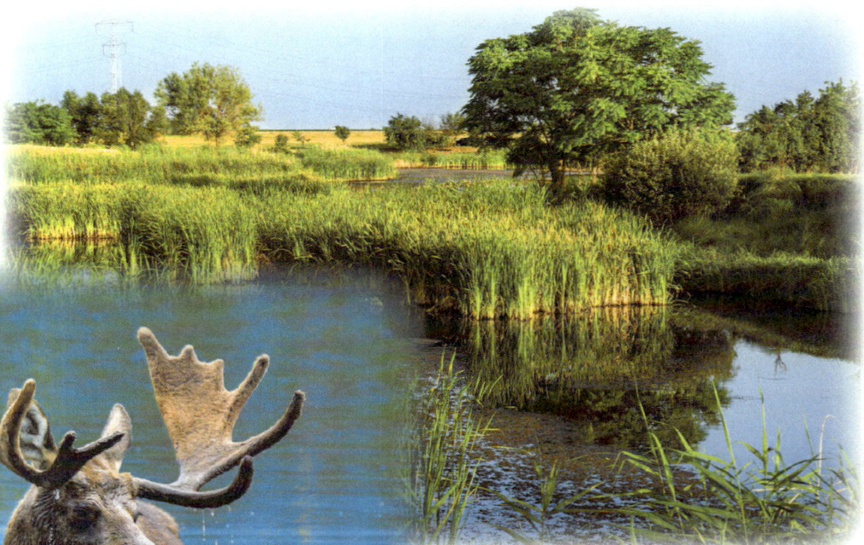

Photographer Constantin Opris, Dreamstime

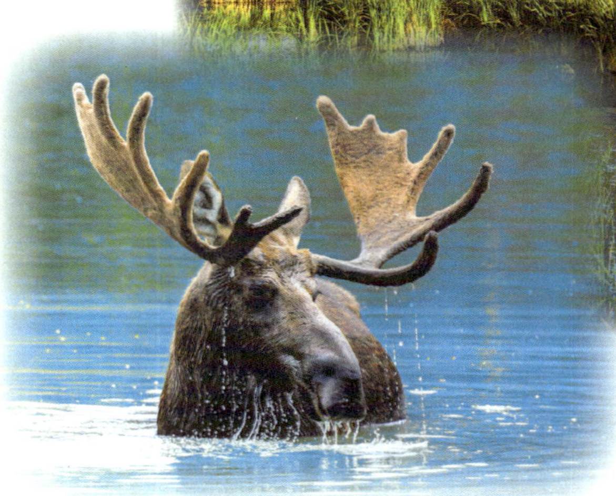

Photographer Gary Gray, Dreamstime

Traditional practices resulted in abundant biodiversity and productivity

II. The Fabric of Life Unfolds in Two Different, Interrelated Ways: Genealogically and Ecologically[15]

Over millennia as species evolve, their lineages form one nested Genealogical Hierarchy (ref. the diagram, next two pages). Each species (living and extinct) and its lineage has one place in the hierarchy. In contrast, the ecological organization of life encompasses a multiplicity of structures; wherein, species perform roles in more than one ecological structure, in one or more ecosystem. Over geologic time, species constitute the fundamental unit of the Genealogical Hierarchy and the many ecological structures that comprise ecosystems.

Genealogical

Classifying and Naming Life Forms

The scientific (genealogical) classification of life forms (systematics) entails classifying and naming (taxonomy) species and clades (taxa). Carolus Linnaeus began this system which he published in the *Systema Naturae* in 1735. Further developed, this classification system is still used today. Systematics is inherently interdisciplinary, involving experts from the fields of paleontology; geology; physics; comparative morphology, anatomy, and physiology; embryology; genetics; molecular biology; and evolutionary biology. The most complete and authoritative list of the world's species is maintained by hundreds of global taxonomists in the Catalogue of Life.[16]

Clades

Clade means kládos or branch – as in branches on the 'tree of life.'

Example Classification of a Species – Artichoke

Like nested Russian dolls, each species fits into a set of progressively broader clades: genus, family, order, class, phylum, kingdom, and domain. For example, artichokes (Genus and species: *Cynara cardunculus*) are in the *Aster* Family, *Asterales*, which is in the *Caryophyllales* Order of succulents, which is in the *Magnoliopsida* Class of primitive flowering plants, which is in the *Tracheophytes* Phylum of 300,000+ vascular ('windpipe') plants, which is in the *Plantae* Kingdom, which is in the *Eukaryota* Domain.

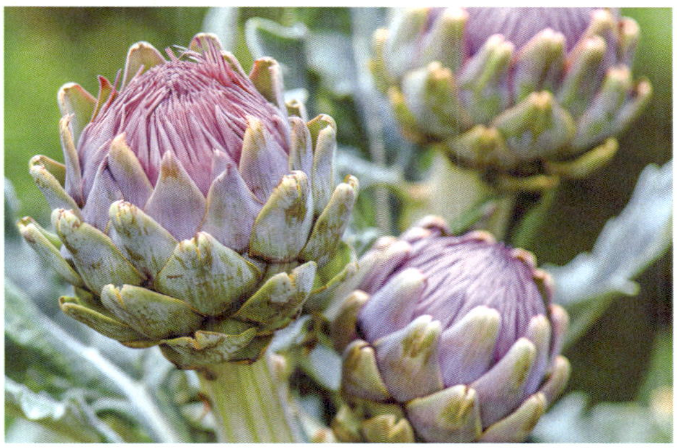

Photographer Ylivdesign, Dreamstime

The *Plantae* (plant and red and green algae foods), *Animalia* (animal foods), *Chromista* (brown algae foods), and *Fungi* (mushrooms and probiotic micro-fungi) Kingdoms occur under the *Eukaryota* Domain; and probiotic bacteria exist under the *Bacillati* Kingdom within the *Bacteria* Domain.

Natural Foods in the Genealogical Hierarchy

KINGDOM - *Phylum*
(food group)

BACILLATI - *Bacillota*
(bacteria)

PLANTAE - *Chlorophyta* and *Rhodophyta*
(green and red algae)

CHROMISTA - *Phaeophyta*
(brown algae)

FUNGI - *Ascomycota*
(micro-fungi)

ANIMALIA - *Chordata*
(sea animals)

PLANTAE - *Tracheophytes*
(plants)

FUNGI - *Ascomycota*
(mushrooms)

ANIMALIA - *Chordata*
(land animals)

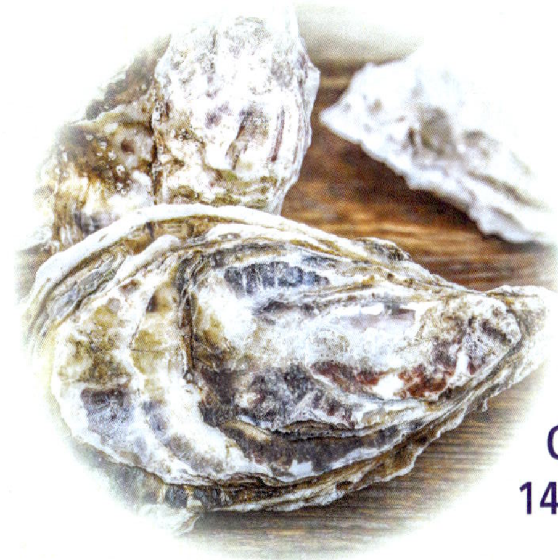

Oysters date back to 145 million years ago

Evolutionary Timeline of the Kingdoms and Phyla of Natural Foods (Examples)

MACRO–EVOLUTION

Species and Other Clades - Examples of Eight Natural Foods

KINGDOMS	BACILLATI (Probiotic bacteria)	PLANTAE (Green and red algae)	CHROMISTA (Brown algae)	FUNGI (Micro-fungi)	ANIMALIA (Sea animals)	PLANTAE (Plants)	FUNGI (Mushrooms)	ANIMALIA (Land animals)
Phylum*	*Bacillota*	*Chlorophyta*	*Phaeophyta*	*Ascomycota*	*Chordata*	*Tracheophytes*	*Basidiomycota*	*Chordata*
Class*	*Bacilli*	*Ulvophyceae*	*Phaeophyceae*	*Eurotiomycetes*	*Actinopterygii*	*Magnoliopsida*	*Agaricomycetes*	*Mammalia*
Order*	*Lactobacillales*	*Bryopsidale*	*Laminariales*	*Eurotiales*	*Scombriformes*	*Malpighiales*	*Hymenochaetales*	*Artiodactyla*
Family*	*Lactobacillaceae*	*Caulerpaceae*	*Lessoniaceae*	*Aspergillaceae*	*Scombridae*	*Malpighiaceae*	*Hymenochaetaceae*	*Bovidae*
Genus species*	*Lactobacillus*	*Caulerpa lentillifera*	*Eisenia bicyclis*	*Aspergillus oryzae*	*Scomber scombrus*	*Malpighia emarginata*	*Inonotus obliquus*	*Bison bison*
* Clades								
Species' Common Name	*Lactobacillus acidophilus*	Sea Grape	Arame	Koji	Mackerel	Acerola	Chaga	Bison
	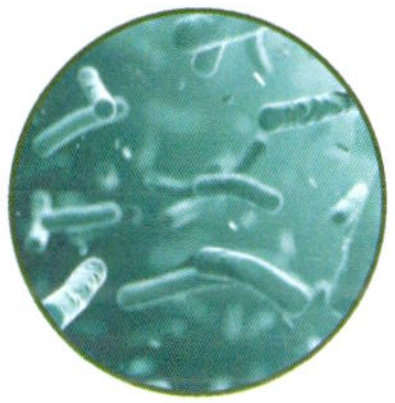	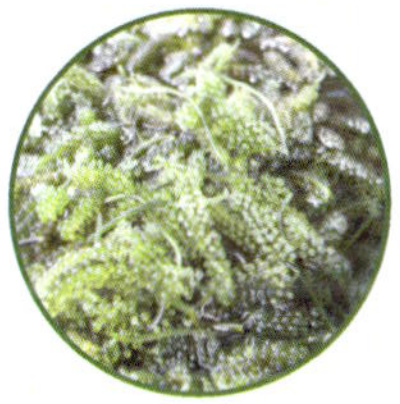	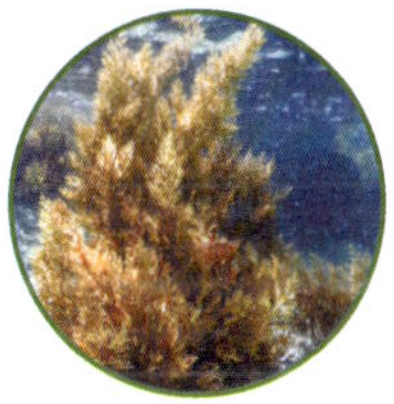	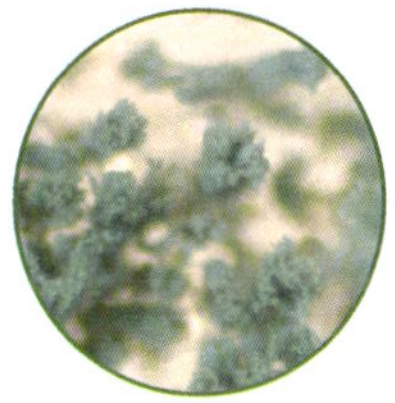	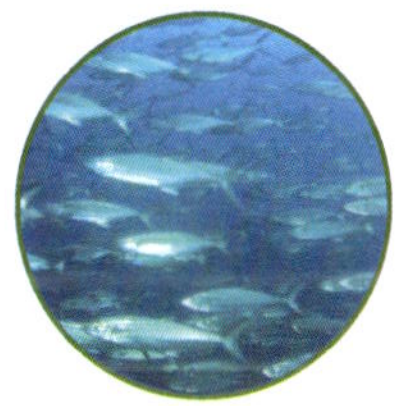	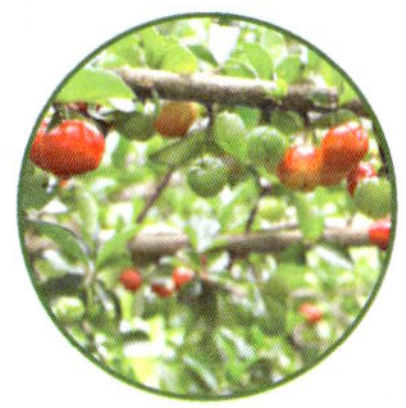	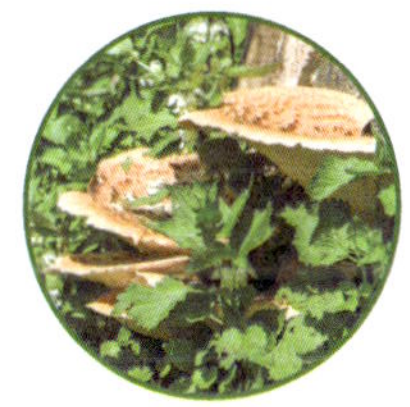	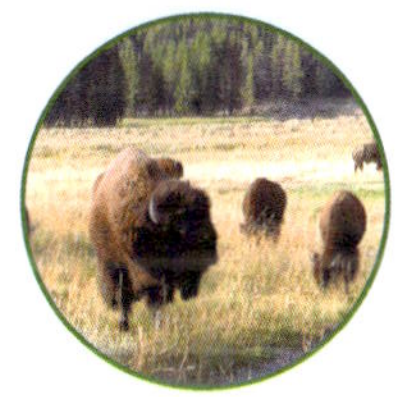

MICRO-EVOLUTION

Organisms and their Genes

Micro-evolution occurs when organisms reproduce and pass on new genetic combinations and variation to their offspring. Bacteria (*Bacteria* Domain) also exchange some genes 'horizontally' while maintaining species integrity. Presently, bacteria comprise 26,000+ classified species[1] and perform crucial roles in most of life's processes. The *Bacteria* Domain is vital to the persistence of every species and ecosystem on Earth.

Design Concept by Amy J. Wing and Sandra L. Jones with Dreamstime images- credited in Acknowledgements

Reference

[1]COL. *Domain: Bacteria Woese et al.*, 2024. Catalogue of Life. (Retrieved 2026, March 2) https://www.catalogueoflife.org.

Threads in the Genealogical Hierarchy

The lineages in the Genealogical Hierarchy are comprised of genealogical units. In micro-evolution, the units are organisms (and their genes) and they adapt over generations. In macro-evolution, the genealogical units are species and the clades that occur above them in the Genealogical Hierarchy. They evolve over millions of years. Each successively higher level of clades is a monophyletic group, sharing a single common ancestor. Since organisms only breed with individuals of their own species (with rare exceptions), reproductive isolation keeps each species and the other clades distinct and separate. In this way, reproductive boundaries maintain the structure of the Genealogical Hierarchy and the integrity of biodiversity overall.

Many isolating mechanisms act as barriers to breeding between closely related species, for example, the species may: 1) occupy the same habitat at different times of the year, 2) be active at different times, one species during the day and the other at night, and/or 3) have behavioral incompatibilities, for instance in avian species, subtle differences between birds' songs keep them from interbreeding.

The Laws of Physics and Species Adaptations

Organisms' genotypes (genome) and phenotypic expression (physical traits and other characteristics) equip organisms with the body design and functionality needed to live and reproduce. Their genotypes enable a certain degree of phenotypic plasticity, the ability to acclimatize (physiologically adjust) to minor changes in the environment. Over thousands of generations, at the species level, genotypes and phenotypic expression evolve, adapting to significant changes in the environment. If species do not adapt to these changes, they may go extinct.

D'Arcy Wentworth Thompson (1860 – 1948) theorized that physical forces largely govern biological form and impose constraints on the forms that might emerge. Thompson demonstrated in his voluminous book, *On Growth and Form*, published in 1917, that the laws of physics direct the process of evolution toward efficiency. For example, using mathematical formulas, he detailed how the branching of blood vessels evolved to optimize the ease of

Example of a Species and Genus Vulnerable to Extinction

The Federally-Listed Endangered Alabama Cavefish

The Alabama cavefish, *Speoplatyrhinus poulsoni*, is one of the rarest species of freshwater fish in the world. Classified as a new species in a new genus, the only population lives in a fragile cave ecosystem of underground pools sustained by the nutrient-rich guano of the gray bat, *Myotis grisescens*. The cave is protected as part of the Key Cave National Wildlife Refuge. Since the Alabama cavefish is the only species in this genus, if it were to go extinct, the genus, too, would go extinct. Nevertheless, both the species and genus would remain in the Genealogical Hierarchy because the hierarchy includes a record of the lineages of all known species and clades, living and extinct–the entire history of life.[17]

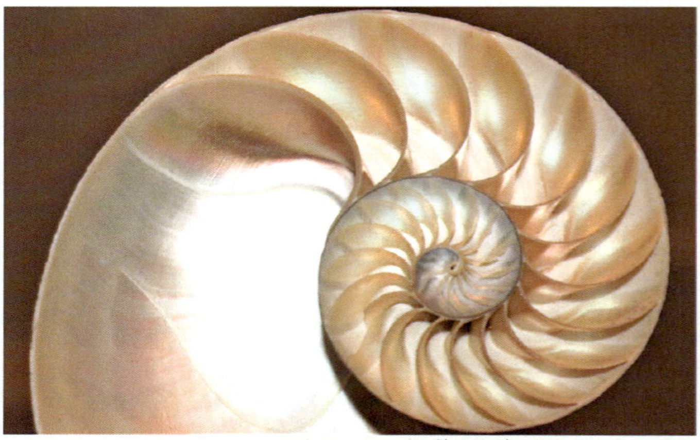

Photographer Lorna Jane, Dreamstime

Bryozoa Shell

blood flow, factoring in the balance of fluid pressure, tension on the vessel walls, and radius of the vessel curvature. He stated that "... even the amount of oxygen which enters and leaves the capillaries is such that the work involved in its exchange and transport is a minimum."[18] Thompson observed reoccurring designs across the kingdoms of life that demonstrate efficiency. For instance, equiangular spirals are present in:[19]

- *Bryozoa* fossils, an aquatic invertebrate with corkscrew shaped helix
- *Foraminifera*, micro-organisms with a miniature shell, known as the 'armored *amoeba*'
- snails' shells
- cats' claws
- beavers' teeth
- the coil of the chameleon tail and elephant tusk
- the spiral flight path of insects toward the light

Spiral Path of Insects
In describing the flight path of insects, Thompson wrote, "Owing to the structure of their compound eyes, these insects do not look straight ahead but make for a light which they see abeam, at a certain angle. As they continually adjust their path to this constant angle, a spiral pathway brings them to their destination ..."[20]

An organism's existing form, function, and life requirements limit their potential for evolution. Since Thompson's prolific writing, evolutionary biologists continue to study constraints in nature that may act as 'side bars' to the evolution of species. To be viable, any new traits must be congruent with the rest of an organism's form and function.

Organisms – Micro-Evolution

Micro-evolution occurs as organisms reproduce and pass on new genetic combinations and variation to their offspring. Charles Darwin in his renowned book, *Origin of Species*, published in 1859, described this phenomenon as 'descent with modification.'[21] Many factors, including adequate nourishment, affect the phenotypic expression of genes throughout an organism's lifetime.

Micro-evolution in bacteria (*Bacteria* Domain) takes place both 1) vertically, through successive generations of offspring and 2) horizontally, through horizontal gene transfer, along with trading metabolites.

Species – Macro-Evolution

Over geologic time, each species encompasses generations of organisms that are reproductively-isolated (with rare exceptions) and occur in populations that are distributed throughout the species' range.

Speciation

Through the process of evolution, new species emerge through speciation, wherein, a new species branches off (diverges) from the original species (such as when one or more of a species' populations become isolated and adapt to different envirionmental conditions).[22]

Punctuated equilibrium

In researching the fossil record, paleontologists and evolutionary biologists Niles Eldredge and Stephen J. Gould demonstrated that the pace of evolution, at geologic time scales, has occurred over long periods of stasis, with minimal change, followed by sudden change. They named this pattern in evolution 'punctuated equilibrium.'[23]

Mountain micro-habitats and biodiversity

Environmental gradients can result in habitat partitioning among species and specialization (where species adapt to different micro-habitat conditions). Worn-down mountains are often exceptionally varied in topography, creating a multitude of micro-habitats. South-facing and north-facing mountainsides provide environmental differences, too, offering different sun exposure. Life zones, delineated by C. Hart Merriam in 1889, display different plant communities that correlate across altitude and latitude (ref. diagram below).[24]

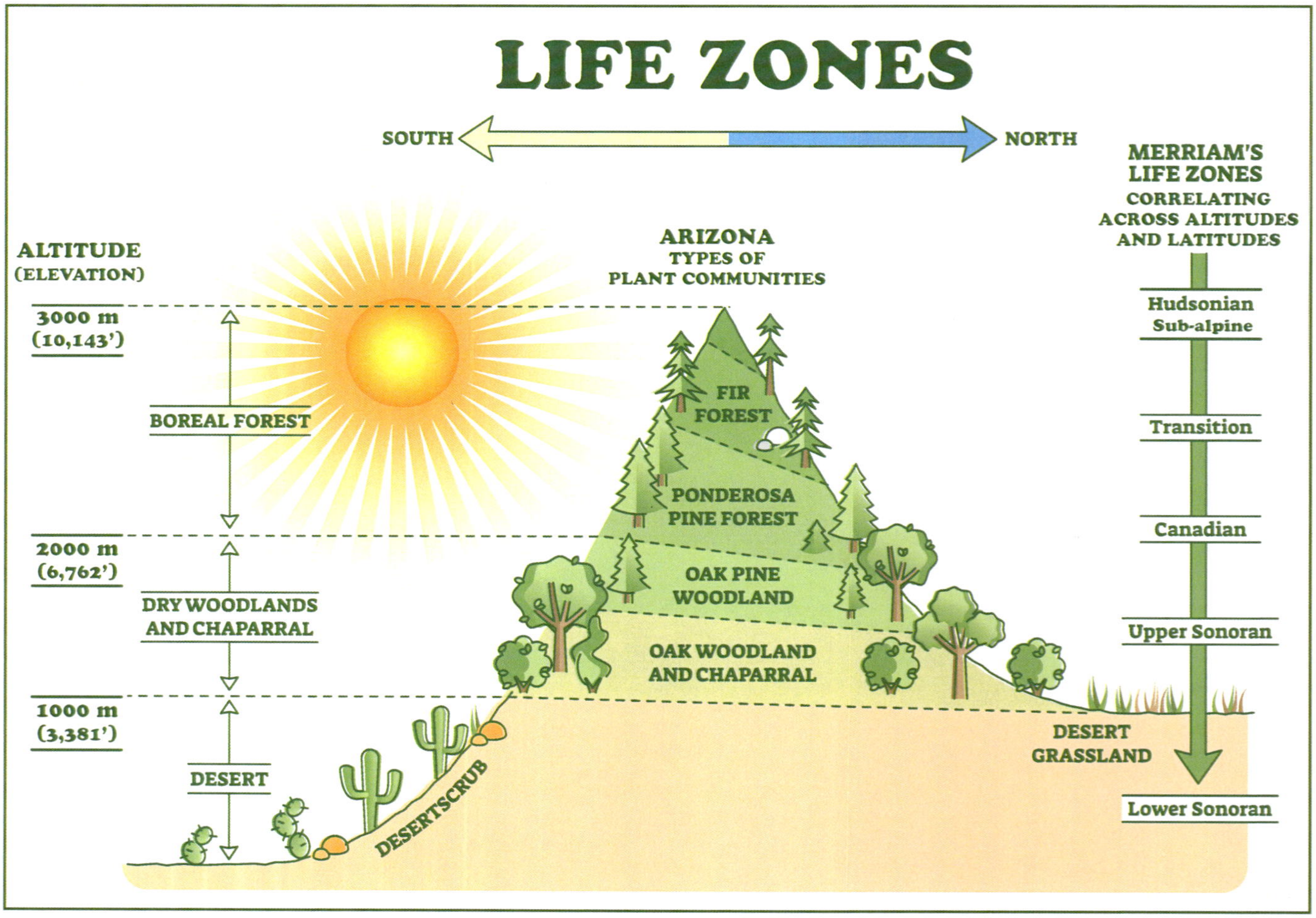

Composed by Sandra L. Jones
Diagram Illustrator VectorMine, & Sun Illustrator Mr E J Wilde, Dreamstime

Ecotones

Across the landscape, ecostones are the places where one ecosystem transitions into another ecosystem. Species ranges often overlap in ecotones, resulting in high biodiversity. Additionally, species adaptations, speciation, and extinctions occur more often in ecotones because ecotones often comprise the outer limits of species' ranges (their peripheral populations).

Adaptive radiation

The abundance of unique species inhabiting islands are often the result of adaptive radiation. When species newly discover and settle on an island this can cause accelerated speciation, with the emergence of multiple species from one ancestral species. Irby Lovette, Cornell Lab of Ornithology at the University of Cornell, New York, offers an example of avian adaptive radiation in the remote islands of the Hawaiian archipelago, where, from a single ancestor, more than 50 endemic honeycreeper species evolved with "... an incredible variety of bill shapes and feeding behaviors..."[25] 'Island biogeography' is the study of populations that become separated (like on an island) from the rest of the species, usually due to a geographic barrier, which causes high rates of speciation and extinction.

'I'iwi or Scarlet Honeycreeper (*Drepanis coccinea*)

The 'i'iwi, scarlet honeycreeper, is endemic to the Hawaiian Islands and federally-listed as a threatened species. While 'i'iwi eat spiders, moths, and other insects, their bill is specialized for feeding on the nectar of native lobelia and mint flowers.[26]

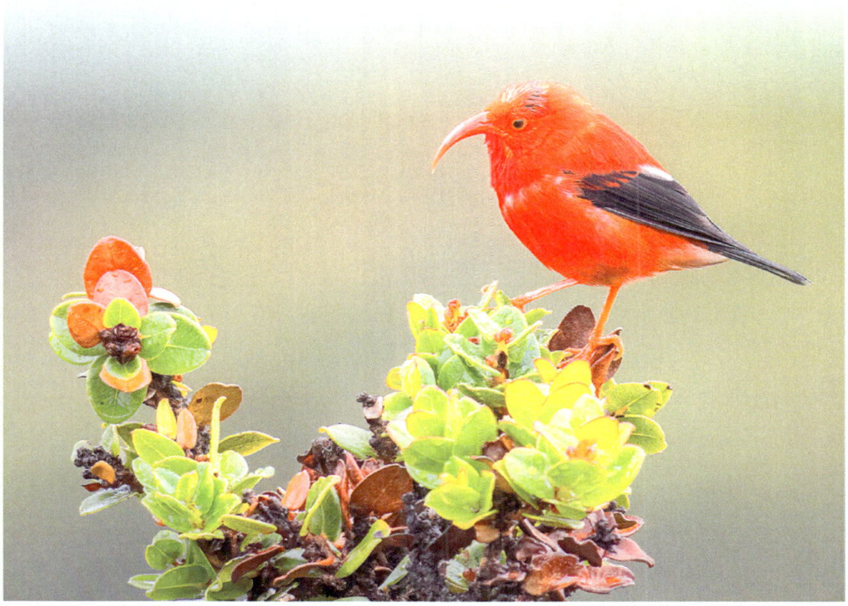

Photographer Satheesh Rajh Rajagopalan, Dreamstime

Clades – Macro-Evolution

Above the Species Level

Clade evolution occurs when some or all members of a clade, such as a genus of insects, undergo evolutionary changes, adapting to their environment. This type of diversification occurs at a broader scale than speciation and may result in many new ecological niches. In a *Journal of Ecological Letter*s article, authors P. Catalina Chaparro-Pedraza, Gregory Roth, and Ole Seehausen discuss adaptive radiation at the clade level. They illustrate that "While most resources usually exist prior to adaptive radiation, novel niches associated with novel resources can be created as a clade diversifies."[27] The authors found an interplay of ecological factors either increased or decreased clade biodiversity.

Ecological

Trophic Organizations – Food Chains Occur in Biological Hierarchies

Trophic Structures

Species, residing in and migrating through terrestrial and aquatic ecosystems, organize into trophic organizations (food chains) that include:

Illustrated by Sandra L. Jones

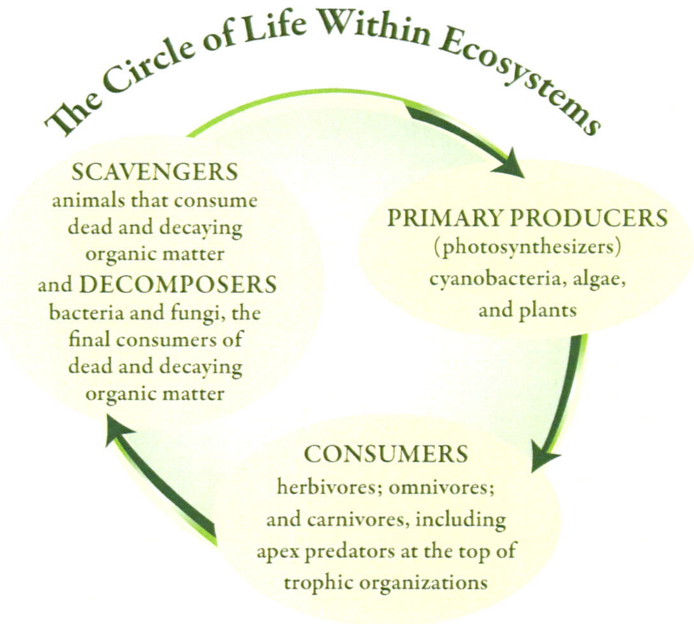

PRIMARY PRODUCERS – cyanobacteria, algae, and plants

Cyanobacteria, green algae, and plants are the primary producers in ecosystems, nourishing nearly all other forms of life. As autotrophs, they produce their own energy through photosynthesis from sunlight, carbon dioxide, water, and nutrients from the soil and sediment. Most live in the euphotic (sunlit) zone, including: the atmosphere; top millimeters of soil; and upper layers of rivers, lakes, and the ocean. In terrestrial ecosystems, freshwater algae, lichens (micro-fungi, cyanobacteria, and/or green algae), and particularly plants, are the primary food source for mushrooms and animals (heterotrophs) that cannot produce their own food. Plants connect above and below-ground ecosystems, as David Wardle at the Swedish University of Agricultural Sciences explains, "They generate the carbon that drives the aboveground (foliage-based) food web and the root-based and detritus-based food webs in the soil[28] (ref. The Soil Food Web diagram page 74).

In the oceans (marine ecosystems), covering seventy percent of the Earth, cyanobacteria and green algae are widespread photosynthesizers. They mostly inhabit the upper, sunlit layers. Only the longer wavelengths of sunlight reach the mesopelagic 'twilight zone' where brown and red algae grow. At deeper depths, their color pigments facilitate the absorption of sunlight for photosynthesis. Red algae and cyanobacteria contain phycobilin pigments, which may include: phycoerythrin (crimson), phycocyanin (blue), and allophycocyanin (indigo blue). Many species of algae have a holdfast that anchors them to the bottom substrate or rocks on the shore; a long stem-like stipe, leaf-like blades, and an air bladder to help them stay afloat and receive sunlight.

Sunlight in the Ocean

In the deepest region of the ocean, the bathypelagic zone, there is no light. Species here emit their own light (bioluminescence). Using parts of their body that are bioluminescent as 'lanterns' and 'searchlights,' they attract mates, search for prey, and engage in schooling communication.

CONSUMERS – animals and mushrooms

The deep ocean and polar regions are especially rich with wildlife. Ocean currents and storms cause upwellings that bring enormous quantities of nutrients up from the ocean floor, making the nutrients available to a wide array of species in the upper layers of the ocean. For example, filter-feeding baleen whales, such as humpback, fin, and blue, migrate from tropical mating and calving grounds to colder waters to feed on an abundance of crustaceans, including krill, and small fish.

Blue Whales (*Balaenoptera muscularis*) in Touch Across Oceans

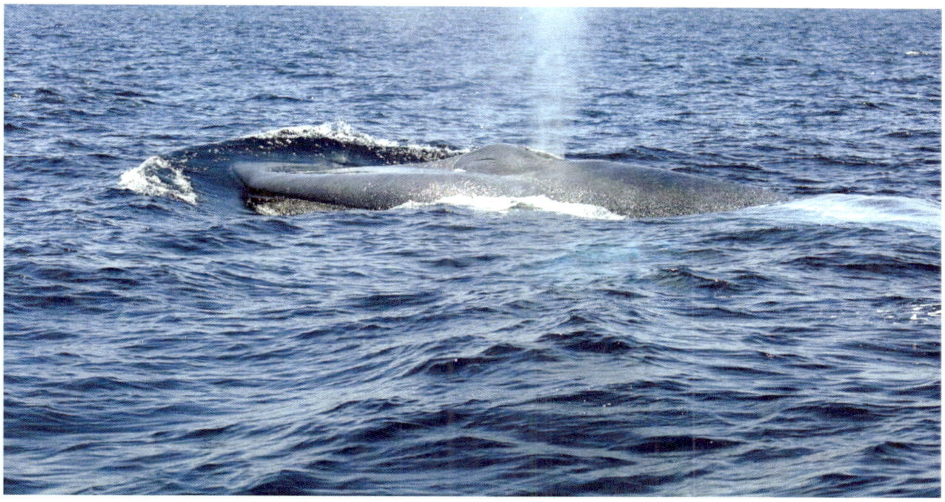

Photographer Sbure, Dreamstime

Blue whales are the largest known species to have ever lived on Earth, growing up to ~100 feet in length (30 meters) and 160 tons. While communicating with one another in the vast ocean, sometimes over thousands of miles, they send their vocalizations below the thermocline where the temperature remains constant and speed of sound is greatest.

In terrestrial ecosystems, mushrooms depend on plants for their sustenance and are themselves food for animals. Some species of mushrooms, for example, absorb nutrients from standing or fallen, decaying trees. In the forests of the Pacific Northwest in the United States, truffles, living underground, provide food for more than 350 species of animals, including: elk, deer, bear, small mammals, slugs, and insects. The truffles emit alluring scents that attract animals throughout the forest to dig them up. The animals often carry them off to eat them elsewhere. Once the animals have consumed the truffles and defecated, the truffle spores will germinate in these new areas, increasing truffle populations throughout the forest.[29]

As consumers, top predators maintain balance in the trophic organizations of ecosystems by causing a 'trophic cascade.' A classic example of this is sea otters (top predators) that maintain underwater kelp forests along the coast by consuming sea urchins that would have otherwise overgrazed the kelp. Likewise, sharks (top predators) consume algivorous (algae-eating) fish, safeguarding the integrity of coral reef ecosystems in the oceans. In a similar fashion, wide-ranging wolves, lions, and cheetahs, as top predators, consume grazing and foraging herbivores, such as elk and zebras, ensuring the continuance of grasslands and savannahs.

Scavengers and decomposers

Performing a crucial role in aquatic and terrestrial ecosystems, scavengers and decomposers consume animal remains and fungal, algal, and plant material, developing it into humus–fertile, organic sediment and topsoil. Animals that scavenge for food include: seagulls, sharks, lobsters, crabs, vultures, ravens, African jackals, coyotes, raccoons, dung beetles, and millipedes. Decomposers complete the process of decomposition by consuming the remains left by scavengers. The decomposers are either: 1) detritivores that eat dead matter and digest it in their intestinal tract (such as some species of starfish, snails, worms, and beetles) or 2) saprotrophs which are largely bacteria and micro-fungi (including yeasts and molds) that secrete digestive enzymes externally to break down organic matter.

Coming full circle, the primary producers (photosynthesizers–cyanobacteria, algae, and plants) depend on the decomposers. For example, bacteria and micro-fungi break down nitrogen into ammonia, nitrate, and nitrite which are key nutrients for plants.

Soil food web

Underground soil food webs support ecosystems and contain several kingdoms and domains of life. This includes:

- the five kingdoms that encompass natural foods: *Animalia, Chromista, Fungi, Plantae* Kingdoms (of the *Eukaryota* Domain) and single-celled organisms in the *Bacillati* Kingdom (of the *Bacteria* Domain)
- single-celled organisms in the *Protozoa* Kingdom (of the *Eukaryota* Domain) and *Archaea* (of the *Archaea* Domain)[17]

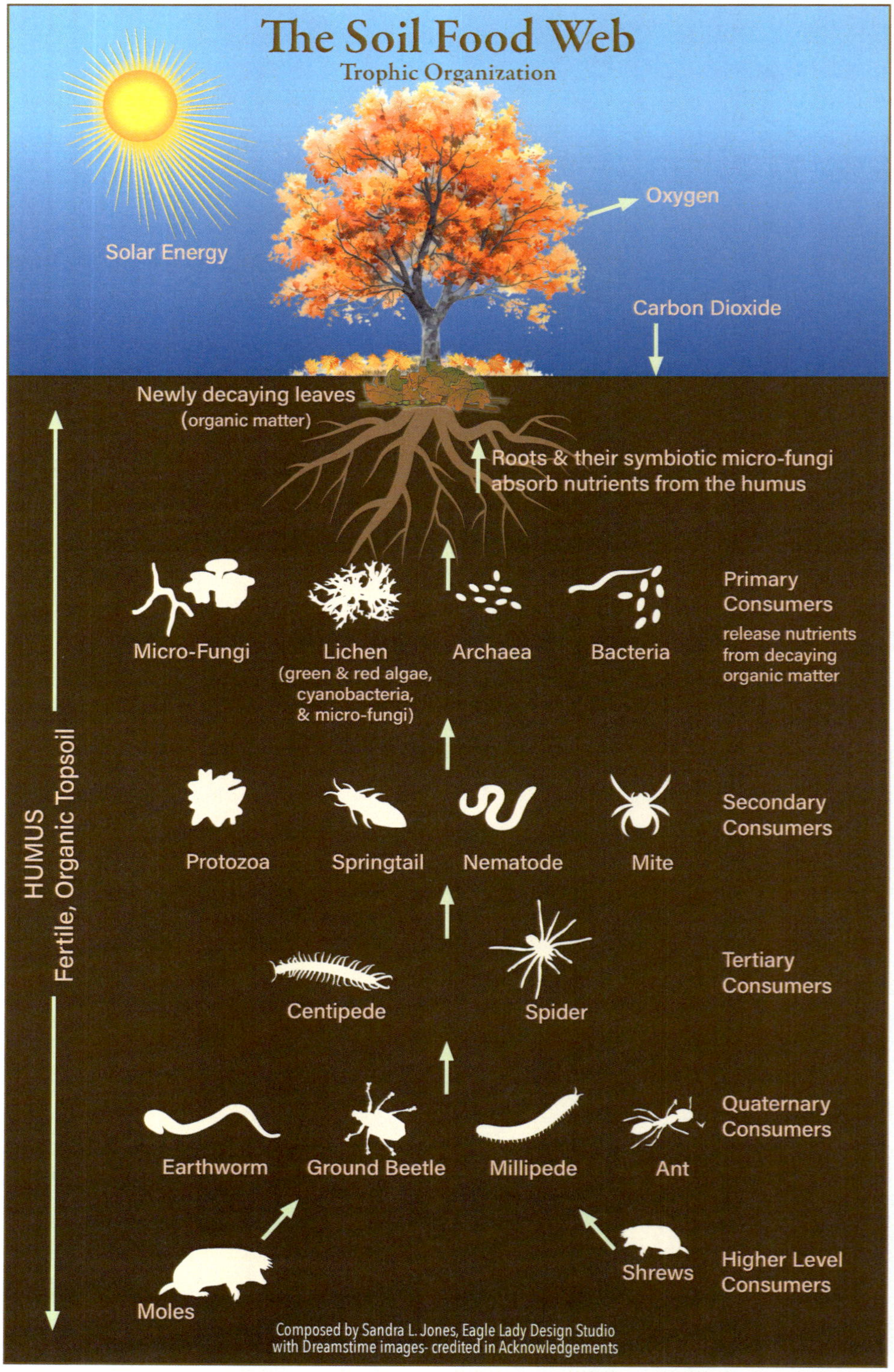

Intra-Species Associations

Green Frogs (*Rana clamitans*)

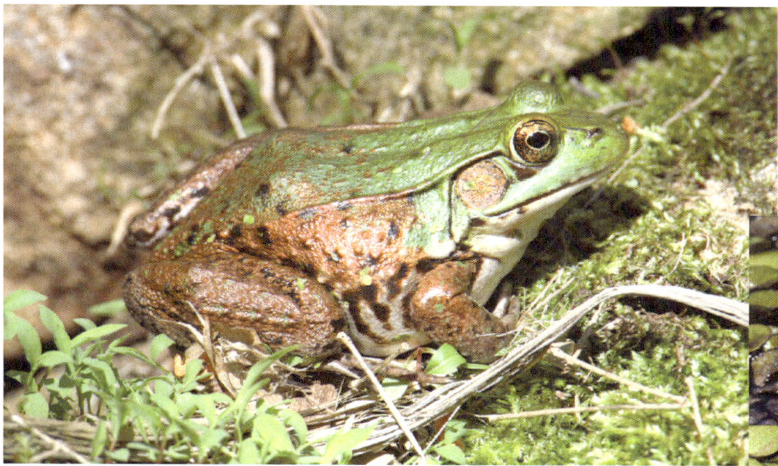

Photographer Steve Byland, Dreamstime

Sunning on a grassy rock

Species Associations

Intraspecies – within species
Interspecies – between species

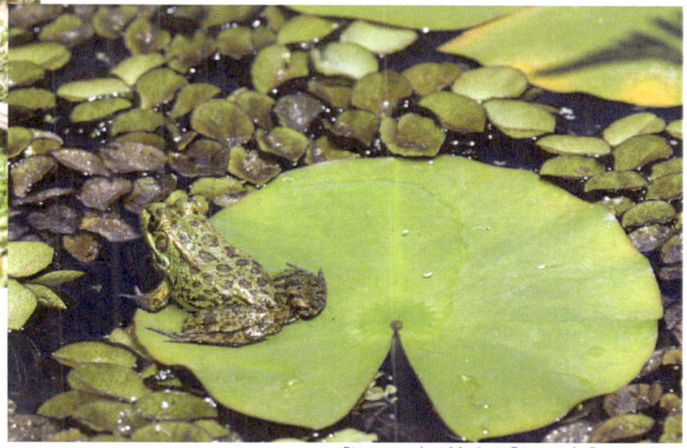

Photographer Mariusz Prusaczyk, Dreamstime

On a water lilly pad

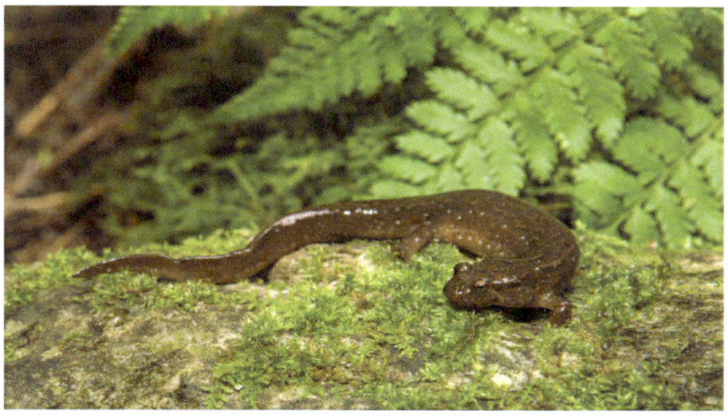

Photographer Jason Ondreicka, Dreamstime

Northern Dusky Salamander (*Desmognathus fuscus*) Resting in a cluster of moss

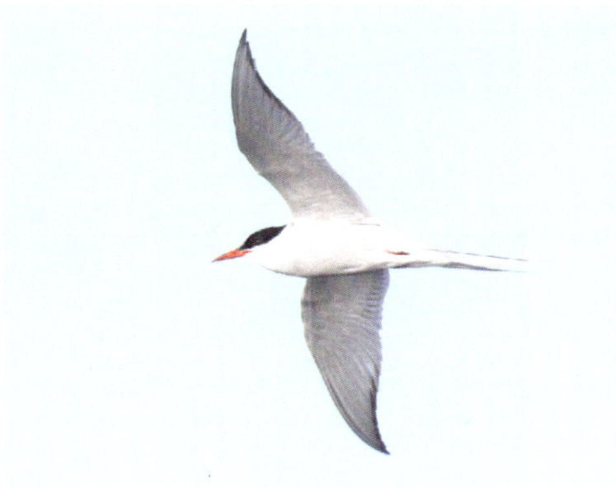

Photographer Pascal Halder, Dreamstime

Arctic Tern (*Sterna paradisaea*) Migrating

Resting

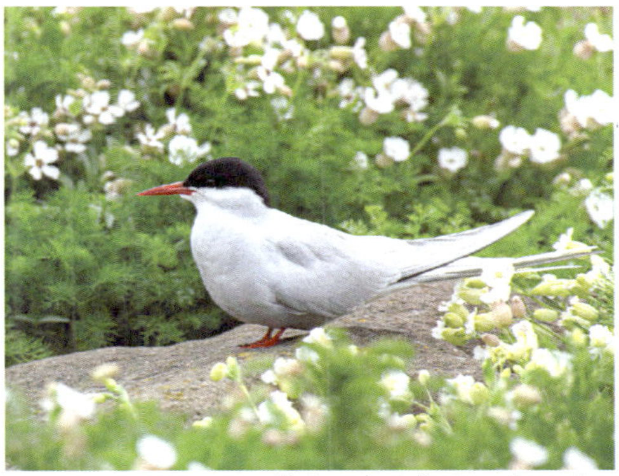

Photographer Julian Popov, Dreamstime

Individual home ranges comprise species' ranges

Each organism carries out its life cycle on discrete patches of habitat throughout its home range. Some organisms are relatively solitary; for example, amphibians, including frogs and salamanders, spend most of their time independently on small patches of land and water. For instance, northern dusky salamanders, inhabiting a limestone stream and sandstone creek, were found to have home ranges between 1.4 to 48.4 square meters (1.5 to 5.2 yards).[30] In contrast, the individuals of other species are more interactive and have overlapping home ranges. For instance, the home ranges of arctic terns, encompassing their vast migration routes, extend from the Arctic to Antarctica. Arctic terns are gregarious and collaborate in flight, undertaking the longest annual migration of any species.

The home ranges of all the organisms of a species comprise the species' range.

Coordinated movements within species

Organisms of the same species often coordinate together. Skeins of geese flying in formation and schools of fish synchronizing their movements, with great agility, work with the laws of physics to save energy and increase their efficiency. Interbreeding between dispersed populations of organisms–of the same species–helps maintain diversity throughout the species' gene pool. In many cases, the young move out on their own (natal dispersal) and establish themselves in new territory or join other populations.

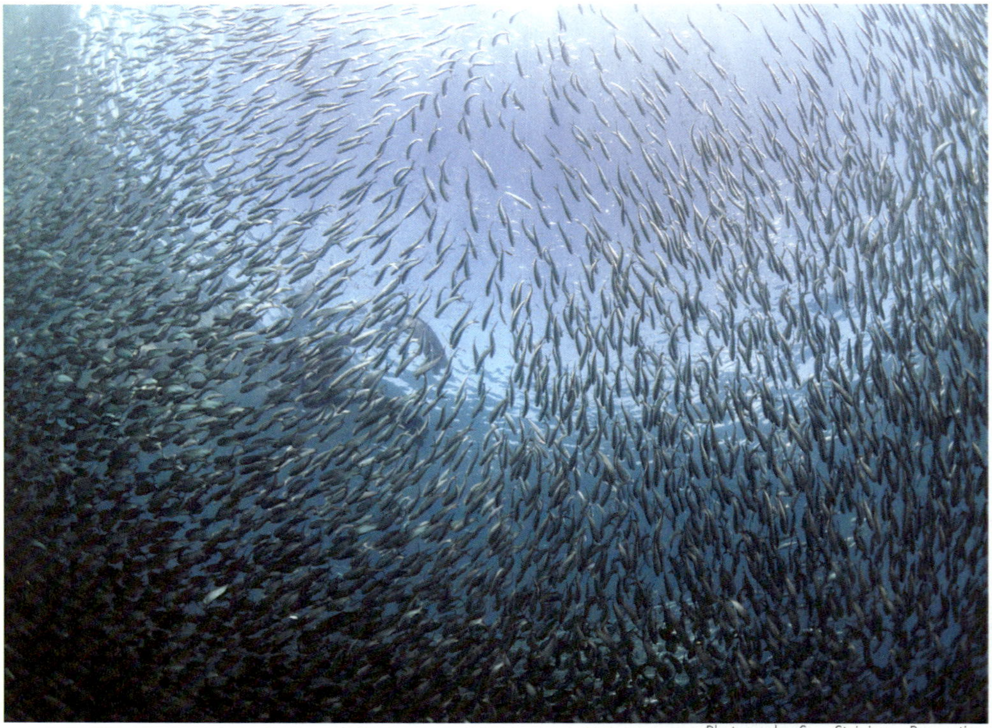

Photographer Sean Steininger, Dreamstime

School of Sardines (*Sardinella tawilis*) near the Philippine Islands

Inter-Species Associations

There are no set barriers to species forming ecological relationships, unlike the barriers to interbreeding between species that keep species distinct and separate in the Genealogical Hierarchy. Co-evolution occurs when different species have long-term ecological relationships that affect the evolution of each species involved. Over millennia, inter-species ecological associations provide cohesiveness and stability to these species and to the ecosystems of which they are a part.

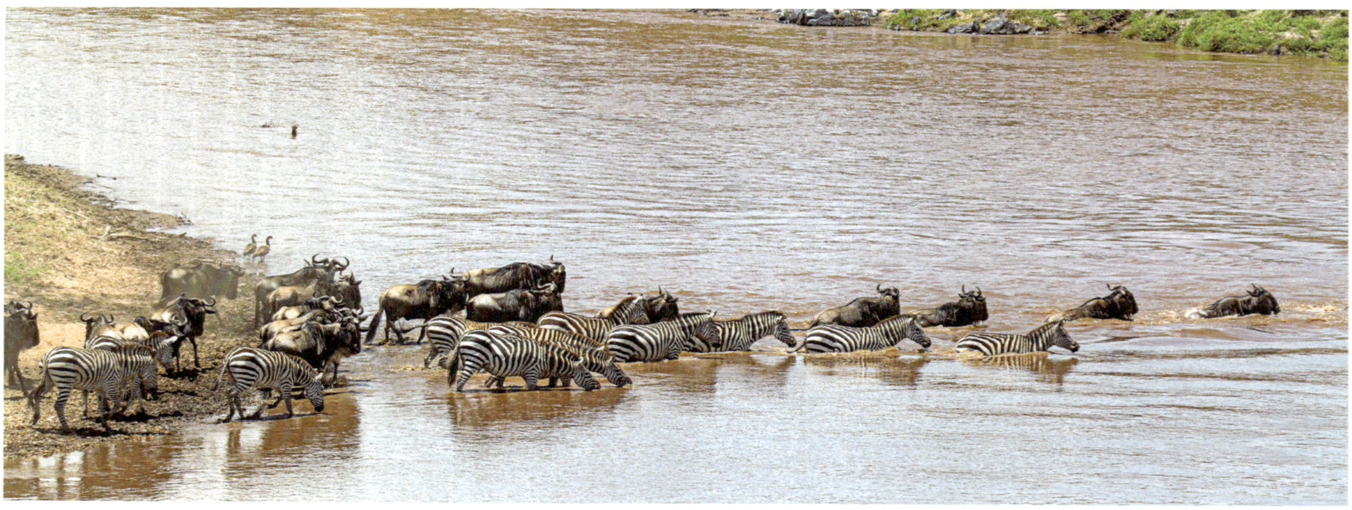

Photographer Adogslifephotov, Dreamstime

Zebras (*Equus burchelli*) and wildebeests (*Connochaetes taurinus*) crossing the Serengeti-to Maasai Mara

Migrating together

Zebras and wildebeests graze side-by-side as they follow the seasonal greening of African grasslands and savannahs, regenerating these ecosystems. Annually, zebras and wildebeests cross the Serengeti to the Maasai Mara in Kenya. One of the ways they are compatible is that their food preferences complement, zebra selecting tall grasses and wildebeests preferring the shortgrass. Additionally, each species benefits from the keen senses of the other (the zebras' vision and wildebeests' hearing), assisting them in jointly protecting their herds from lions, cheetahs, leopards, and other predators.

Habitat associations

Gophers share the extensive dug-out rooms and tunnels of their burrows with other species, such as indigo snakes, eastern diamondback rattlesnakes, burrowing owls, opossums, gopher frogs, and gopher crickets that come in seeking protection from extreme temperatures, wildfires, and predators.

Reproduction

Plants, algae, and mushrooms depend on a wide variety of animals to disperse their seeds, propagules, and spores; for instance, tropical trees in the Pacific Islands of Fiji, Philippines, Polynesia, and Samoa depend on fruit-eating flying foxes (bats) to disperse their seeds. Displaying inviting colors, shapes, and scents, flowering plants rely on nectar-feeding insect, bird, and bat pollinators for reproduction. Once pollenated, many of these plants grow seeds enveloped by colorful, aromatic fruits and vegetables–which attract a wide diversity of animals that consume the fruits and vegetables and disperse the seeds.

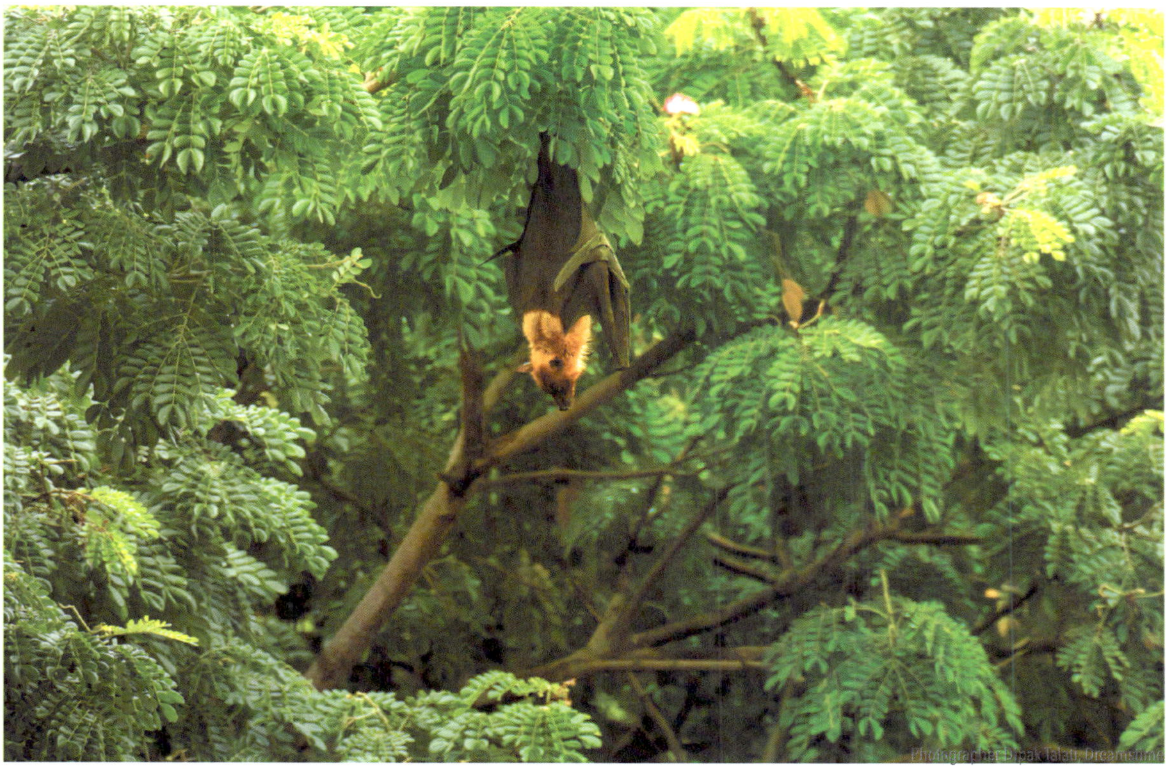

Golden-mantled flying fox (*Pteropus pumilus*) on an island in the Philippines

Generalists and specialists

Species that are generalists, such as wolves and coyotes, have the adaptive advantage of being versatile, able to live in a variety of habitats and feed on a wide array of prey; whereas, species that are adapted to highly specialized relationships benefit from mutualism (symbiosis/reciprocity) and reduced competition.

Symbiosis in Richly Diverse Tropical Rainforests

Specialized Relationships Between Brazil Nut Trees, Orchid Bees, Bucket Orchids, Arboreal Ants, and Agoutis

Brazil nut trees (*Bertholletia excelsa*) are entirely dependent on orchid bees of the *Euglossa, Eulaema, and Euplusia* genera to pollinate their flowers. The male bees of these genera cover themselves in the nectar scent of the bucket orchid (*Coryanthes horichiana*) to attract a mate; and bucket orchids only grow in the arboreal nests of *Azteca, Campanotus, and Crematogaster* ants. These genera of ants feed on the bucket orchid nectar, fertilize the soil by the orchid roots with their feces, and defend the orchids against herbivores.

Brazil nut trees also depend on agouti (*Dasyprocta variegata*) to harvest their nuts. When ripe, the Brazil nuts drop to the forest floor where the agouti find them, crack them open with their strong jaws and sharp teeth, eat some, and bury some for later. The nuts that germinate and grow into Brazil nut trees sustain this elaborate ecological symbiosis in the Amazon rainforest.[31]

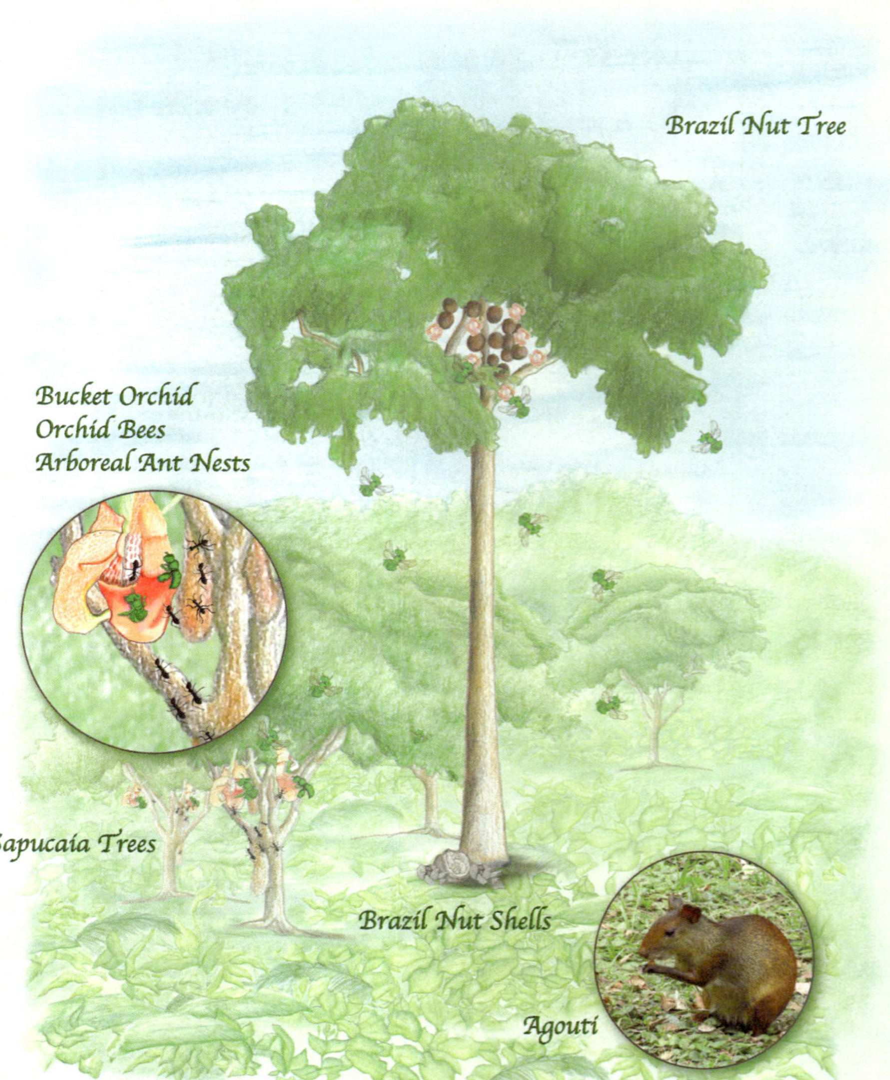

Caution:
Brazil nuts are high in selenium; therefore, it is important to limit the amount consumed per day.

Illustrated by Sandra L. Jones, Eagle Lady Design Studio
Photography by Cleverson Felix, © Dreamstime.com
Ants illustrated by Andjelka Simic, © Dreamstime.com

The Intertwined Biotic and Abiotic Components of Ecosystems

Bog Lakes with Smalls Islands in Soomaa National Park, Estonia

Long-tailed ducks (*Clangula hyemalis*)

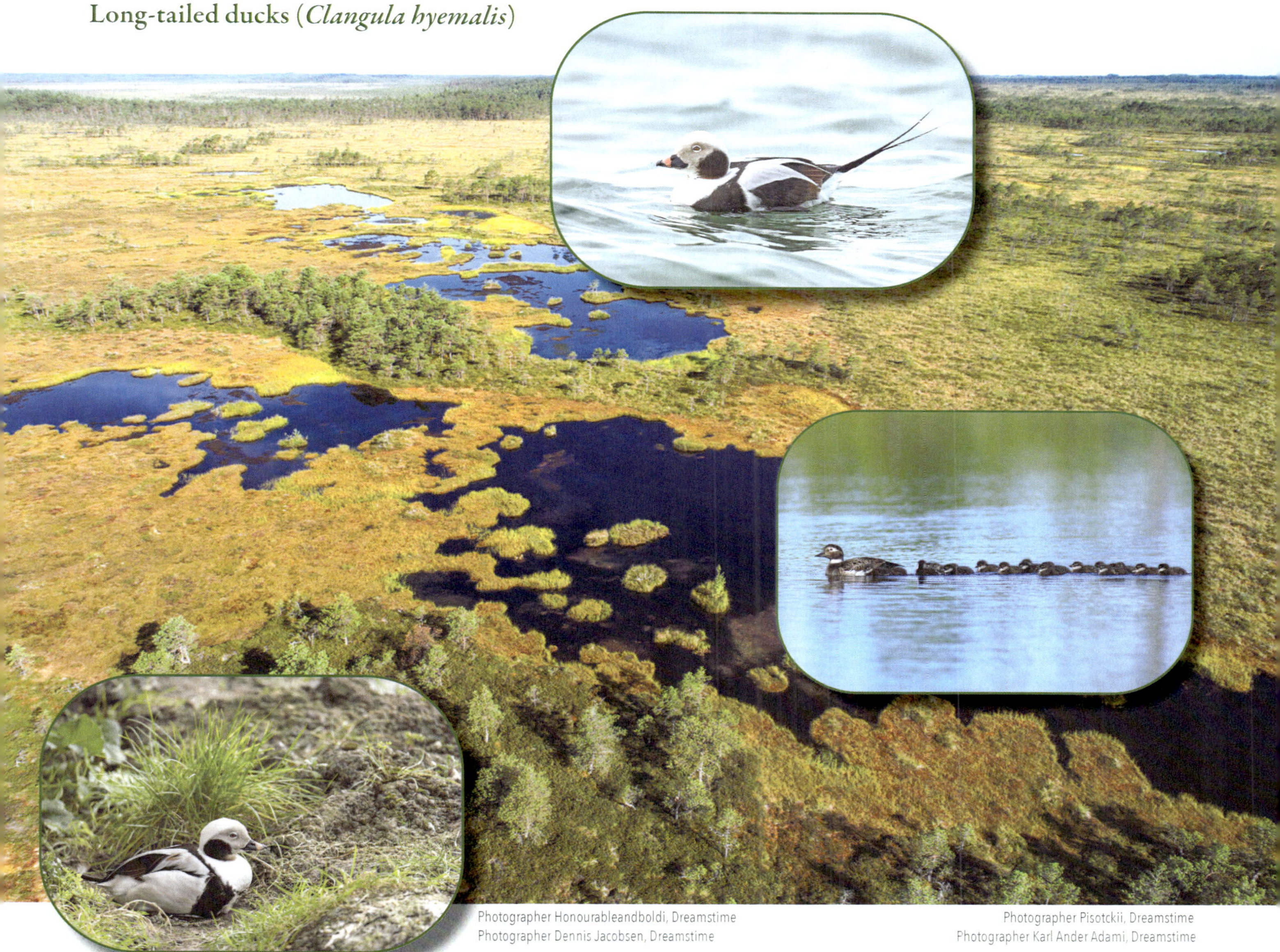

Photographer Honourableandboldi, Dreamstime
Photographer Dennis Jacobsen, Dreamstime

Photographer Pisotckii, Dreamstime
Photographer Karl Ander Adami, Dreamstime

Niches

Species' niches encompass the resources they need throughout their life cycle. Ducks, geese, and swans depend on both aquatic and terrestrial environments. During the breeding season, for instance, long-tailed ducks nest and raise their ducklings in places where there is an intermix of open water (where they feed) and upland habitat (where they nest). In the Soomaa National Park of Estonia, their populations spread out across a broad expanse of wetlands.

Resource partitioning and guilds

Resource partitioning facilitates the coexistence of species with similar ecological requirements

Resource partitioning occurs where species living in close proximity tend to co-evolve adaptations that enable them to partition (use) resources differently. The partitioning of resources may be clearly divided or have significant overlap.

Guilds encompass species that perform similar ecosystem functions. Insectivore guilds, for example, include: ground-feeders, flower-feeders, and air-feeders (catch insects in the air). The redundancy of guild species (performing similar ecological functions) enhances ecosystem stability and resilience, enabling ecosystems to adjust to changes in species composition (such as when species come and go with the seasons).

Resource Partitioning Among Cavity-Nesting Birds in Standing Dead Trees

Standing coniferous dead trees (snags) support forest birds that nest, forage and store food, perch, and drum on the bark–as a means of communicating. Partitioned over time and space, woodpeckers and sapsuckers are the main excavators, creating nests for themselves and their young. When the young are fledged and the nests are abandoned, then they may be used by secondary cavity nesters, as outlined below.

'Primary cavity nesters guild' (main excavators)[32]

- Lewis's woodpeckers carve a hole in a snag. Then, they build their nest inside and raise their young at a distance 4-15 m (13-50 ft) above the ground
- Williamson's sapsuckers make a hole and nest at a distance 3-18 m (10-55 ft) above ground

'Secondary cavity nesters guild'
select their nest sites and move in after the woodpeckers and sapsuckers have left their nests:

- flammulated owls which prefer a nest height of 8-15 m (25-50 ft) above ground
- pygmy nuthatches nest in a somewhat lower part, 3-15 m (10-50 ft) above ground
- mountain bluebirds select nest cavities that are the lowest at 3 m (10 ft) above ground

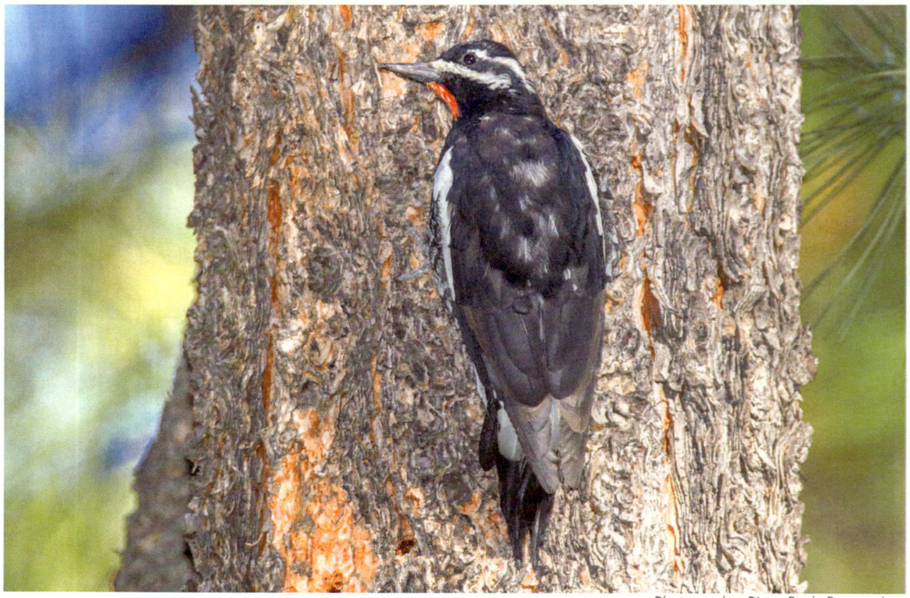

Williamson sapsucker (*Sphyrapicus thyroideus*) carving a hole to build a nest for his family in a ponderosa pine tree

Photographer Rinus Baak, Dreamstime

Natural Succession and Disturbance Regimes Create Mosiacs of Habitat

Natural succession occurs when the species composition substantially changes in 'seral' stages. In terrestrial ecosystems, for example, when trees move into a prairie, they may eventually develop the area into a woodland, and then a forest. Natural disturbance regimes, such as wildfires and flooding, 'set back' succession to earlier seral stages. Examples include:

1) Spreading unevenly across a prairie, woodland, or forest, wildfires create a patchwork (mosiac) of habitats at various seral stages, enhancing biodiversity. New plant growth may follow a wildfire that burns vegetation and re-mineralizes the soil. After the wildfire sweeps through, grasses and forbs may be the first to re-establish, then shrubs, then trees. In the Great Plains, wildfires, grazing, mound-building, and badger and prairie dog digging maintained prairies in early-successional seral stages for thousands of years.

2) In a freshwater pond, the succession of plants may start with herbaceous plants that are submerged, then others that are floating, then emergent plants; then shrubs; and then trees, the pond becoming a swamp. A flood regime could then return the area to an open pond.

Plants often change the environment in ways that enable other plants to move in and grow in the area, supporting the development of an ecosystem. Three separate examples: 1) nitrogen-fixing legumes might make way for plants that depend on fixed nitrogen, 2) shade-dependent plants follow plants that flourish in the sun and provide shade, and 3) grasses that stabilize sand dunes may be followed by plants that require the dune stability that the grasses provide.

A 'Nested Ecosystem' Embedded Within a Broader Ecosystem

Redwoods Nested Ecosystem Example

An ancient redwood forest ecosystem thrived along the coast of northern California and the Pacific Northwest in the United States for thousands of years. While most of the redwood trees have been cut down, remnant patches of protected redwood forest persist today and encompass some of the tallest trees on Earth. As the trees transpire, water lifts from their leaves into the cool air and condenses, coinciding with incoming fog from the Pacific Ocean. In this moist climate, hundreds of feet above the forest floor, aerial 'nested ecosystems' evolved on the upper branches of the redwood trees. Thickets of huckleberry bushes, ferns, and the seedlings of conifer trees (some large enough to bear cones) grow and build soil, which in some places is one meter (~3.3') thick.[33] Like soil on the forest floor, canopy soil absorbs and holds water and nutrients which nourishes the redwood trees and their arboreal inhabitants.

Species living in aerial redwood ecosystems include: invertebrates; *Crustacea*, including *Copepoda* that migrate up the tall trees from forest streams; amphibians, including the wandering salamander (*Aneides vagrans*); mammals, for example, the yellow-checked chipmunk (*Neotamias ochrogenys*); and birds, including the Steller's Jay (*Cyanocitta selleri*) and federally-listed endangered marbled murrelet (*Brachyramphus marmoratus*)–a seabird that nests in the redwoods and flies back and forth to the Pacific Ocean where it hunts for fish.[33] Huckleberries are common canapy plants, such as the evergreen huckleberry (*Vaccinium ovatum*).

A keystone species in the redwood canopy, the leatherleaf fern (*Rumohra adiantiformis*), forms mats around the canopy soil. This enables the soil to hold a tremendous amount of water and provides habitat for spiders, centipedes, crickets, and other insects.[34] In their research, Cal Poly Humboldt professor Stephen Sillett, who discovered the redwood canopy ecosystems, and research associate Marie Antoine found that the fern mats only occur in the largest and oldest redwood trees. The old growth (elder) redwood trees, and their canopy nested ecosystems, are fundamental to sustaining the biodiversity, complexity, and health of the ancient redwood forest–supporting the resilience, regeneration, and extent of the forest, which is needed for this ecosystem's survival over the long term.[34]

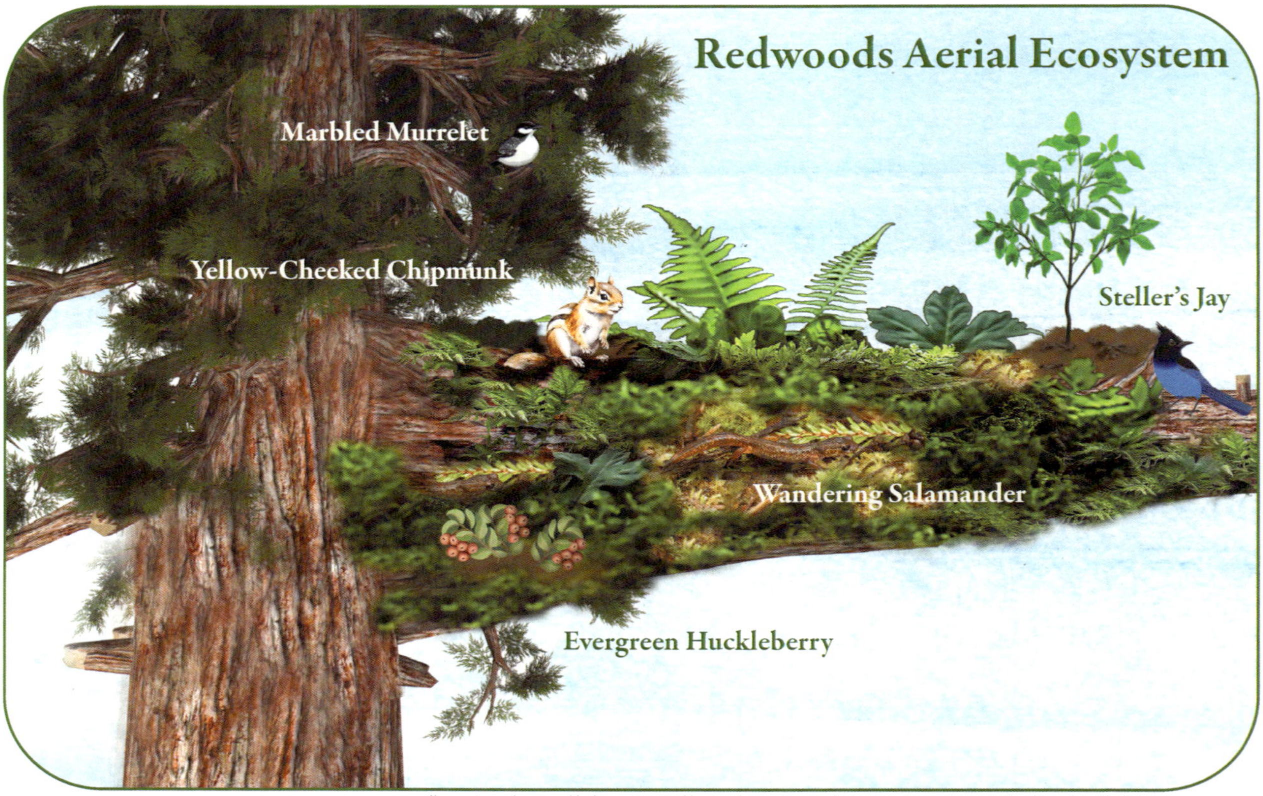

Illustrations above and below composed by Sandra L. Jones with Dreamstime images- credited in Acknowledgements

On a large branch, high in the canopy of old-growth forests composed of red and yellow cedar, hemlock, fir, and spruce trees, female marbled murrelets lay a single egg on a mat of moss, lichen, and organic debris. They also spend much of their time resting and foraging in marine waters near the coast in the Pacific Ocean.

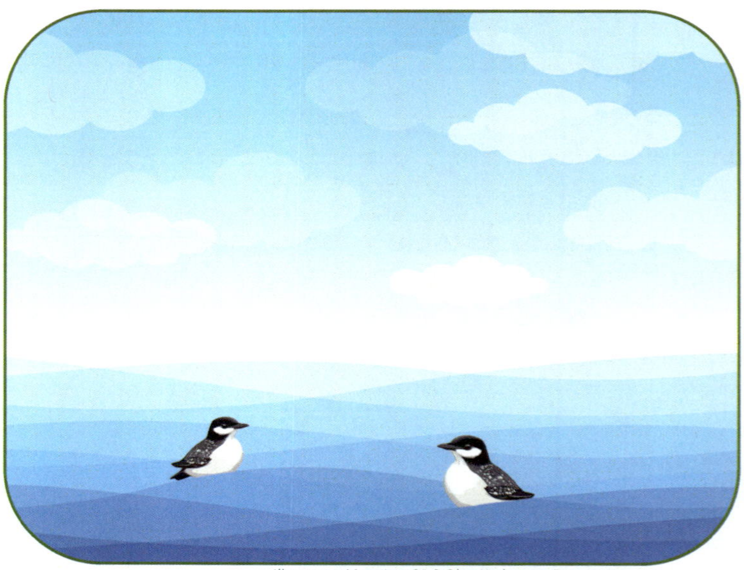

Marbled Murrelet (*Brachyramphus marmoratus*) resting on the surface of the Pacific Ocean

Illustrators Mappingz01 & Olga Kurbatova, Dreamstime.com

III. Life Transformed the Earth into An Embroidery of Rich Colors and Textures

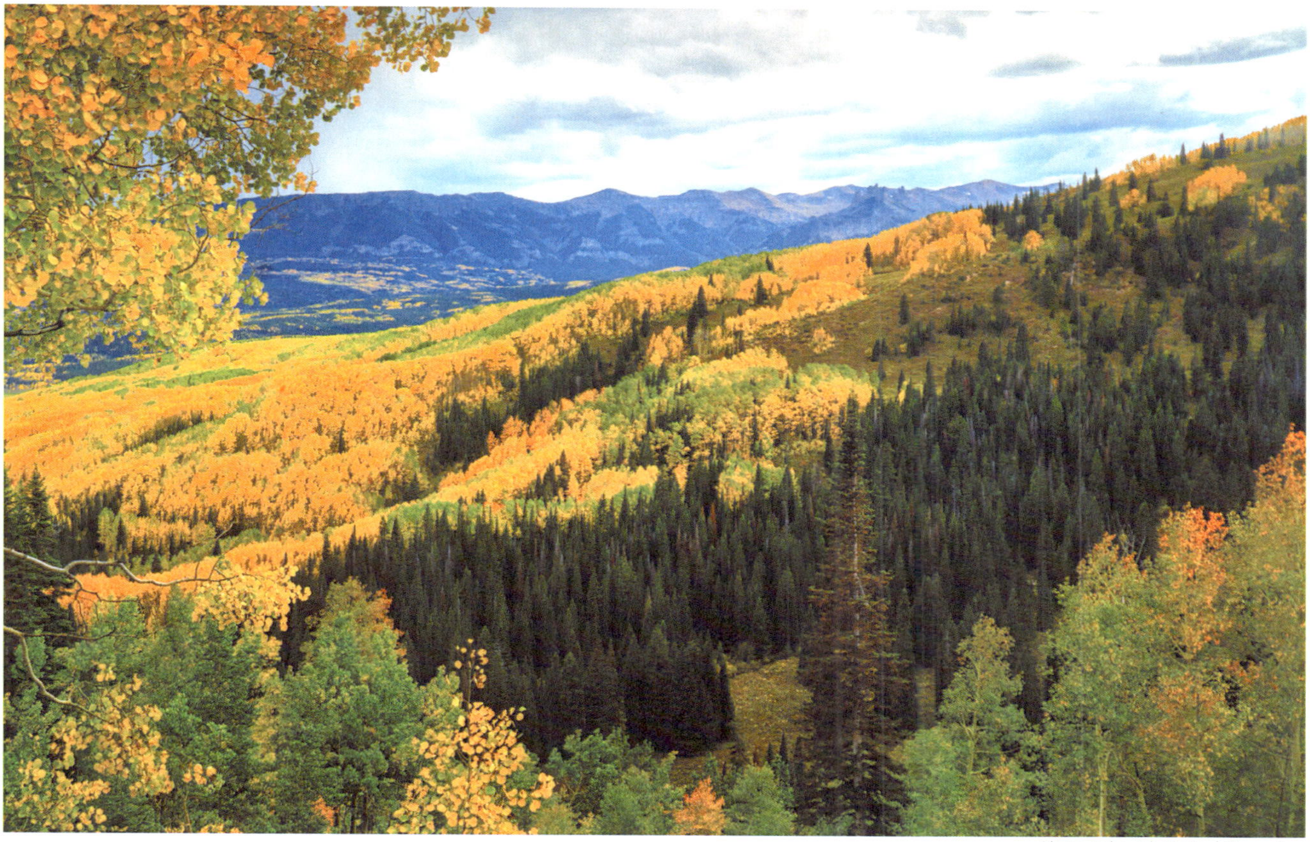

Photographer John DeBord, Dreamstime

Autumn Colorado Landscape

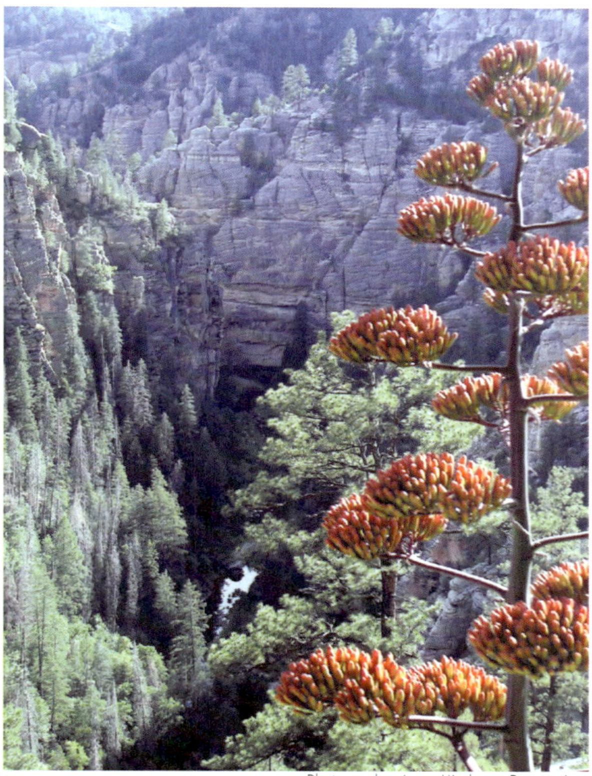

Photographer Jason Hindman, Dreamstime

Century plant (*Agave americana*) blossoms in Clear Creek, northern Arizona

Homeostasis in the Biosphere

The upper parts of the Earth's crust, oceans, and atmosphere are the product of living organisms or have been massively modified by their presence, astrobiologist and geochemist James Lovelock explains in his book, *The Ages of Gaia: A Biography of Our Living Earth*.[35] Life's transformation of the environment and adaptations to it are inseparable.[36] Significant environmental conditions produced by organisms include: breathable air, fertile soil and sediment, lush vegetation, and ecosystems with highly complex and inter-dependent species diversity.

Example of atmospheric homeostasis

Biological processes produce many life-sustaining conditions in the biosphere. Early on in the history of life, oxygen was only a trace gas in the atmosphere. Once plants were established on Earth, the additional oxygen they produced opened a giant new niche; whereupon, oxygen-consuming animals, fungi, and bacteria evolved to fill the niche; in turn, the carbon dioxide (CO_2) these animals, fungi, and bacteria released supplied the plant, algae, and cyanobacteria photosynthesizers. Oxygen levels continued to rise until ~two million years ago, when oxygen production and consumption in the biosphere reached an equilibrium and continued to maintain this steady state ever since. "Organisms keep the percentage of the earth's oxygen in the atmosphere at 21 percent and the mean temperature at 20 Celsius."[37]

The chemistry of the atmosphere balances out at the highest genealogical level, the domains and kingdoms of life. Ernst Mayr, Professor Emeritus, Museum of Comparative Zoology, Harvard University, in his book, *What Evolution Is*, reflected on this, stating that "Increased CO_2 production by a flourishing animal population will permit an increased CO_2 uptake by the plant world."[38]

Organisms Modify their Environment

The first inhabitants on Earth were micro-organisms and they remained the sole inhabitants for an estimated three billion years; and they continue to have fundamental roles in abiotic and biotic processes. The earliest anaerobic bacteria, for instance, still run ". . . vital and extensive ecosystems of the anoxic zones beneath the sea floor, wet lands and marshes, and in the guts of nearly all consumers including ourselves."[39] In the oceans, coral micro-organisms secrete a substance that forms a thin layer on the water's surface; this changes the surface tension of the water, reducing the size and energy of the waves which protects the reef and its inhabitants.[40]

On land, micro-organisms effectively break down rock much faster than wind or water (flooding, freezing, and thawing).[41] With powerful enzymes and acids, fungi, for example, break down rock into soil and consume the mineral nutrients that are released. In his book, *Entangled Life*, mycologist Merlin Sheldrake explains that calcium and silica, released by the work of fungi, react with carbon dioxide in the atmosphere. The resulting compounds, including carbonates and silicates, once they make it to the oceans, are used by marine organisms to make their shells. When these organisms die, their shells sink and pile up, hundreds of meters thick, on the ocean floor.[42]

The origin of soil

The first soil builders were photosynthesizing algae, the ancestors of plants. They moved out of shallow pools onto land millions of years ago. Author Merlin Sheldrake reveals that the sunlight, unfiltered by water, and more accessible carbon dioxide in the air drew early photosynthesizing algae to venture onto desolate, rocky landscapes.[43] Before the algae ancestors of plants developed roots, they exchanged nutrients with bacteria and micro-fungi, collaborating in breaking down and dissolving rock and creating the first soils that eventually gave plants a place to establish roots. These partnerships persisted; more than ninety percent of all plant species today depend on rhizobacteria ('root bacteria') and mycorrhizal fungi ('root fungi').[44] As soil creators with their bacterial and fungal partners, plants make up ~80 percent of the mass of all life on earth and are the foundation of terrestrial ecosystems.

Mycorrhizal Defined

Mycorrhizal fungi: the word 'myco' means fungus and 'rrhizal' means root.

Plant partnerships in the soil

"To the question of "How can we improve the soil? The answer must be, "Ultimately, plants improve the soil on their own. They do this through the symbiosis between plants, bacteria, and fungi. Plants are really the only soil improvers."[45]

–Pius Floris and Freek Van Haagen

Partnering for millions of years, plants and their symbiotic bacteria, micro-fungi, and invertebrates (such as worms and beetles) develop and continually enrich the organic soil that sustains the wetland, grassland, forest, tundra, and desert ecosystems throughout the world. Soil biologists Pius Floris and Freek Van Haagen, in their film titled, *Soil is a Living Organism: a Short Film on How to Restore Soil Health*, illustrate how plant roots develop more easily in soil when there are passageways left by the decomposing roots of plants that lived there before them.[45] Traveling through historic passageways, roots navigate more deeply and build more fertile soil. In reciprocity, rhizobacteria deliver nearby nutrients to the plant roots. The presence of the rhizobacteria around the roots forms a protective barrier for the plants against disease. Mycorrhizal fungi can travel much farther than plant roots, delivering as much as seven times more nourishment to plants than the plants could have obtained on their own. Mycorrhizal fungi's thin filaments move into the soil micro-pores in search of water molecules and mineral micro-nutrients, which they absorb and transport back to the plant roots. Like the rhizobacteria, mycorrhizal fungi feed on the glucose produced by plants they support.[45]

Aggregated soil structures made by terrestrial organisms

Soil organisms make their home in the earth, building the structures and bringing together the resources they need to sustain themselves. Soil scientist Mary-Howell R. Martens, in her article, "The Soil Food Web: A World Beneath Our Feet," explains how soil micro-organisms retain nitrogen, phosphorous, potassium, sulfur, and calcium in their bodies, preventing these and other micro-nutrients from being leached or removed from the soil by water runoff.[46] Martens also details how microbial waste products form a glue that sticks soil particles and organic matter together in small, loose clumps. This aggregated soil structure resists compaction and erosion and provides space for the movement of air, water, and the organisms themselves.[46] Well-constructed soil acts as a sponge, soaking in rainwater that supports a diversity of soil life. Once established, plants hold the soil in place with their roots; and, through evapotranspiration, bring rainfall to the area, replenishing the groundwater, springs, and streams. In these freshwater ecosystems, organic debris filters to the bottom where benthic communities decompose it, making nutrient-dense sediment.

The formation and bioturbation of sediment by marine organisms

Long before the formation of the soil by plants and their microbial partners on land, the decaying remains and waste products of early sea life, settling to the bottom, produced sediment on the ocean floor that furnished nutrition for prehistoric marine life. Living organisms disturb soil and sediment (bioturbation) in many ways. On land, bioturbation occurs when plant roots displace the soil and when animals scurry across or dig in the ground; whereas, in aquatic environments, the activity of bioturbators may alter the chemical properties of the sediment. This happens, for example, when bioturbators build and irrigate their burrows, introducing fresh oxygenated water. Their activity increases the exchange of solutes between the sediment and water column, extending the oxic/anoxic interface deeper into the sediment layers which benefits an array of nitrogen-cycling microbial communities. As a result, the abundance and diversity of micro-organisms is generally far greater in burrow wall sediment than in the surrounding sediment.

Invertebrate architects in the soil support tropical forest ecosystems

Edward O. Wilson, former Curator of Entomology at the Museum of Comparative Zoology at Harvard University, emphasized the fundamental role of invertebrates in ecosystems worldwide. For instance, Wilson portrays how in Central and South America, "The leaf-cutting ants excavate vertical galleries and living chambers as deep as five meters into the soil. They and other kinds of ants, as well as bacteria, fungi, termites, and mites, process most of the dead vegetation and return its nutrients to the plants to keep the great tropical forests alive."[47]

IV. Life Blankets the Earth

"Ecosystems are open to the flow of energy and materials. As they develop, they increase their nutrient retention and recycling capacity."[48] –Gilberto Cintrón-Molero

The Earth has a great capacity for sustaining life; and life is continually renewing itself. In many ways, the organisms in ecosystems self-organize from the bottom up–the smallest species and nutrient-rich particles ever-regenerating the foundation of ecosystems. Conservation biologist and entomologist Edward O. Wilson describes how "A rain of planktonic bacteria, fungus spores, small seeds, and insects, spiders, and other small creatures falls continuously on most parts of the Earth's land surface."[49]

Global abiotic and biotic disturbance regimes support ecosystems across the world

Ancient grassland and wetland ecosystems transitioned, as climates changed over geologic time. They become some of the driest mineral-rich deserts that supply nutrients and sustain tropical rainforests. Over millennia, for example, Pacific Ocean Trade Winds have been carrying dust clouds from the Gobi Desert in East Asia to where they fertilize the rainforests in the Hawaiian Islands.[50] Similarly, over thousands of years, the Northeast Trade Winds have blown dust clouds from the Bodélé Depression ancient lakebed in Chad, Africa, to the Amazon basin.[51] While the Hawaiian and Amazon rainforests depend on desert wind-driven, trans-continental nutrients, their hydrological systems largely stay in place. Plumes of water vapor lift off tropical forests (facilitated by sulfur compounds emitted by micro-organisms) and form clouds above the forests, keeping the forests cool and moist.

Biologically-rich ecosystems have been degrading over the last century

Historically, the diversity and abundance of species and the ecosystems they inhabited were more complex, robust, and resilient than they are today. The Sonoran Desert ecosystem is an example, having once supported 2,000 species of plants, over 1,000 species of bees, and 100 endemic species of reptiles found nowhere else in the world. In many places, millions of fish schooled in rivers, lakes, and oceans; millions of migrating birds filled the sky; and millions of grazing and foraging animals roamed the grasslands and savannahs.

In the 1950s, Rachel Carson began documenting how the pesticide DDT was causing genetic damage and poisoning wildlife, accumulating up the food chain wherever it was applied. She showed how DDT weakened the shells of birds' eggs, causing them to thin and break, including the eggs of bald eagles. In 1962, Carson's book, *Silent Spring*, including a fable of the arrival of spring without bird songs, inspired the environmental movement and enactment of natural resources conservation statutes in the United States, including: the Clean Air Act of 1963, as amended; National Environmental Policy Act of 1969, as amended; Clean Water Act of 1972, as amended; and Endangered Species Act of 1973, as amended (ref. Appendix A, pages 282 - 289).

NEPA: A broad national framework for protecting the environment

The National Environmental Policy Act (NEPA) is a 'sunshine' (transparency) statute, requiring all federal agencies to inform and involve the public before taking major federal actions. For instance, under NEPA, an agency proposing a major federal action, such as reintroducing wolves into a national park or building a dam, is required to publish the proposed action in the Federal Register–describing the need for the proposed action; the authorities under which the agency would be acting; and how the proposed action meets the purposes of statute(s), such as the Endangered Species Act and Fish and Wildlife Coordination Act. The NEPA process and general timeline should be clearly explained, such as where and when documents will be available, the timeframe of public comment periods, and when open houses will be held in the area where the project is being proposed. The agency then prepares an environmental assessment (EA) or an environmental impact statement (EIS) that includes the proposed action; alternative ways to carry out the proposed action (including the 'no action alternative'); and an analysis of the direct, indirect, and cumulative impacts of the proposed action. In the EA or EIS, the agency responds to substantive public comments and recognizes how specific concerns and recommendations have been addressed and potentially incorporated into revised alternatives or the final decision on the proposed action.

Ecosystems unraveling

Ecosystems continue to be fragmented, degraded, and destroyed when they are converted to industrial agriculture, urban development, and related infrastructure (including roads, dams, and power plants). Under these circumstances, ecosystems may degrade insidiously; wherein, their reduced capacity may be hidden by compensations for the stresses. For example, when species are extirpated (no longer exist in a particular area), some of the remaining species may fill gaps in the food chain or take over other ecological roles. These degraded ecosystems that are 'hollowed out' have lost their species diversity and ecological complexity. Reaching a threshold of change, ecosystems may rapidly decline to a deteriorated state.

In recent decades, the conversion of ecosystems and associated air, water, and soil pollution has significantly impaired species' habitats and the human environment worldwide. Conservation biologists Reed Noss, Florida Institute for Conservation Science; Edward T. LaRoe, III, National Biological Service, Washington, D.C.; and J. Micheal Scott, University of Idaho, wrote a comprehensive report on the status of ecosystems titled "Endangered Ecosystems of the United States: A Preliminary Assessment of Loss and Degradation." The authors documented critically-endangered (>98% decline), endangered (85-98% decline), and threatened (70-84% decline) ecosystems. Old-growth forests, vernal pools, and free-flowing rivers were found to be especially degraded (excerpts below).[52]

48 conterminous U.S. states

- 95-98% of virgin forests destroyed by 1990
- 53% loss of wetlands from 1780's to 1980's
- 98% of an estimated 5.2 million km of streams are degraded enough to be unworthy of federal designation as wild or scenic rivers

Key to ecological restoration is the conservation of patches of degraded ecosystems that are still intact with the potential to be restored. Also important is protecting: the threatened and endangered species; remnant habitat patches with native soil microbiomes; 'seed banks' with native seeds; and natural springs.

Intact Ecosystems Protect the Complexity of Life

For complex life to persist on Earth, interconnected ecosystems must sufficiently blanket the planet in order for organisms to regulate the biosphere. Without enveloping the Earth, abiotic physical and chemical forces could overtake life's processes.[54] Being highly complex adaptive systems, tropical rainforests require a substantial amount of their historic range to be sustainable and resilient. Like the photosynthesizing algae in the oceans, tropical forests are contributing necessary oxygen that is sustaining life on Earth.[55]

Wolves Brought Life to the Yellowstone Ecosystem

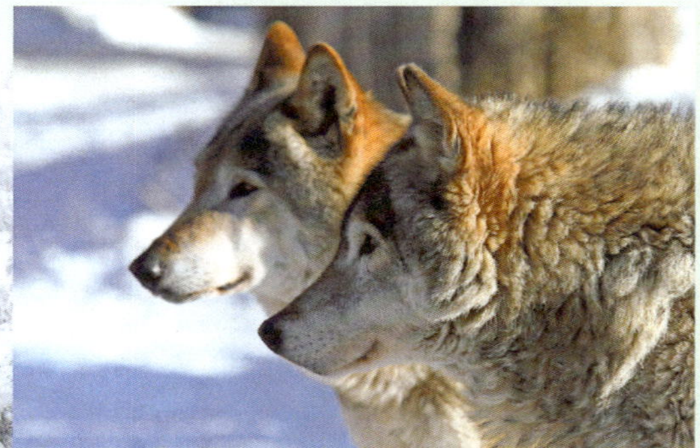

Photographer Tatiana Belova, Dreamstime

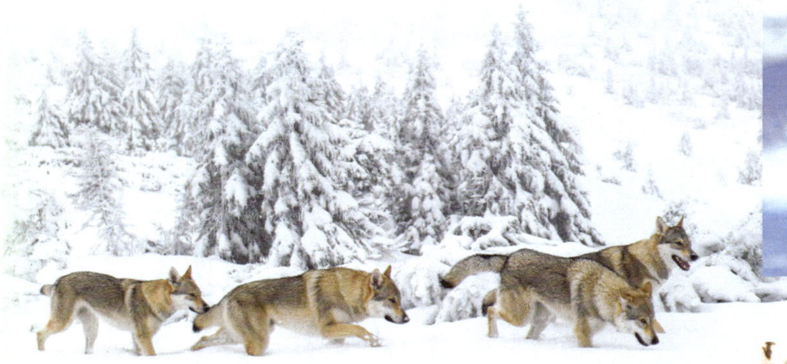

Photographer Jan Havlicek, Dreamstime

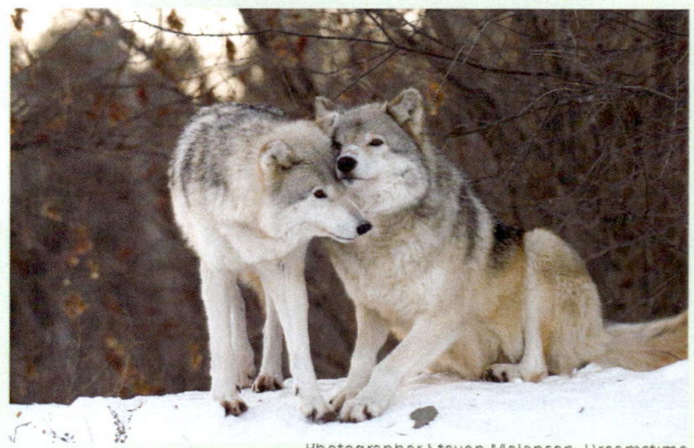

Photographer Steven Melanson, Dreamstime

Gray Wolves (*Canis lupus*) reintroduced to Yellowstone National Park

When gray wolves were reintroduced into Yellowstone National Park in 1995, seventy years after they had been eradicated, they created a more natural balance in the Yellowstone ecosystem.[56] Like other top predators, the wolves caused a 'trophic cascade' of beneficial effects in the trophic organizations (food chains) below them. To avoid the wolves, elk and deer left the valleys and gorges, allowing grasses, bushes, and tree saplings to establish (including willows and cottonwoods). Moving more, the hooves of the elk aerated the soil which then retained more water and encouraged more herbaceous plants. This brought in neotropical songbirds to nest in the regenerating grasslands and woodlands. As the wolves reduced the numbers of coyotes, the numbers of small mammal populations rose. This drew raptors to the Yellowstone ecosystem, including eagles, hawks, and osprey. With plants stabilizing the banks and providing shade, which cooled the water near the banks, the rivers meandered less, flowed more, and supported more aquatic species, including: muskrats, beavers, otters, waterfowl, fish (including the Yellowstone cutthroat trout), and amphibians.[56]

Muskrats (*Ondatra zibethica*) swimming

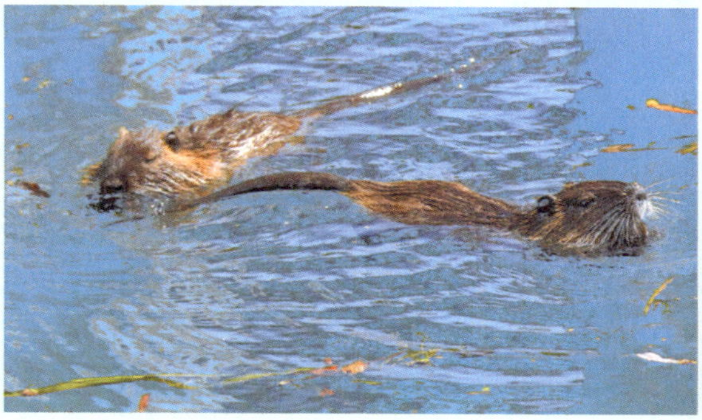

Photographer Erik Zunec, Dreamstime

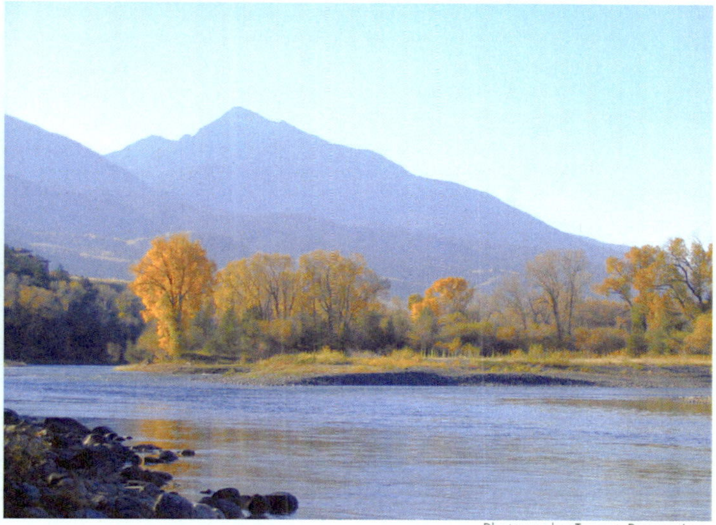

Cottonwood Trees Along the Yellowstone River

Photographer Taseret, Dreamstime

The return of the wolves improved the river habitat, benefiting aquatic species, such as muskrats.

V. Seamlessly Conserving Species, Habitats, and Ecosystems

"The return of Nature in swaths of wildland across the continents is morally compelling for what it provides future generations. It is ultimately the best way to protect native faunas and floras, and to add both physical and biological stability to the global environment."[57] –Edward O. Wilson

'Monarch Butterfly Waystation Program'

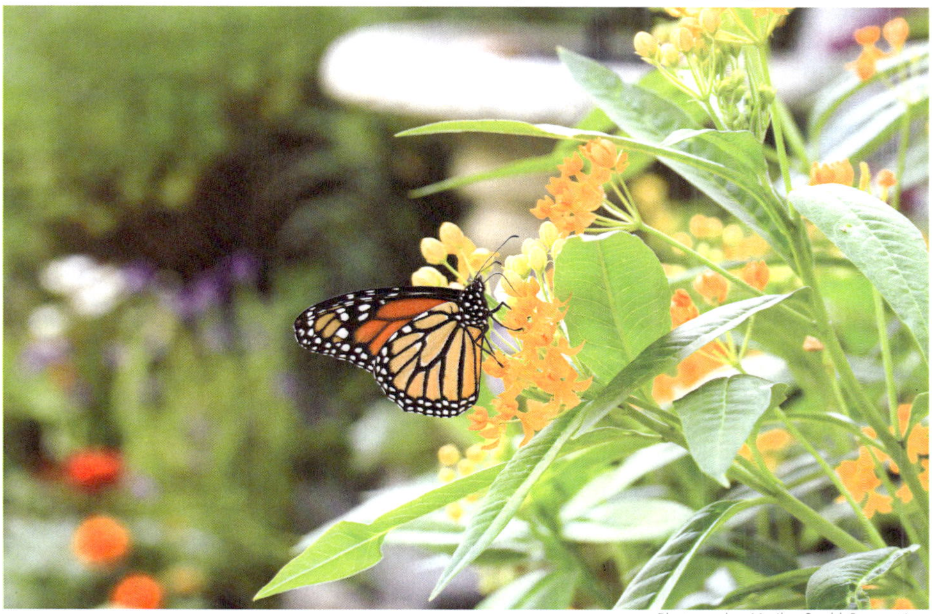

Photographer Marilyn Gould, Dreamstime

Monarch Butterfly (*Danaus plexippus*) Feeding on Milkweed (*Asclepias*)

The 'Monarch Butterfly Waystation Program' engages a network of individuals and communities that provide habitat for hundreds of millions of monarch butterflies migrating from their breeding grounds in the United States and Canada to where they winter in central Mexico. When conditions are favorable, the butterflies make their return flight home in the spring.[58]

'Coastal First Nations Great Bear Sea Initiative' and 'North Coast Integrated Marine Area Initiative'

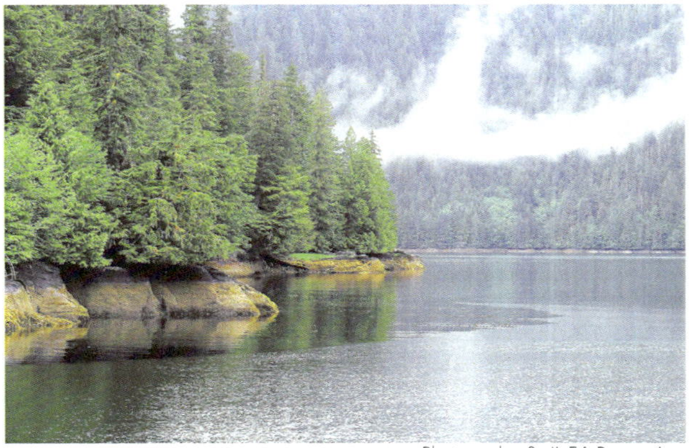

Photographer Serjio74, Dreamstime

Great Bear Sea Coast

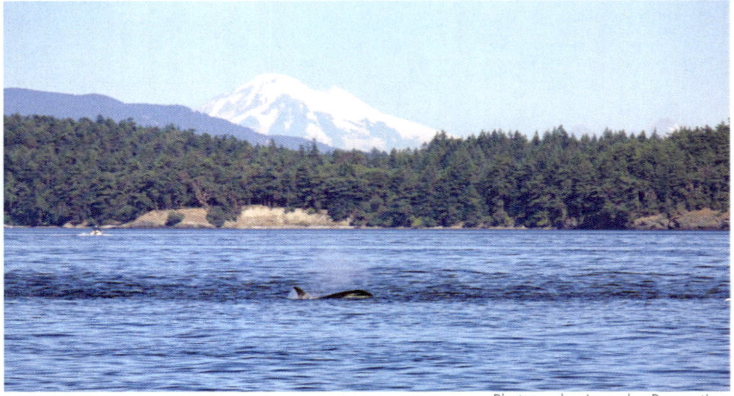

Photographer Ivansabo, Dreamstime

Orca (*Orcinus orca*)

Seventeen First Nations in the Province of British Columbia and other entities in Canada founded: 1) the 'Coastal First Nations Great Bear Sea Initiative,' protecting more than 6.4 million hectares (~15.8 million acres) of ancient coastal temperate rainforest and 2) the 'North Coast Integrated Marine Area Initiative,' encompassing a marine protected area network for the Northern Shelf Bioregion.[59]

'Florida Wildlife Corridor'

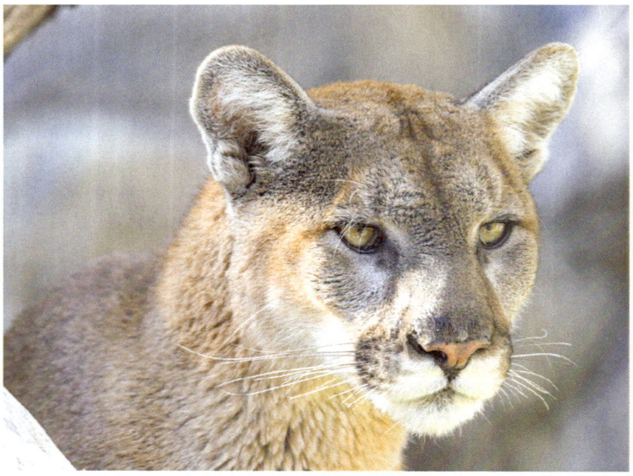

Photographer Chon Kit Leong, Dreamstime

Florida Panther, (*Puma concolor coryi*)

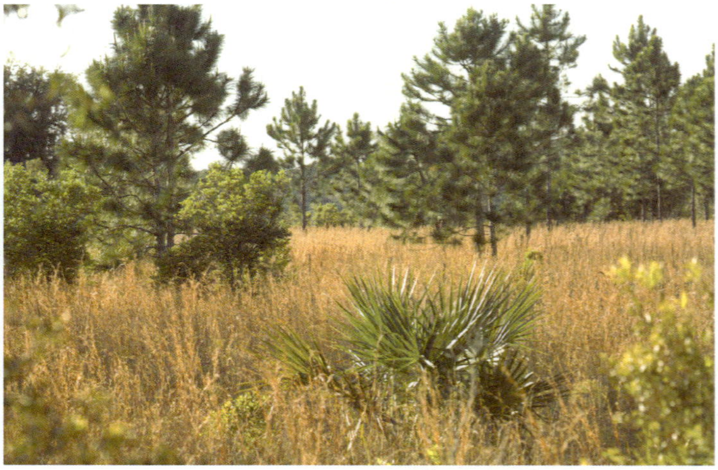

Photographer Jeffrey Holcombe, Dreamstime

Florida Scrub Habitat

The 'Florida Wildlife Corridor' conservation program was established under the Florida Wildlife Corridor Act of 2021. It comprises nearly 18 million acres of contiguous wilderness and working lands crucial to the survival of many of Florida's 131 imperiled species, including the wide-ranging, top predator Florida panther that roams the subtropical hardwood hammocks, scrub habitats, pine forests, and freshwater swamps.[60]

'Necanicum Wildlife Corridor Conservation Plan'

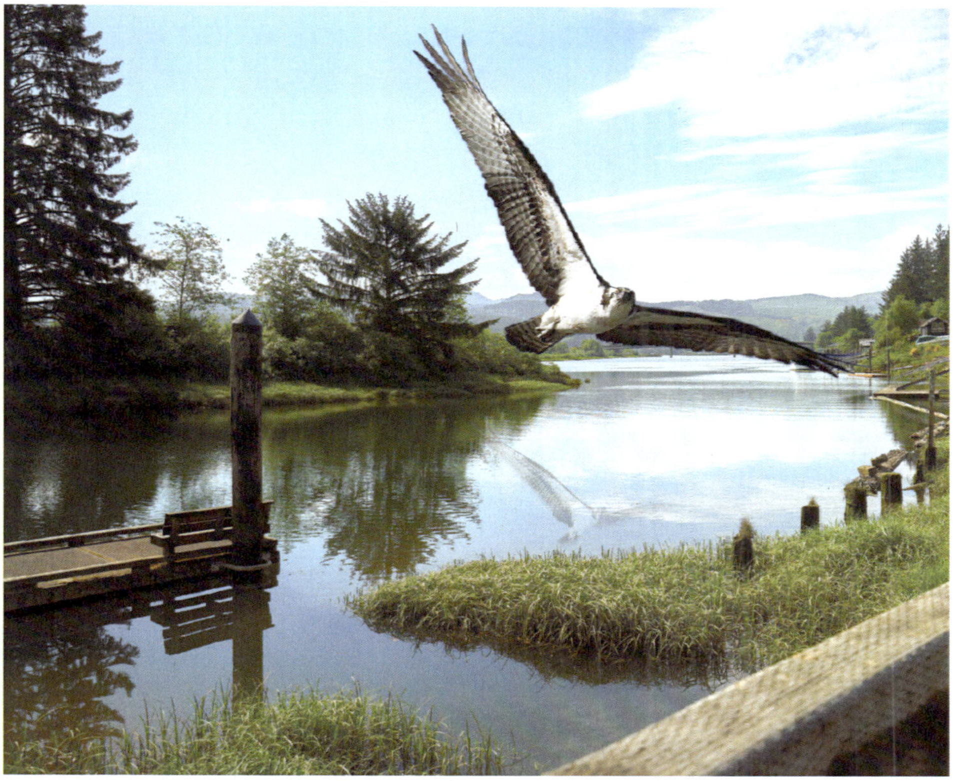

Photographer Vismax, Dreamstime Photographer Mark Hryciw, Dreamstime

Oregon Osprey (*Pandion haliaetus*) in the Necanicum River Watershed

The 'Necanicum Wildlife Corridor Conservation Plan' of the North Coast Land Conservancy protects the nearly 49,000-acre Necanicum River watershed. Floodplain restoration, conservation priorities, and land protection are planned for mountain, forest, and stream habitat from the Coast Range headwaters of the Necanicum River and its tributaries to the Pacific Ocean.[61, 62]

VI. Gathering Partners to Restore Ecosystems

The Lomakatsi Restoration Project

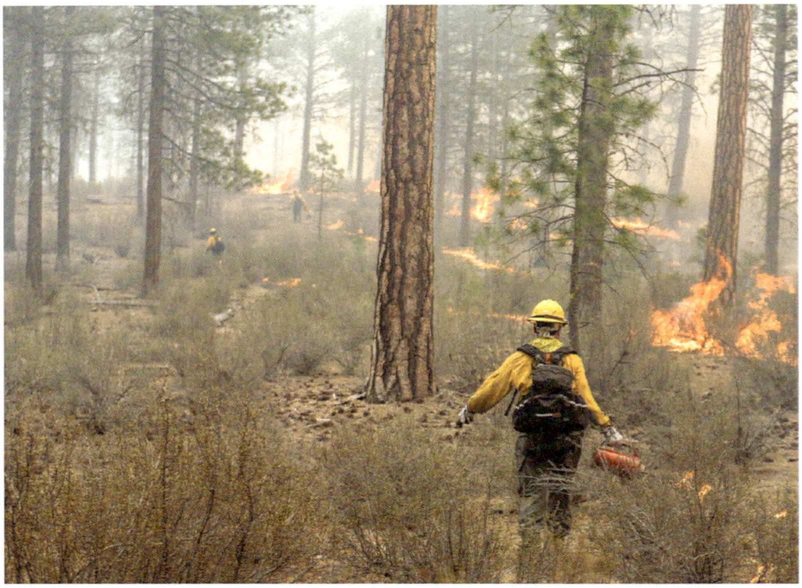

Photography by Lomakatsi Restoration Project

Lomakatsi Restoration Project develops and implements forest and watershed restoration projects throughout Oregon and northern California. Their specialists engage with tribal and rural communities to restore and protect forests, streams, and cultural resources through ecological thinning, prescribed fire, and riparian restoration, including planting native shade plants for salmon and other aquatic species.[63,64]

An understory prescribed burn supported by Lomakatsi inter-tribal crew members in the Ashland, Oregon, watershed.

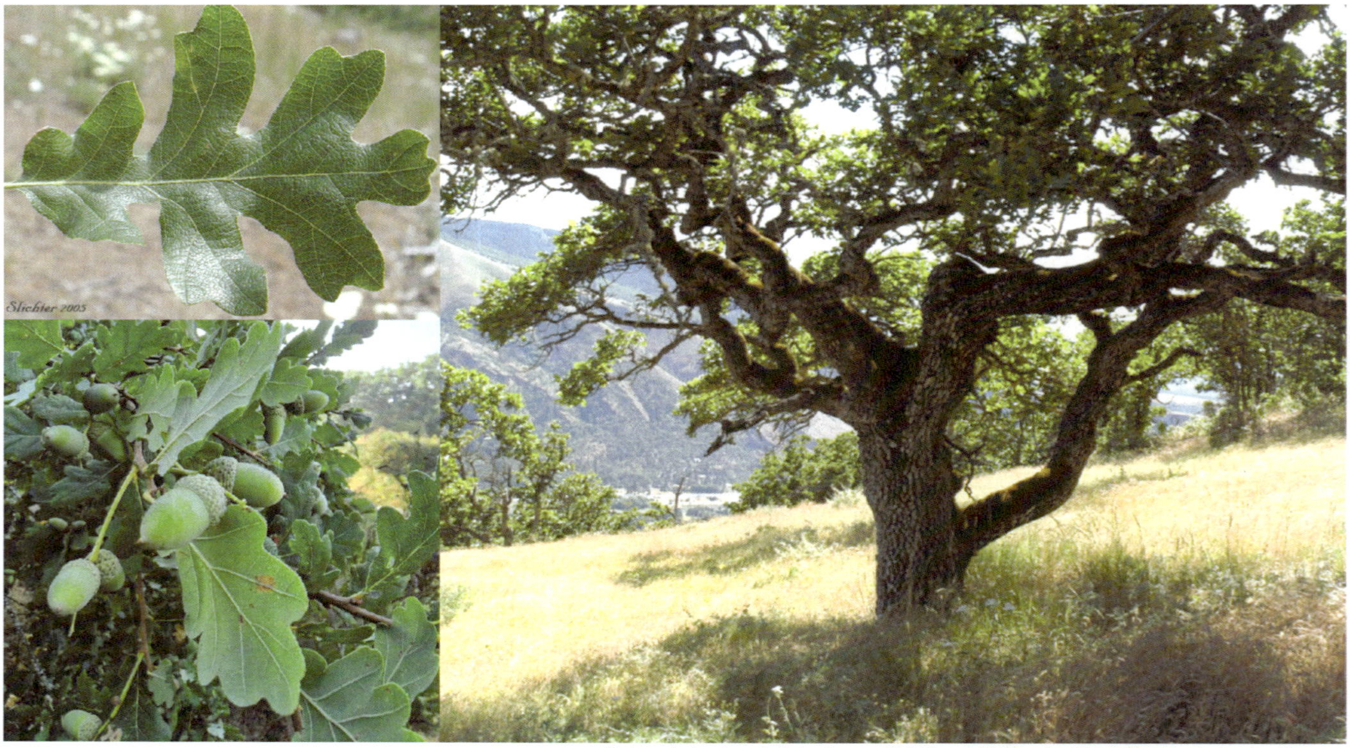

Photography by science.halleyhosting.com, Phil J Savage Photography at dreamstime.com, heritageseedlings.com

Oregon White Oak Tree and Acorns (*Quercus garryana*)

Oak woodlands are fire-adapted, having historically grown in frequent-fire environments. By restoring the natural fire regime and ecological functions across the landscape, the Lomakatsi Restoration Project applies fire to maintain oak habitats and promote acorn production.

'Ecocultural Stewardship and Riparian Restoration at Hat Creek' Example of a Lomakatsi Restoration Project

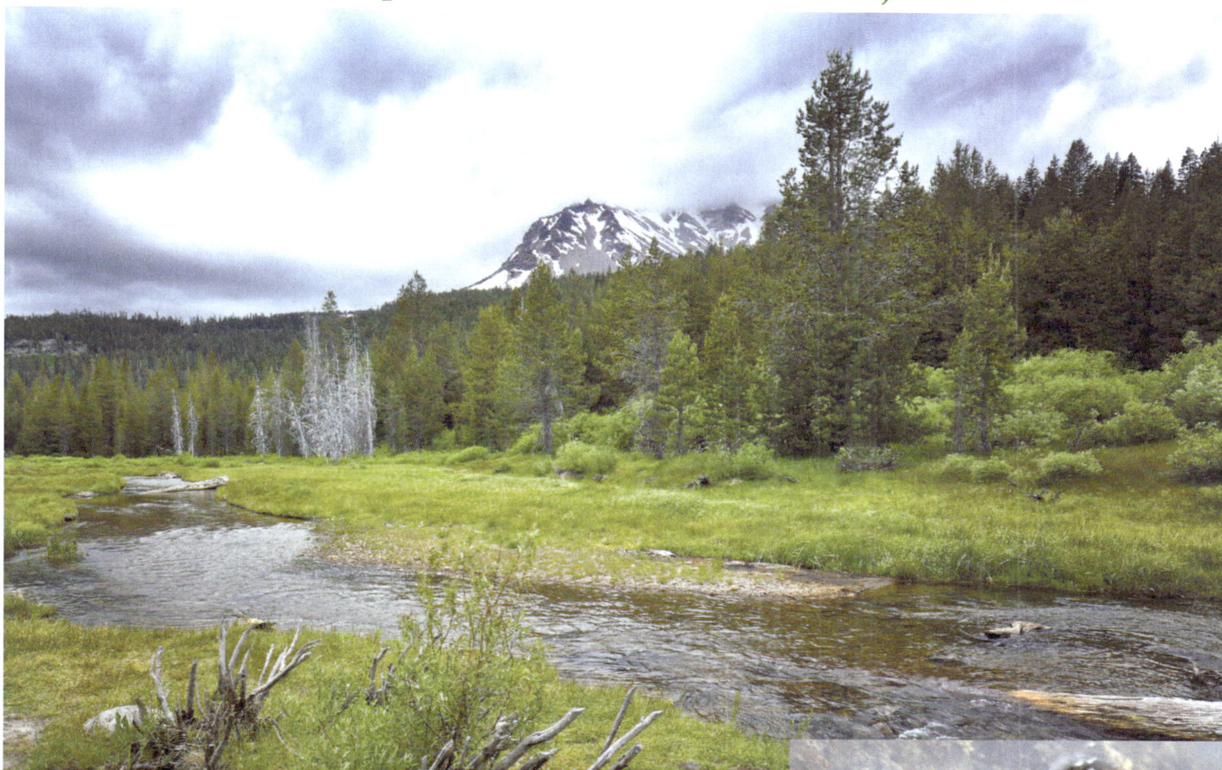

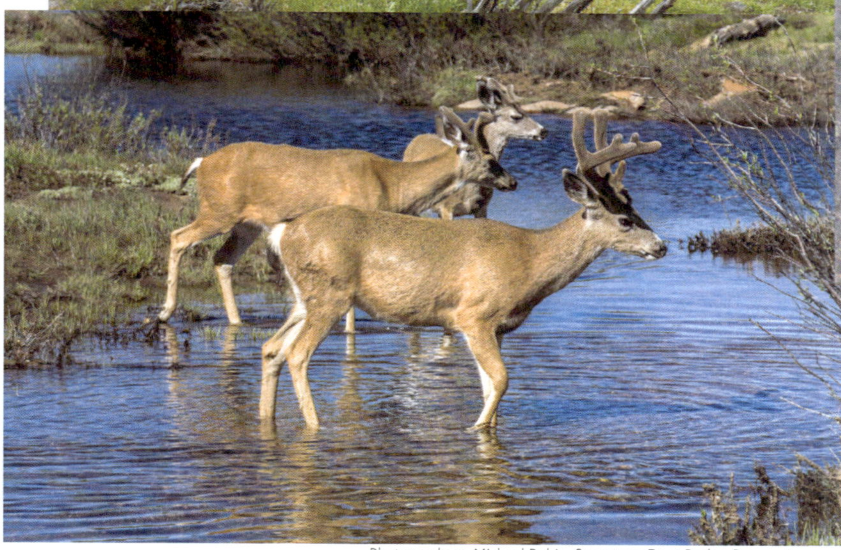

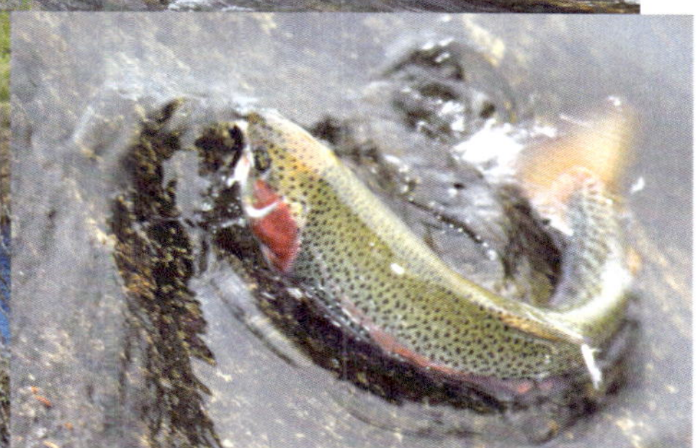

Hat Creek and Riparian Habitat, Wild Rainbow Trout and Mule Deer

Photographers: Michael Rubin, Straystone, Trout Dodos, Dreamstime.com

The Ilmawi people have been living alongside spring-fed, cold-water Hat Creek and the broader Pit River area since time immemorial. They are one of the eleven bands comprising the Pit River Nation and speak Palaihnihan-Hokan, the indigenous language spoken in the Shasta region of California. Fishing, hunting, foraging, and gathering, and life along Hat Creek is central to the Ilmawi people and is of tremendous ecological importance, including the diversity of native foods they subsist on. Their knowledge of the ecosystem guided the Hat Creek Riparian Restoration; and youth education opportunities, involving cultural and ecological aspects, were integral to the project (ref. https://lomakatsi.org).

Photo collages courtesy of Southern Oregon Fire Ecology Education and compiled by Sofia Maciel with Southern Oregon Forest Restoration Collaborative, pages 99 -101

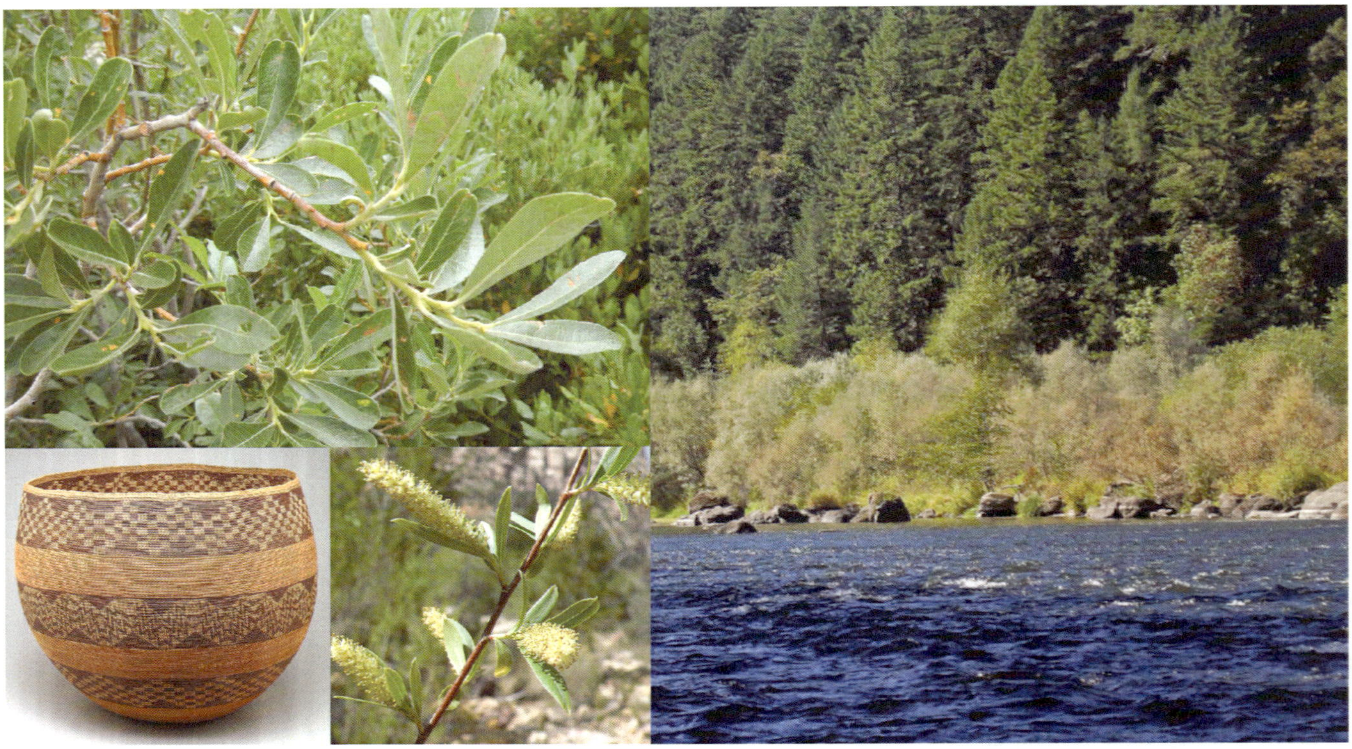

The Pit River Tribe Uses Willow Shoots to Weave Baskets

On Ilmawi ancestral lands, the Pit River Tribe, California Trout, and Lomakatsi Restoration Project collaborated in restoring the ecological functions of this culturally-important ecosystem. Through this partnership project, some of the more than 200 plant species of cultural significance to the Pit River Tribe were planted throughout the Hat Creek riparian corridor, including: willow, tule, and dogbane (weaving) and wild rose, camas, and yapa (edible and medicinal). Once these plants established their dense root systems and aboveground structural diversity, they have continued to protect fragile low terrace soils, stabilize the banks, and provide essential shade habitat that supports local populations of trout and a wide variety of other aquatic life.

Lomakatsi Restoration Project
(ref. https://lomakatsi.org)

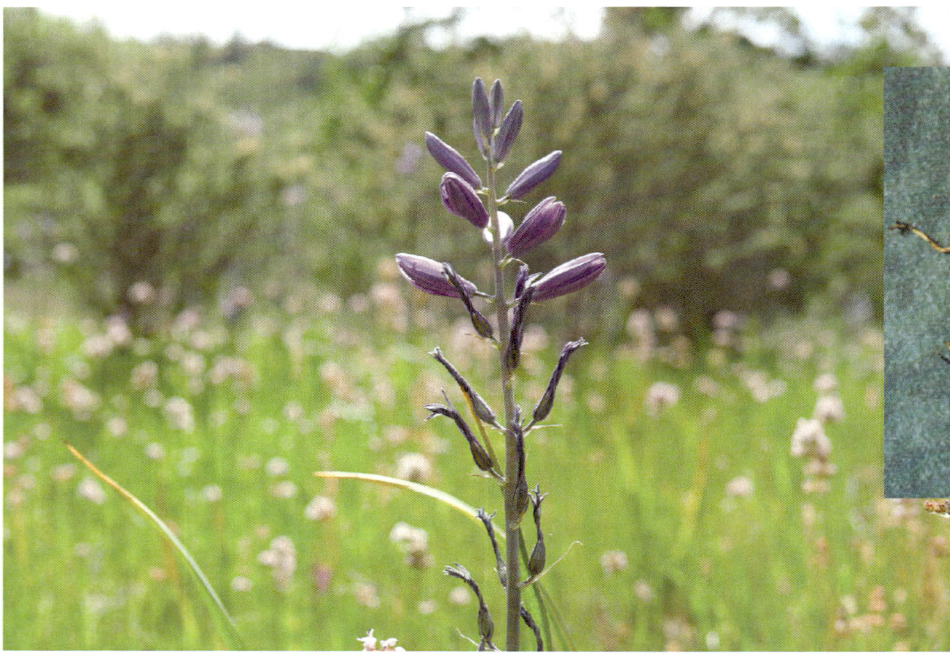

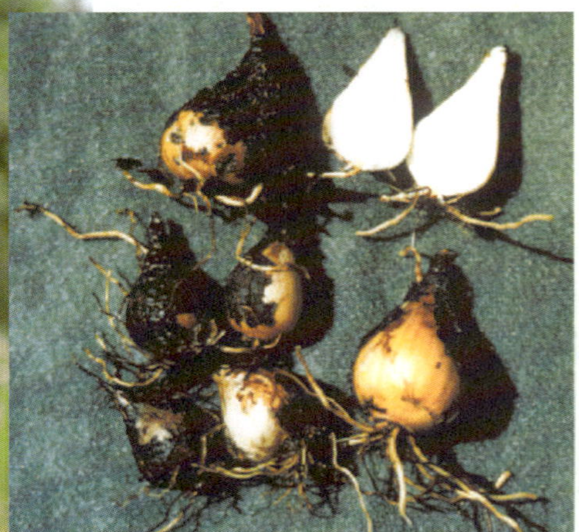

Photography by Nancy Turner & Katherine Turner

Camas Lily and Edible, Medicinal Bulbs

Photography by Tom Greco, Lomakatsi Restoration Project

Industrial Dam Removal Restores Ecosystems

Worldwide – Industrial Dams, Holding Back Water, Dried the Surrounding Landscapes

Thousands of dams have displaced more than ½ billion people[65] and caused the extinction of dozens of freshwater species.[66] Water diversions and pumping stations on a large scale have depleted groundwater and aquifers, dried landscapes, and degraded grassland, woodland, forest, and desert ecosystems.

In Nature, Beaver Dams Bring More Water and Wildlife to the Surrounding Landscapes

When beaver families build dams, they create pond and wetland habitat that recharges groundwater and aquifers and supports a wide array of aquatic and terrestrial species.

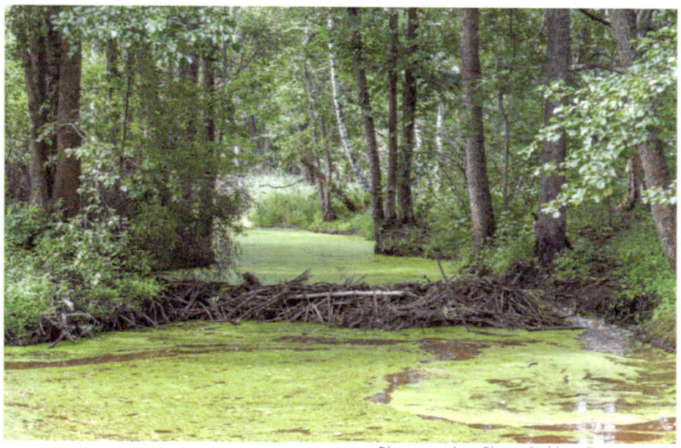

Photographer Chase Dekker, Dreamstime

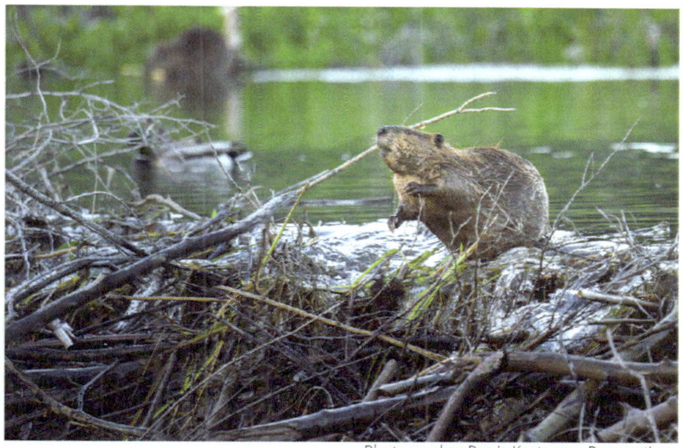

Photographer Denis Kostroma, Dreamstime

With ecological restoration, industrial dams are removed, allowing water once again to move through the surrounding watershed:

- supplying water to the rivers and streams
- recharging the groundwater (including aquifers)
- furnishing water to pastoralists, gardeners, farmers, hunters, and fishers (people who harvest fish) in rural communities, enabling them to grow and harvest their own food

Certain species require an intact continuum between terrestrial, freshwater, and marine ecosystems to complete their life cycles, including anadromous fish, such as salmon and trout. By removing industrial dams, rivers become free-flowing again (resuming their flood regimes), enabling fish passage, and sustaining river life. Thereupon, plants flourish in the riparian zone, providing the shade habitat that many species depend on; fish return to their upstream spawning grounds; and, when no longer stagnant and low in oxygen, water quality improves throughout the entire river system.

Berms and Swales Capturing Rainwater Support Regenerative Gardens and Farms

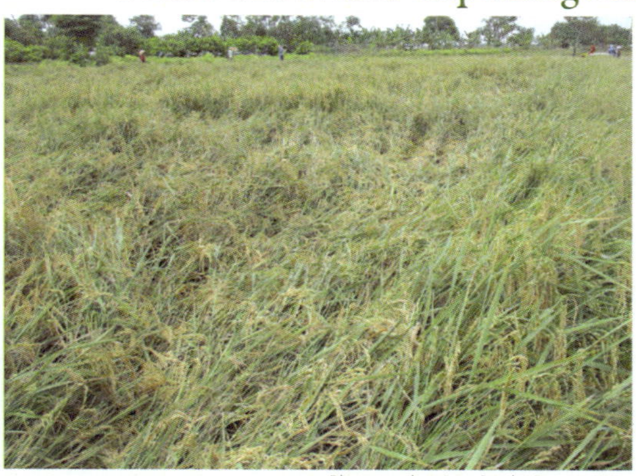

Photographer Azot Susila, Dreamstime

Permaculture practitioners build berms and swales to replenish water in degraded ecosystems and to develop regenerative gardens and farms. On hillsides, this is done perpendicular to the natural slope of the land. The swales allow rainwater to seep into the soil.

Permaculture techniques restore ecosystems, such as swales–the arc-shaped depression in the grassland (photo on left)

VII. Human Health Is Closely Tied to Replenishing Nutrient-Rich Soil

Flavorful, nutrient-dense natural foods grow in rich, dark, moist soil (humus) that develops from decomposing organic matter

"... rebuilding and conserving our soils ... [is] the surest guarantee of the future health and strength of the nation."[67]
–Weston A. Price, D.D.S.

Regenerative Gardens and Farms

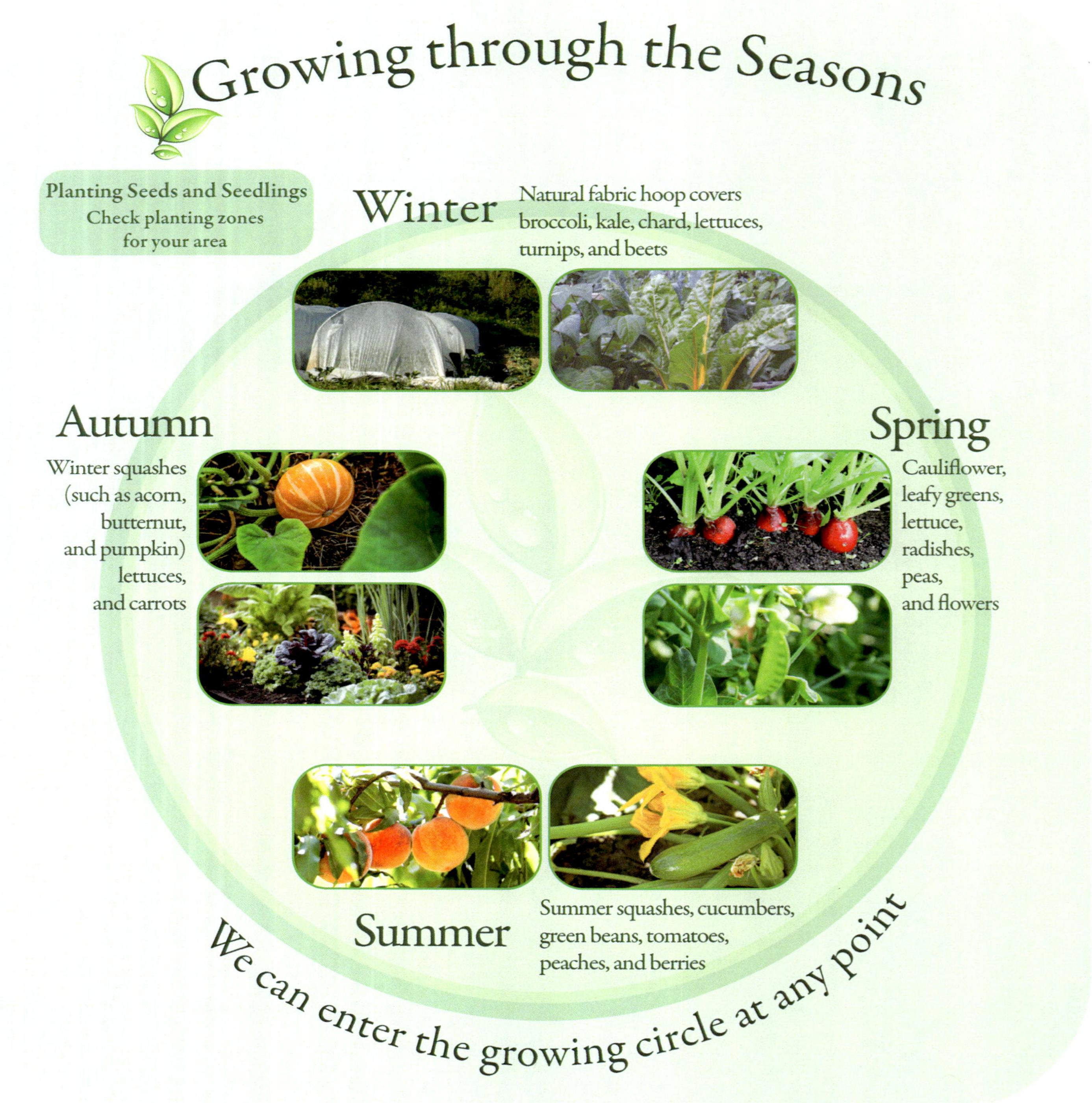

Composed by Sandra Jones, Eagle Lady Design Studio with Dreamstime images- credited in Acknowledgements

GARDENS AND FARMS ARE ENRICHED WHEN THEY ARE CONNECTED TO THE SURROUNDING ECOSYSTEM, SUCH AS ALONG A RIVER WHERE THEY ARE WATERED AND FERTILIZED WHEN THE RIVER FLOODS—SUPPLYING NUTRIENTS AND ORGANIC MATTER.

Five Steps to Grow a Garden

Selecting Food Plants

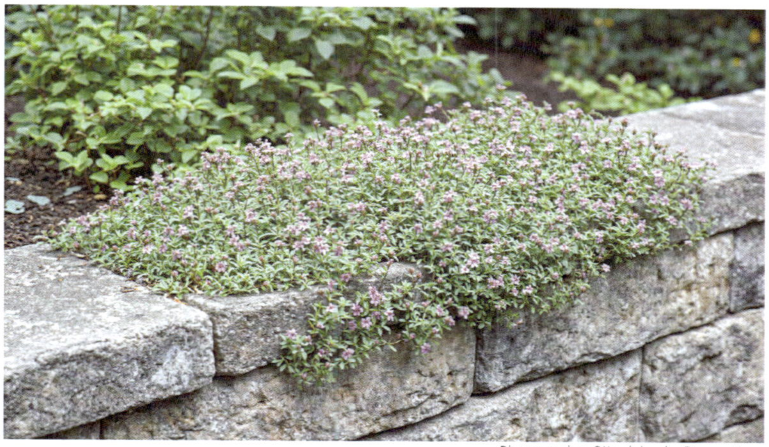

Photographer Gijsvdabeele, Dreamstime

Creeping Thyme

Step 1) Choose food plants to grow in the garden, including window boxes, planters, raised beds, or even along the edge of a rock wall.

In selecting food plants, consider:

- nutritional goals, including colorful phytonutrients
- textures, flavors and, cultural preferences
- diverse plant families to minimize pest pressures
- companion planting based on growing requirements, such as amount of sun or shade for different varieties; seasonality
- whether to plant seeds or grow seedlings indoors (such as under hoop row covers or in a greenhouse) where planting can be started sooner, protected from the elements
- writing a list of seeds and seedlings and procure them (some may be available at farmers' markets)

Designing and preparing beds for window boxes, planters, and/or raised beds

Step 2) Create a spatial layout of the garden

Consider inter-planting – three spatial dimensions are described below:

- in the center – plant the tallest and slowest-growing plants, for example, fruits that need pollinating, such as pea pods, green beans, cucumber, tomatoes, and berries
- out from the center – plant more shade-tolerant or vining plants (cucumber varieties may be bushes or vining, both varieties require full sun)
- at the outer edge, closest to where the gardener can easily reach – plant the lowest and fastest-growing food plants, such as leafy greens, carrots, and radishes

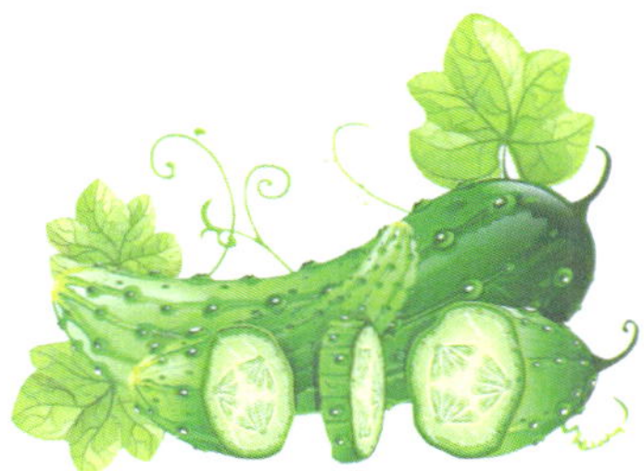

Il ustrator Yaroslav Borysovych, Dreamstime

Step 3) Prepare the garden bed

Soil preparation

- start with native soil and amend it with quality cured compost
- supplement amendments in layers

Amendments to consider:

green manure (cover crop planted before the growing season), animal manure, fish meal, seaweed, compost and compost teas, rock powder, and woody plant material (chipped branches)

Seed Catalogs

Seed catalogs (in-hand or online) provide descriptions of different varieties of plant foods; their qualities, such as whether they are better eaten fresh or used for cooking; growing requirements; and other resources.

Watering and Harvesting

Step 4) Water the garden daily and monitor the soil health and plants' readiness for harvest

- consider mulch to hold in moisture and suppress weeds
- if see signs of distress, the soil may need attention (aeration or more amendments) – refer to gardening resources
- if pests arrive, they may need to be removed or deterred; and there may be a need to attract pollinators
- research beneficial species for the bioregion

Step 5) Harvest through the season, cutting outer leaves or ripe fruits or vegetables and leaving the rest to grow. As needed, plant more seeds or seedlings

Once organic matter decays, it turns into humus–fertile, nutrient-rich, moist, productive soil. Compost (food scrapes); vegetation, wood (dead branches), rock powder, manure, seaweed, and fish meal are potential sources to develop humus in the topsoil. Rotating the planting of different food plants each season or year naturally returns nutrients to the soil that had been taken up by the plants previously. Alfalfa, rye grass, and other deep-rooted plants bring up minerals to the topsoil. Organic mulches can be shredded and layered over soil, such as *brassica* species, clover, and/or vetch; they will then inhibit unwanted plants from coming up, allow the desired food plants to grow through. As the mulch breaks down, it turns into soil.

Ollas

Ollas, porous pots made of baked clay, are used for watering especially in arid climates. They have been used as an ancient water method throughout Asia, Africa, and the Americas. They are filled with water with the drain hole sealed if necessary. Placed beneath the soil, the water inside slowly seeps out into the surrounding soil, watering the plants nearby.

Composting – Creating Fertile Soil with the Decomposition of Organic Matter

During meal prep, collect unwanted food trimmings

Step 1) in kitchen, place in a container with a lid and take outside to compost bin at least every other day

Outside, 2 compost bins or piles

Step 2) Build your compost with in the 1st bin with **BROWNS** and **GREENS** until full. Then, let cure/decompose. While 1st bin cures, start building compost in the 2nd bin.

- bins should have air space, such as between boards of wood
- ideal bin size is ~one meter (3.3 feet) by ~one meter (3.3 feet)[68]
- connect to natural soil on the ground with a bin open at the bottom or add a layer of soil with soil micro-organisms to the bottom of a bin[68]

Compost during the 'curing' process, transforming into soil

- compost warms as the micro-organisms metabolize (break down) the organic matter. For soil health, inhabited by probiotic soil organisms, and for adequate break down of the compost into humus (fertile soil), the temperature should reach 130° F (54° C) to 160° F (71° C); steam may be visible rising from the compost as it cures. In the center of the compost, place a compost thermometer to read the temperature.[68]

Compost turns into soil

- in ~12 weeks, the temperature cools and the compost should have turned into rich, dark soil with a healthy, earthy scent
- ready to use as soil amendments in garden beds, window boxes, and flower and herb pots[68]

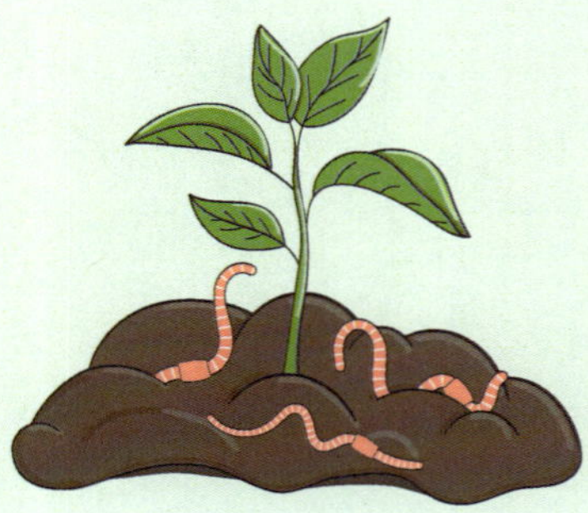

Healthy plants, like people, have their own natural resistance to pathogens (malnourished and stressed plants are the ones that become susceptible to disease). When wildlife come to feed on healthy plants, exclusion structures may be useful or vacuum collection of insects. Pest-repelling herbs, such as thyme, oregano, and rosemary can be planted around vegetables or fruit trees and be harvested as fresh-cut herbs.

Backyard Composting – Layer Browns and Greens

PROVIDE ACCESS TO AIR; CHECK NATURAL MOISTURE CONTENT[70]

- alternate brown and green layers (brown always on top, and overall add 3x as much brown material than green)
- add food from kitchen to the center of the pile
- while curing/decomposing (naturally heating up), turn compost with shovel or pitch fork (once per week, or at least once every other week)[70]
- check compost moisture – compost should feel damp
- at this point, compost is ready to use

Browns (carbon)	Greens (nitrogen)
fireplace wood and tree branches	shrub trimmings
wood chips	spring and summer leaves
autumn leaves	vegetables, leafy greens, tea bags
hay, straw	hair and fur
nut shells	algae (kelp or other seaweeds)
egg shells	manure – chicken, cow, horse

Pastureland is often integral to the organic, regenerative farm ecosystem. Grazing and foraging animals aid in water percolation, aerate the soil, and add nutrients back to the land through manure. As they walk, they naturally work decaying plant matter and seeds into the earth. Consuming the tender tops of plants, grazing and foraging animals activate new healthy plant growth, making the pasture more productive. Chickens, guinea hens, and quail, foraging for sprouting seeds, tender shoots, and leaves, and may consume unwanted pest insects.

Saving Seeds and Nurturing Flowering Plants and Pollinators

Allowing food plants to go to seed (bolt) on a farm or in a garden is 'seed-saving.' Each new generation of seeds changes a little through the process of evolution, creating new varieties. This naturally produces genetically diverse, open pollinating seeds that are adapted to local conditions. Organic and regenerative gardeners and farmers save and plant the seeds of natural foods that are valued for their flavor, color, and other traits. Sharing food plant seeds with the community is an excellent way to create heirloom varieties. Additionally, when plants go to seed they provide food for pollinators. Drying in the sun, plants left in place through the non-growing seasons may also furnish nest sites for small pollinators, such as: bees, butterflies, moths, and beetles. Bird and bat pollinators may inhabit standing dead trees (snags) in the area while reptile and mammal pollinators may live in the nearby meadows, woodlands, and forests.

Bats are especially farm-friendly pollinators. Being of the *Chiroptera* order (meaning 'hand' and 'wing'); they use their thumb on their wings for climbing and eating. Bats are nocturnal and some species fly one-half to two miles (8,000 acres/3,240 hectors) in search of food each night.[71] A colony of anywhere between 80 to 800 forest bats can live under the bark and in the crevices of one standing dead tree. In one summer, big brown bats may consume up to 18 million or more potentially unwanted root worms; and a nursing little brown bat may eat more than 4,500 insects each night, including mosquitoes.[69]

'Organic, Regenerative Gardening Based on Micro-Climates'

'Agriscaping – Elegant Edible Landscaping'

"Agriscaping's mission is to improve local food access & sustainability by transforming landscapes into elegant, edible food gardens easily managed with the help of online tools, education and professional support."[70]

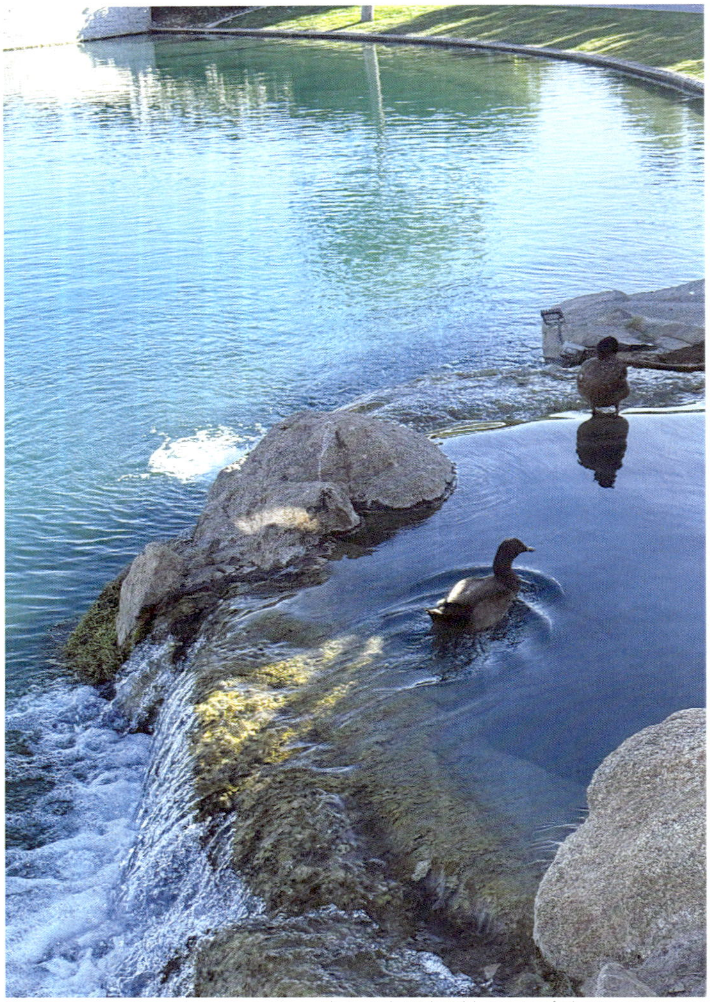

Photographer Juli Walsh, Director of Education, Agriscaping

Agriscaping

The term agriscaping is the act of creating elegant, productive, and sustainable landscapes for the betterment of health and humanity.

Regenerative Irrigation System

Agriscaping specialists put in place an irrigation system for Pecan Lake at the Queen Creek Botanical Gardens; wherein, they cultivate 'living water' with the organic debris from the fish and other aquatic organisms in the lake–circulating it through the botanical gardens and surrounding landscapes.

Water flows in and out of Pecan Lake at the Queen Creek Botanical Gardens

<u>Apply aesthetic, health-giving, and ecological principles</u>

1) Educate people on the science and art of agriscaping, principles and practices
2) Assess the productive capacity of landscapes and the needs and wishes of those who live there, which includes a Water-Harvesting Assessment of available rainwater and greywater resources
3) Create a Custom Micro-Climate Zone map to identify the prime growing locations for desired foods and medicinal plants–special processing is used to obtain the medicinal properties
4) Complete Edible Planting Charts to align optimal plants for each zone
5) Design a beautifully-integrated landscape for ease of implementation and maintenance
6) Cultivate healthy, organic soil structure with supporting regenerative irrigation systems that produce nourishing fresh natural foods for families and communities

Increase the growing capacity of landscapes by establishing new micro-climates

- construct additional micro-climates (micro-habitats), for example, by excavating the earth to develop open-air, subterranean gardens and walipini (earth-sheltered structures for growing plants)
- terrace hillsides
- put in shade structures, such as tree canopies
- devise trellises, for instance, making use of existing fences
- build wall gardens, some with shelves–each level providing a different micro-climate

Companion planting and pruning for plant health and creating beautiful floral patterns

- place plants next to each other that offer harmonious color combinations and that complement by adding mutually beneficial nutrients to the soil and/or release scents that avert common pests
- prune bushes, such as rosemary and myrtle berry, into hedges for attractive landscaping and use the edible trimmings (the top tier in freshness and quality) for making fresh (raw) and cooked meals, fodder for animals, and the remaining for compost.

Edible Mature Plants Can Be Especially Rich in Nutrients

Intentionally letting plants fully mature allows for more nutrient-rich and tender leaves, stems, buds, flowers, and seeds. Along their journey to maturity, plants support an abundant array of pollinators, develop soil structure, and furnish nutrient-dense natural foods that taste as good as they look.

Photography by Amy J. Wing

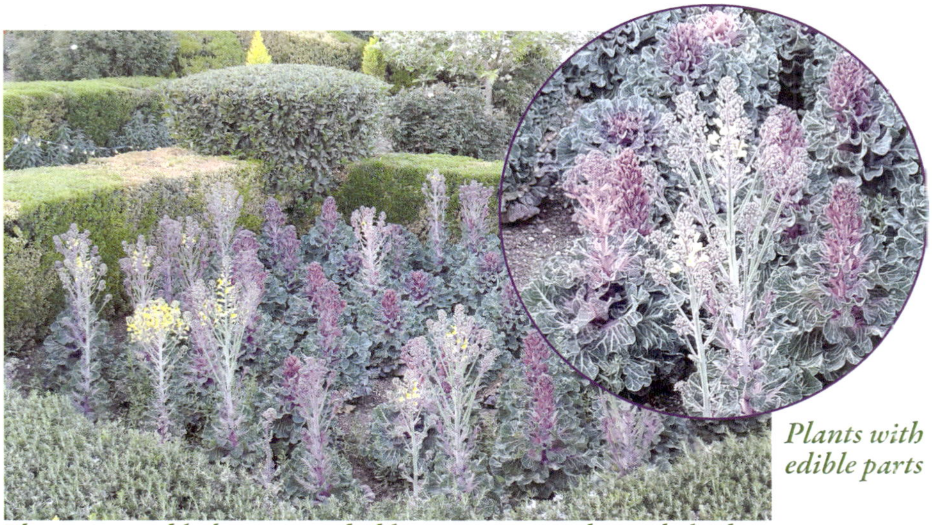

Plants with edible parts

Flowering red kale surrounded by rosemary and myrtle hedges

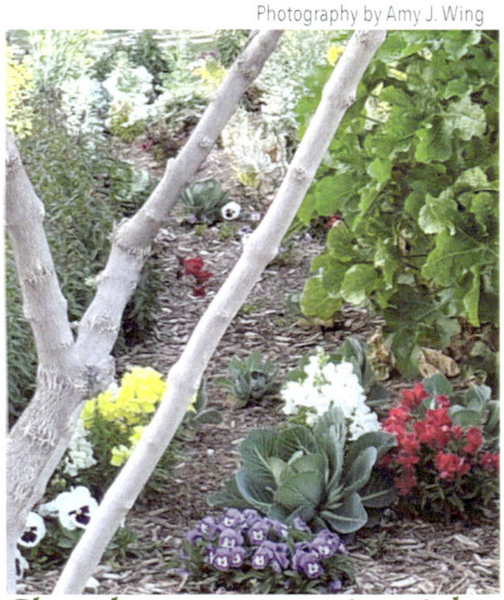

Chasteberry tree, pansies, violas, cabbage, and snap dragons

Water wheel used to shell pecans, chasteberry in bloom hollyhock–completely edible (roots, leaves, flowers, and seeds)

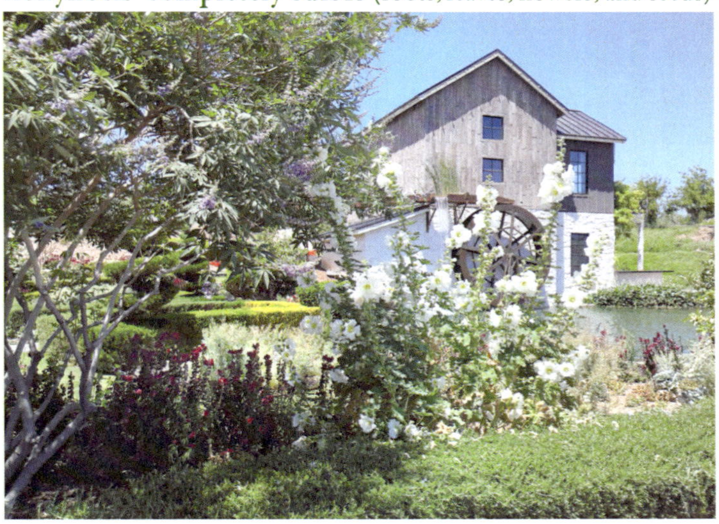

Flowering white kale and snap dragons

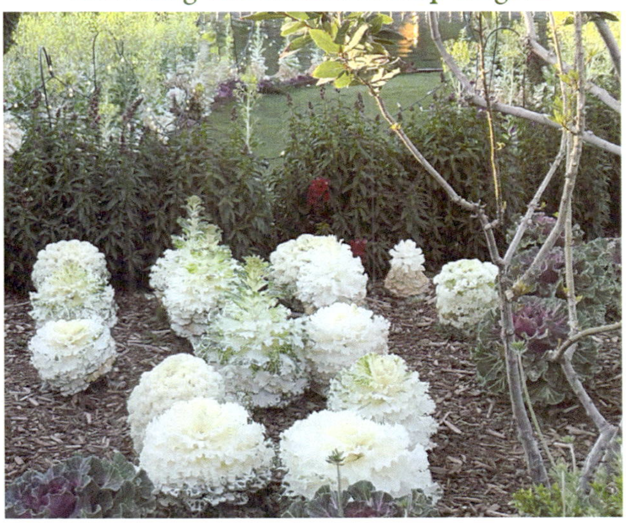

Harvesting Wild Foods from Nature

Wild foods were traditionally harvested in pristine ecosystems–fishing, hunting, foraging, and gathering. Across the Earth's grasslands and savannahs, pastoralists migrated with water buffalo, antelope, camels, reindeer, sheep, goats, cows, and other grazing animals, obtaining meat and milk. In terrestrial environments, edible plants and mushrooms were harvested. And various kinds of edible algae were gathered along the coasts of the continents.

Wild Foods that Nourish Humans and Other Animals in a Northern Hardwood Forest

In the northern hardwood forests of North America, some of the predominant native trees are: sugar maple (*Acer saccharum*), beech (*Fagus grandifolia*), and yellow birch (*Betula alleghaniensis*). Under the canopy of the large, deep-rooted sugar maple, one can often find wild ginger (*Asarum canadense*) and wood leeks (*Allium tricoccum*). Wild columbine (*Aquilegia canadensis*), with edible flowers, grows on the outer edge of the shade provided by the sugar maple and, on the sunnier side, blackberry bramble (*Rubus allegheniensis*).

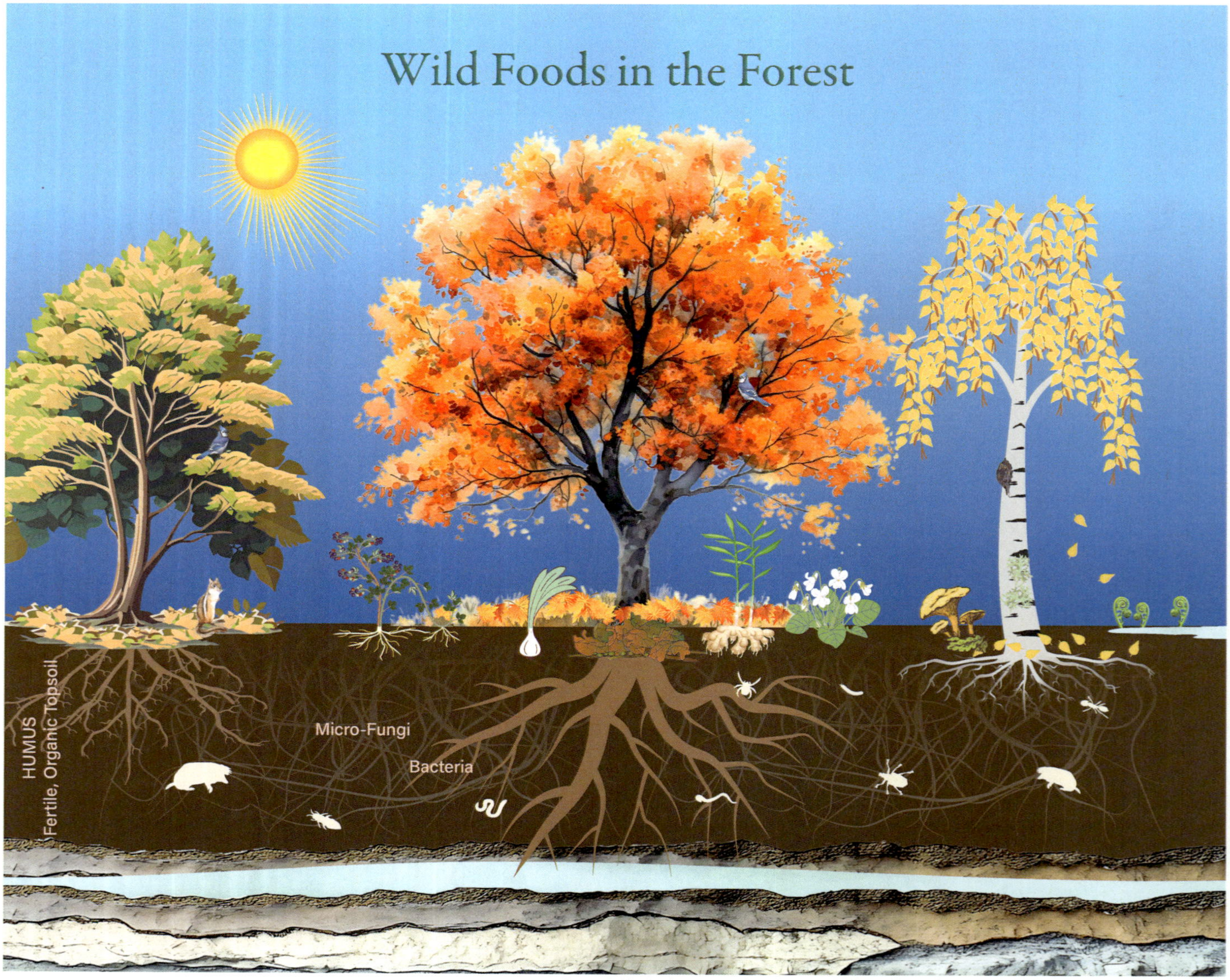

Composed by Sandra Jones, Eagle Lady Design Studio with Dreamstime images- credited in Acknowledgements

Beech tree nuts are a preferred food source by many species, including: black bear (*Ursus americanus*); red fox (*Vulpes vulpes*); raccoon (*Procyon lotor*), eastern chipmunk (*Tamias striatus*); and birds, including the blue jay (*Cyanocitta cristata*). More than one hundred species of caterpillars consume the nuts too, and seek refuge in the dry autumn leaves on the forest floor. The early hairstreak (*Erora laeta*) is a rare caterpillar entirely dependent on the nuts and leaves of the beech tree and beaked-hazel shrub (*Corylus cornuta*) for their sustenance. The birch tree is inhabited by wild chaga (*Inonotus obliquus*) and lichen (*Usnea species*) on the trunk and wild chanterelle mushrooms (*Cantharellus lateritius*) at the base. Fiddlehead ferns (*Matteuccia struthiopteris*) grow alongside the brooks and streams.

Falling leaves, twigs, and branches lying above the ground protect the soil structure that provides air space for the movement of soil life and the absorption and storage of water. Below ground, the micro-fungi and bacteria break down organic matter into rich, dark humus (fertile soil), releasing nutrients that are taken up by plants, mushrooms, and animals into the broader food web.

Soil species include:

- *Protozoa* kingdom–*protozoa* (single-celled organisms) feed on micro-fungi and bacteria and also consume decaying organic matter
- *Animalia* kingdom
    - *Annelida* phylum – earthworms
    - *Arthropoda* phylum – arthropods (invertebrates with jointed legs), including: mites centipedes, millipedes, springtails, spiders, ground beetles, and ants
    - *Nematoda* phylum – nematodes (round worms)
    - *Chordata* phylum (*Mammalia* class) – moles and shrews

The nutrients that build human health can only be found in nature

Wild-harvested or cultivated in organic, regenerative gardens and farms

VIII. Weaving Together a Bright Future

Our Earth, Our Home

It took more than four billion years for organisms to develop the complex and interconnected ecosystems that comprise the Earth's biosphere. As conservation journalist Swati Thiyagarajan eloquently stated, ". . . it's an ancient biological system that sustains life."[71]

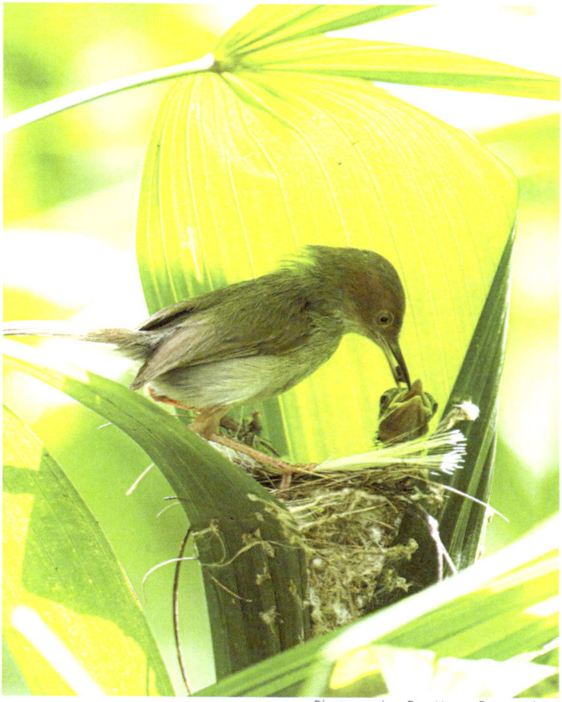

Photographer Duc Hong, Dreamstime

Protecting nature safeguards the continuity of life

Tailorbirds (***Orthotomus***)
Living in the Tropical Forests of Asia

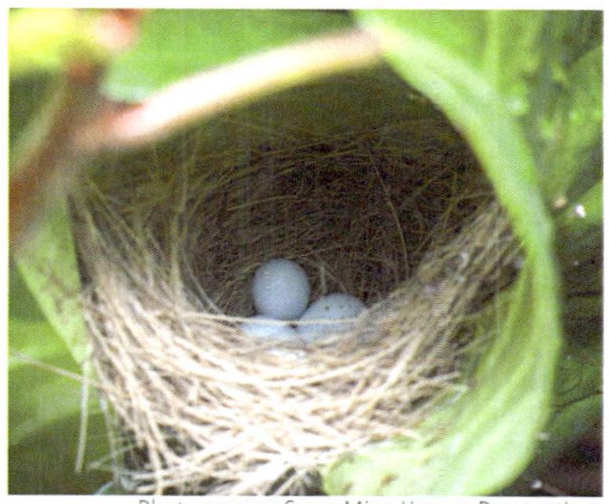

Photographer Swee Ming Young, Dreamstime

Resourcefully, a tailorbird sews together the sides of a broad, strong, and supple leaf to make a cradle for the nest. She wraps the leaf around herself to check its size. Then, she curls the leaf, twisting spider web strands around it. She makes tiny holes in the edges with her bill and, through the holes, laces plant fiber or silk from spider webs or caterpillar cocoons that her mate brings her. After sewing 150 to 200 stitches, she folds part of the leaf from above to make a roof. Afterward, her mate lines the cradle with soft material, such as grass, feathers, fur, and plant down to complete the nest.[72]

Ecological Mapping of the Earth Helps Us Understand and Conserve Nature

Landform, soil, water, climate, and biota of the interrelated ecosystems and bioregions of the coterminous United States are depicted on maps by the U. S. Geological Survey.[73,74]

References

[1]Lovelock, J. (1995). *The Ages of Gaia: A Biography of Our Living Earth* (p. x). New York, NY: W.W. Norton & Company, Inc.

[2, 3, 4]Hazen, R. M. (2005). *Genesis: The Scientific Quest for Life's Origins* (pp. 155, 21, 112–113). Washington, D.C.: Joseph Henry Press.

[5]Glasser, R. J. (1979). *The Body Is the Hero* (p. 15). New York, NY: Random House, Inc.

[6]Pollack, G. H. (2013). *The Fourth Phase of Water* (pp. 49–70). Seattle, WA: Ebner and Sons Publishers.

[7]USFWS. Coachella Valley National Wildlife Refuge – Our Species. U.S. Fish and Wildlife Service. Retrieved 11/24/2024: https://www.fws.gov/refuge/coachella-valley/species.

[8, 9]USFWS. (1984). *Coachella Valley Fringe-Toed Lizard Recovery Plan* (p. 10). Portland, OR: U.S. Fish and Wildlife Service.

[10]NPS. (2017, November 2). *Bison bellows: What's wallowing all about?* Fort Collins, Colorado: National Park Service. https://www.nps.gov/articles/bison-bellow-1-28-16.htm#:~:text=As%20bison%20roll%20and%20lay,vertebrates%20and%20invertebrates%20as%20well.

[11]Augustine, D., Davidson, A., Dickinson, K., & Van Pelt, B. (2019). Thinking like a grassland: challenges and opportunities for biodiversity conservation in the Great Plains of North America. *Rangeland Ecology & Management*. Retrieved from: https://www.sciencedirect.com/science/article/pii/S1550742419300697?via%3Dihub.

[12]Anderson, M. K. (1996). Tending the wilderness (p. 160). *Restoration & Management Notes.*

[13]Stewart, O. (Edited and with introductions by Henry T. Weis and M. Kat Anderson). (1908). *Forgotten Fires: Native Americans and the Transient Wilderness* (p. 3). (Editors Lewis, H. T., Anderson, M. K.). Norman, OK: University of Oklahoma Press.

[14]Anderson, M. K. (1996). Tending the wilderness (p. 156). *Restoration & Management Notes.*

[15]Eldredge, N. (1998). *Life in the Balance: Humanity and the Biodiversity Crisis* (p. XIII). Princeton, NJ: Princeton University Press.

[16]Species 2000, Integrated Taxonomic Information System, Global Biodiversity Information Facility, and the Alliance for Biodiversity Knowledge. (2020). *Catalogue of Life*. Virtual organization: Global Core Biodata Resource. https://www.catalogueoflife.org.

[17]Cooper, J. E. & Kuehne, R. A. (1974, June 13). *Speoplatyrhinus poulsoni*, A new genus and species of subterranean fish from Alabama. Copeia. 2, 486–493.

[18, 19, 20]Thompson, D. W. (1917). *On Growth and Form* (pp. 147, 206–214, 212). USA: CPSIA. www.ICGtesting.com.

[21]Eldridge, N. (1999). *The Pattern of Evolution* (pp. 80–81). New York, NY: Niles Eldridge.

[22]Gould, S. J. (1992, December). What is Species? (p. 41). Commentary. Discover.

[23]Brockman, J. (Editor and Publisher). (2023). *Conversation with Stephen Jay Gould; Chapter 2 The pattern of life's history.* (2023). Edge Foundation, Inc. https://www.edge.org/conversation/stephen_jay_gould-chapter-2-the-pattern-of-lifes-history.

[24]NAU. Biotic communities of the Colorado Plateau: C. Hart Merriam and the Life Zones Concept. Biota. (2001, August 8). Flagstaff, AZ: Northern Arizona University. https://nrm.dfg.ca.gov/FileHandler.ashx?DocumentID=7647.

[25]Lovette, I. (2018, December 20). *Why evolution goes wild on islands: The science of adaptive radiation.* Cornell Lab of Ornithology. Ithaca, NY: Cornell University. https://www.allaboutbirds.org/news/why-evolution-goes-wild-on-islands-the-science-of-adaptive-radiation.

[26]DLNR. (2024). *'I'iwi. Native Birds of Hawai'i.* Hilo, HI: Division of Forestry and Wildlife: Wildlife Program, Department of Land and Natural Resources, State of Hawaii. https://dlnr.hawaii.gov/wildlife/birds/iiwi.

[27]Chaparro-Pedraza, P. C., Roth, G., & Seehausen, O. (2022, April 25). The enrichment paradox in adaptive radiations: Emergence of predators hinders diversification in resource rich environments. *Journal of Ecological Letters.* (4):802–813. https://www.ncbi.nlm.nih.gov/pmc/articles/PMC9303570.

[28]Wardle, D. A. (Editors, Terborgh, J. & Estes, J. A). (2010). *Trophic Cascades: Predators, Prey, and the Changing Dynamics of Nature* (p. 203). Washington, D.C.: Island Press.

[29]Trappe, J. M. Molina, R., Luoma, D. L., Cázares, E., Pilz, D., Smith, J. E., Castellano, M. A., Miller, S. L., Trappe, M. J. (2009, April). *Diversity, ecology, and conservation of truffle fungi in forests of the Pacific Northwest* (pp. 1–15). Pacific Northwest Research Station, U.S. Forest Service, Department of Agriculture, General Technical Report PNW-GTR-772.

[30]VHS. (2024). *Northern dusky salamander (Desmognathus fuscus)*. Virginia Herpetological Society. https://www.virginiaherpetologicalsociety.com/amphibians/salamanders/northern-dusky-salamander/index.php.

[31]Nature and More. (2024, September). *A story of ants, bees, and orchids: the bucket orchids.* 582 Notes. https://libutron.tumblr.com/post/98322480262/a-story-of-ants-bees-and-orchids-the-bucket.

[32]Casey, D., Altman, B., Stringer, D., & Thomas, C. (2015). *Land managers' guide to cavity-nesting bird habitat and populations in ponderosa pine forests of the Pacific Northwest*. American Bird Conservancy. https://abcbirds.org/wp-content/uploads/2015/05/PonderosaPinebirdguide.pdf.

[33]Bourne, Jr. J. K. (2009, October). Forests in the air. National Geographic, p. 54–55. *Journal of the National Geographic Society. 216*(4).

[34]CPH. (2024, March 11). *Research reveals how to reinvigorate canopy biodiversity in regenerating redwood forests*. Humboldt Now. Arcata, CA: Cal Poly Humboldt. https://now.humboldt.edu/news/research-reveals-how-reinvigorate-canopy-biodiversity-regenerating-redwood-forests.

[35, 36, 37]Lovelock, J. (1995). *The Ages of Gaia: A Biography of Our Living Earth* (pp. 32, 11, 32). New York, NY: W.W. Norton & Company, Inc.

[38]Mayr, E. (2001). *What Evolution Is* (p. 42). New York, NY: Basic Books.

[39, 40, 41]Lovelock, J. (1995). *The Ages of Gaia: A Biography of Our Living Earth* (pp. 90, 117–118, 217). New York, NY: W.W. Norton & Company, Inc.

[42, 43, 44]Sheldrake, M. (2021). *Entangled Life* (p. 131, 123–124). New York, NY: Random House.

[45]Floris, P. & Haagen, F. V. (2017). Soil is a living organism: a short film on how to restore soil health (11:55 minutes). *Plant Health Cure*. Retrieved from: https://www.youtube.com/watch?v=8ugaL6wsXME.

[46]Martens, M. R. (2000). *The soil food web: a world beneath our feet*. Acres U.S.A. Magazine, https://www.ecofarmingdaily.com/build-soil/soil-life/soil-microbes/soil-food-web.

[47]Wilson, E. O. (1987, December). The little things that run the world (pp. 344–346). *Journal of Conservation Biology.1*(4).

[48]Cintrón-Molero, G. (2012, August 22). Personal communication, International Affairs, U.S. Fish and Wildlife Service.

[49]Wilson, E. O. (1999). *The Diversity of Life* (p. 20). New York, NY: W. W. Norton & Company.

[50]Kurtz, A. C., Derry, L. A., & Chadwick, O. A. (2001, January 25). Accretion of Asian dust to Hawaiian soils: Isotopic, elemental, and mineral mass balances (p. 1971). *Geochimica et Cosmochimica Acta, 65*(12). http://www.geo.cornell.edu/eas/PeoplePlaces/Faculty/derry-new/publications/1-s20-s0016703701005750.pdf.

[51]Washington, R., Bouet, C., Cautenet, G., & Tegen, I. (2009, December 8). Dust as a tipping element: The Bodélé Depression, Chad. *Proceedings of the National Academy of Sciences. 106*(49), 20564–20571.

[52]Noss, F. R., LaRoe, E. T., & Scott, J. M. (1995, January). *Endangered eco-systems of the United States: A preliminary assessment of loss and degradation.* 266 Publications. https://www.researchgate.net/publication/246063035_Endangered_eco-systems_of_the_United_States_A_preliminary_assessment_of_loss_and_degradation.

[53]Cintrón-Molero, G. (2015, June 11) Personal communication, International Affairs, U.S. Fish and Wildlife Service.

[54, 55]Lovelock, J. (1995). *The Ages of Gaia: A Biography of Our Living Earth* (pp. 72, 226). New York, NY: W.W. Norton & Company, Inc.

[56]Dowser, T., Waldman, S. P., Voorhis, C., & Fishing 4, Greater Yellowstone Coalition, and Roadtrippers (2022). *The trophic cascade: How wolves change rivers* [Film]. Westcliffe, CO: Mission Wolf. https://missionwolf.org/trophic-cascade.

[57]Wilson, E. O. (2000, Spring). Special Issue: The Wildlands Project (p. 1–2). *WildEarth.10*(1).

[58]Monarch Watch. *Monarch Waystation Program*. Retrieved 11/24/2024: https://www.monarchwatch.org/waystations.

[59]CFN. Our Great Bear Sea: *A historic agreement, Coastal First Nations – Sea Legacy* [Film]. Retrieved 11/24/2024: https://ourgreatbearsea.ca/pfp-closing.

[60]FWCF. *About the corridor*. St. Petersburg, FL: Florida Wildlife Corridor Foundation. Retrieved 11/24/2024: https://floridawildlifecorridor.org/about/about-the-corridor.

[61]NWC. *Necanicum Plan*. Seaside, OR: Necanicum Watershed Council. Retrieved 11/24/2024: https://www.necanicumwatershed.org/our-watershed.

[62]NCLC. (2014, September). *Necanicum Wildlife Corridor Conservation Plan*. Seaside, OR: North Coast Land Conservancy. https://nclctrust.org/wp-content/uploads/2024/03/NecanicumPlan_1-16-15.pdf.

[63]LRP. (2025). Lomakatsi Restoration Project. https://lomakatsi.org.

[64]USFWS. *Oak Habitat Restoration, Oregon* [Film]. U.S. Fish and Wildlife Service. https://youtu.be/nAsHfTdERDc.

[65]Minard, A. (2010, June 4). *Dams cutting off 400 million people from food and income*. National Geographic. https://www.nationalgeographic.com/science/article/100604-dams-economic-impact.

[66]ARA. (2024). Dams. Alabama Rivers Alliance. https://alabamarivers.org/dams.

[67]Price, W. A. (2019). *Nutrition and Physical Degeneration* (p. 414). (8th ed.). Lemon Grove, CA: Price-Pottenger.

[68]SCDHEC. *Composting: recycling naturally – simple steps for starting at home*. South Carolina Department of Environmental Services. Retrieved January 7, 2025: https://scdhec.gov/sites/default/files/Library/OR-1705.pdf.

[69]USFS. (2002, December). *Bats and Dead Trees* [Brochure]. Kaibab National Forest, Williams, AZ: U.S. Forest Service.

[70]Agriscaping (2025). http://www.Agriscaping.com.

[71]Sanctuary Nature Foundation. (2020, June). Meet Swati Thiyagarajan. *Sanctuary Asia*. *40*(6). https://sanctuarynaturefoundation.org/article/meet-swati-thiyagarajan.

[72]Begum, T. *Tailorbirds: The little birds that stitch their nests*. London: Natural History Museum. Retrieved 11/24/2024: https://www.nhm.ac.uk/discover/the-bird-that-stitches-its-home.html.

[73]Sayre, R., Comer, P., Warner, H., & Cress, J. (2009). *A New Map of Standardized Terrestrial Ecosystems of the Conterminous United States*. Professional Paper 1768. U.S. Department of the Interior, U. S. Geological Survey.

[74]Cress, J. J. & Sayre, R. (2017, July 14). *Global Terrestrial Ecosystems*. U.S. Department of the Interior, U. S. Geological Survey. https://www.usgs.gov/centers/geosciences-and-environmental-change-science-center/science/global-ecosystems.

PART IV
Nutrient Library

Examples: natural foods, their nutrients and health benefits

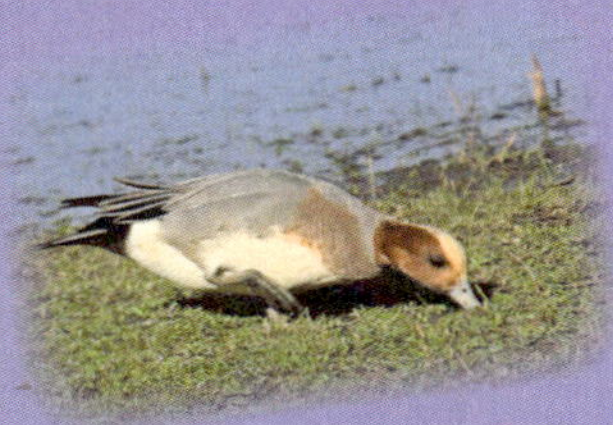
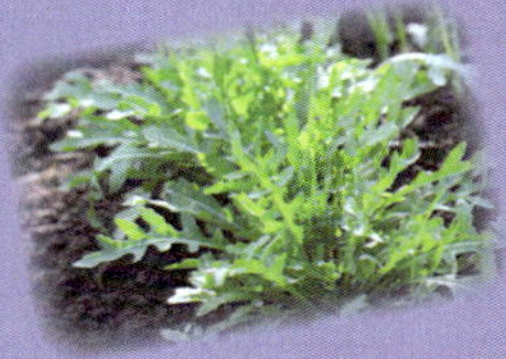
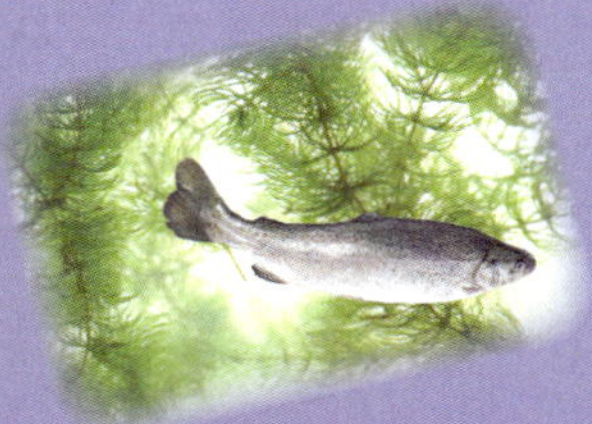
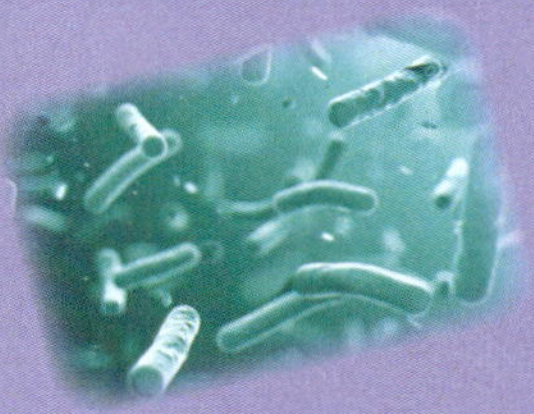
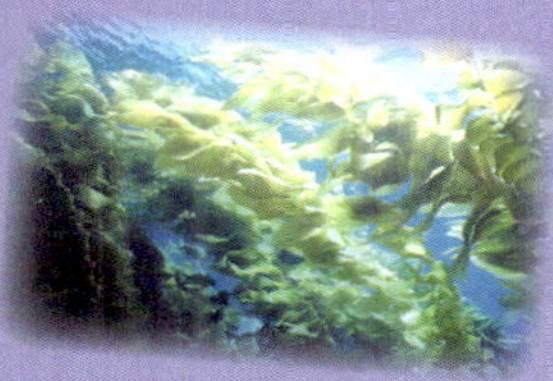
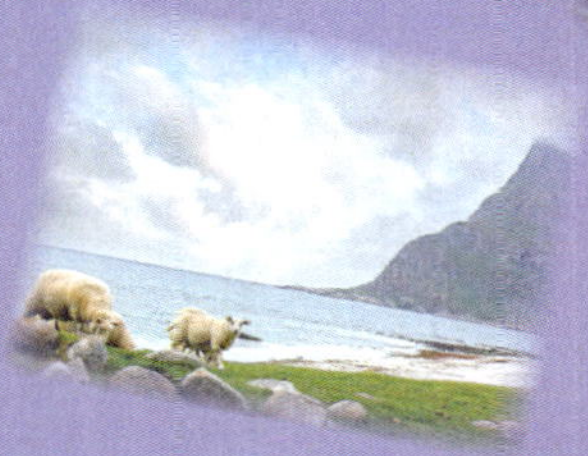
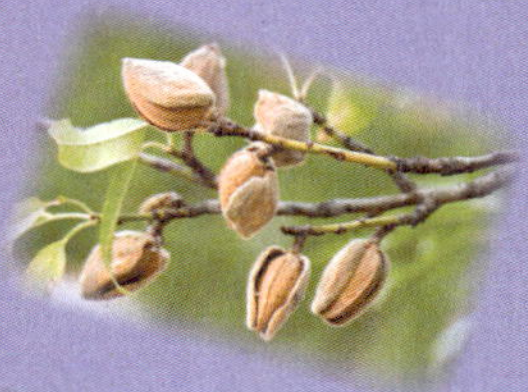
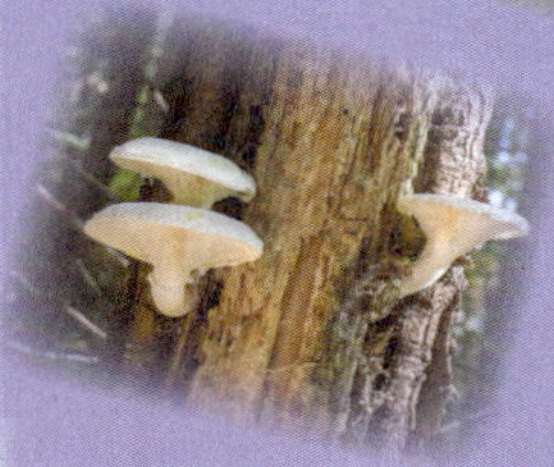

Five Kingdoms of Life

Animal Foods
Animalia Kingdom

Plant Foods
Plantae Kingdom

Mushrooms
Fungi Kingdom (Macro-Fungi)

Algae Foods
Plantae Kingdom (Green & Red Algae Foods)
Chromista Kingdom (Brown Algae Foods)

Probiotics
Bacillati Kingdom (Bacteria)
Fungi Kingdom (Micro-Fungi)

Across All the Kingdoms

Macro Nutrients

Protein

Lipids

Carbohydrates

Micro Nutrients

Vitamins

Enzymes

Vital Molecules

Minerals

Animal Food Nutrients

KINGDOM: *ANIMALIA* | **NUTRIENTS** | **HEALTH BENEFITS**

Animal foods are the best or only sources of these nutrients, in the most bioavailable form, and present in essential quantities (pages 1, 2, 3 of this chart)

Seafoods

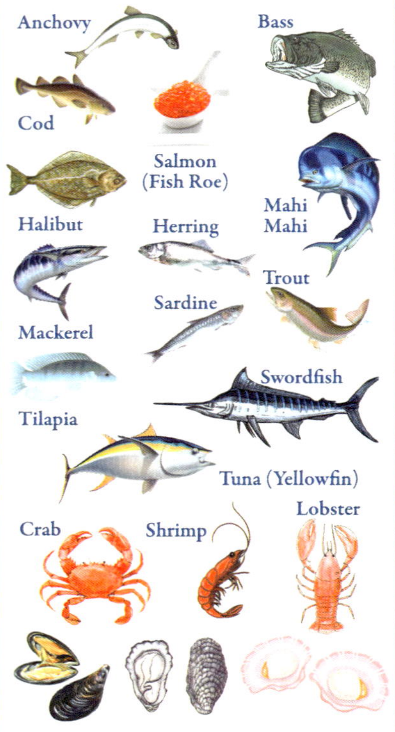

Meats

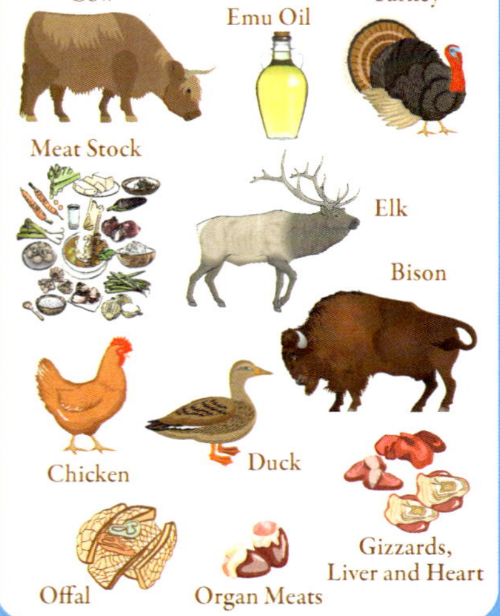

Eggs

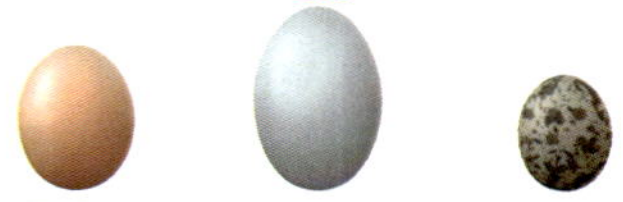

Nutrients	Health Benefits
Docosahexaenoic acid (DHA) *Animal foods are a direct source of DHA. Less efficiently, plant sources must be converted from alpha-linolenic acid (ALA) to DHA*[1]	Essential for cognitive, neurological, and cardiovascular health
Conjugated linoleic acid (CLA)	Protects against atherosclerosis and osteoporosis; anti-tumor
Arachidonic acid (AA) *Animal foods are a direct source of DHA. Less efficiently, plant sources must be converted from alpha-linolenic acid (ALA) to DHA*[1]	Provides structure to cell membranes and protects the intestinal lining; critical to initiating and resolving inflammation
Saturated animal fats *Only present in animal foods*	Needed for digesting, absorbing, and assimilating protein,[2] minerals, and the fat-soluble vitamins A, D_2, D_3, E, K_1, K_2; anti-microbial; and supports brain function[3]
Cholesterol *Only present in animal foods*	Integral to neuron synapses, supports the nervous system, precursor of all hormones and bile, protects the intestinal wall and arteries
Fat-soluble vitamin A *Although less efficient, the body can make vitamin A using enzyme reserves and carotenes from non-animal foods* *Vitamin A retinol and retinyl esters only present in animal foods*	Required for healthy bones, skin, vision, hearing, and fighting infections; supports the thyroid and heart health; and needed for assimilating protien, minerals, and water-soluble vitamins[4]
Fat-soluble vitamin D_3 *When the skin absorbs UV B sunlight, 7-dehydrocholesterol converts it into vitamin D_3, with vitamin A playing a critical role* *Only present in animal foods, mushrooms growing in sunlight, and algae*	Activates the absorption of calcium and phosphorus in the process of bone regeneration
Fat-soluble vitamin K_2 *All forms of vitamin K_2 are produced by probiotic bacteria except K_2 MK-4, which is especially nourishing and comes from animal sources.* *K_2 MK-4 is abundant in emu oil, poultry liver, and egg yolk (ref. bottom of page 12)*	Supports energy production, the integrity of the skin, and bone development and repair; neuro-protective; and protects against calcification of the arteries[5]
Water-soluble vitamin B_{12} *Comprised of co-enzymes methyl cobalamin and adenosyl cobalamin, which are produced by probiotic bacteria in ruminant animals* *Only present in animal foods*	Required for producing red blood cells; with folate, manufactures DNA Adenosyl cobalamin protects mitochondria and the myelin sheath surrounding nerve cells
Complete protein, with easily absorbable essential amino acids *The fat-soluble vitamins present in animal fats aid in assimilating protein*[2] *Only present in animal foods*	The body uses proteins and saturated fats to manufacture DNA and to produce and maintain cells, tissues, enzymes, hormones, and neurotransmitters
Heme iron *Only present in animal foods*	As a key component of the hemoglobin in red blood cells, heme iron carries oxygen from the lungs to all parts of the body

Continued...

Animal Food Nutrients

KINGDOM: *ANIMALIA*	NUTRIENTS	HEALTH BENEFITS
Bone Broth (with gelatin-rich cartilage) 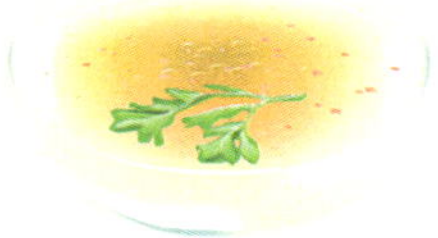 The gelatin in bone broth is a 'water-loving' (hydrophilic), colloidal substance that lubricates and soothes the intestinal lining and supports digestion. Seafood Bone Broth 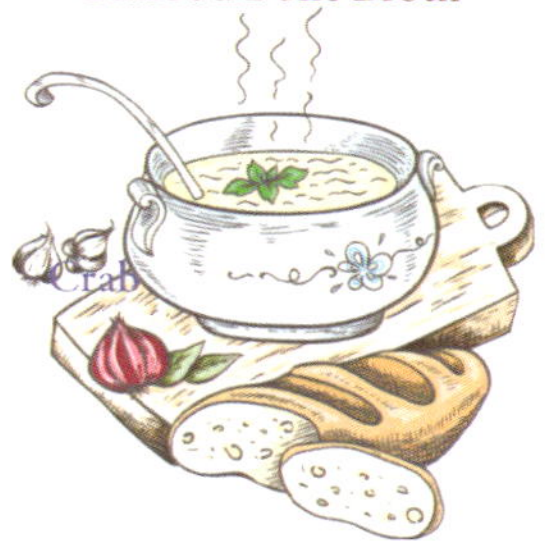	**Collagen** *Only found in animal foods*	Builds strong and flexible bones, cushions joints, maintains supple arteries and corneas, and reduces inflammation, and used by the body to restore connective tissue and heal wounds
	Hyaluronic acid *Only found in animal foods*	Nourishes cartilage as a constituent of synovial fluid, and lubricates joints
	Chondrocytes *Only found in animal foods*	Produces proteoglycans and collagenous fibers, regenerating cartilage
	Chondroitin and keratan sulfates *Only found in animal foods*	Hydrating by attracting and holding water (negatively charged)
	Glucosamine *Only found in animal foods*	Regenerates intervertebral discs and joints, repairs intestinal musca, and supports the immune system[7]
	Glycine, proline, glutamine, alanine *Amino acids also found in non-animal foods*	Needed for digestive health, and supports the immune system[7]
	Major Minerals *Calcium, chloride, magnesium, phosphorus, potassium, sodium, and sulfur*	Available in their "... ready-to-use ionized form as a true electrolyte solution ..."[8]
Bone Marrow *(soft, fatty tissue in bones, produces blood cells)* 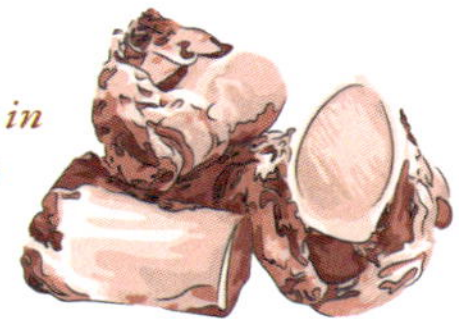	**Hematopoietic cells and marrow adipose** Differentiates and becomes connective tissue cells of any organ as needed	Produces new blood cells, increases the flow of oxygen in the blood, prevents infections, and neuro and cardioprotective
Seafood 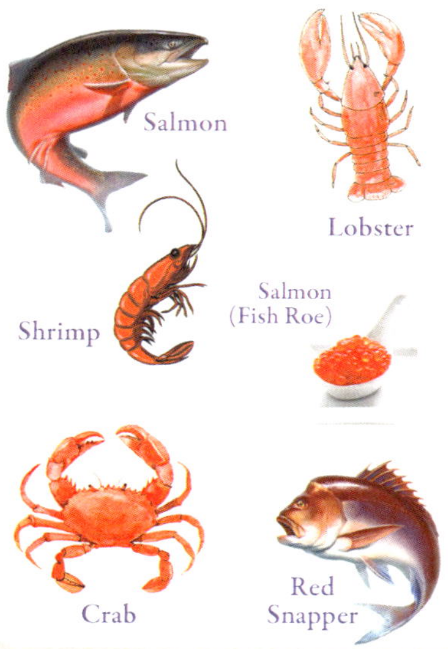	**Astaxanthin** *An orange-pigmented carotene in algae that is consumed by sea animals and accumulates up the food chain*	Anti-oxidant *(one of the most effective)*, boosts cognitive function, protects the heart, improves vision, and supports the immune system

Continued...

Animal Food Nutrients

KINGDOM: *ANIMALIA*

RAW WHOLE MILK PRODUCTS[6]

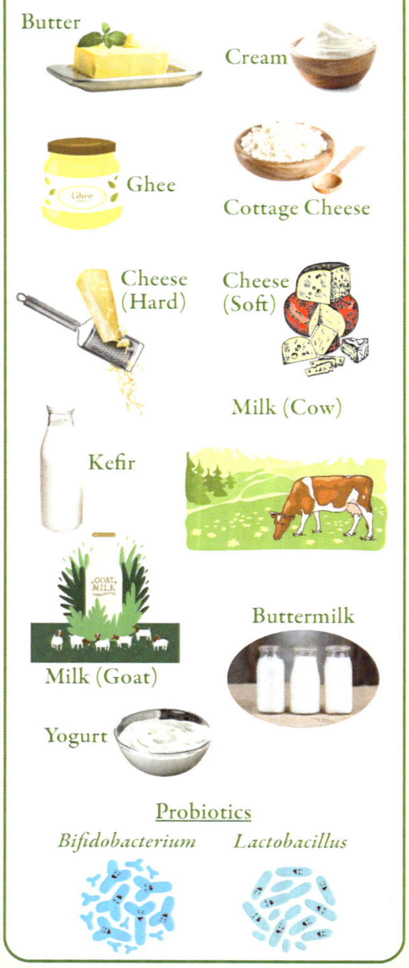

NUTRIENTS	HEALTH BENEFITS
Fat soluble vitamin K_2 *Known as activator X[3], produced by bacteria*	Mineralizes the teeth, destroys pathogens; reduces risk of cataracts; prevents calcification and stiffness in pineal gland, arteries, and joints
Glycosphingolipids	Supports digestion and guards against gastro-intestinal infection
Myristic acid	Used in the myristylation process of cell membranes and mitochondria which is important for kidney function[7] and cardiovascular health
Lactoferrin	Facilitates iron absorption, anti-inflammatory
B-lymphocytes and macrophages, lysozyme enzymes	Anti-microbial
Immunoglobulins, neutrophils, and lymphocytes	Builds and strengthens the immune system
Polysaccharides	Prebiotics that feed the microbiome
Oligosaccharides	Protects nutrients from being destroyed by stomach acids and the intestinal lining from pathogens
Phospholipids	Guards against absorption of pathogens or toxins
Hormones and growth factors	Stimulates the maturation of cells and prevents leaky gut
Mucins	Prevents pathogens from adhering to intestinal lining
Fibronectin	Repairs damaged tissues, anti-microbial
Lactobacilli, *Bifidum*, and other probiotics	Produces lactic acid, anti-microbial

RAW HONEY BEE PRODUCTS

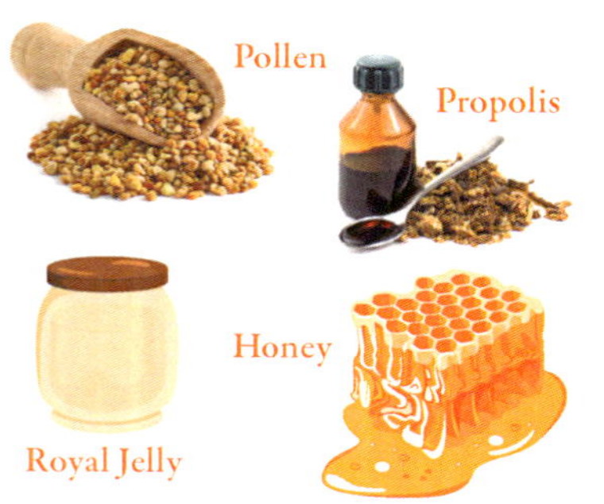

Not for infants until at least one year old. Many people are allergic to bee products.

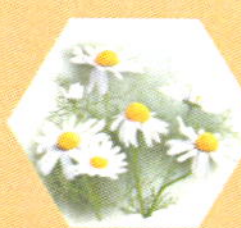

Floral origin phytonutrients in bee products: lycopene, resveratrol, ellagic acid, beta carotene, lutein, zeaxanthin, kaempferol, quercetin

NUTRIENTS	HEALTH BENEFITS
Nutrient dense; vitamin D metabolites	Increases nutrient absorption, improves cognition, supports bone health
Flavonoids and polyphenols	Enhances immunity, reduces allergies, reduces pain, wound healing
Apisimin and jelleine	Anti-bacterial, anti-fungal, anti-oxidant, strengthens the immune system
Phenolic compounds	Supports a health microbiome, anti-inflammatory, cardio-protective

References

[1, 5, 7]Fallon Morell, S. (2017). *Nourishing Fats* (pp. 93, 117, 173). New York, NY: Grand Central Life & Style.

[2, 3, 4, 8]Fallon Morell, S. (2001). *Nourishing Traditions* (pp. 29, 39, 37, 41). Washington, D.C.: NewTrends Publishing, Inc.

[6]A Campaign for Real Milk. (2015). *Pastured, unprocessed, full-fat real milk: Nature's perfect food* [Film]. Washington, D.C.: The Weston A. Price Foundation https://www.realmilk.com/audio-and-video.

Colorful and Protective Plant Nutrients

KINGDOM: *PLANTAE*		PHYTONUTRIENTS	HEALTH BENEFITS
 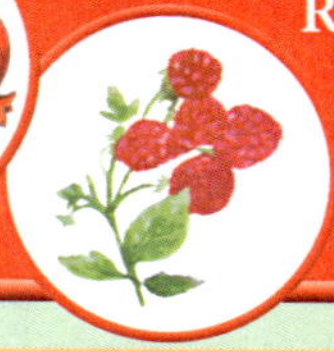	**RED** Pomegranate & raspberry	Ellagic acid Lycopene	Ellagic acid: anti-viral, anti-cancer, protects skin from UV exposure Lycopene: antioxidant, lowers blood pressure, supports vision, may help reduce pain
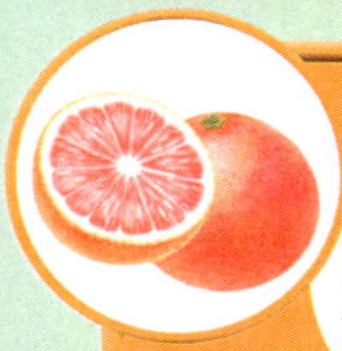 	**ORANGE** Grapefruit & peach	Beta carotene Flavonoids	Beta caratene: antioxidant, used by the body to make vitamin A Flavonoids: strengthens the immune system, blood vessels, and connective tissue
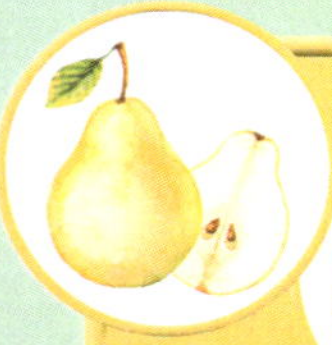 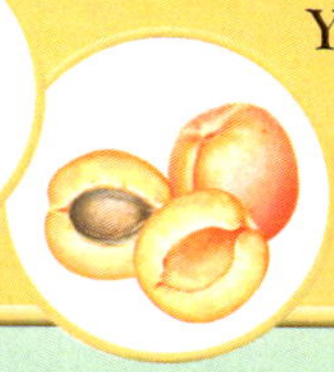	**YELLOW** Pear & apricot	Kaempferol Zeaxanthin	Kaempferol: anti-inflammatory, anti-cancer, and protects bone and nerve tissue Zeaxanthin: supports cognitive function and key to eye health, especially the macula and retina
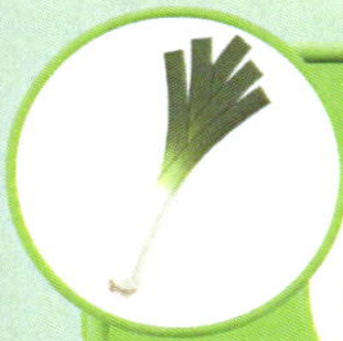 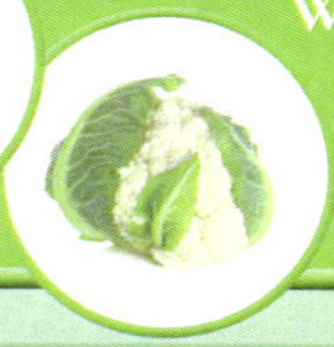	**WHITE & GREEN** Leek & cauliflower	Allyl sulfides Quercetin	Allyl sulfides: antibiotic, anti-viral, anti-fungal, anti-mutagenic, and helps the body detoxify Quercetin: anti-oxidant, anti-inflammatory, reduces blood pressure
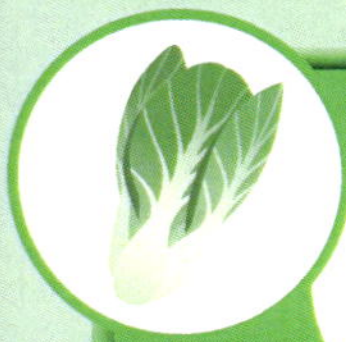 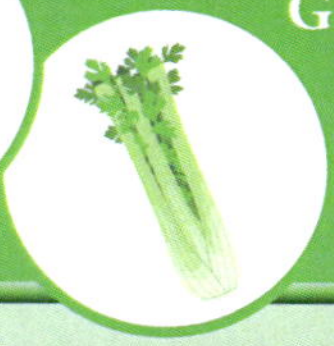	**GREEN & WHITE** Bok choy & celery	Indoles Lutein	Indole: anti-inflammatory, stimulates liver detoxification, protects against DNA damage Lutein: antioxidant, protects eyes and skin from UV light
 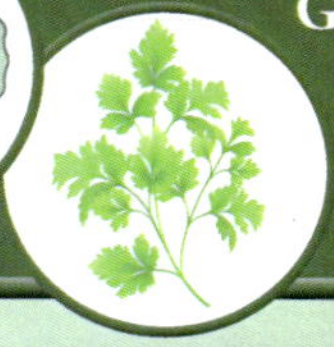	**GREEN** Green cabbage & parsley	Chlorophyll Folate	Chlorophyll: detoxifies and helps build red blood cells Folate: supports healthy cell growth and fetal development
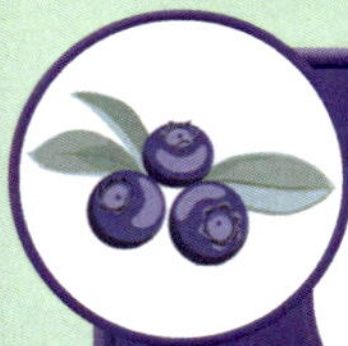 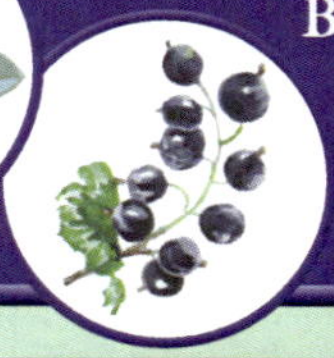	**BLUE & PURPLE** Blueberry & currant	Anthocyanins Pterostilbene	Anthocyanins: involved in the production of vitamin C, protects connective tissue Pterostilbene: anti-inflammatory, anti-tumor, anti-cancer
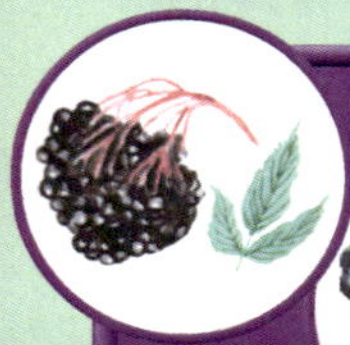 	**RED & PURPLE** Elderberry & blackberry	Resveratrol Betacyanin	Resveratrol: antioxidant; protects the cardiovascular system, brain, and nervous system Betacyanin: supports liver detoxification

Designers Cyd Ceres Card & Sandra L. Jones, Eagle Lady Design Studio

Five Example Plant Families

Natural foods that are closely related, such as in the same family, often have similar characteristics including nutrients and health effects.

Cruciferous *(Brassicaceae)*
Grass *(Poaceae)*
Nightshade *(Solanaceae)*
Onion *(Alliaceae)*
Rose *(Rosaceae)*

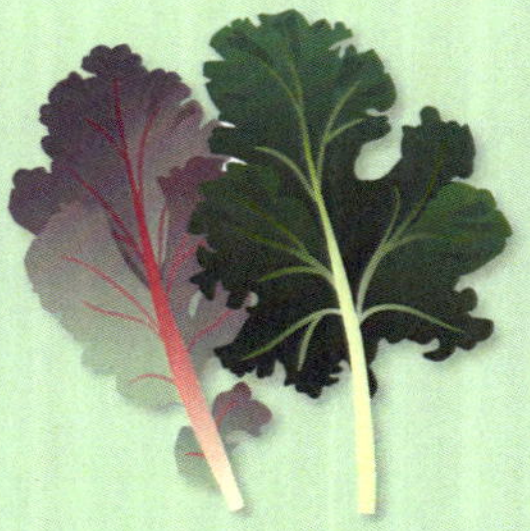

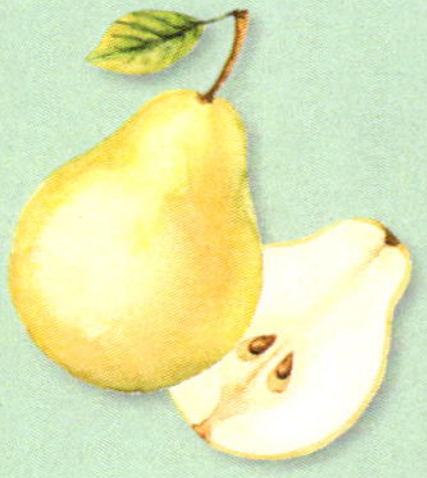

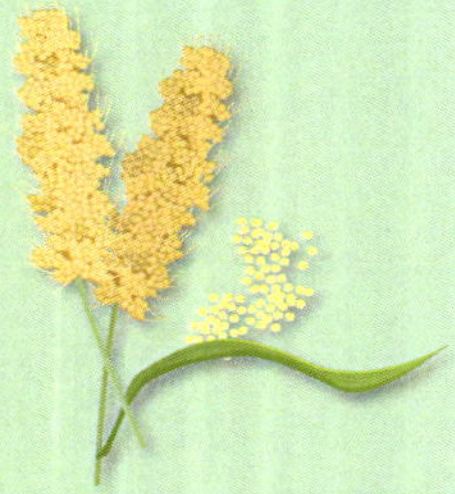

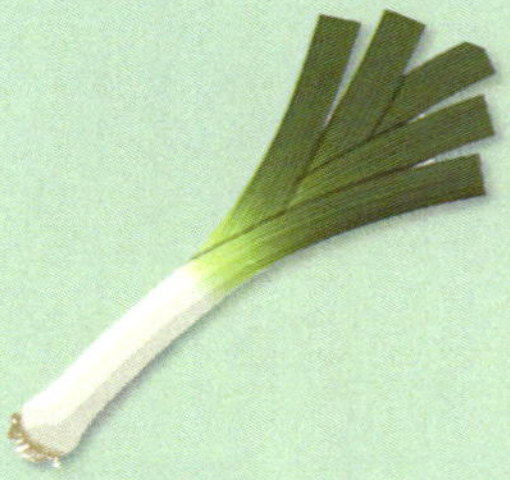

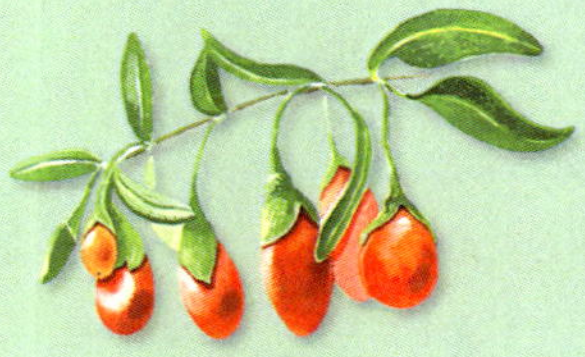

Cruciferous Family *Brassicaceae*

The *Brassicaceae* family of vegetables and leafy greens contains sulfur compounds, such as sulforaphane, indole, and-3-carbinal, that have anti-cancer properties. However, these foods also contain goitrogens, natural toxins that the plants use to defend themselves against insects and other predators. Goitrogens may block the absorption of iodine, an important mineral for the thyroid gland. Cooking *Brassicaceae* vegetables reduces this effect. Fifteen members of the *Brassicaceae* family are displayed below.

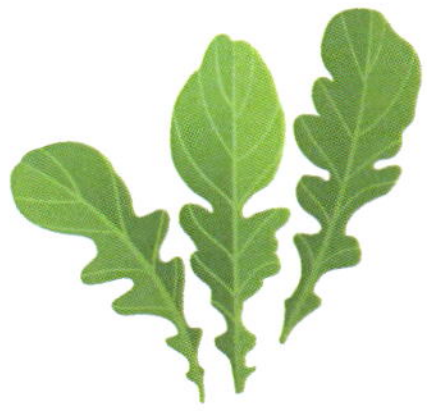
Arugula

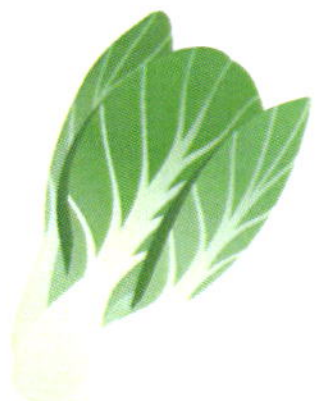
Bok Choy

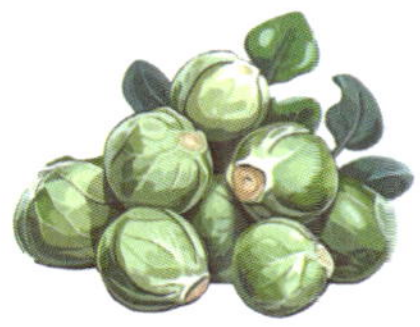
Brussels Sprouts

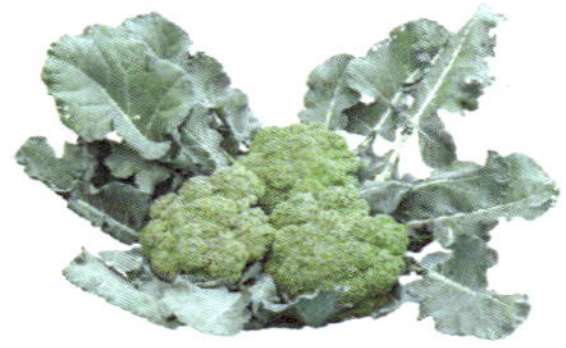
Broccoli

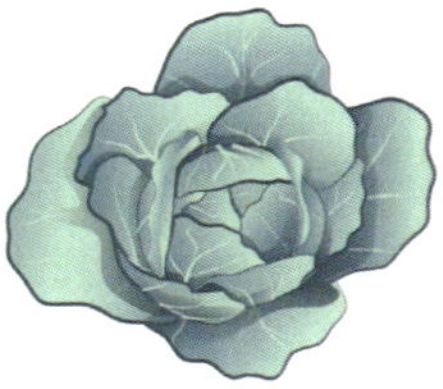
Cabbage (green)

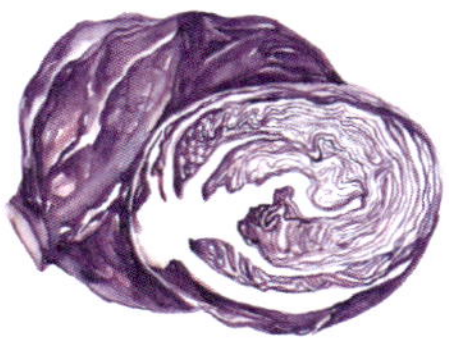
Cabbage (purple)

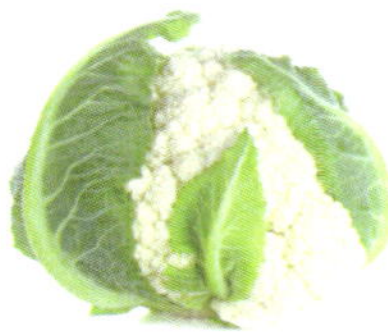
Cauliflower

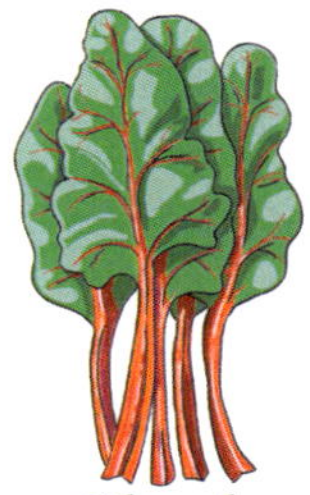
Chard

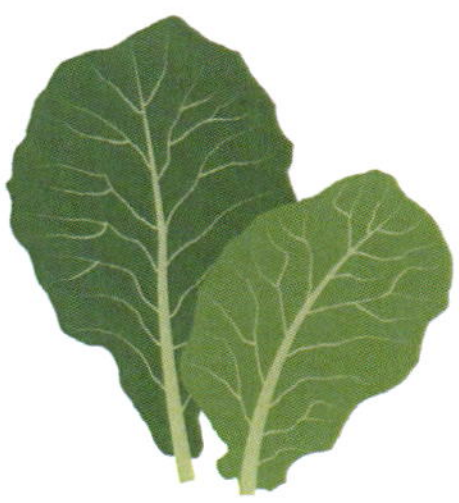
Collard Greens

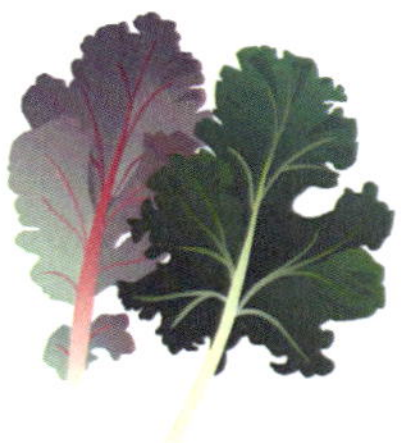
Kale

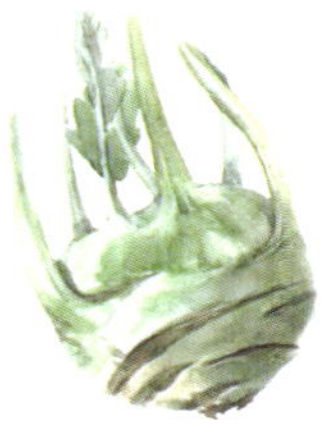
Kohlrabi

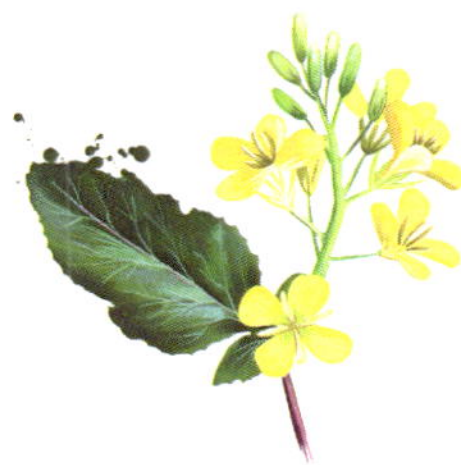
Mustard Greens

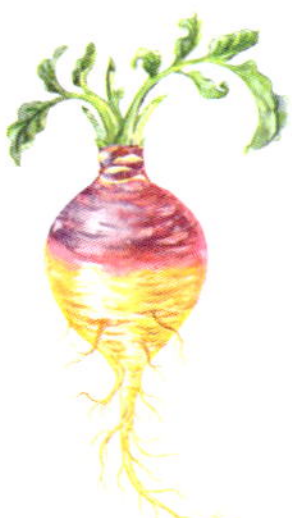
Rutabaga

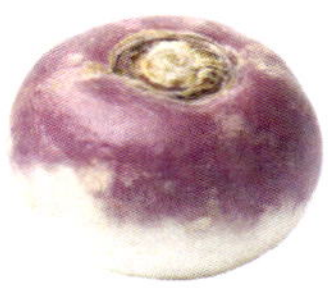
Turnip

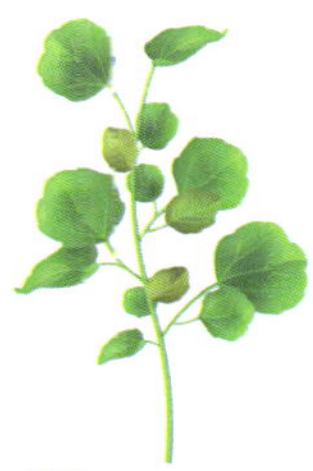
Watercress

Grass Family
Poaceae

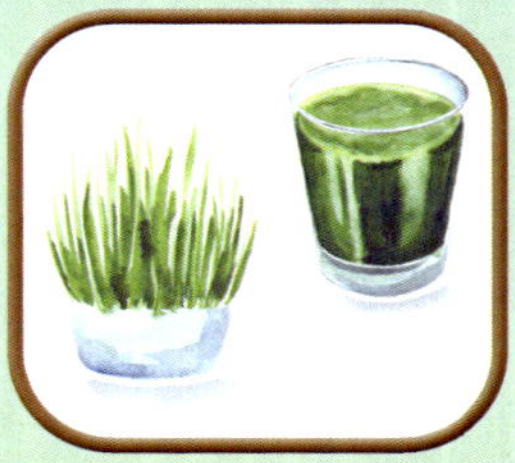

Leaves (Grass)

The thin leaves of edible *Poaceae* grasses, when freshly juiced (or milled, dried, or powdered), promote excellent health. Barley, oat, rye, and wheat grasses are an example. Their chlorophyll and enzymes detoxify and oxygenate the blood, improving cardiovascular, respiratory, and immune function. Juiced or milled, these raw grasses are strongly anti-cancer, anti-parasite, and anti-fungal.

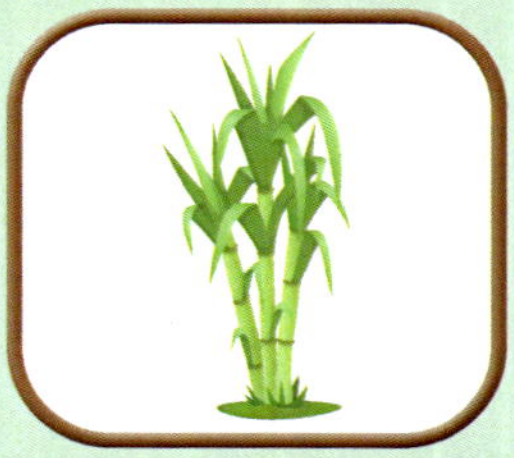

Stalk (Cane)

Molasses and sorgo grass juices extracted from the stalk (or cane) of sweet sorghum are high in anti-oxidants, minerals, and vitamins.

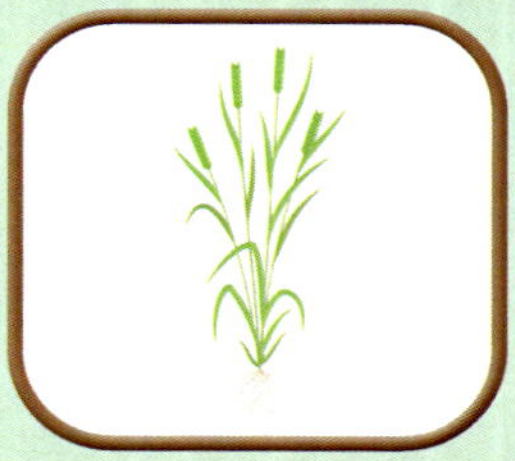

Seeds (Grains)

The edible seeds (grains) of the *Poaceae* plant family have three main parts:

- Germ – the seed's embryo, which germinates and sprouts into a new plant
  Protein, vitamin E; lecithin, folate and other B vitamins; phosphorus and magnesium
- Endosperm – the tissue that surrounds and nourishes the embryo during germination
  Carbohydrate polysaccharides, including hemicellulose and beta-glucan fiber, B vitamins, minerals
- Bran – the outer covering (coat) of the seed
  B vitamins, minerals, soluble (oat) and insoluble (rye) fiber that supports the microbiome and digestion

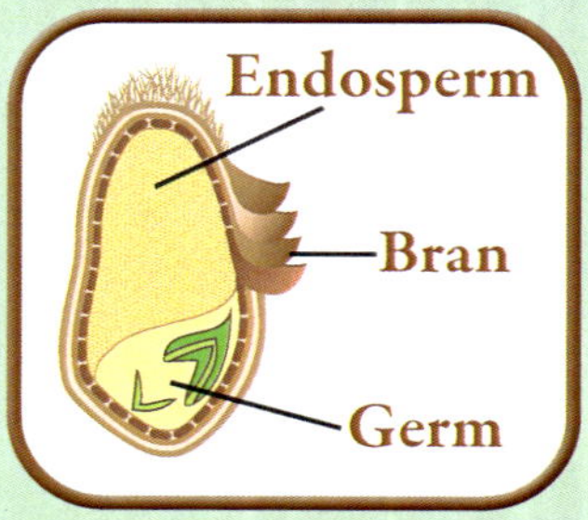

Traditionally, grains and other seeds were soaked, sprouted, and fermented. This initiates germination; whereupon, enzymes break down proteins into amino acids, lipids into fatty acids; and carbohydrates into simple sugars (making the nutrients available to the plant embryo). Preparing seeds this way significantly increases the digestibility and bioavailability of the nutrients. Ten members of the *Pinaceae* family are depicted below.

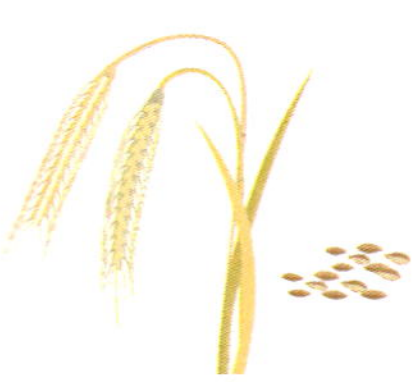
Barley

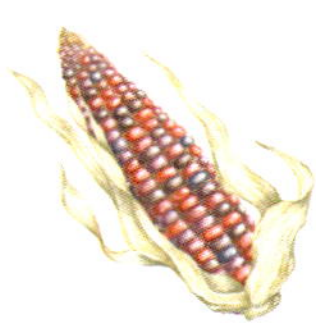
Maize/Corn

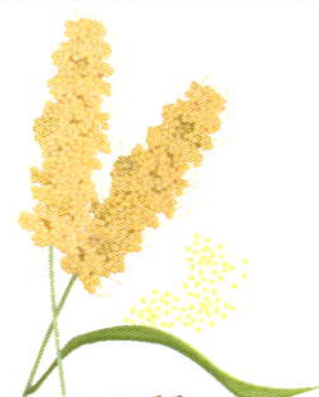
Millet

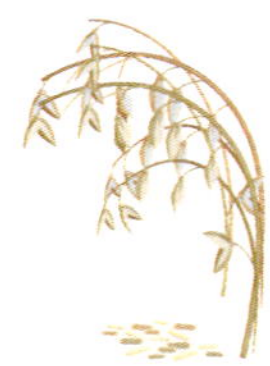
Oat

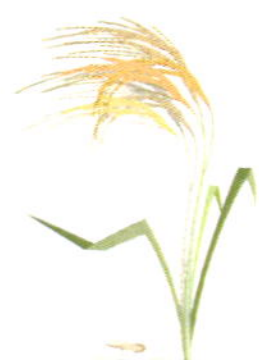
Rice

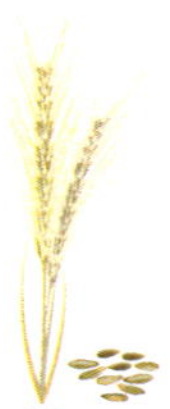
Rye

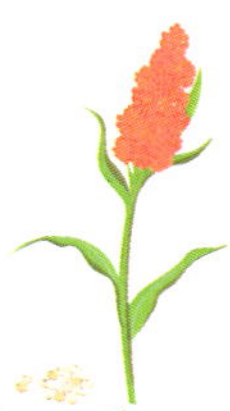
Sorghum

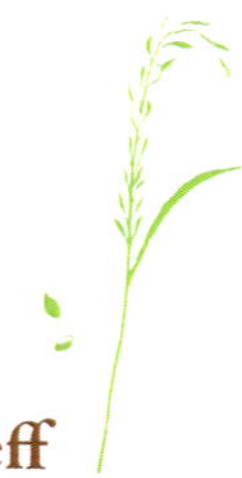
Teff

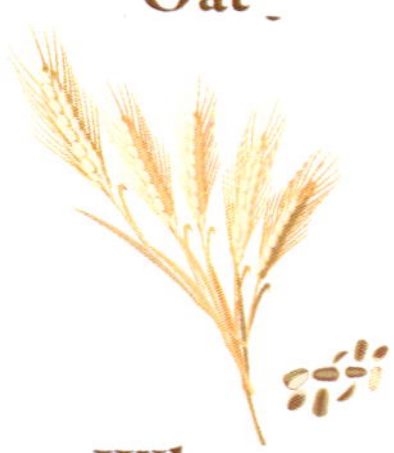
Wheat

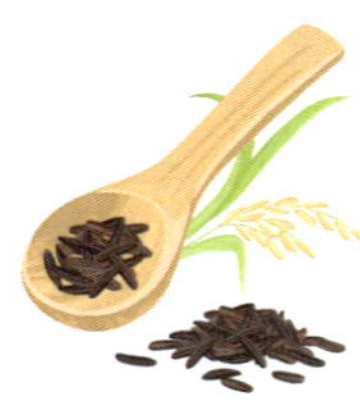
Wild Rice

Nightshade Family
Solanaceae

Natural foods of the nightshade (*Solanaceae)* family are nutritious and provide many health benefits. However, they contain toxic alkaloids, including: solanine (primarily in white potatoes), tomatine (primarily in tomatoes), capsaicin (primarily in peppers), and nicotine (found in most of these foods). Depending on the person's sensitivity, any of these foods can cause irritation, especially of the gastrointestinal system, or inflammation, such as joint pain. These alkaloids are quite thermo-stable so that cooking does little to reduce their effects. Solanine may be stored in the body and released during times of stress. Not everyone has this sensitivity. To explore this possibility, a person can remove these foods from their diet to see results. It may take a few weeks to notice a difference, allowing the body time to eliminate the harmful substances and recuperate, before experiencing relief from conditions, such as gastrointestinal discomfort or osteoarthritis. Nine members of the *Solanaceae* family are displayed below.

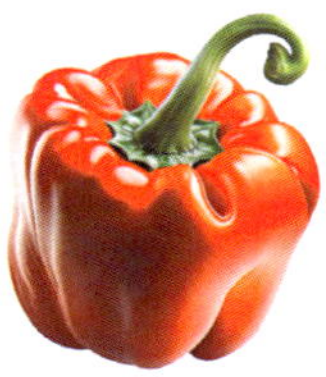

Bell Pepper

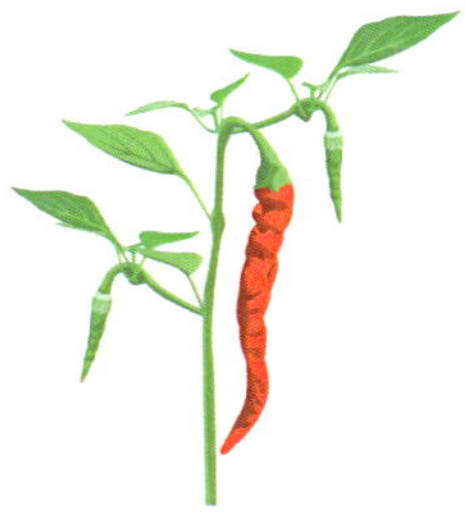

Cayenne Pepper

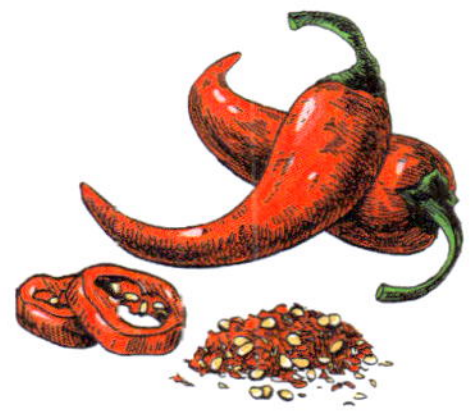

Chili Pepper

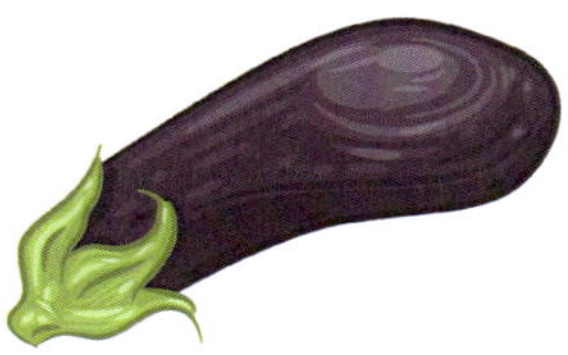

Eggplant

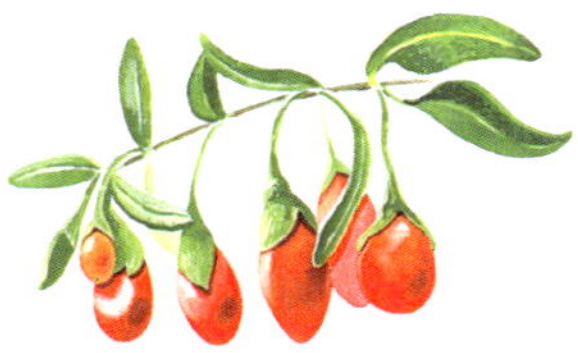

Gogi Berry

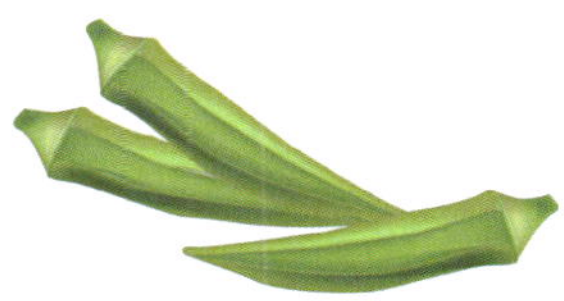

Okra

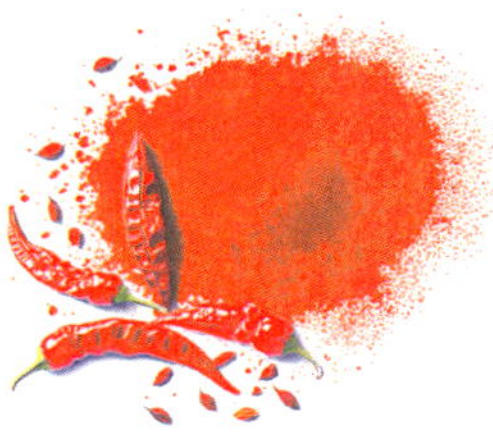

Paprika

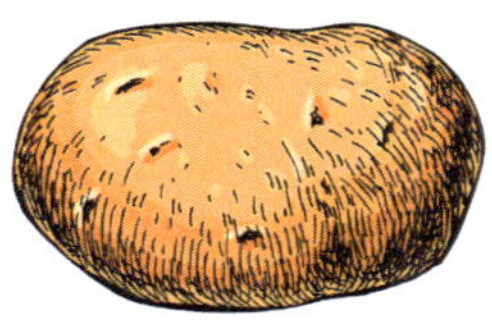

Potato

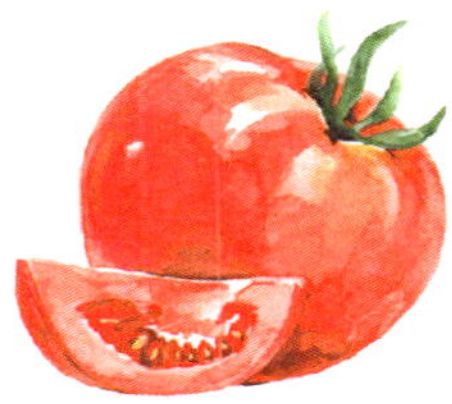

Tomato

Onion Family
Alliaceae

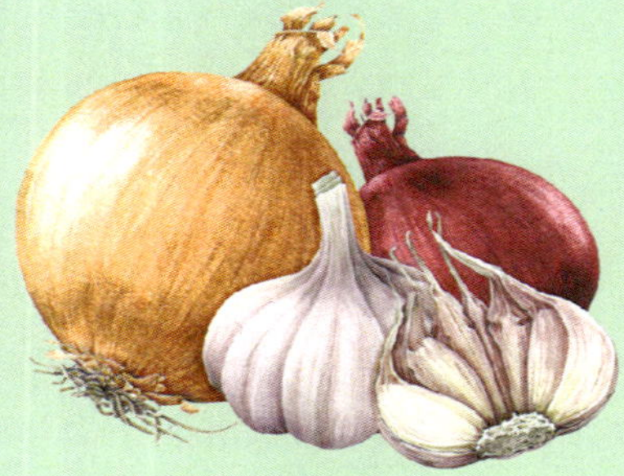

The Onion Family (*Alliaceae*) includes plant foods with leaves that grow from a bulb at their base. The most common are from the genus *Allium*. They furnish a suite of nutrients, including: allicin, potassium, selenium, manganese, B vitamins, vitamin C, bioflavonoids (especially quercetin), phenolic acids, and saponins. When crushed, *Alliums* release the enzyme alliinase which converts their sulfur compounds and other volatile oils into pungent scents. These robust compounds provide exceptional health benefits, including: anti-oxidant, anti-inflammatory, anti-tumor, anti-viral, anti-bacterial, anti-fungal, and anti-parasite properties. Seven *Alliums* are depicted below.

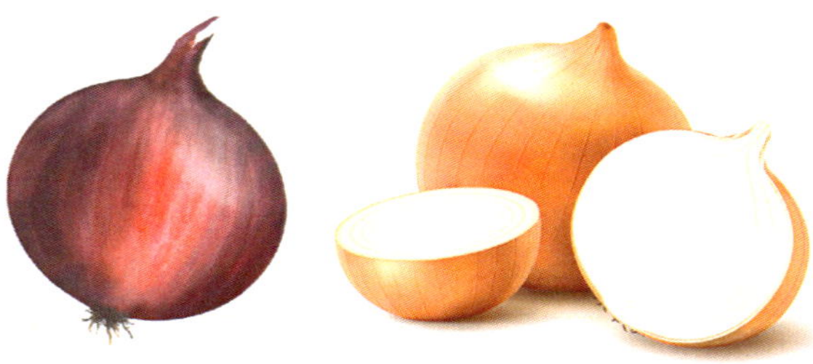

Red and White Onions

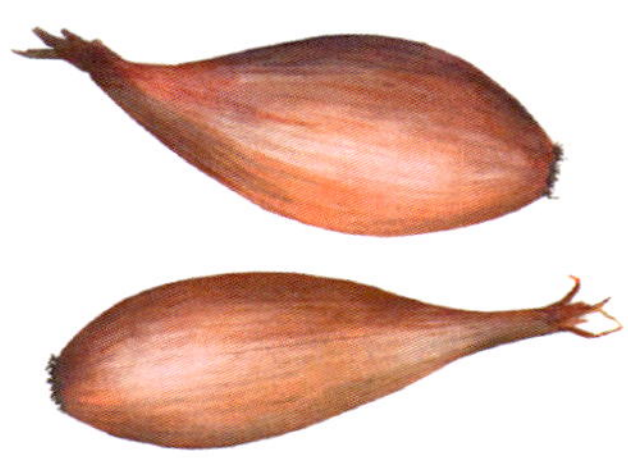

Shallots

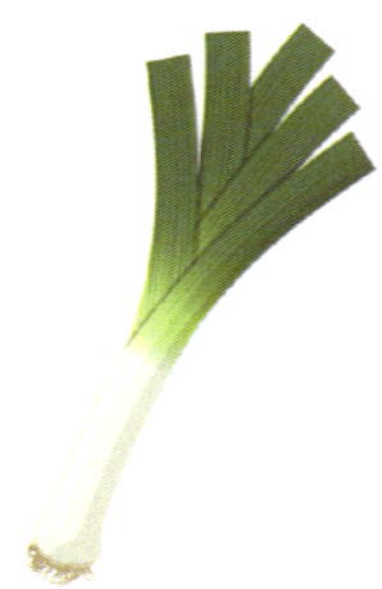

Leeks

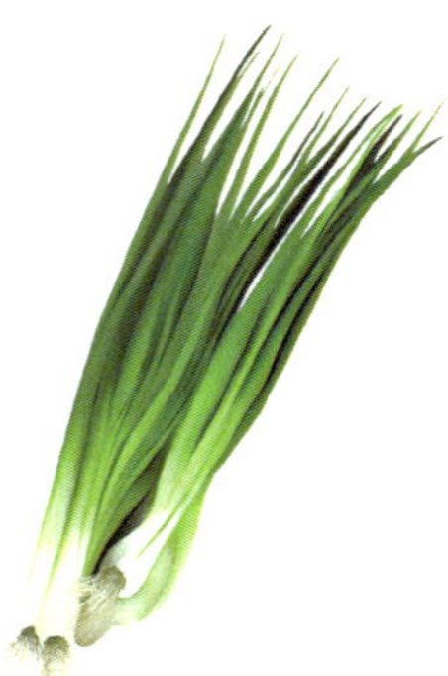

Scallions

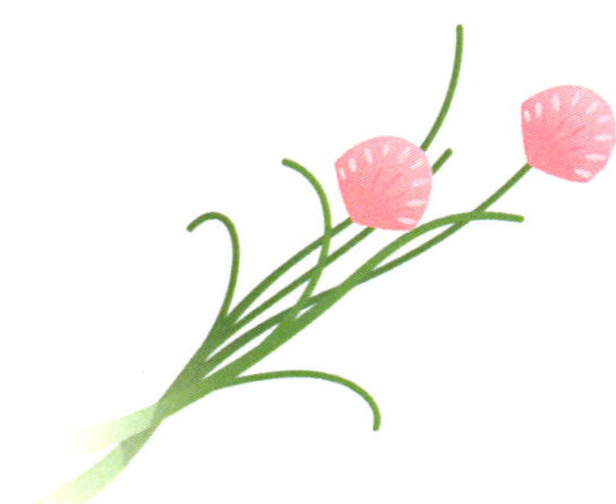

Chives

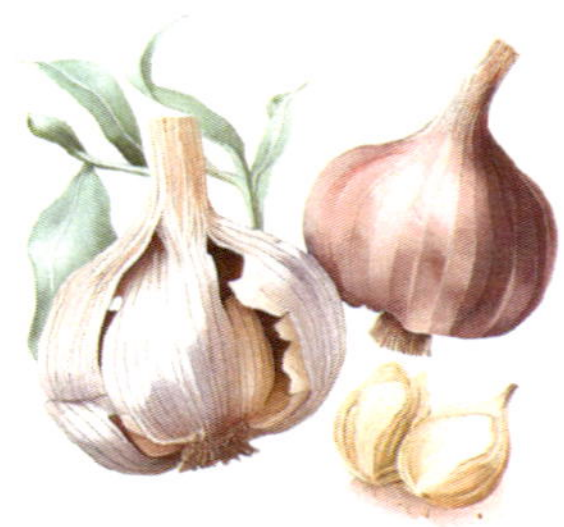

Garlic

Rose Family
Rosaceae

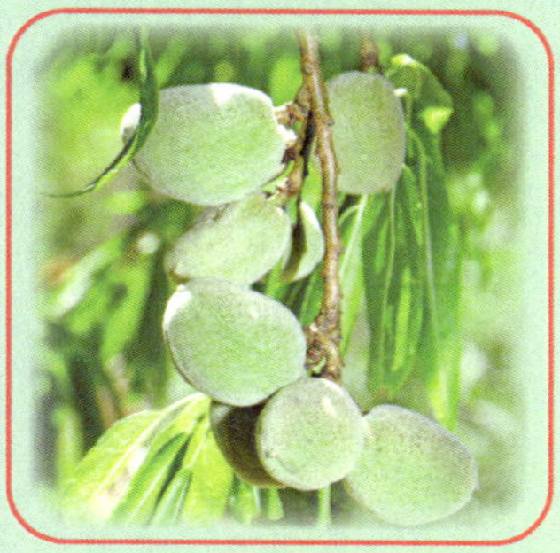

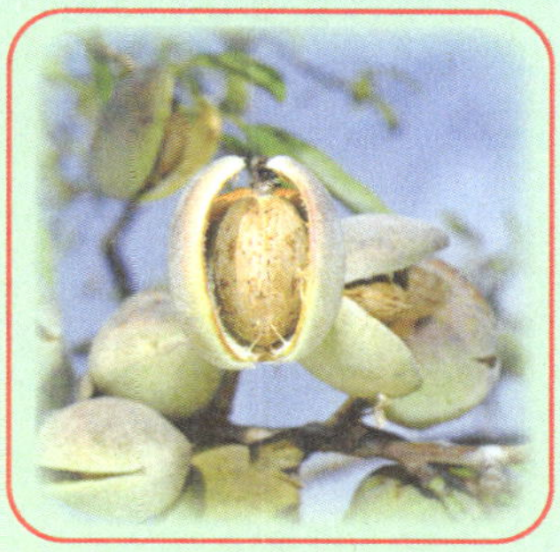

The *Rosaceae* family encompasses hundreds of colorful fruits high in antioxidants. Apricots, cherries, nectarines, peaches, and plums are examples of drupes or 'stone fruits' (with a single inedible seed encased in a hard shell or pit). Druplets are aggregated fruits, like blackberries and raspberries. Apples and pears contain ample amounts of pectin that promotes healthy digestion and boosts the immune system, however, their seeds are toxic. On the other hand, almonds are an example of an edible *Rosaceae* seed. They contain beneficial fatty acids, vitamin E, magnesium, and fiber. Ten of the *Rosaceae* family foods are depicted below.

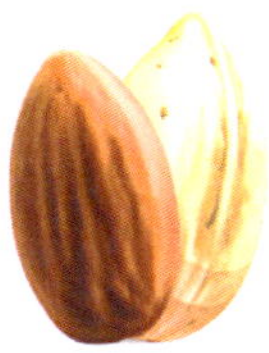

Almond

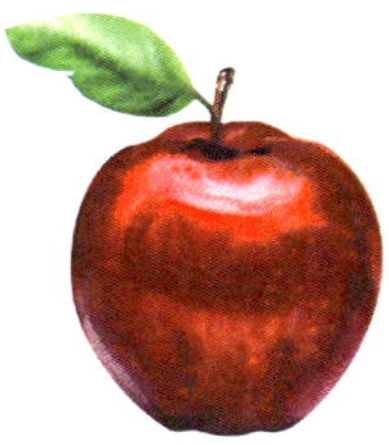

Apple

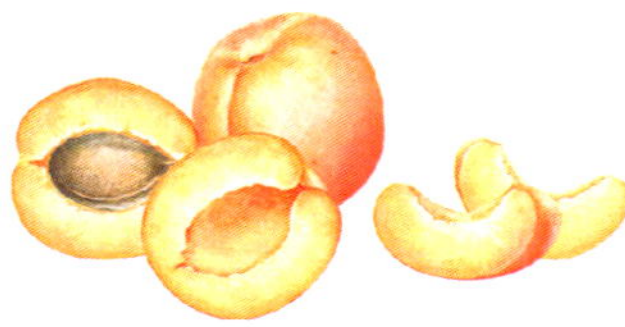

Apricot

Blackberry

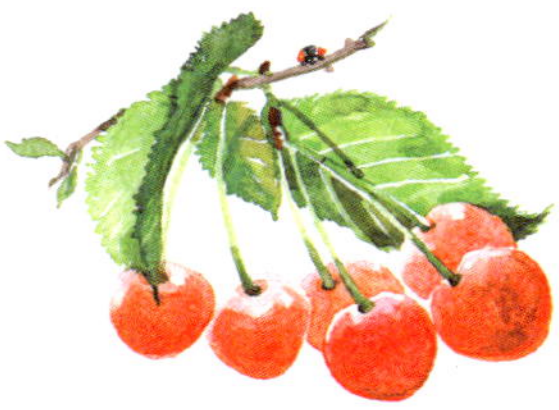

Cherry

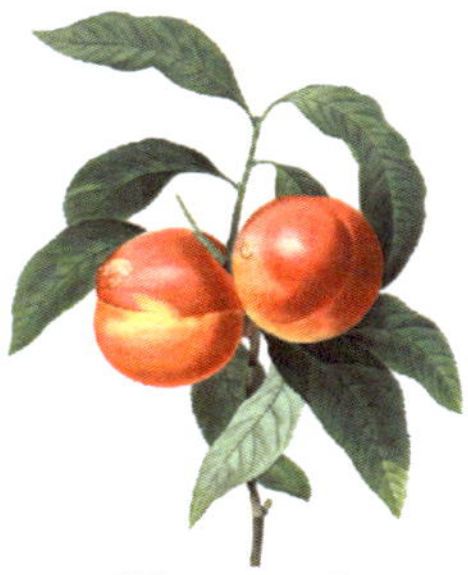

Nectarine

Peach

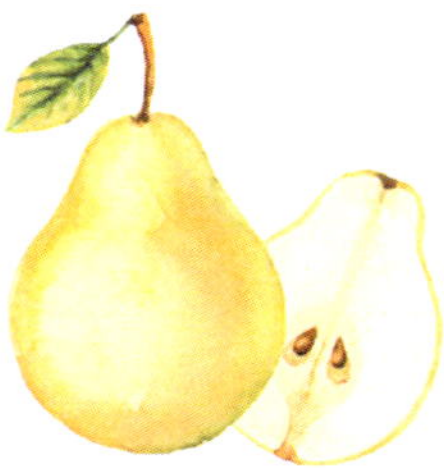

Pear

Plum

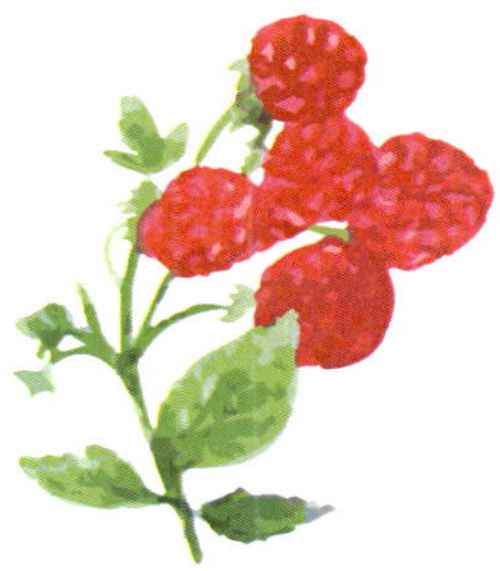

Rasberry

Edible Parts of Plants

Their Nutrients and Health-Giving Properties

Botanical Nutrition

Roots

Plants store nutrients, including complex carbohydrates and starches, in their roots to carry them through the winter.

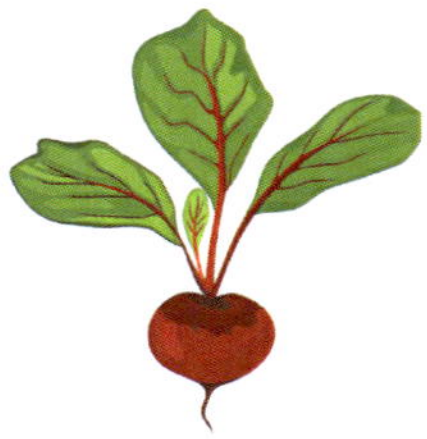

Beet

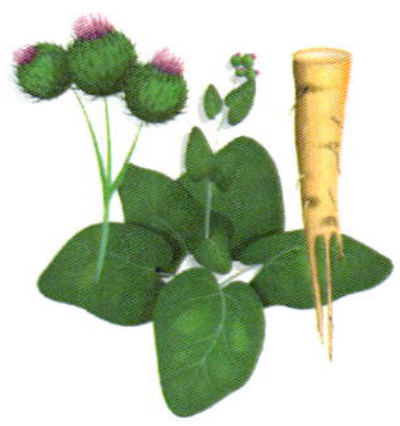

Burdock

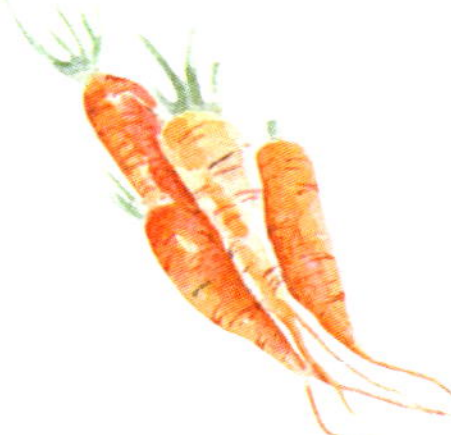

Carrot

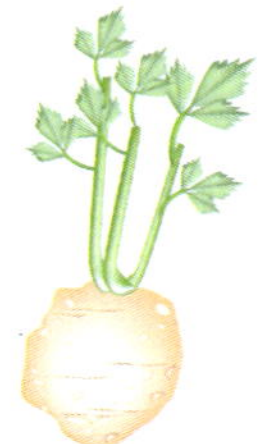

Celeric

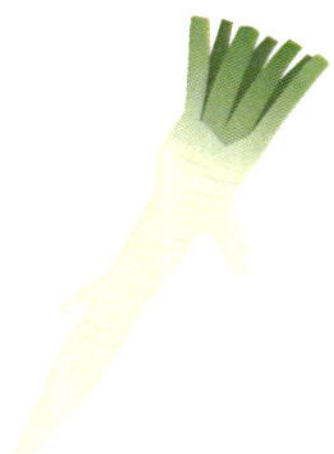

Horseradish

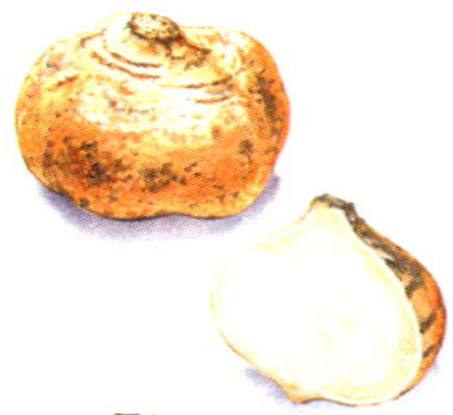

Jicama

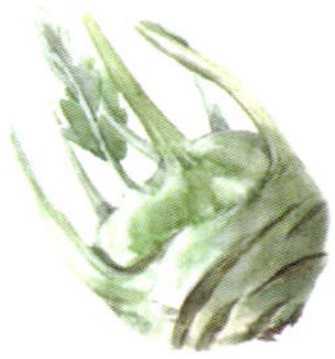

Kohlrabi

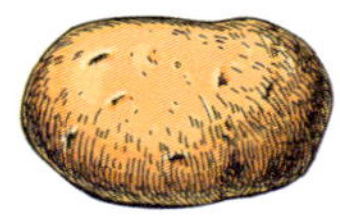

Potato

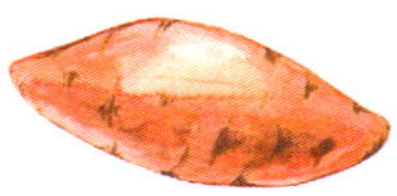

Sweet Potato

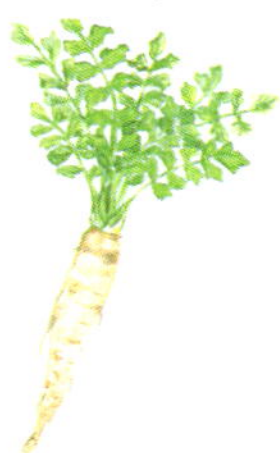

Parsnip

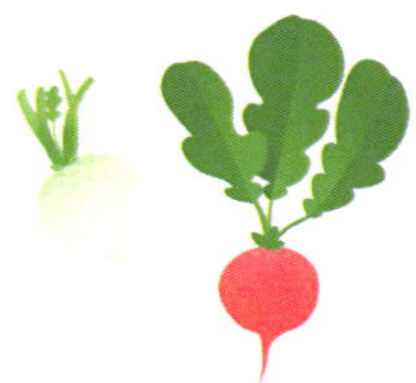

Radish

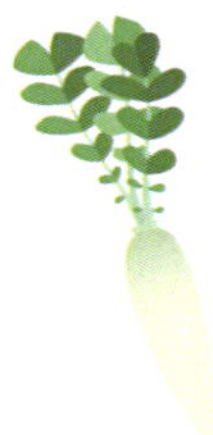

Daikon

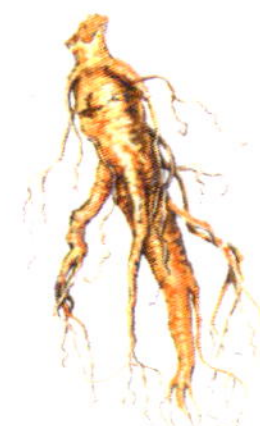

Ginseng

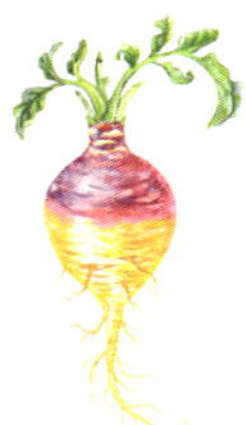

Rutabaga

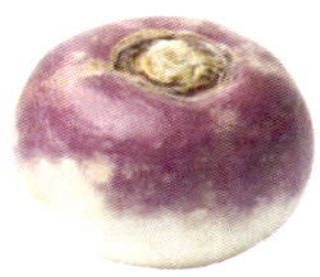

Turnip

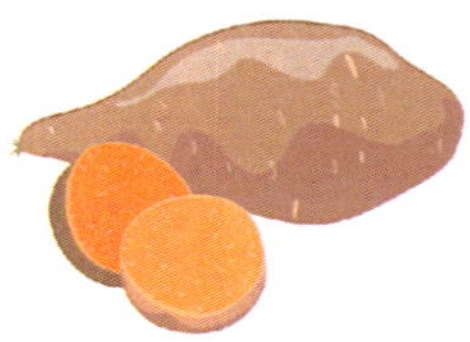

Yam

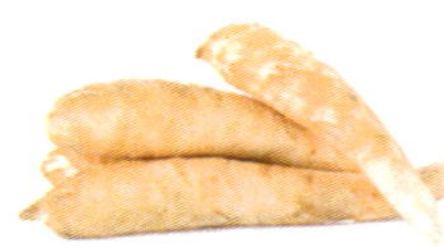

Arrowroot

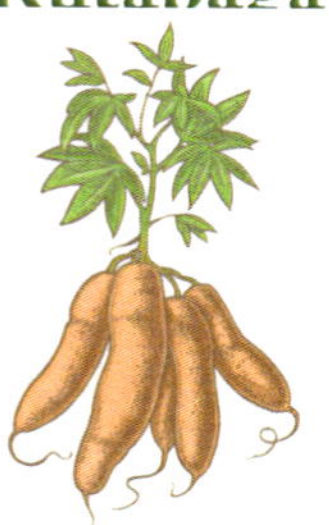

Casava

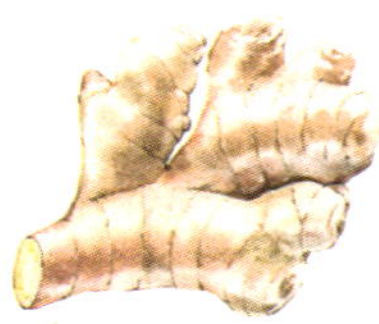

Ginger

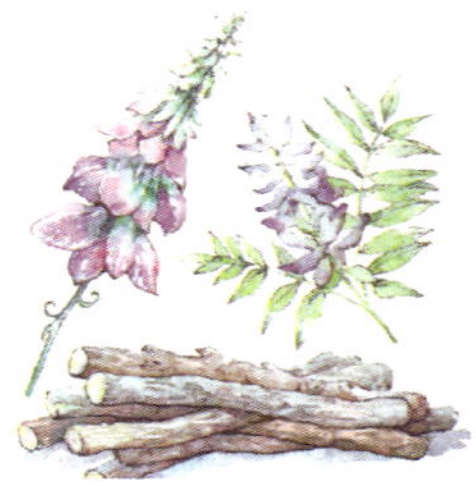

Licorice

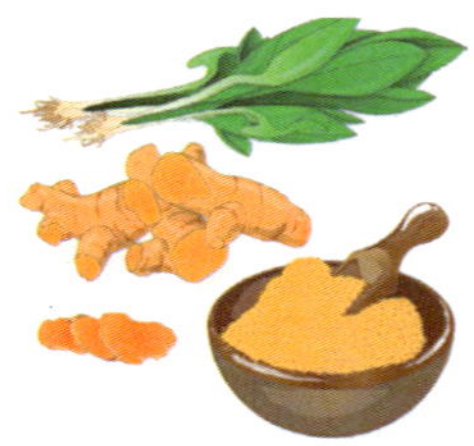

Turmeric

Continued...

Botanical Nutrition

Bulbs with Leaves

Quercetin offers strong anti-inflammatory and antihistamine benefits.

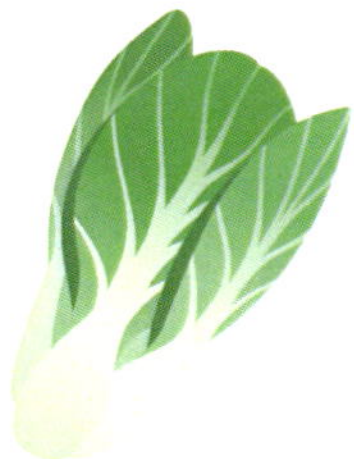

Bok Choy

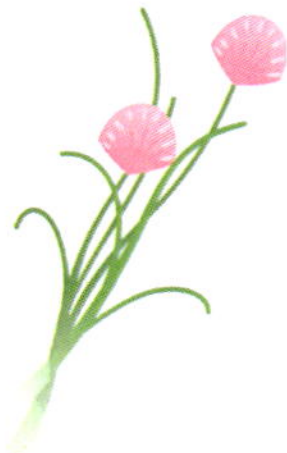

Chives

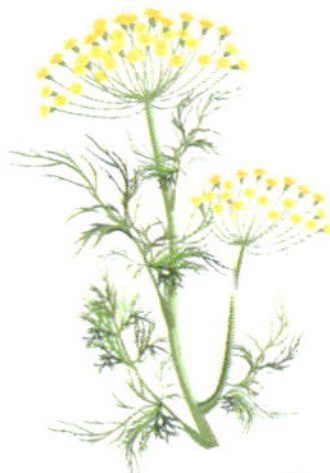

Fennel

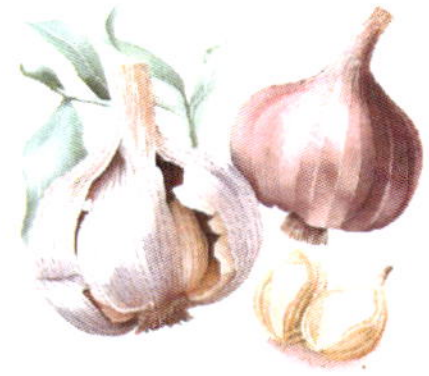

Garlic

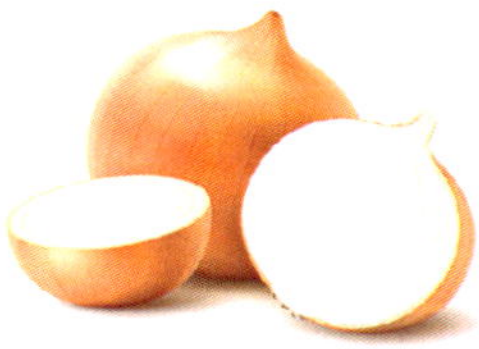

Onion

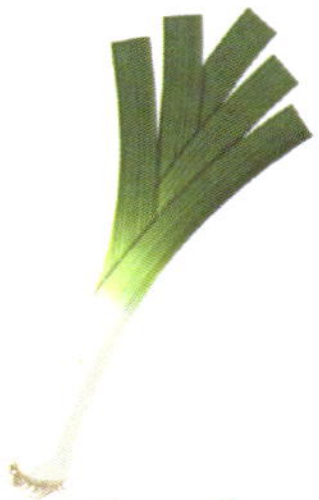

Leek

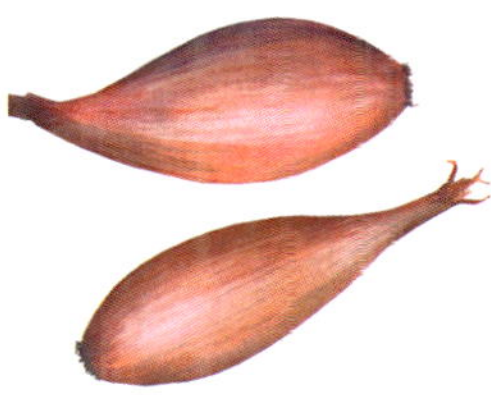

Shallot

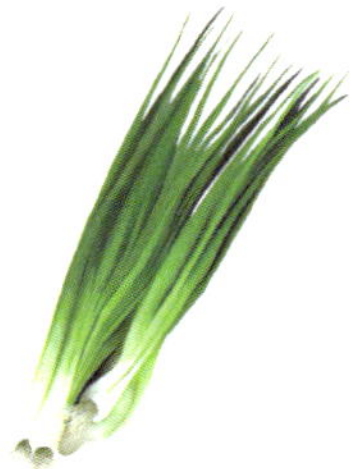

Scallion

Stalks, Canes, Stems, and Leaves

Glutathione (powerful anti-oxidant) and inulin (prebiotic food for probiotic bacteria) are present in asparagus and cabbage. Natural sodium in celery supports the nervous system and balances intracellular and intercellular fluids with potassium. Molasses and sorgo syrup, with concentrated minerals and vitamins, are extracted from the segmented stalk (cane) of sorghum.

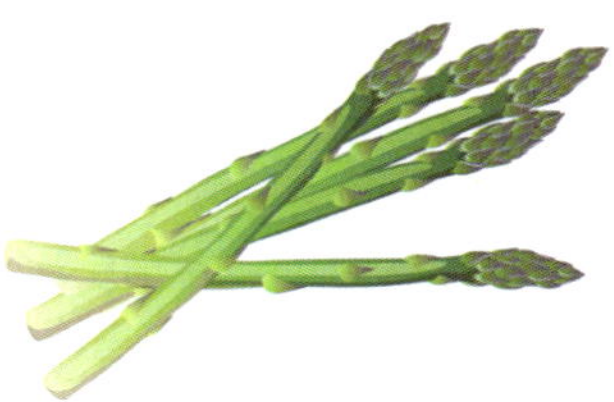

Asparagus

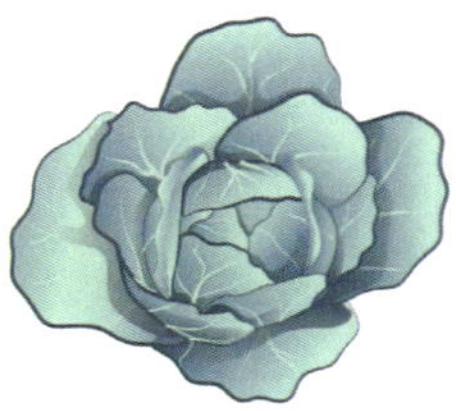

Cabbage

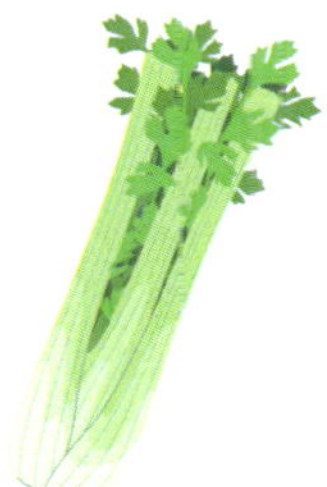

Celery

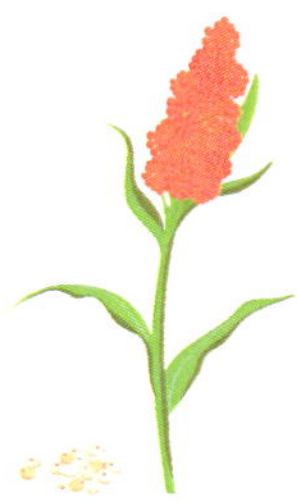

Sorghum

Continued...

Botanical Nutrition

Bark

As the outer covering of various species of cinnamon trees, cinnamon bark protects the inner tree with anti-microbial compounds that are imparted to us when we consume them. Cinnamon is anti-oxidant, anti-inflammatory, anti-diabetic, and anti-cancer.

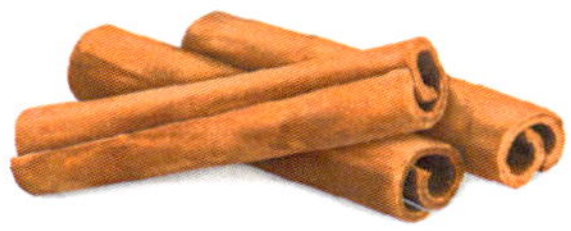

Cinnamon

Flowers

Chamomile is calming. Chrysanthemum has quercetin, an anti-oxidant and anti-histamine. Lavender improves melatonin levels, promoting restful sleep. Saffron, comprised of the thread-like stigmas of the *Crocus sativus* flower, contains safranal which increases circulation and supports cognitive function.

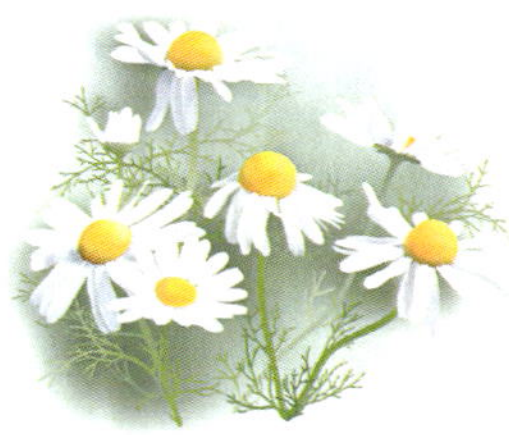

Chamomile

Chrysanthemum

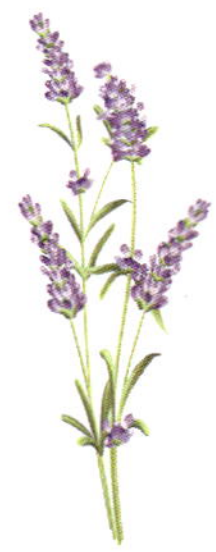

Lavender

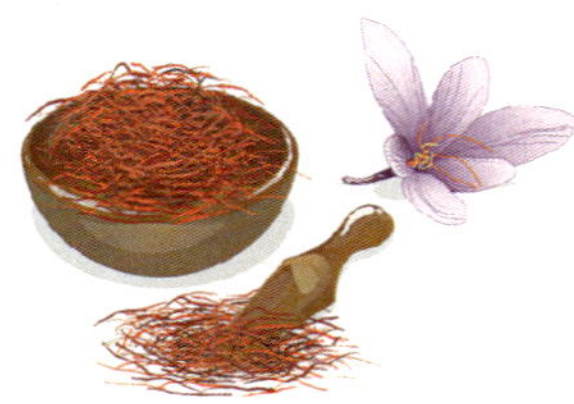

Saffron

Flower Buds

Artichoke, broccoli, Brussels sprouts, and cauliflower are renowned for their anti-cancer properties. Cloves are soothing, anti-inflammatory, anti-septic, and fight gum disease.

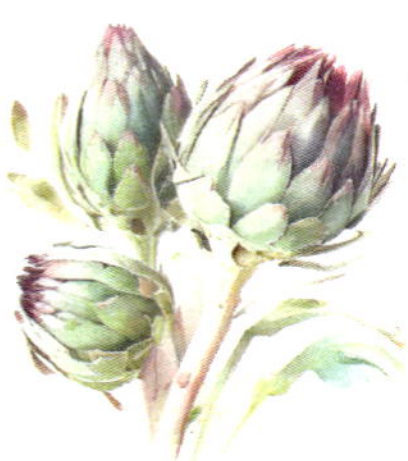

Artichoke
(flower petals & stalk)

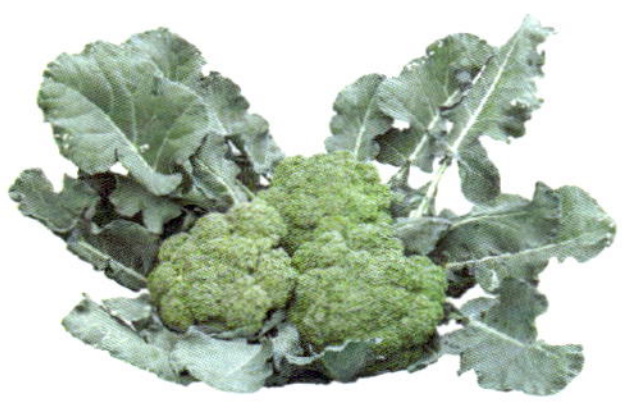

Broccoli

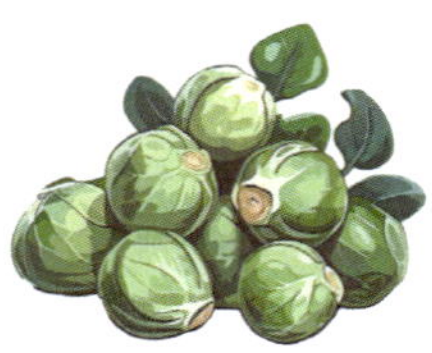

Brussels Sprouts

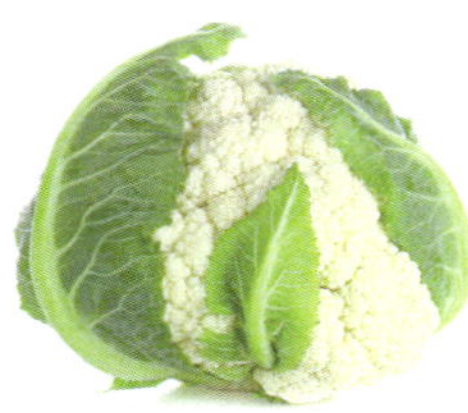

Cauliflower

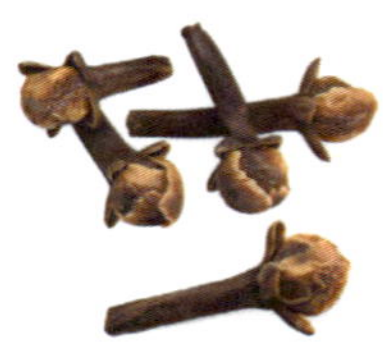

Clove

Continued...

Botanical Nutrition

Fruits

Fruits encompass a full array of colorful phytonutrients, including: lycopene, beta-carotene, zeaxanthin, chlorophyll, folate, anthocyanins, and resveratrol. The colors and sweetness of fruits and the nectar in their flowers attract symbiotic bat, insect, and bird pollinators. However, their fruits also attract predators, such as insects and pathogenic microbes. As a defense against these predators, some plants defend themselves by producing anti-bacterial, anti-fungal, and anti-parasite substances (for example, limonoids in citrus fruits). These plant foods and their anti-microbial properties may confer this immune system benefit to us when we consume them.

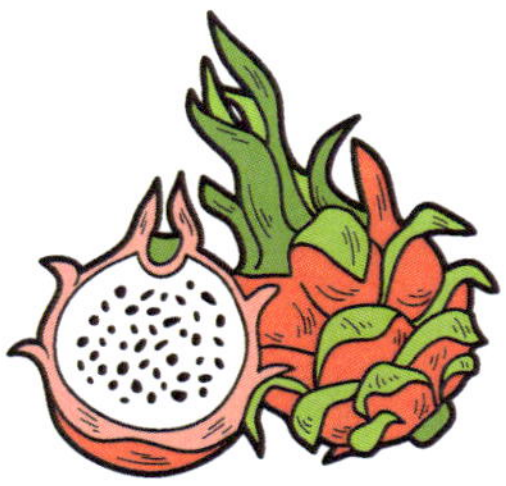

Dragon Fruit

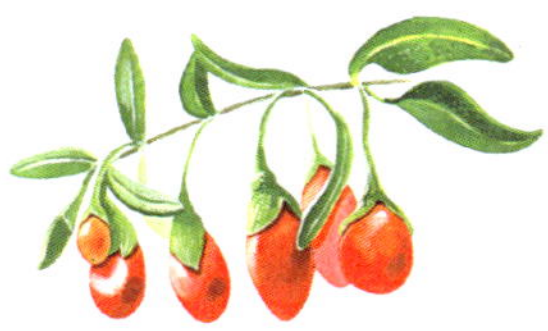

Goji Berries

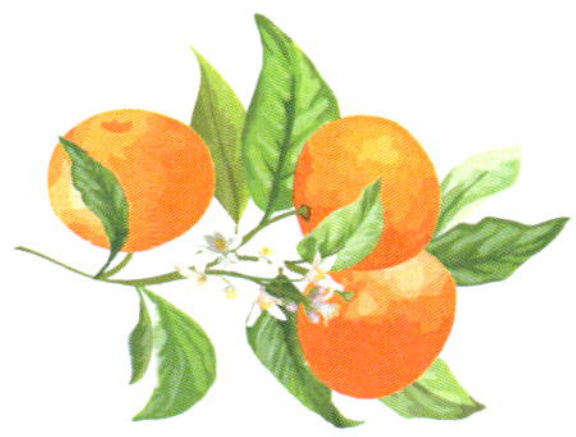

Orange (mandarin)

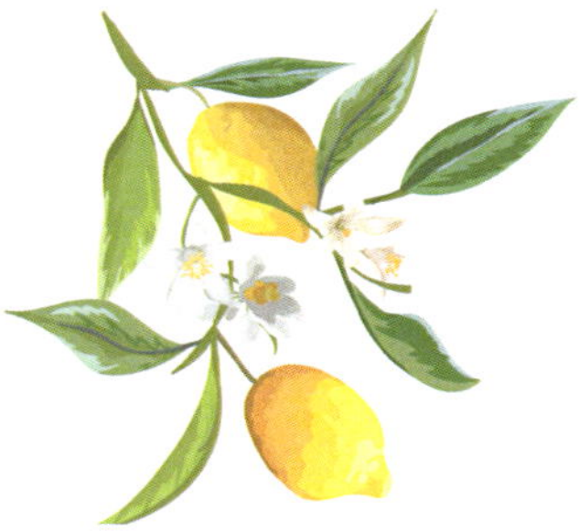

Lemon

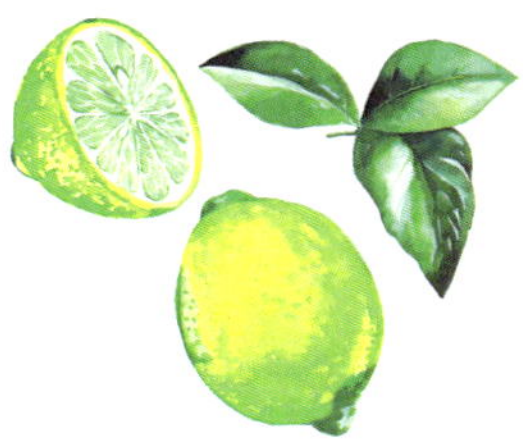

Lime

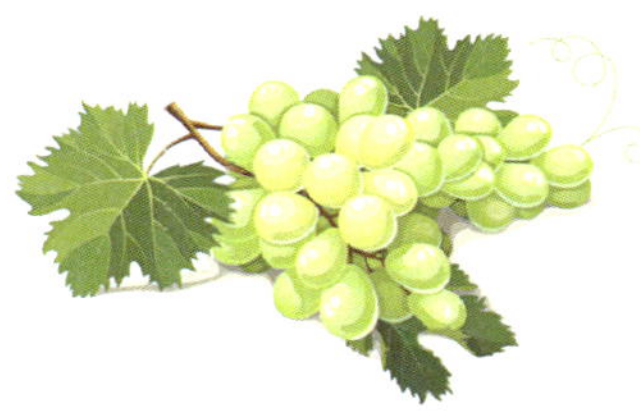

Grapes (green)

Blueberry

Plum

Continued...

Botanical Nutrition

Refreshing, Non-Sweet Fruits

From the standpoint of botany, these refreshing and piquant (lively tasting pepper) foods are fruits; and they encompass the plant's seeds. However, lacking sweetness, they are commonly thought of as vegetables or, in the case of peppercorn, as a seasoning. Black peppercorn's piperine gives it pungency; and for those who do not find pepper to be irritating, this food may support a healthy metabolism and aid in wound healing.

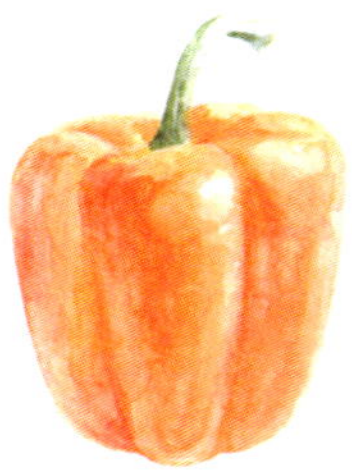

Bell Pepper

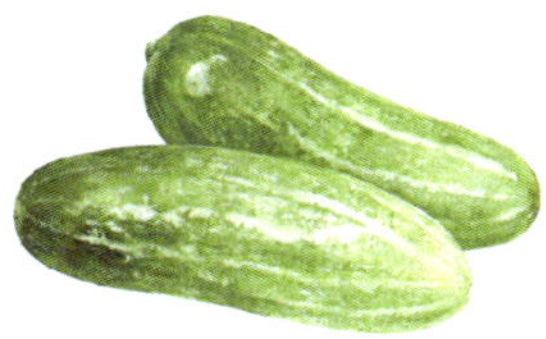

Cucumber

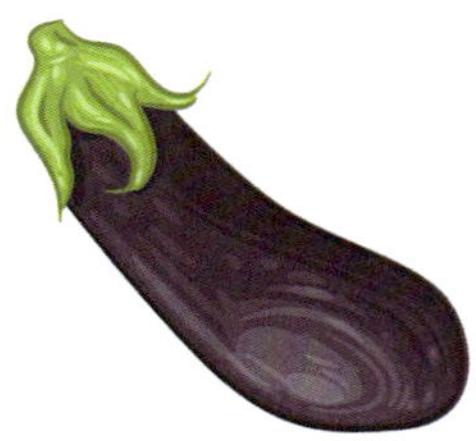

Eggplant

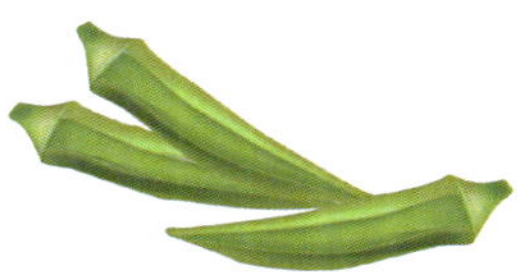

Okra

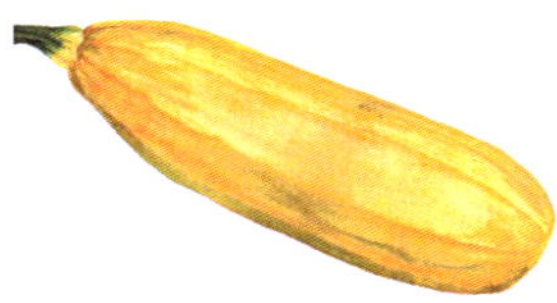

Yellow Squash
(Summer)

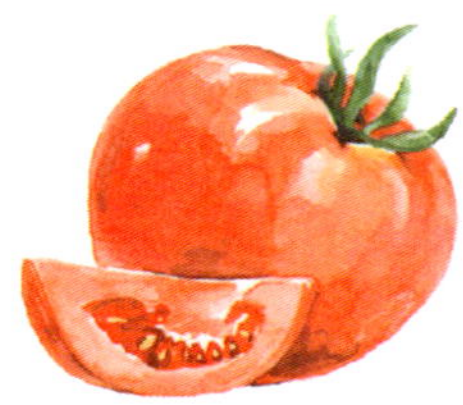

Tomato

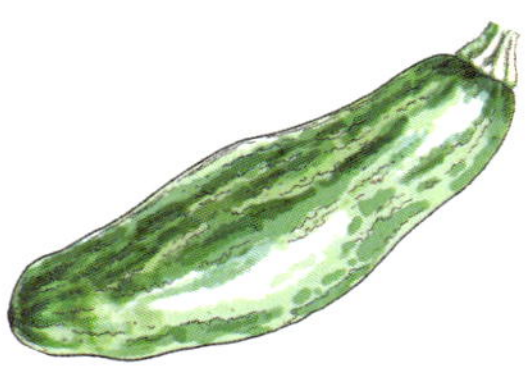

Zucchini

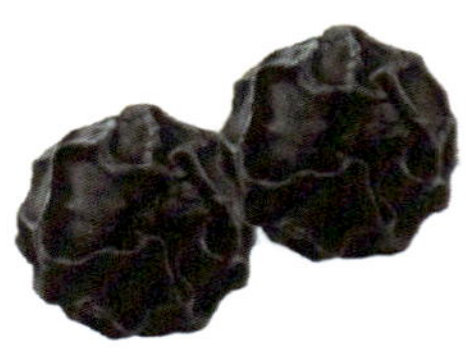

Peppercorn (black)

Continued...

Botanical Nutrition

Seeds in Pods (fresh and dried)

Seeds, protected in pods, contain B vitamins, phosphorus, fiber, protein, carbohydrates, and fatty acids.

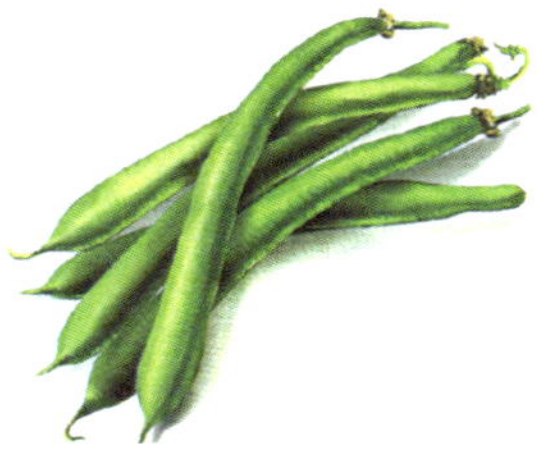

Green Bean (fresh)
Legumes

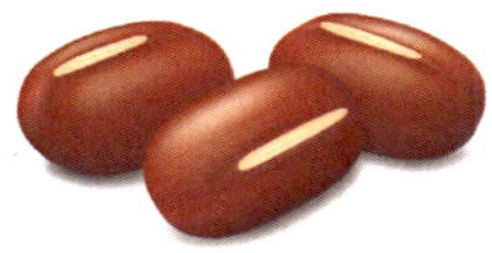

Legumes

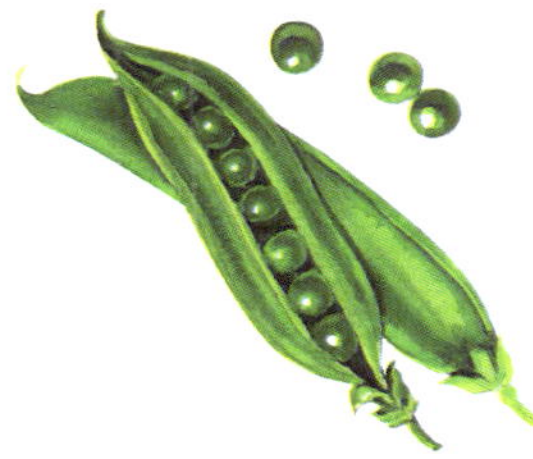

Peas (fresh)
Legumes

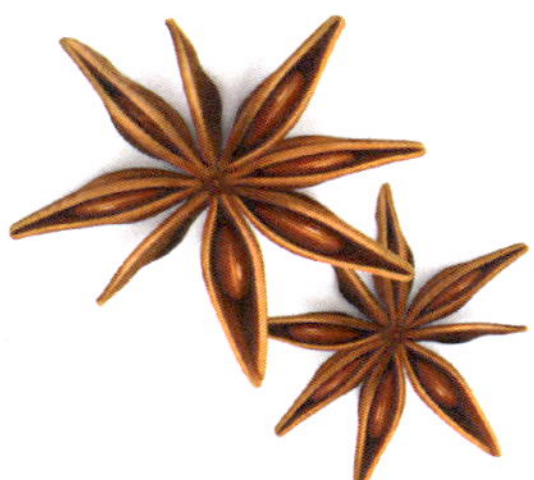

Star Anisse

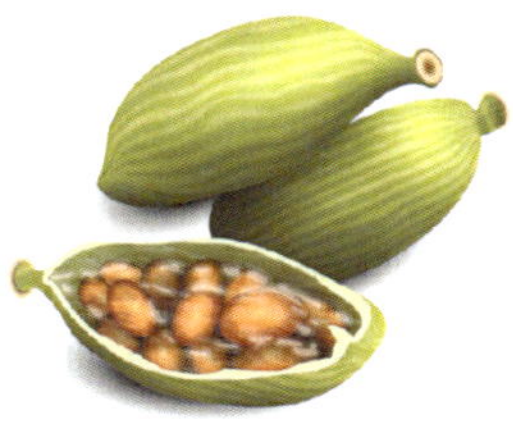

Cardamom

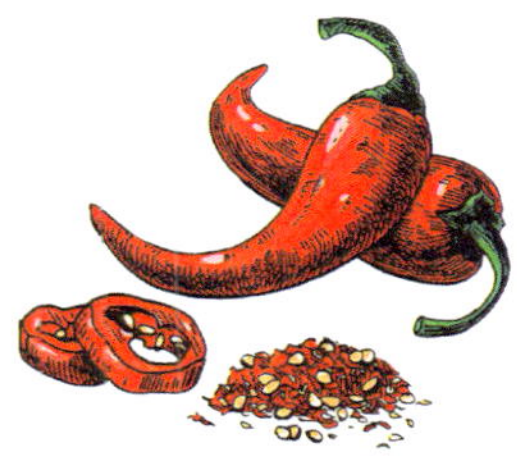

Chili

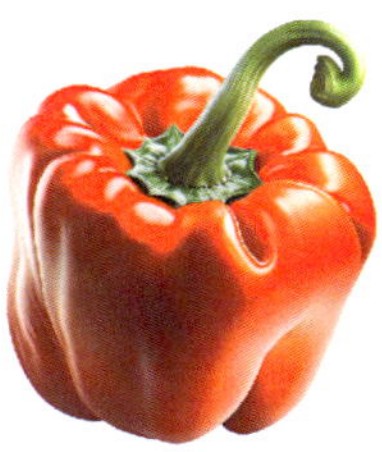

Peppers

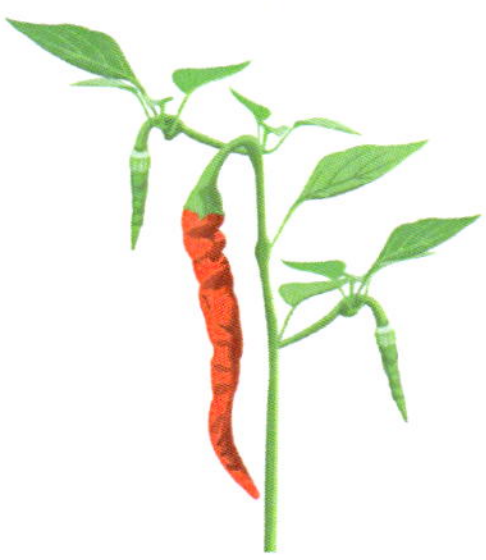

Cayanne Pepper

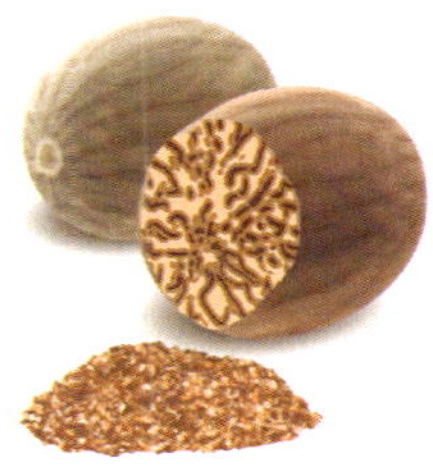

Nutmeg

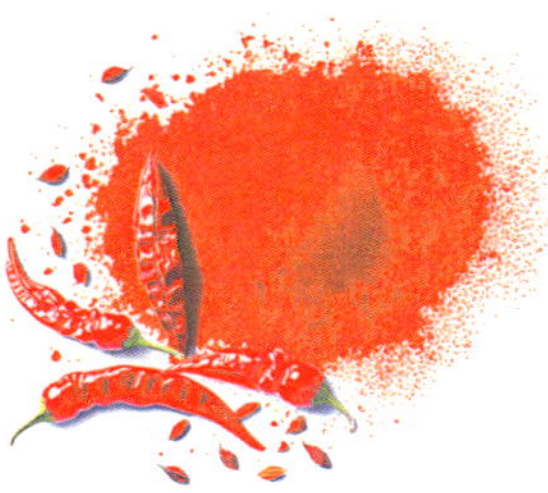

Paprika

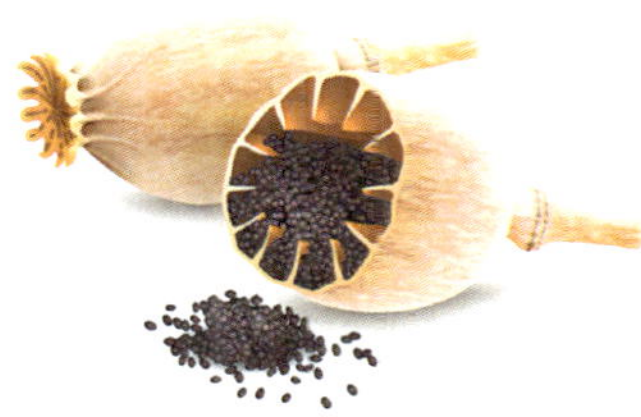

Poppy

Continued...

Botanical Nutrition

Seeds (fresh and dried)

Seeds are embryos that develop into plants. They contain the necessary nutrients to sustain them through germination, until the plant can send up green sprouts to catch the sunshine and send down roots to draw water and nutrients from the soil. They are high in vitamins, minerals, protein, fatty acids, and fiber.

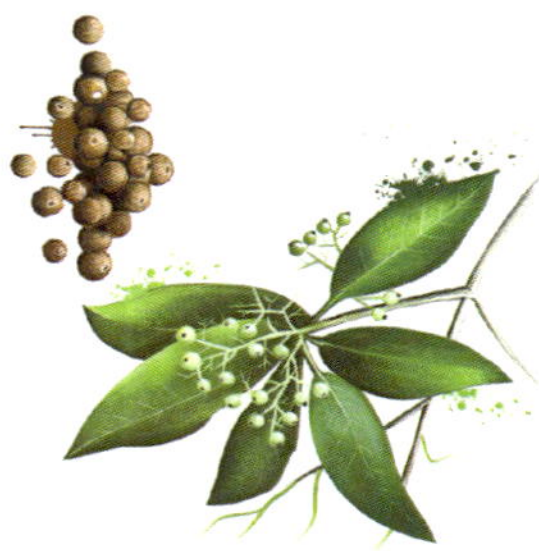

Allspice

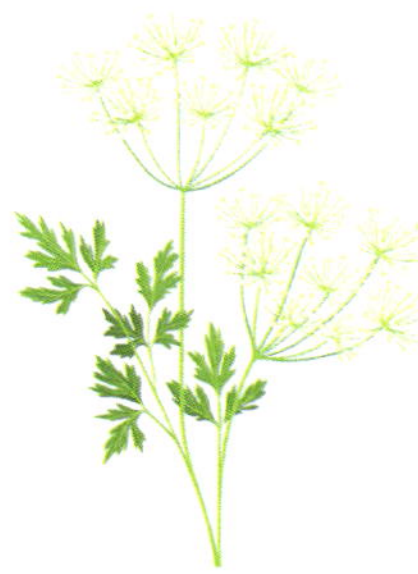

Anise

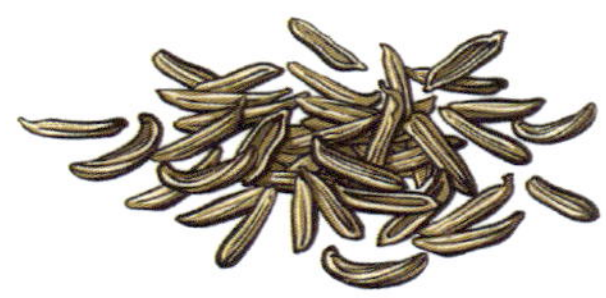

Caraway

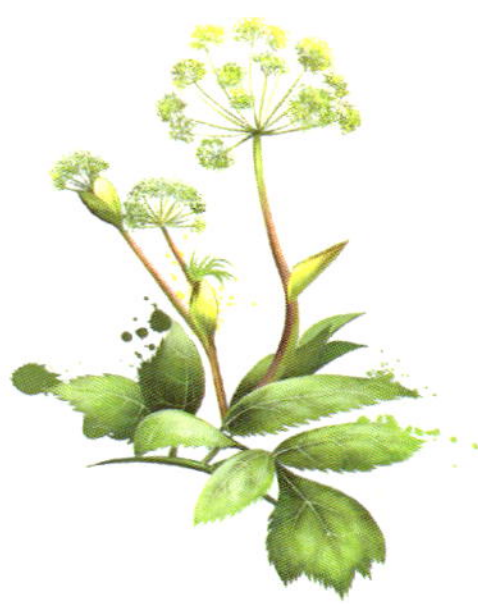

Celery

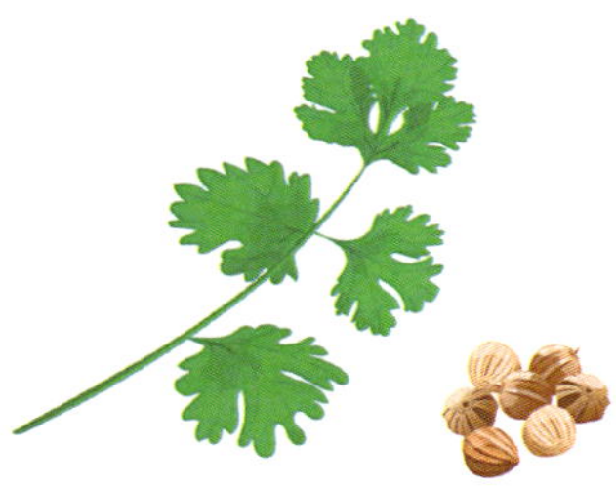

Coriander

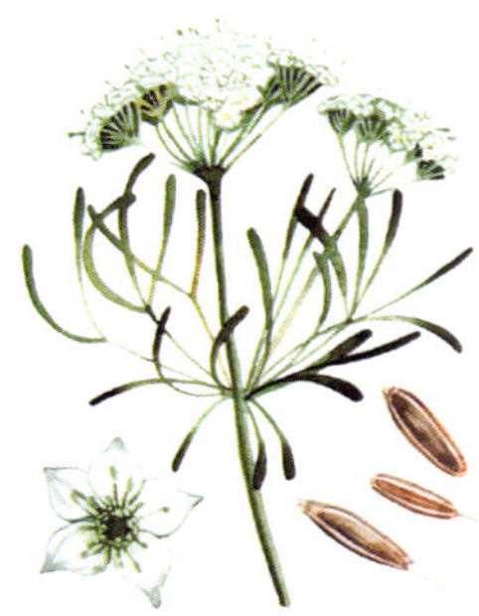

Cumin

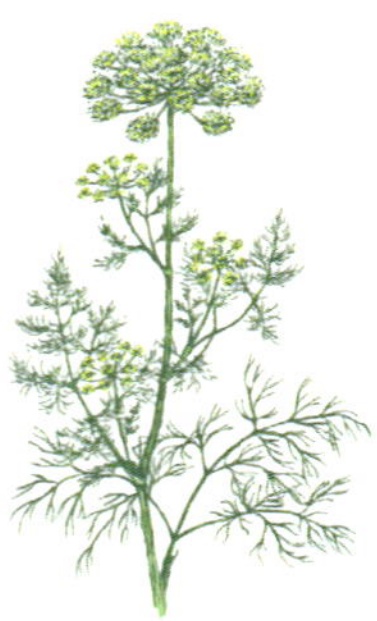

Dill

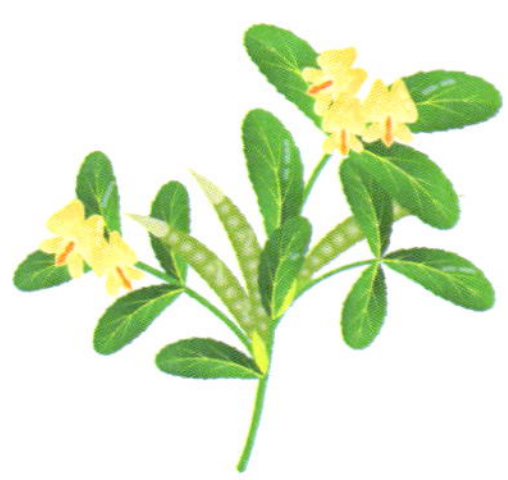

Fenugreek

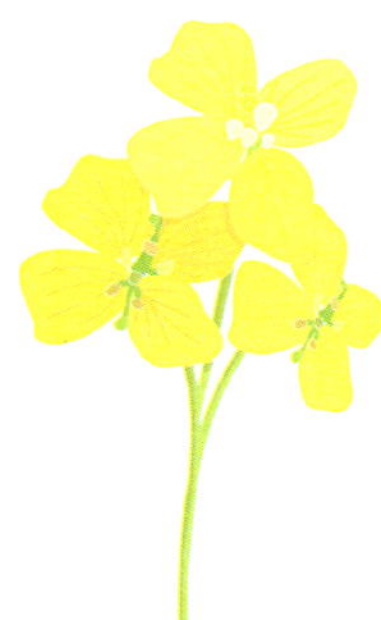

Mustard

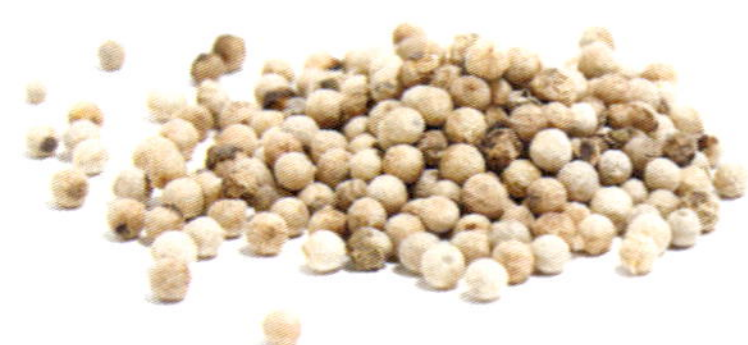

Peppercorn (white)

Continued...

Botanical Nutrition

Leaves (leafy greens)

The green pigment chlorophyll in leafy greens is molecularly similar to hemoglobin. The significant difference is that the chlorophyll molecule is built around a magnesium ion, whereas, hemoglobin (necessary to bind oxygen in the blood) is constructed around an iron ion. Given their notable molecular similarity, leafy greens (and other natural foods that contain chlorophyll) superlatively facilitate the body in regenerating (cleansing/detoxing and rebuilding) the blood. Folate in leafy greens is essential for proper cell and tissue development and is used in protein metabolism.

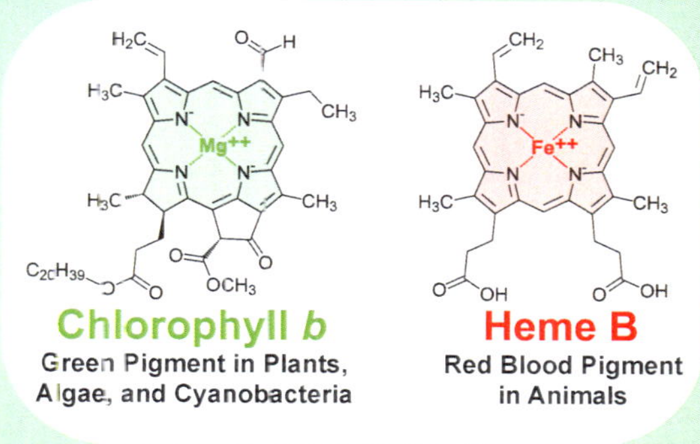

Illustrator Peter Hermes Furian, Dreamstime

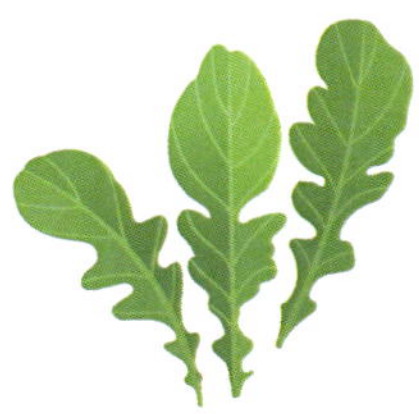

Arugula

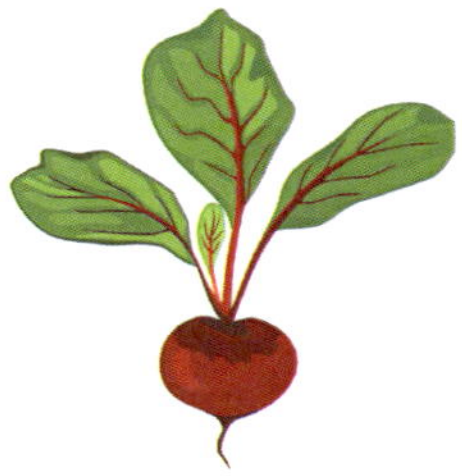

Beet Greens

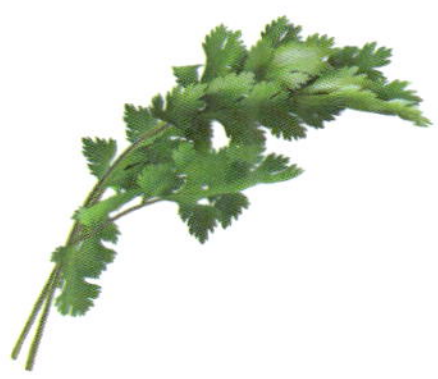

Cilantro

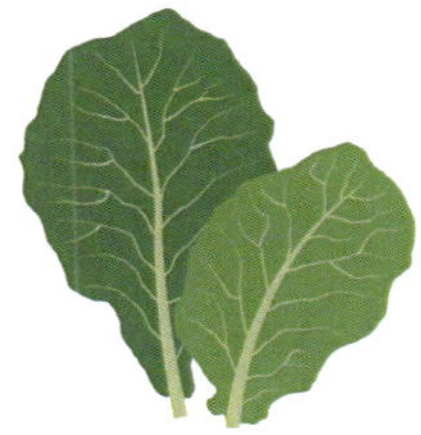

Collard Greens

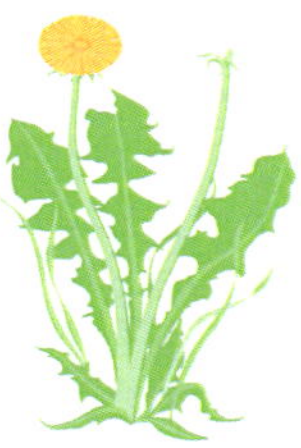

Dandelions

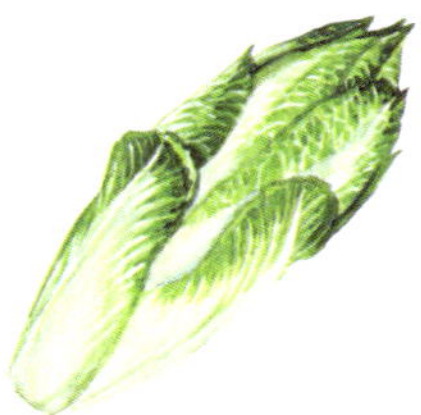

Endive

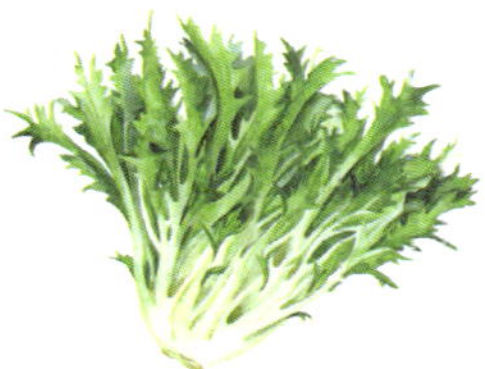

Escarole

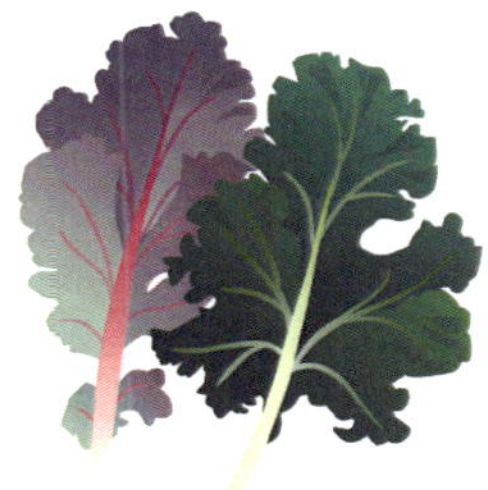

Kale

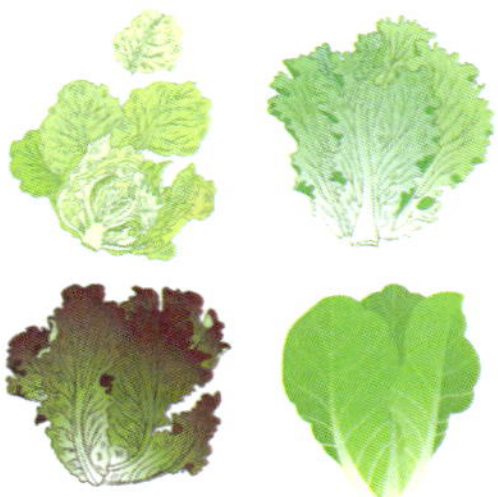

Lettuce (Butter, Green Leaf, Red Leaf, Romaine)

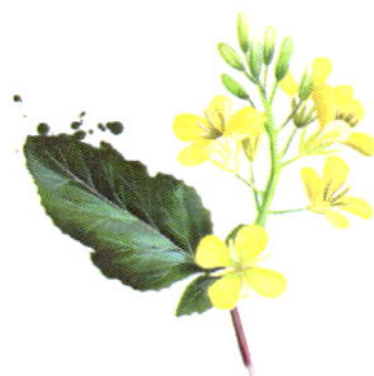

Mustard Greens

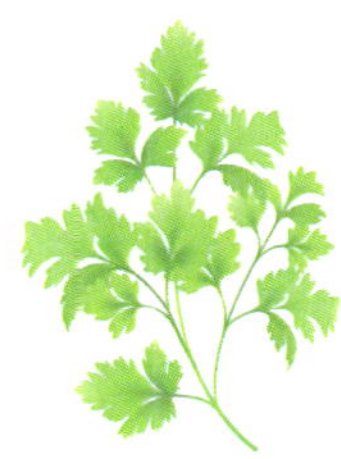

Parsley

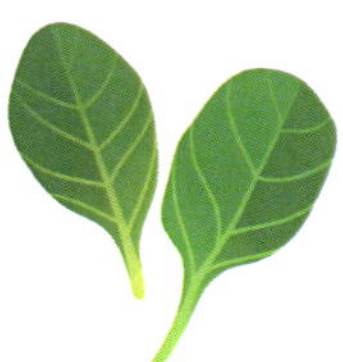

Spinach

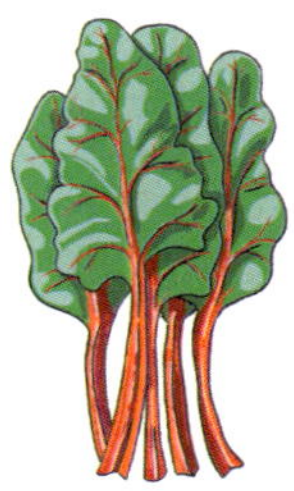

Swiss Chard

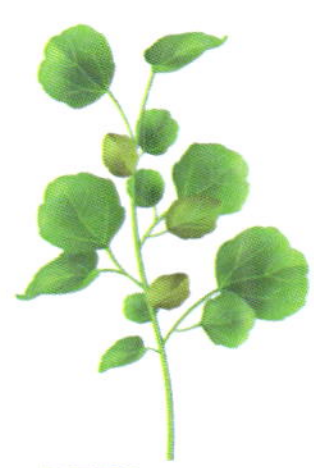

Watercress

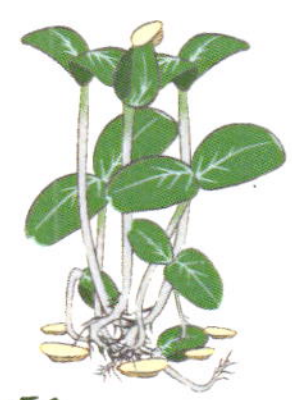

Microgreens (Sunflower)

Continued...

Botanical Nutrition

Leaves (leafy greens)

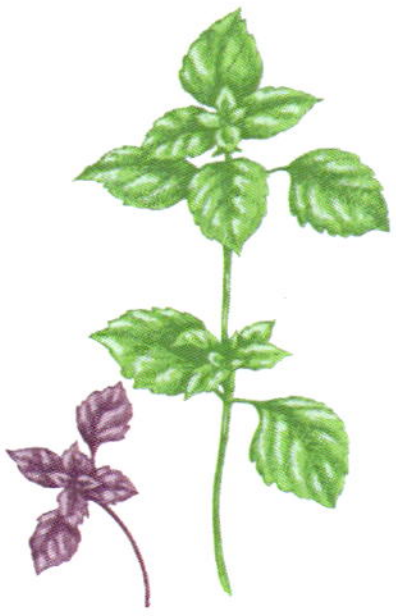
Basil

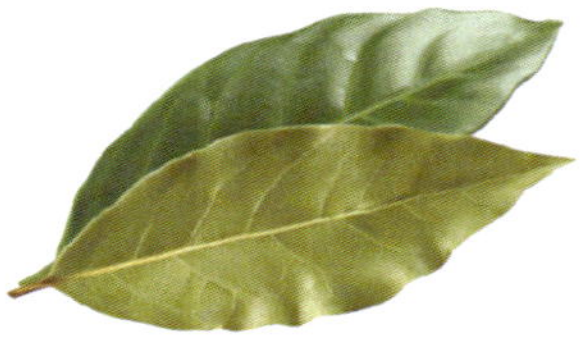
Bay Leaf

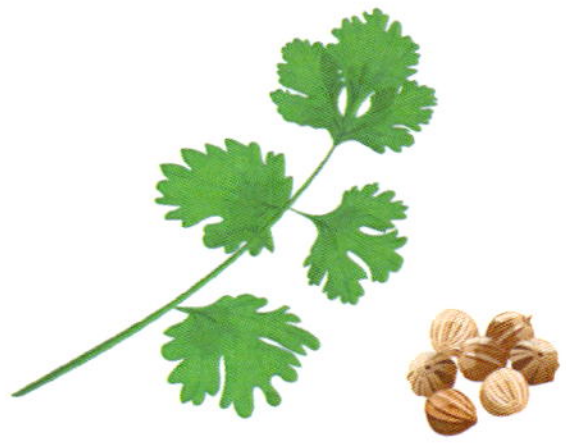
Coriander

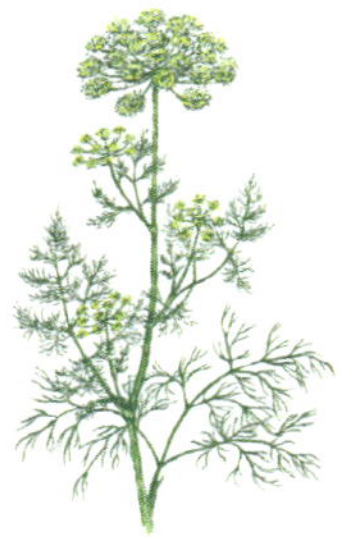
Dill

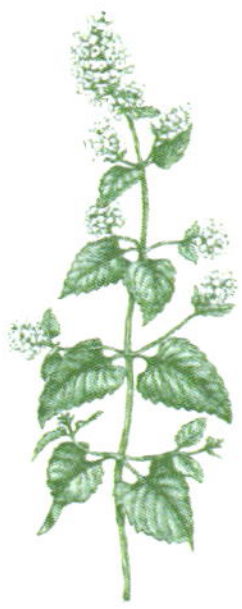
Lemon Balm/Melissa

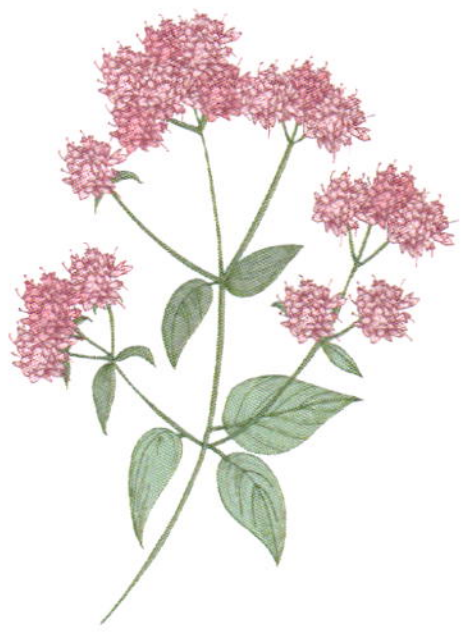
Marjoram

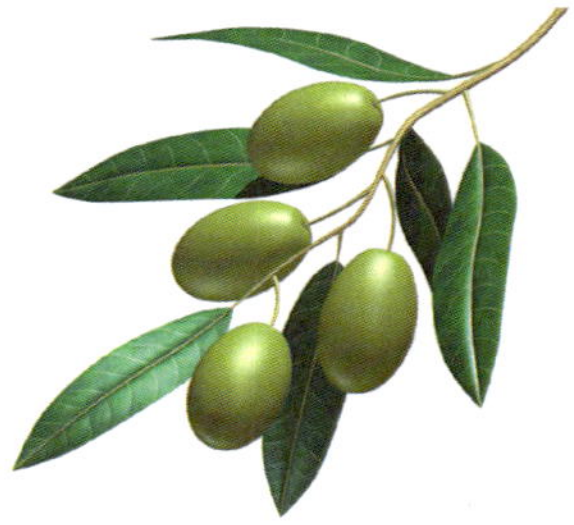
Olive

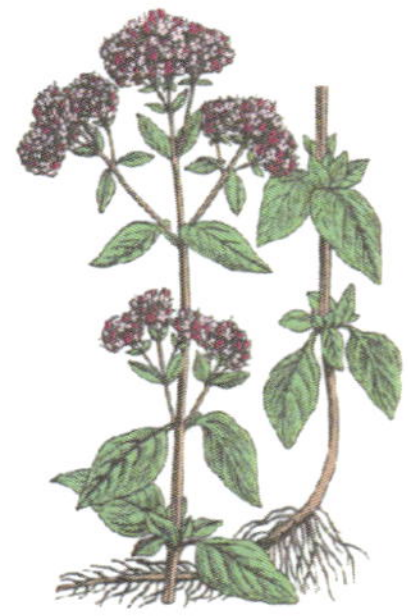
Oregano

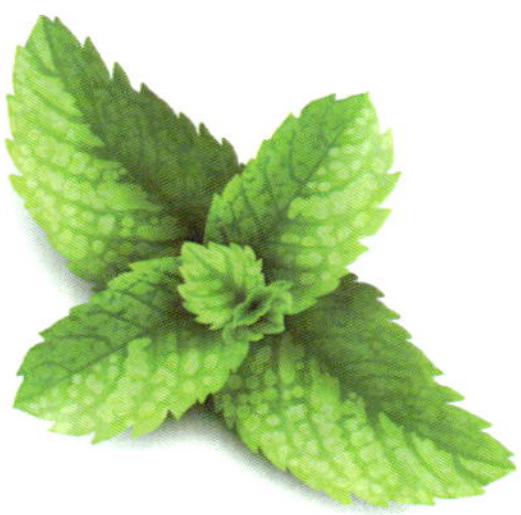
Peppermint

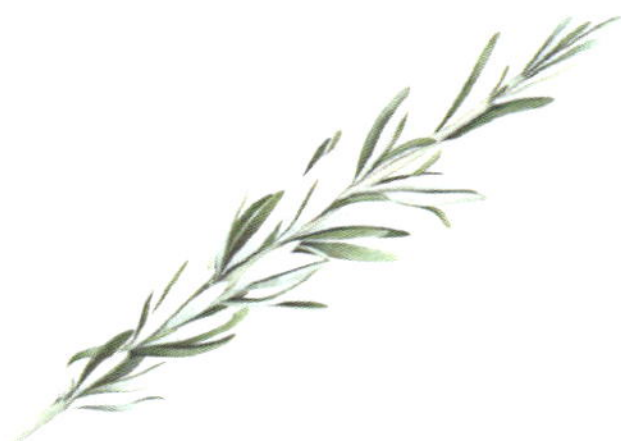
Rosemary

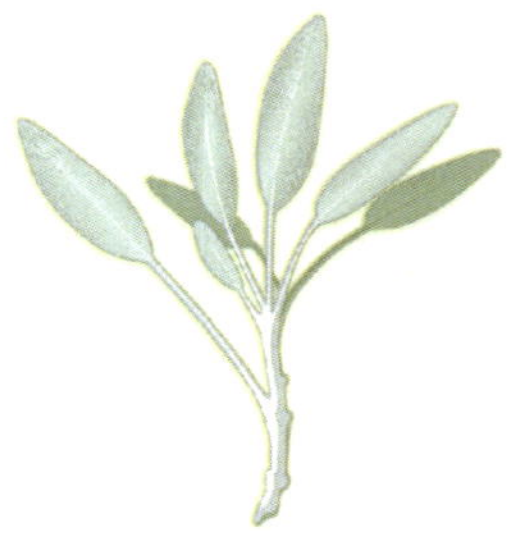
Sage

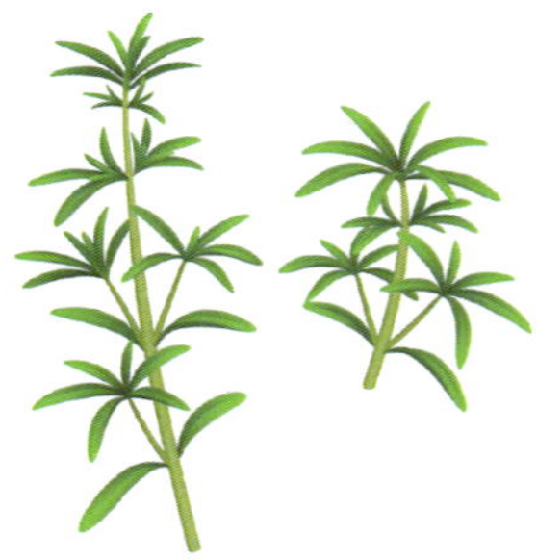
Savory

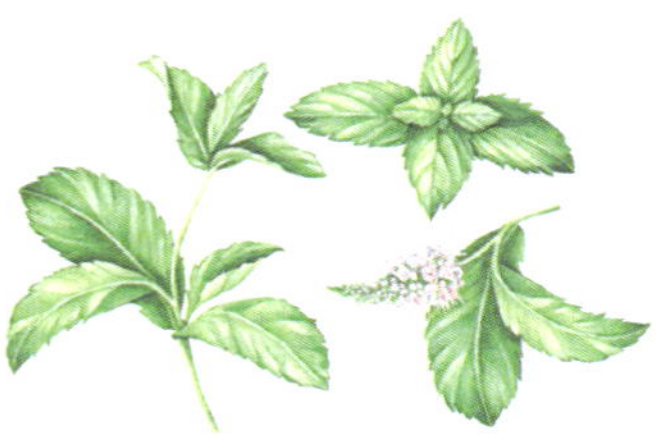
Spearmint

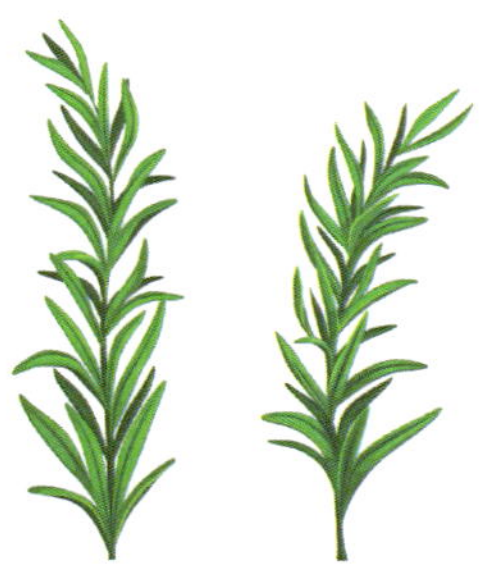
Tarragon

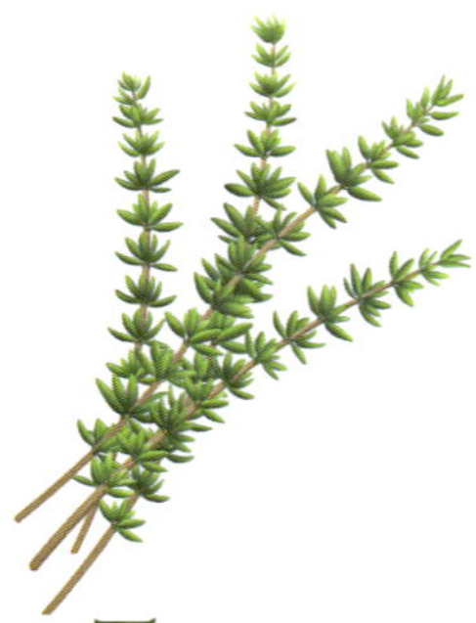
Thyme

Healing Properties of Herbs

Herbs can rejuvenate the body. Special processing is often used to obtain their medicinal properties.

HERBS	PROPERTIES	HEALTH BENEFITS
Dandelion, Burdock Root, Licorice	Alterative	Neutralizes toxins, cleanses the blood
Turmeric, Lavender, Clove	Analgesic	Relieves pain
Chamomile, Fennel Seed, Kelp	Antacid	Reduces excess acidity
Elderberry, Fenugreek, Caraway Seed	Anti-catarrhal	Decreases mucus
Pineapple, Basil, Lemon Balm	Antipyretic	Cools, reduces fever
Garlic, Oregano, Sage	Antiseptic	Kills pathogenic microbes
Anise, Cumin, Fennel	Carminative	Relieves flatulence
Artichoke, Beet, Gentian	Cholagogue	Promotes discharge of bile into the small intestine
Slippery Elm, Sea/Irish Moss, Flax	Demulcent	Mucilage soothes damaged or inflamed tissue
Peppermint, Cardamom, Turmeric	Digestant	Aids digestion
Parsley, Burdock Root, Dandelion	Diuretic	Increases the flow of urine
Licorice, Ginger, Gentian	Sialagogue	Stimulates the flow of saliva, aiding the digestion of carbohydrates
Star Anis, Dulse, Ginger	Stimulants	Warms, increases energy and circulation
Fenugreek, Rosemary, Thyme	Vulnerary	Supports the recovery of wounds

Mushroom Nutrients

Cooking Mushrooms
Mushrooms should be well-cooked to destroy any pathenogenic bacteria and to enhance digestibility and nutrient absorption.

Edible and Poisonous Mushroom Look-Alikes
There are many edible mushrooms that look like poisonous mushrooms; therefore, it is very important to accurately identify them before consuming them. Poisonous mushrooms are still poisonous when cooked.

Kingdom, Phylum Edible Mushroom	Myco Nutrients	Health Benefits
Fungi, Basidiomycota Common Name	*All have beta-glucan polysaccharides that support the immune system*	
Chaga 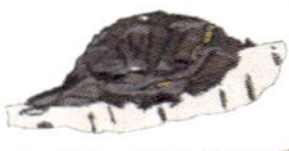	Triterpenes (botulin) Superoxide dismutase, zinc, melatonin	Supports skin, hair, and eye health
Chanterelle 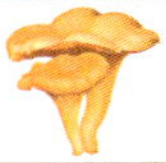	Chitosan Pyrogallol acid	Strengthens bones, increases blood circulation Reduces inflammation, wound healing
Cremini / Baby Bellas Portobello (when mature) 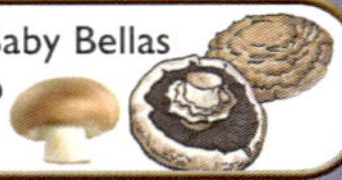	Gallic acid phenols Protcatechuic acid phenols	Decreases oxidative stress, anti-inflammatory Enhances the immune system, anti-tumor
Enoki	Proflanin Flammulin	Anti-oxidant, repairs sun-damaged skin Anti-viral, anti-inflammatory
Lion's Mane 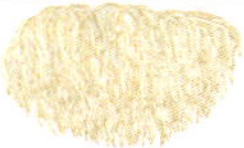	Erinacenes Hericenones	Neuro-protective, improves cognitive function Alleviates digestive problems, anti-tumor
Maitake 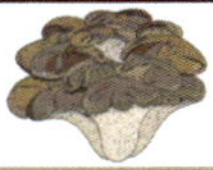	Grifolan Proteoglucan	Adaptogenic, anti-viral, anti-tumor Aids in metabolism and regulation of blood sugar
Oyster 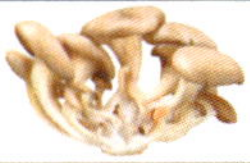	Lovastatin Pleuran	Calms the nervous system Anti-tumor, anti-inflammatory
Porcini 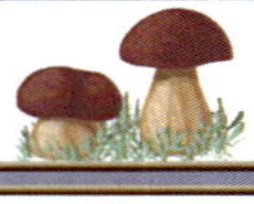	Ergothioneine Glutathione	Protects mitochondria from oxidative stress Detoxes tissues, inter-cellular anti-oxidant
Reishi 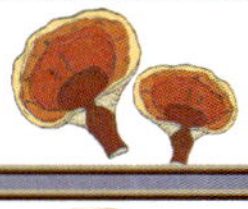	Triterpenes Ganoderans	Improves circulation, sleep, and mental capacity Supports respiratory system
Shiitake 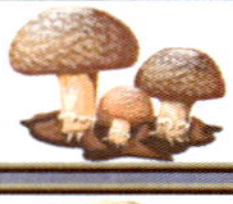	Lentinan Eritadenine	Detoxifies, guards against infection Protects cardiovascular system
Turkey Tail Blue 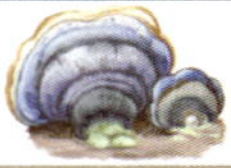	Krestin polysaccharides Peptide polysaccharides	Supports bone marrow regeneration, anti-tumor Heals infections, kidney and liver tonic

Fungi, Ascomycota Common Name	*All have beta-glucan polysaccharides that support the immune system*	
Morel 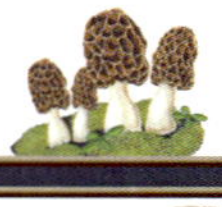	Ergosterols and tocopherols Succinic acid	Maintains digestive health, resists infection Cardiovascular-protective, anti-inflammatory
Truffle 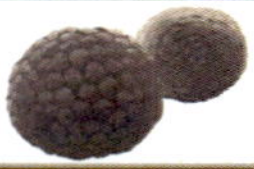	Phenolics, terpenoids Anandamide	Anti-oxidant, neurotransmitters, Endocannabinoid enzymes support homeostasis

Colors and Hues of Protective Algae Nutrients

Algae Color Groups Kingdom, Phylum	Algal Nutrients	Health Benefits
GREEN *Plantae, Chlorophyta*	**Chlorophylls a & b**, **Betalain**, **Siphonoxanthin**, Beta carotene	Builds and detoxifies the blood, anti-tumor, wound healing
	Indole alkaloids (caulerpin, hordenine)	Anti-viral, anti-tumor, anti-spasmodic, anti-inflammatory, reduces chronic pain
	Oligosaccharides	Nourishes the microbiome
	Sulphated polysaccharides (ulvans, galactans, xylans, mannans)	Enhances glucose metabolism, reduces hypertension
BROWN *Chromista, Phaeophyta*	**Fucoxanthin**, Chlorophylls a & c, Beta carotene, Xanthophylls	Supports the immune system, anti-tumor, reduce blood coagulation
	Alginic acid (colloidal polysaccharide in algae cell walls)	Moisturizes, enhances the elasticity of the skin
	Laminarin, fucoidan, phlorotannin (only found in brown algae)	Protects against skin damage by UV sunlight, sleep aid, neuro-protective, enhances memory
RED *Plantae, Rhodophyta*	**Phycobilin**, Chlorophylls a, Beta carotene	Supports cardiovascular function, anti-oxidant, anti-inflammatory
	Phycobilins (in red algae and cyanobacteria)	Strengthens the immune system, neuro-protective, anti-viral
	Sesquiterpenes, diterpenes, triterpenes	Anti-fungal, anti-parasitic, anti-viral, reduces glucose in the blood
	Carotenoids, ascorbic acid, tocopherols	Anti-inflammatory, anti-oxidant, anti-tumor, reduces hypertension

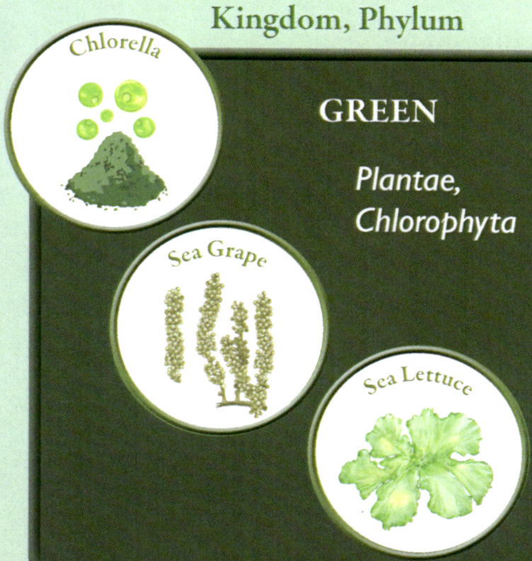

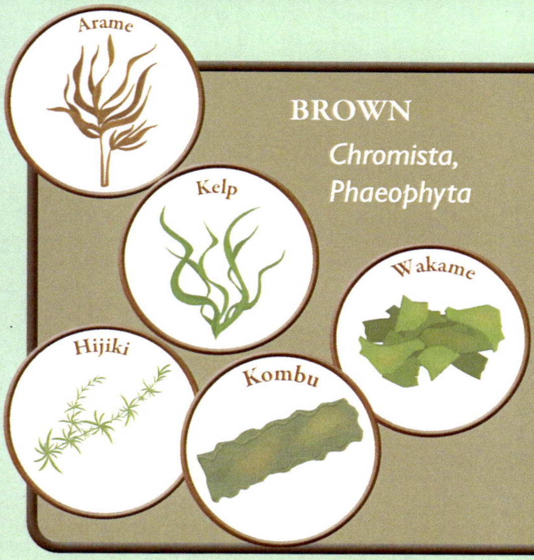

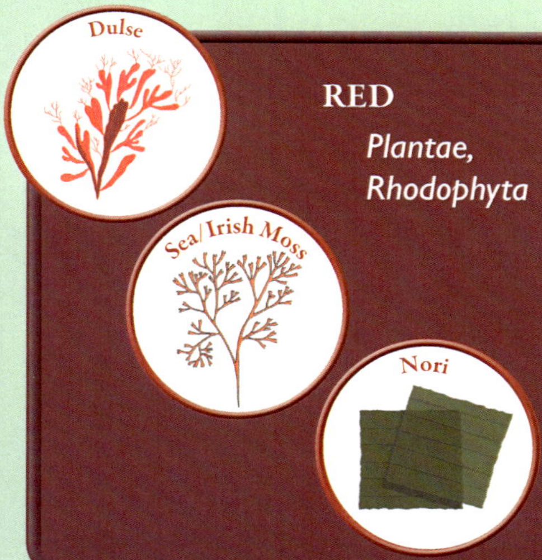

Conceptual Designer J. Kristin Little

Bacteria and Micro-Fungi Probiotics

Probiotic bacteria and micro-fungi break down natural foods and release their nutrients, aiding in digestion. They also guard against pathogenic microbes, protecting the musca lining of the intestinal tract, preventing gastrointestinal diseases, and supporting our immune system.

Kingdom, Phylum Probiotic Microbe	Nutrients	Health Benefits
BACTERIA in lacto/milk and wild ferments 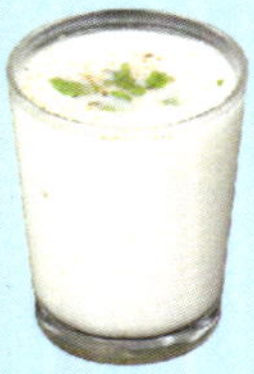 Buttermilk 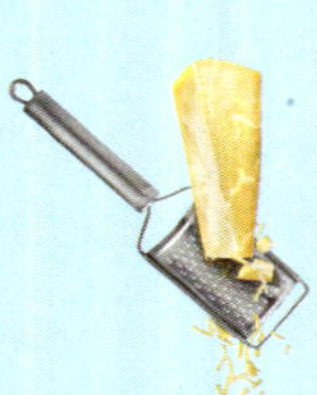 Hard Cheese 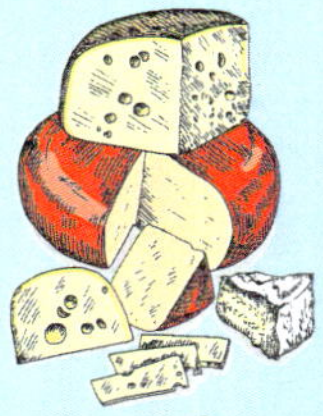 Soft Cheese 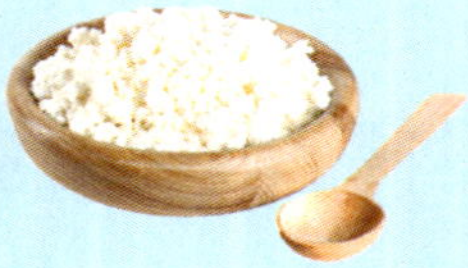 Cottage Cheese 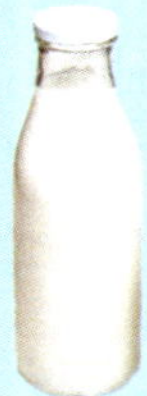 Kefir 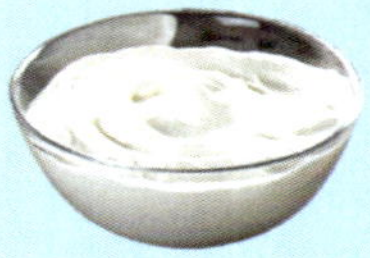 Yoghurt	Lactic acid *The enzyme lactase breaks down lactose (milk sugar) into lactic acid* 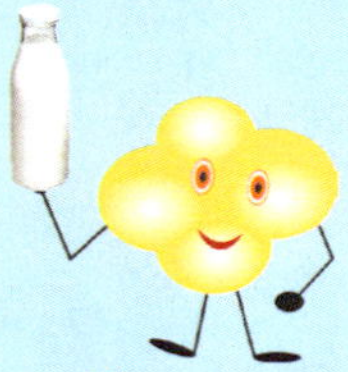	Protects and restores the integrity of epithelium (outer cells of tissues), including the intestinal lining; supports digestion, relieves diarrhea, guards against infection, degrades and helps eliminate metabolic waste
Kingdom: *Bacillati* (*Bacteria* Domain) Phylum: *Bacillota* *Lactobacillas* (many species) 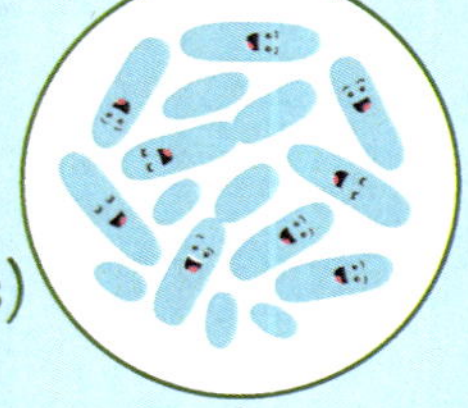	Bacteriocins	Inhibits pathogenic bacteria, fungi, viruses
Kingdom: *Bacillati* (*Bacteria* Domain) Phylum: *Actinomycetota* *Bifidobacterium* (many species) 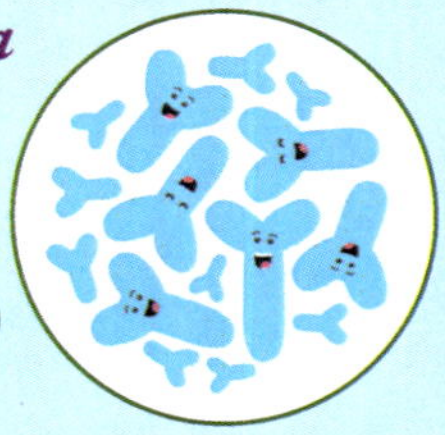	Acetic, butyric, propionic acids	Anti-tumor; cardiovascular, liver, and neuro-protective; supports the integrity of the intestinal lining; maintains healthy glucose levels

Continued...

Bacteria and Micro-Fungi Probiotics

Kingdom, Phylum Probiotic Microbe	Nutrients	Health Benefits
BACTERIA – starter culture for natto soybean ferment Kingdom: *Bacillati* (*Bacteria* Domain) Phylum: *Bacillota* *Bacillus subtilis* 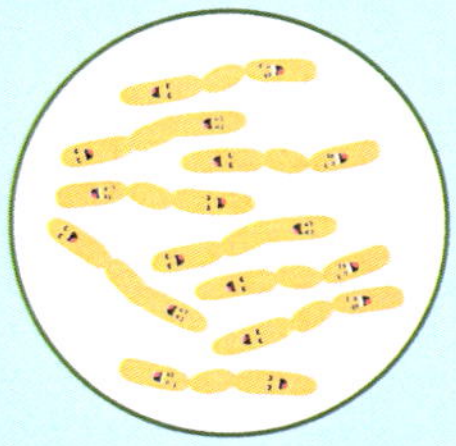 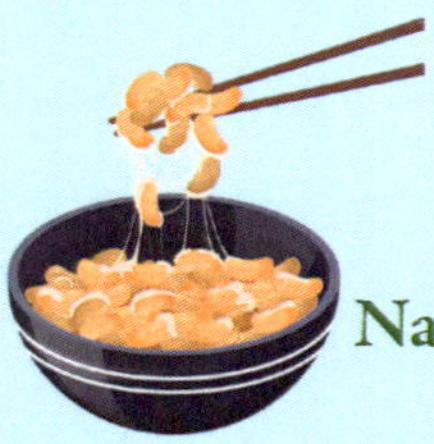 Natto	Nattokinase	Supports the respiratory system (breaks up mucus and clears bronchial tubes and sinuses), strengthens blood vessel walls, anti-coagulant (dissolves blood clots), improves circulation, lowers blood pressure - *too much can cause bleeding or hemorrhaging*
MICRO-FUNGI and BACTERIA starter culture for kefir and kombucha (Kefir naturally contains probiotic bacteria, such as generas *Lactobacillas and Bifidobacterium*) Kingdom: *Fungi* Phylum: *Ascomycota* *Saccharomyces cerevisiae* 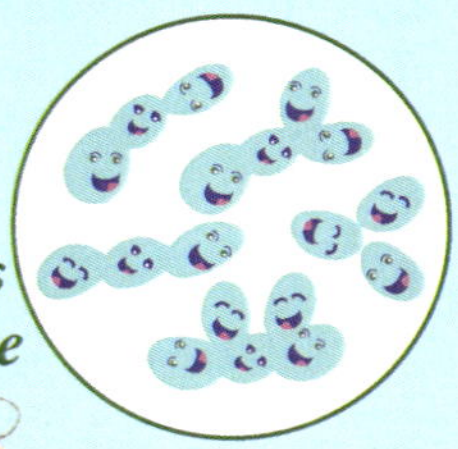 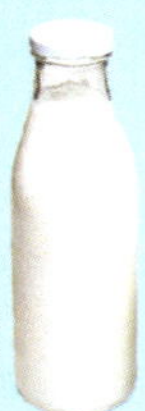 Kefir 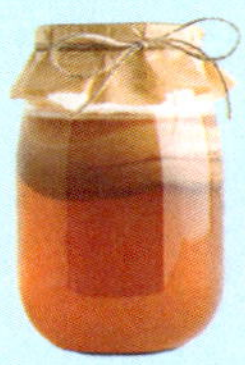 Kombucha	Acetic, gluconic, tartaric acids	Anti-oxidant; anti-inflammatory; inhibits the growth of harmful micro-organisms, including pathogenic bacterial and viruses
MICRO-FUNGI – starter culture for miso and tamari soybean ferment Kingdom: *Fungi* Phylum: *Ascomycota* *Spergillus oryzae* (Koji) 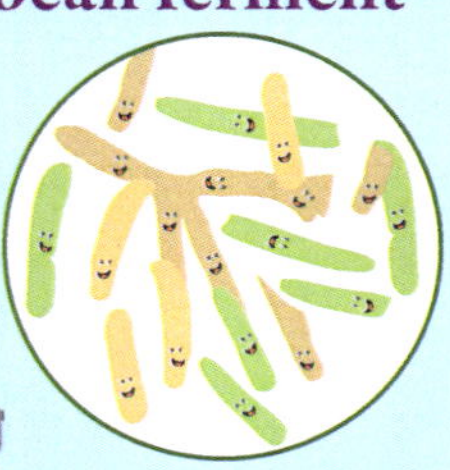 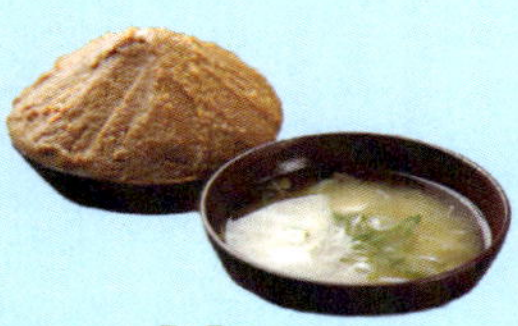 Miso 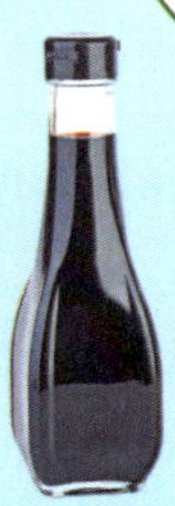 Tamari	Glucosylceramide	Improves cardiovascular and cognitive functions, reduces inflammation, protects the intestinal lining

Protein – Amino Acid Nutrients

 Our body is mostly made of protein. Once the protein we consume is broken down into its component amino acids, the body uses these free amino acids to construct the protein needed to build and repair RNA, DNA, cells, tissues, organs, hormones, and enzymes.

AMINO ACIDS — **ROLE IN THE BODY**

Amino Acids the Body CANNOT Produce

The body cannot produce these amino acids; they must be consumed in our diet.

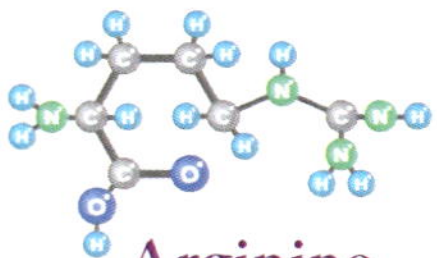
Arginine

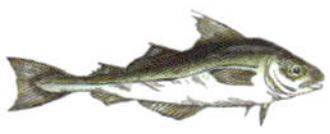
Haddock

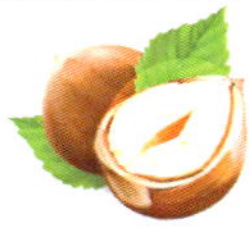
Hazelnuts

Essential for growth and development

Balanced with lysine, aids in healing wounds; used to produce nitric oxide for expanding the blood vessels and increasing circulation; and needed for the secretion of glucagon and insulin

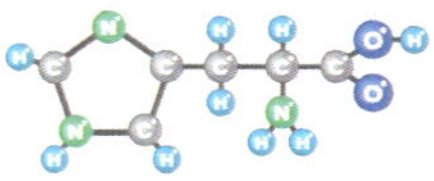
Histidine

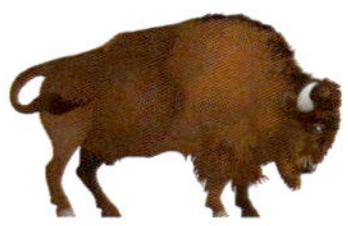
Bison

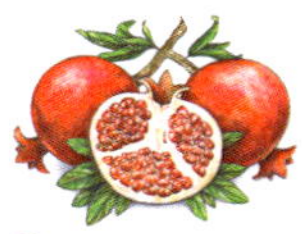
Pomegranate

Essential for growth and development

Provides a protective allergic response to allergens and other irritants, dilating the blood vessels and supporting the immune system; and increases production of HCL in the stomach

BRANCHED-CHAIN AMINO ACIDS

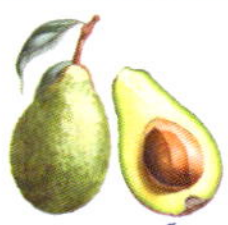
Avocado

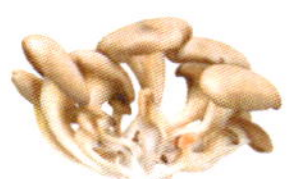
Oyster Mushroom

Maintains and repairs muscle tissue; regulates glucose; protects mitochondria; and helps synthesize glutamate and gamma-aminobutyric acid (GABA)

The three branched-chain amino acids are:

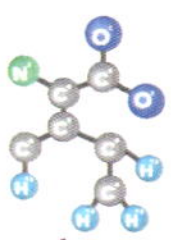
Isoleucine

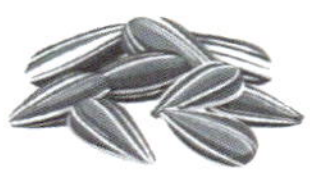
Sunflower Seeds

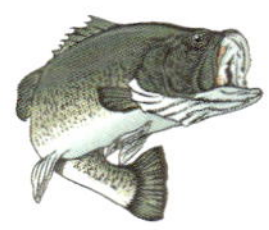
Bass

Acts as the oxygen-carrying pigment inside of red blood cells and is essential for producing hemoglobin

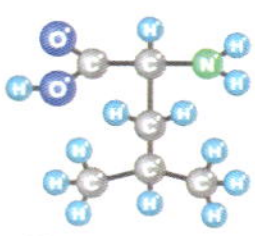
Leucine

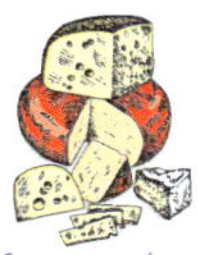
Cheese (soft)

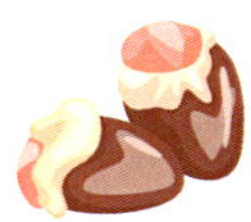
Organ Meats

Protects the cardiovascular system; involved in muscle metabolism; repairs tissue; and helps in wound healing

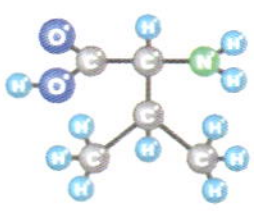
Valine

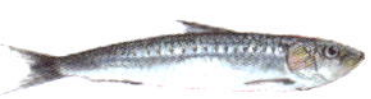
Sardines

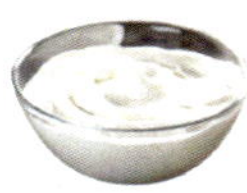
Yogurt

Supports mitochondrial function by reducing oxidative stress; and supplies muscles with glucose for energy production

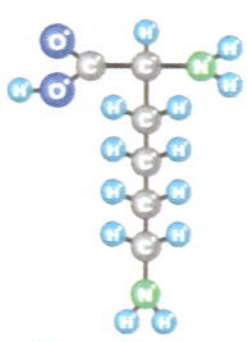
Lysine

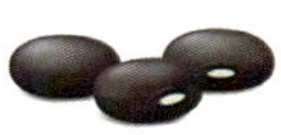
Black Bean

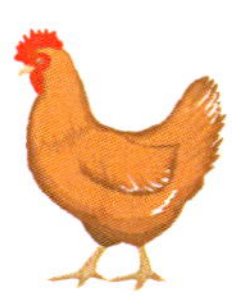
Chicken

Strong anti-viral; required for collagen formation and bone development; builds muscle; and maintains healthy blood vessels

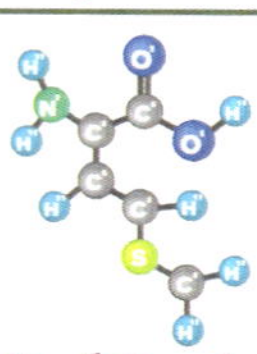
Methionine

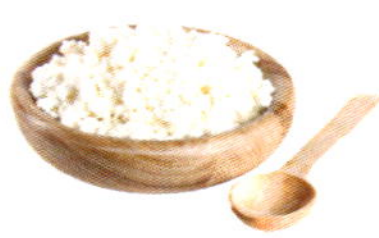
Cottage Cheese

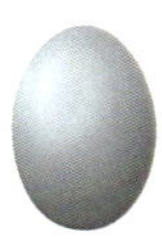
Duck Egg

Required for enzyme synthesis and tissue development; supports brain and nerve function; anti-oxidant; and detoxifies the body

Continued...

Protein – Amino Acid Nutrients

AMINO ACIDS | **ROLE IN THE BODY**

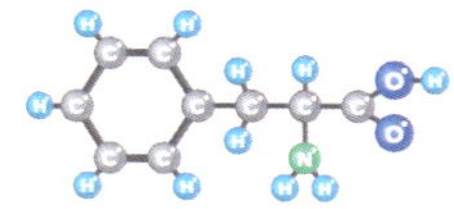

Phenylalanine

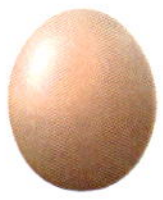

Chicken Egg

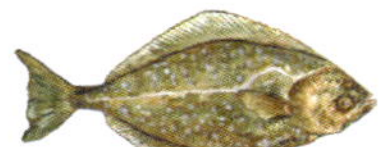

Halibut

Regulates hormones and converts to tyrosine in the liver, which is used to produce dopamine, epinephrine, and norepinephrine

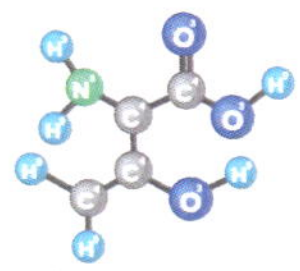

Threonine

Organ Meats

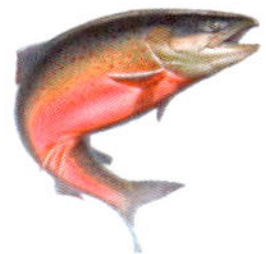

Salmon

Needed for thymus gland function; uses collagen and elastin in producing skin and connective tissue; and helps metabolize fat

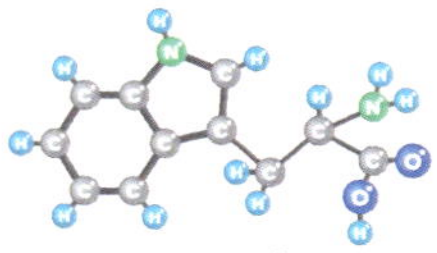

Tryptophan

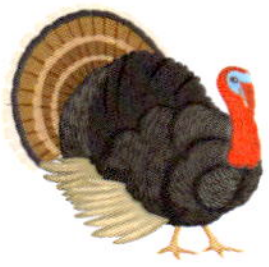

Turkey

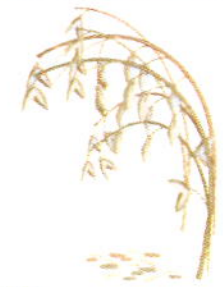

Oats

Involved in producing the neurotransmitter serotonin; regulates sleep; and helps form the pigment melanin

Amino Acids the Body CAN Produce

The amino acids, and foods that contain them, listed below, can be obtained from our diet or they can be made by the body using other amino acids and nutrients

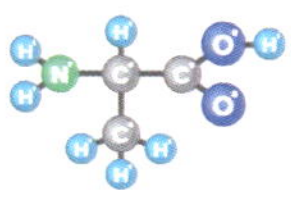

Alanine

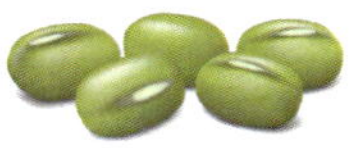

Mung Bean

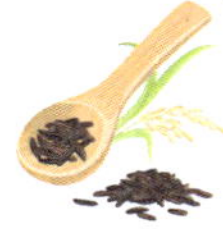

Wild Rice

One of the simplest amino acids, can be made with pyruvate from glucose metabolism as well as by the three branch-chain amino acids

Required for enzyme synthesis, helps provide energy to the muscles, and increases muscle endurance

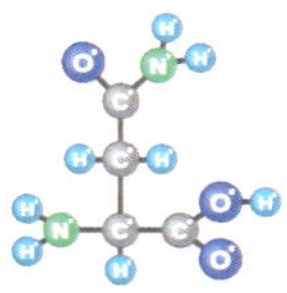

Asparagine

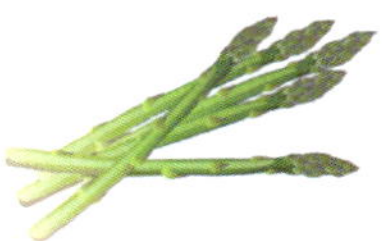

Asparagus

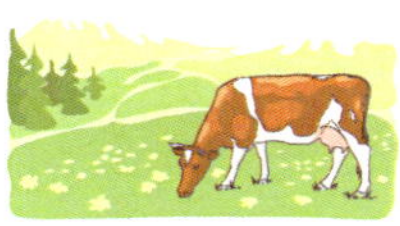

Milk Products

Made from aspartic acid and adenosine triphosphate

Forms part of DNA, essential for brain function and the central nervous system; facilitates mineral absorption

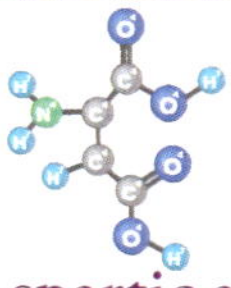

Aspartic acid

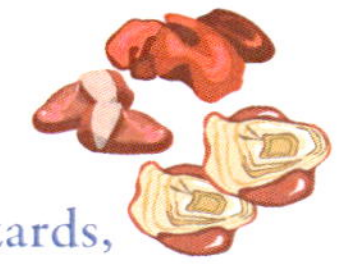

Gizzards, Liver & Heart

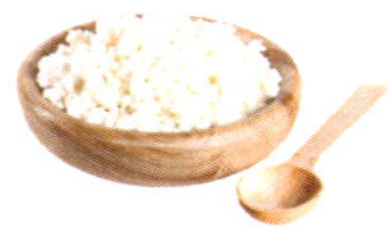

Cottage Cheese

Made with pyruvate from glucose metabolism

Forms part of DNA and RNA, needed for brain activity (memory), and strengthens stamina

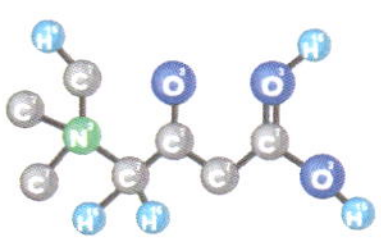

Carnitine

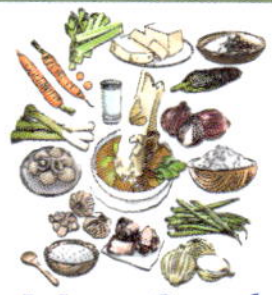

Meat Stock

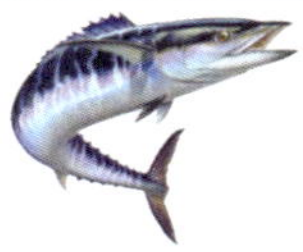

Mackerel

Can be synthesized from lysine and methionine

Transports long-chain fatty acids to the mitochondria for energy production, increases oxygen availability, and heart and lung protective

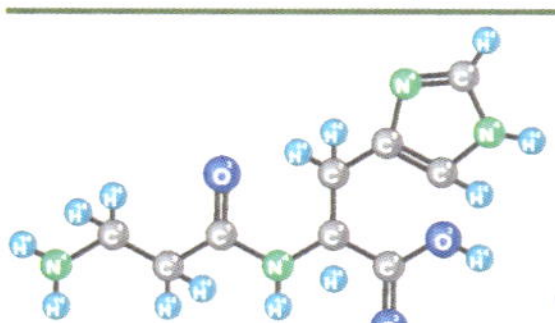

Carnosine

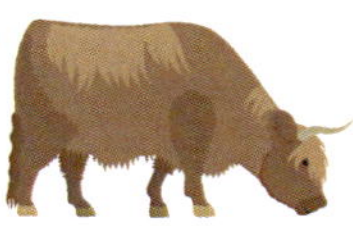

Cow

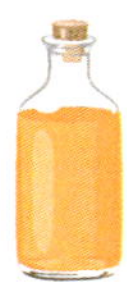

Cod Liver Oil

Made from beta-alanine and histidine

Powerful anti-oxidant; prevents cataracts; protects cellular chromosomes from oxidative damage; and enhances longevity

Continued...

Protein – Amino Acid Nutrients

AMINO ACIDS	ROLE IN THE BODY
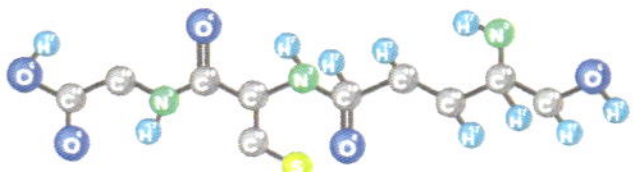 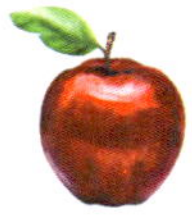 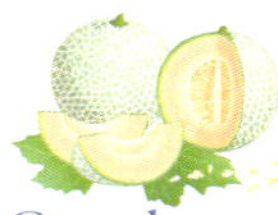 **Glutathione** — Apple — Cantaloupe *A tripeptide composed of the amino acids: cysteine, glutamate, and glycine*	Helps eliminate fat-soluble toxins, such as heavy metals and pesticides; powerful anti-oxidant
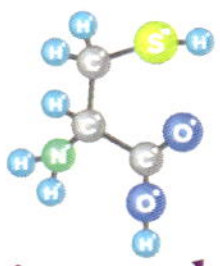 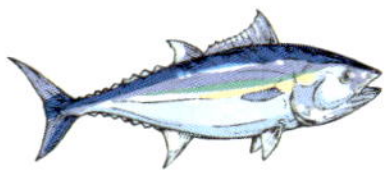 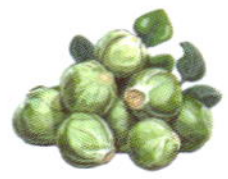 **Cysteine and Cystine** — Tuna — Brussels Sprouts *Made from serine and methionine; two cysteine molecules form Cystine*	Strengthens the immune system; increases growth of hair and nails; and detoxifies, including helping the body remove heavy metals
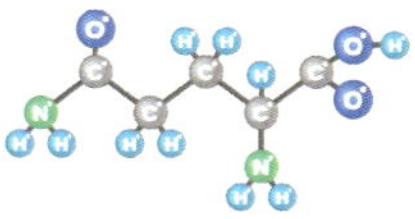 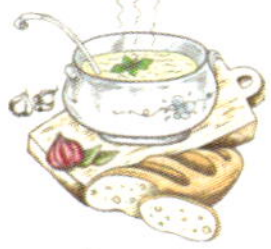 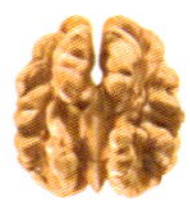 **Glutamine** — Seafood Broth — Walnut *Made from aspartic acid, arginine, proline, and alpha-ketoglutarate*	The most abundant and versatile amino acid in the body; maintains the integrity of the lining of the intestines; as part of the glutamatergic system, glutamine balances the neurotransmitter glutamate, which activates the nervous system with the neurotransmitter gamma-aminobutyric acid (GABA). This calms the nervous system, lowers blood pressure, and enhances sleep.
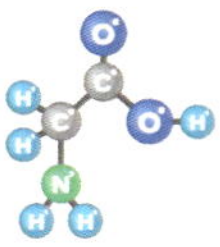 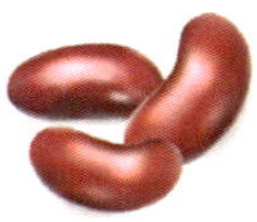 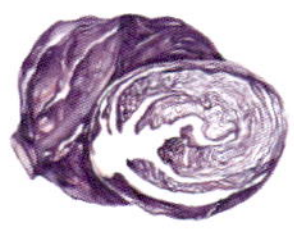 **Glycine** — Kidney Bean — Red Cabbage *Made from serine and methionine; two cysteine molecules form Cystine*	Anti-inflammatory, supports neurotransmitters, has a relaxing effect, and facilitates detoxification
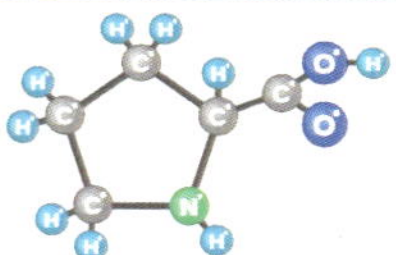 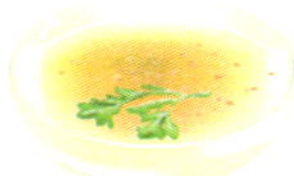 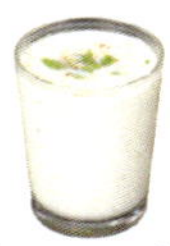 **Proline** — Bone Broth — Buttermilk *Made from glutamate, with vitamin C*	Used to synthesize collagen which maintains and regenerates the arteries and connective tissue, including the skin, ligaments, tendons, and cartilage; supports the joints and promotes wound healing
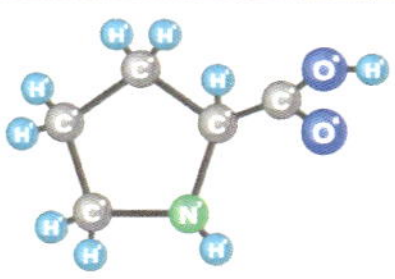 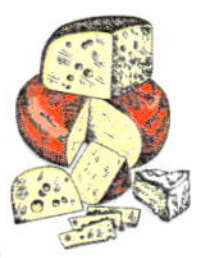 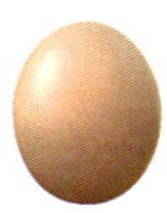 **Serine** — Cheese (soft) — Chicken Egg *Made from glycine, with folate, B_3, and B_6*	Needed for the metabolism of fats, formation of muscle, and development of myelin sheath (sleeves of fatty tissue that spiral around and protect the nerves cells)
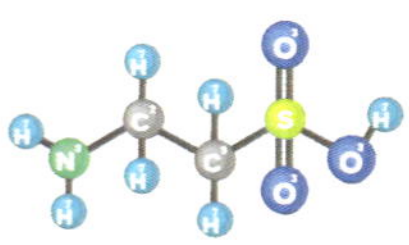 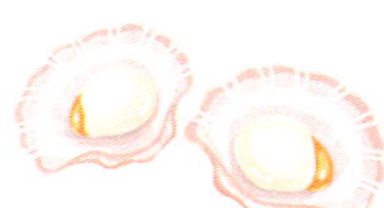 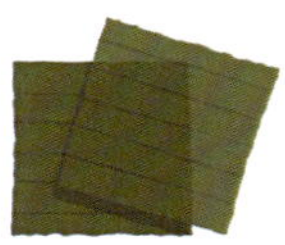 **Taurine** — Scallop — Nori *Sulfur compound made from either cysteine or methionine with B_6*	Neuro-protective; needed for brain, retina, heart, lung, and kidney function; used in the formation of bile; assists in glucose metabolism, increasing insulin receptors
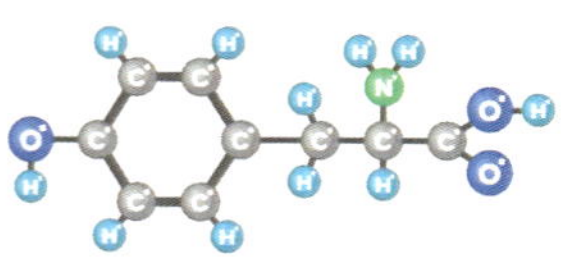 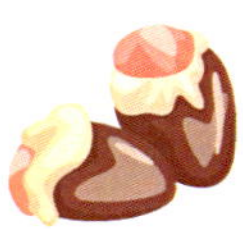 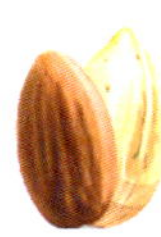 **Tyrosine** — Organ Meats — Almond *Made from phenylalanine*	Required by the adrenal, thyroid, and pituitary glands, production of melanin, and development of the neurotransmitter's norepinephrine and dopamine; improves stamina

Lipids – Fatty Acid Nutrients

Lipids are Insulating, Cushioning, and a Key Source of Energy

Lipids (fats and oils) are energy dense; one gram contains 9 calories. In contrast, one gram of protein or carbohydrates contain 4 calories. Triacylglycerol comprises more than 90% of the lipids in the body. Lipids insulate and cushion the joints, organs, nerves, and skin and keep the tissues and skin moist.

Animal fats and tropical oils contain saturated (stable) lipids. At room temperature, they are in a solid state and resist rancidity, remaining fresh and edible for a long time. This lipid stability occurs when there is molecular saturation of the fatty acids; wherein, all available carbon atoms are bonded (filled) and tightly packed with hydrogen atoms.

Mono-unsaturated lipids (fats and oils) are less stable than saturated lipids; they remain fresh at room temperature for a relatively long time (but less than saturated lipids) before turning rancid. Poly-unsaturated lipids are liquid at room temperature, molecularly unstable, and need to be refrigerated to stay fresh.

FATTY ACID NUTRIENTS	CARBON CHAIN LENGTH	SATURATION AND STATE (liquid or solid) AT ROOM TEMPERATURE	ROLE IN THE BODY
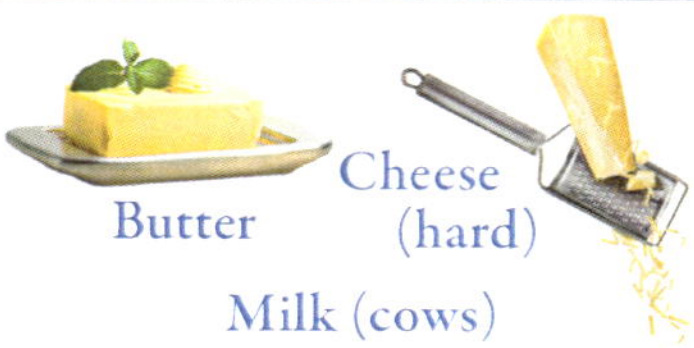 Butter Cheese (hard) Milk (cows) 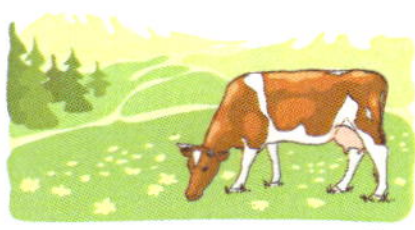 **Butyric Acid** *In the butterfat of cow's milk* Milk (goat's) 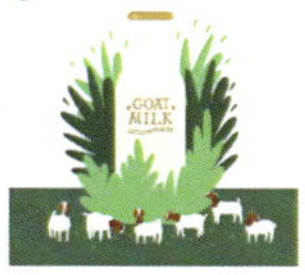 **Capric acid** *In the butterfat of goat's milk*	**Short-chain** *Easily absorbed and assimilated, provides quick energy*	Saturated, solid (stable)	Facilitates the digestion, absorption, and assimilation of fat-soluble vitamins A, D_2, D_3, E, K_1, K_2; increases the number of cell receptors for thyroid hormones; strongly protective against pathogenic micro-organisms Fights fungal infection, including the overgrowth of *Candida albicans* yeast which thrives on sugars in an alkaline environment (such as when there is a betaine and hydrochloric acid deficiency)
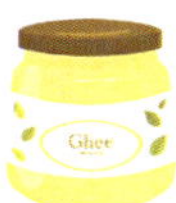 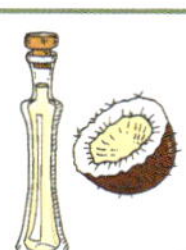 Ghee Coconut Oil **Caprylic/Octanoic acid**	**Medium-chain** *Relatively easy to absorb and assimilate, provides quick energy*	Saturated and unsaturated, solid (stable)	Protects heart function, improves the integrity of the blood vessels; anti-inflammatory; and soothes irritated skin
 Beef Tallow/Suet **Stearic acid**	**Long-chain** *Digestion, absorption, and assimilation is slow and complex (involving bile emulsification), provides sustained energy (mono-unsaturated fats are easier to digest than saturated fats)*	Saturated and unsaturated, solid (stable)	Supports brain, adrenal gland, eye, and ear functions; assists in blood circulation and absorption of oxygen; and reduces plaque build-up in the arteries
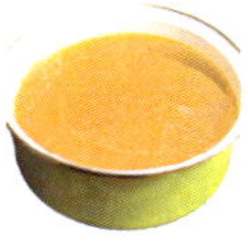 Chicken, Duck, & Goose Fat **Palmitoleic acid**		Mono-unsaturated (relatively stable)	Immune-building, enhances gastrointestinal and cardiovascular health; and strengthens hair, nails, and skin

Continued...

Lipids – Fatty Acid Nutrients

FATTY ACID NUTRIENTS	CARBON CHAIN LENGTH	SATURATION AND STATE (liquid or solid) AT ROOM TEMPERATURE	ROLE IN THE BODY
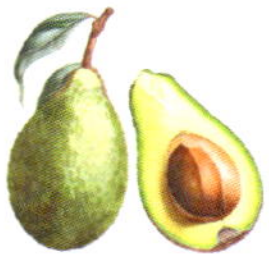 Avocado 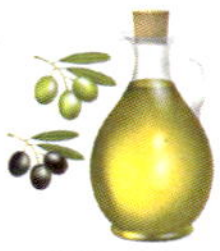 Olive oil **Oleic acid (OA)**	**Long-chain** *Easier to digest than saturated fats, provides sustained energy*	Mono-unsaturated, liquid (saturated fats in avocados make them solid) (relatively stable)	Anti-viral, anti-fungal, lowers blood pressure, improves insulin sensitivity, and protects the skin
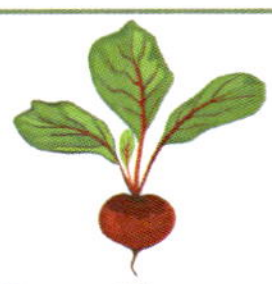 Beet Greens 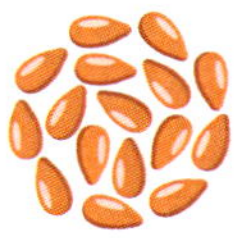 Flax Seed **Alpha-linolenic acid (ALA)** 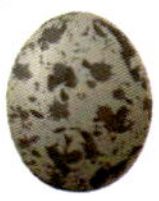 Quail Egg 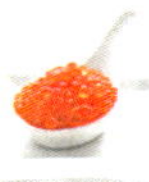 Fish Roe **Docosavhexaenoic acid (DHA)** 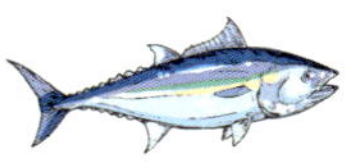 Tuna 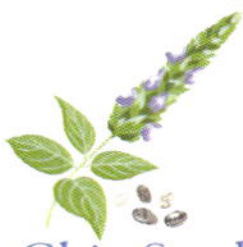 Chia Seed **Eicosatetraenoic acid (EPA)**	**Very long-chain** omega-3 linolenic fatty acids; relatively easy to digest; provides sustained energy	Poly-unsaturated, liquid *(unstable vulnerable to rancidity)*	Reduces plague formation in the arteries, lowers blood sugar, anti-oxidant, and protects the liver and kidneys Crucial for growth and development of the brain, eye, and nerve tissues; cardiovascular protective Reduces pain and swelling, anti-inflammatory, and prevents calcium deposits in the arteries
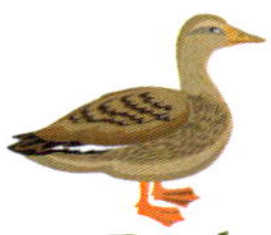 Duck 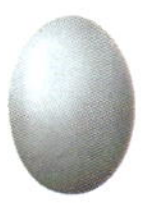 Duck Egg **Arachidonic Acid (AA)** 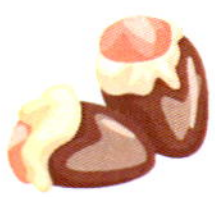 Organ Meats 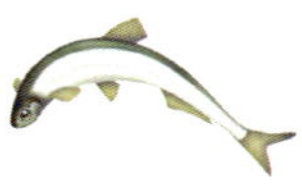 Anchovy **Dihomo-gamma-linoleic acid (DGLA)**	**Very long-chain** omega-6 linolenic fatty acids; relatively easy to digest; provides sustained energy. The body uses omega-6 linolenic fatty acids (LA) to manufacture Arachi-donic Acid (AA).	Poly-unsaturated, liquid *(unstable vulnerable to rancidity)*	Maintains the integrity of cell membranes and is a precursor for prostaglandins (tissue hormones that support cellular processes) Constituent of neuronal phospholipids, supporting peripheral blood flow to the nerves
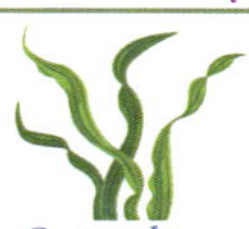 Spirulina 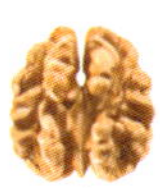 Walnut **Gamma-linoleic acid (GLA)** 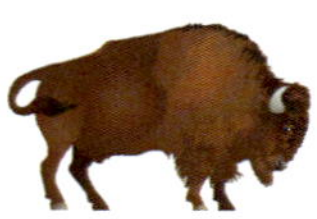 Bison  Kefir **Conjugated linoleic acid (CLA)** *Mostly found in ruminant (grazing herbivore) anima foods*	**Very long-chain** omega-6 linolenic fatty acids; relatively easy to digest; provides sustained energy	Poly-unsaturated, liquid *(unstable vulnerable to rancidity)*	Improves circulation, reduces blood pressure, increases skin moisture, elasticity, and firmness Enhances the development of lean muscle mass, facilitating fat metabolism; anti-inflammatory

Carbohydrates
Simple and Complex

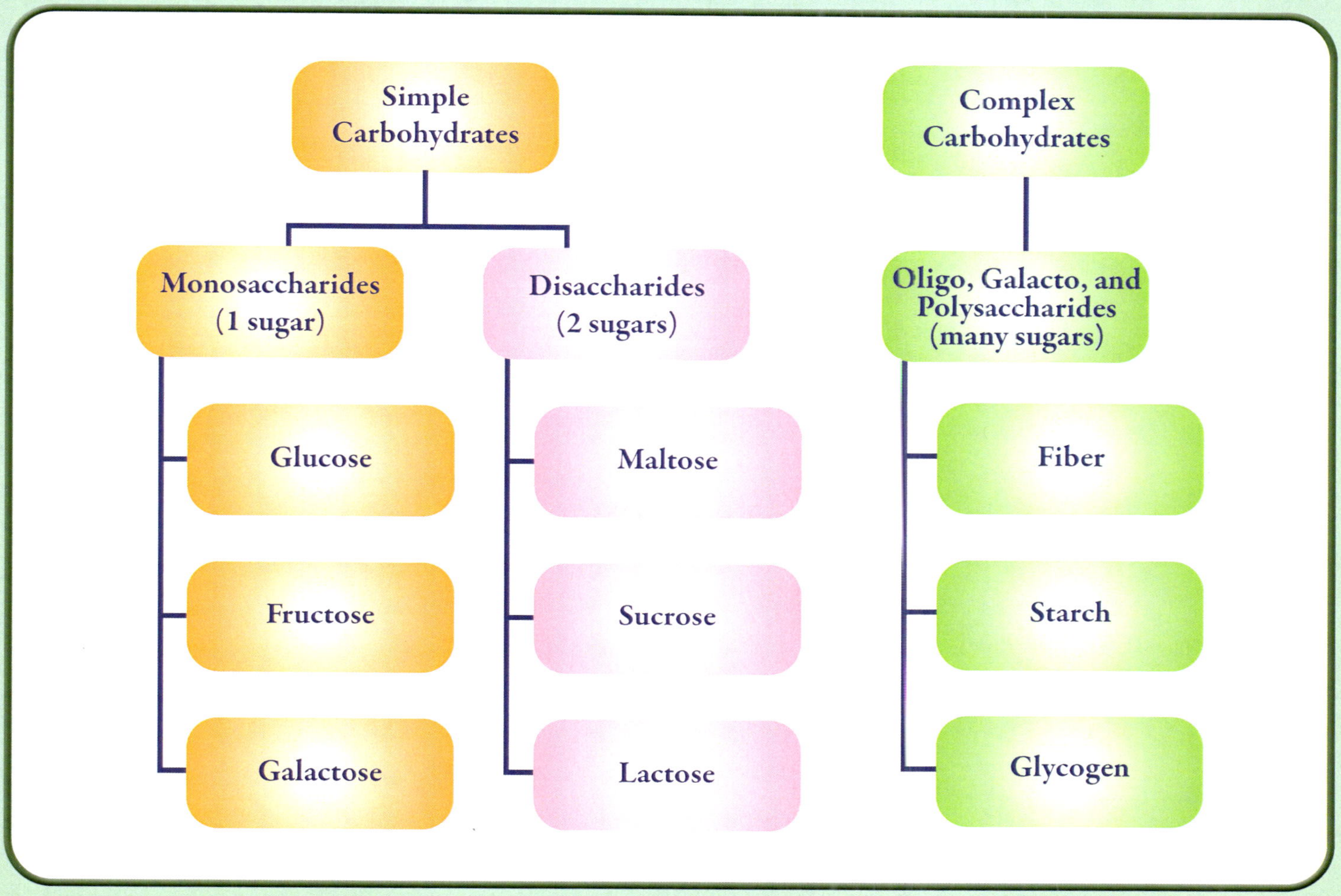

Plant and algae foods, mushrooms, spirulina (cyanobacteria), and lichens (algae, micro-fungi, and cyanobacteria) contain carbohydrates. As primary producers, plants, algae, and cyanobacteria manufacture the precursors to carbohydrates via photosynthesis. With those compounds, they make simple and complex carbohydrates for energy and to grow and develop. Macro-fungi mycelia consume and produce simple and complex carbohydrates, which are present in their fruiting bodies (mushrooms). Animals that live in the sea and on land obtain carbohydrates as food from these sources—plants, algae, cyanobacteria (spirulina and a component of lichens), and mushrooms. Mammals are the only animals that produce carbohydrates (lactose in their milk).

Continued...

Carbohydrates

Simple

There are three main types of carbohydrates: saccharides (sugars), starch, and fiber.

CARBOHYDRATES

SIMPLE CARBOHYDRATES
Mono and Disaccharides

Monosaccharides

The simplest carbohydrates are monosaccharides (single molecules), for example, glucose and fructose. Through digestion, fructose converts into glucose.

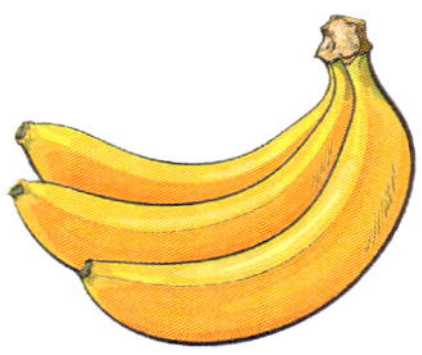

Banana

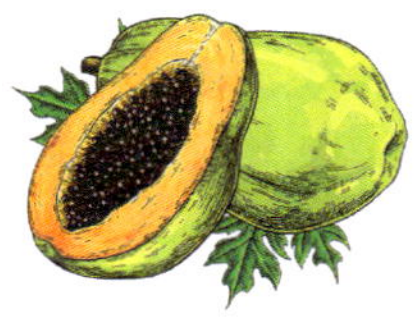

Papaya

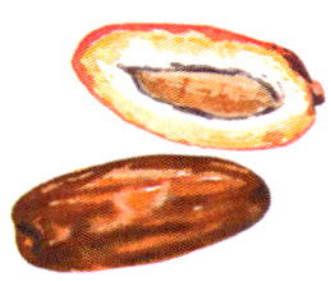

Dates

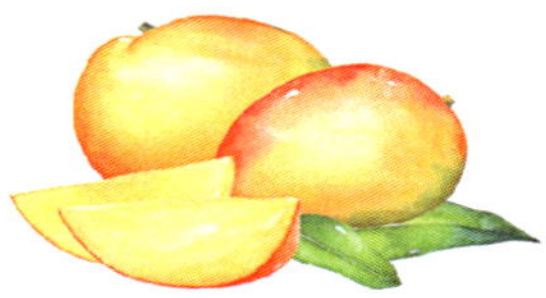

Mango

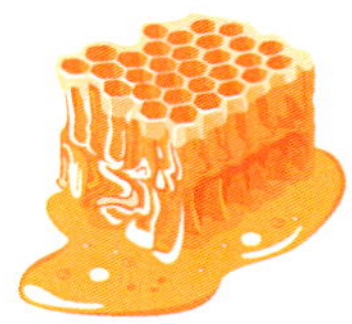

Honey

Fruits contain starch (see page 3) when they are unripe, then the starch turns to mono and disaccharides (sugars) when they ripen.

Disaccharides

Maltose is a disaccharide that breaks down into two glucose molecules.

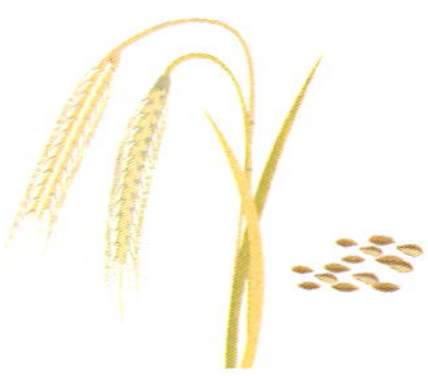

Barley

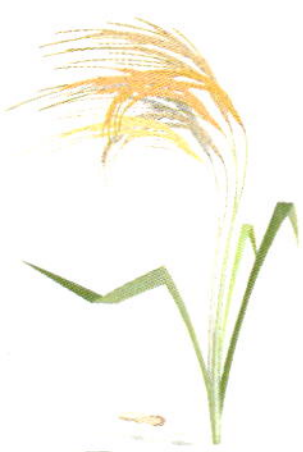

Rice

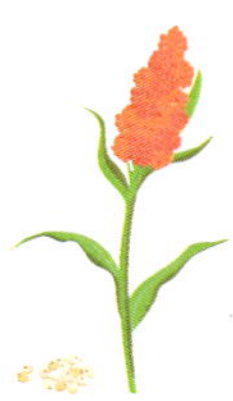

Sorghum

ROLE IN THE BODY

Fructose, maltose, sucrose, and lactose are sugars (mono and disaccharides) that break down into glucose and provide quick energy.

Glucose is the only monosaccharide absorbed directly into the blood where it is carried to the cells.

Insulin from the pancreas and other hormones regulate the amount of glucose in the blood.

Carbohydrates
Simple

CARBOHYDRATES | **ROLE IN THE BODY**

Disaccharides

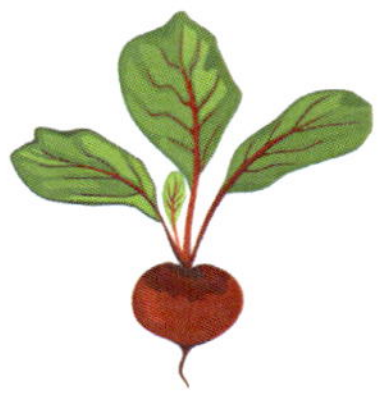
Beets

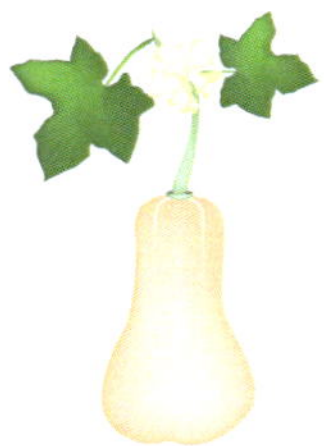
Butternut Squash

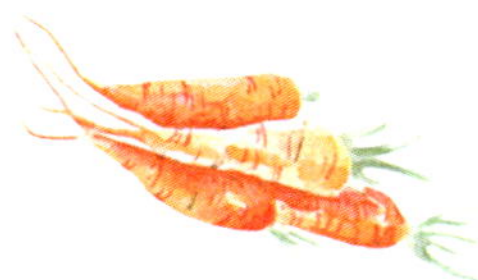
Carrots

Sucrose is a disaccharide that breaks down into one **glucose** molecule and one **fructose** molecule. These six disaccharide foods contain fiber. Some also contain starch (barley, rice, and sorghum).

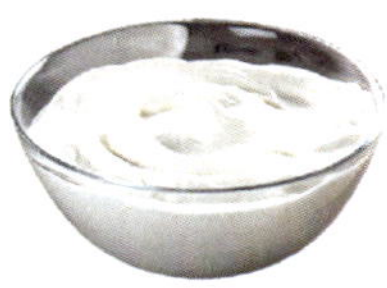
Yogurt

Kefir

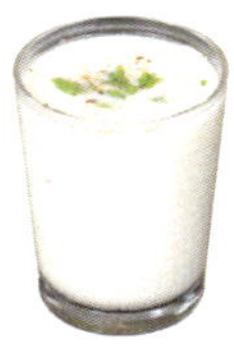
Buttermilk

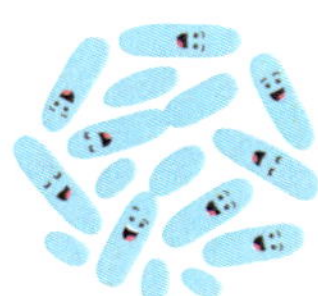
Lactobacillus Bacteria

Lactose (milk sugar) is a disaccharide that breaks down into one **glucose** molecule and one **galactose** molecule. Raw milk from goats or heritage cows, such as, Guernsey or Jersey, containing the original A2 beta-casein protein, most closely resembles human milk and is the easiest to digest. Additionally, raw milk is more digestible when fermented, such as in yogurt or kefir (predigested by lactic acid-producing probiotic bacteria that break down lactose into glucose and galactose). *Milk products have neither fiber nor starch and do not require fiber for digestion.*

Galactose attaches to:

- proteins to form glycoproteins – which become components of nerve cells
- lipids to form glycolipids – which connect cells together to form tissues

Glycoproteins and glycolipids that are present on the surface of red blood cells characterizes blood type O, A, B, or AB.

Continued...

Carbohydrates

Complex

CARBOHYDRATES

COMPLEX CARBOHYDRATES

Oligo, Galacto, and Polysaccharides are Simple Carbohydrates (mono and disaccharides) Linked Together

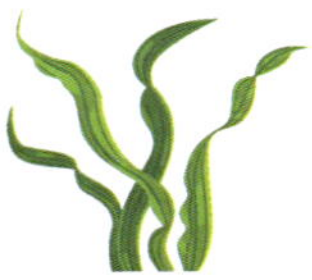

Spirulina

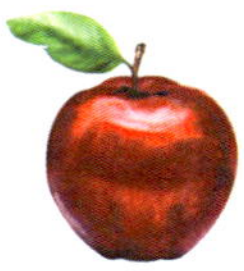

Apple

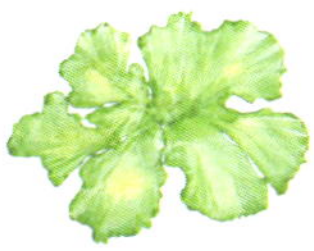

Sea Lettuce

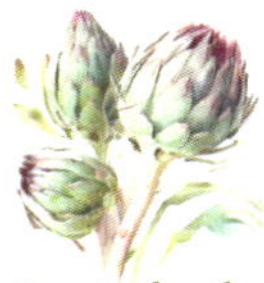

Artichoke

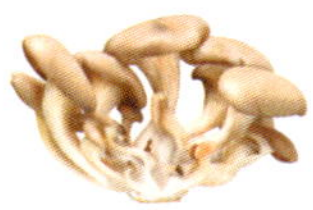

Oyster Mushroom

Fiber is non-starch. It is made of oligosaccharides (three to ten saccharides) and polysaccharides (ten or more saccharides). The foods above contain the following types of fiber: fructo-oligosaccharides (prebiotics), pectin, and cellulose.

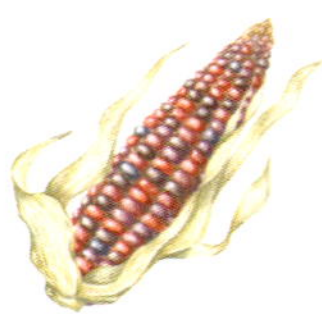

Corn

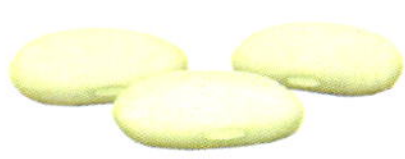

Lima Bean

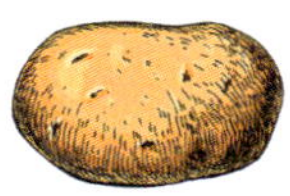

Potato

Starch is composed of **Amylose** and **Amylopectin**. These two compounds are present in grains, legumes, and root vegetables. Amylose comprises 20% to 30% of the starch in these plant foods (α-D-glucose chains) and amylopectin comprises 70% to 80% (α-glucose chains).

ROLE IN THE BODY

Fructo-oligosaccharides (FOS) are prebiotic. They support the microbiome and protect the intestinal lining, enhancing the immune function, slowing digestion, and lowering blood glucose levels that could be raised by the simple saccharides (sugars) or starches in carbohydrate foods.

Amylose passes undigested ("starch resistant") through the small intestine. Then, as a prebiotic, amylose is digested by probiotics in the large intestine. For some people, amylose lowers blood sugar and supports the microbiome; whereas, for other people, amylose aggravates the digestive system and causes inflammation.

Amylopectin has a higher glycemic effect than amylose in raising blood sugar. Additionally, it may cause inflammation.

Humans store **glucose** in the form of **glycogen** within the liver and skeletal muscle. Other animals, fungi, and bacteria also store glucose in the form of glycogen.

Algae and plants store glucose in the form of starch (amylose and amylopectin). They break it down into glucose and release it for energy as needed, such as, during winter when reduced sunlight and temperature limit photosynthesis.

Continued...

Protective Fiber in Edible Plants, Algae, and Mushrooms

Fiber and the digestive enzymes that break them down support digestion, detoxification, and elimination.

Alginate
Present in algae cell walls; broken down by lyase

Provides for a sense of satiety; protects against acid reflux; helps excrete excess cholesterol and bile

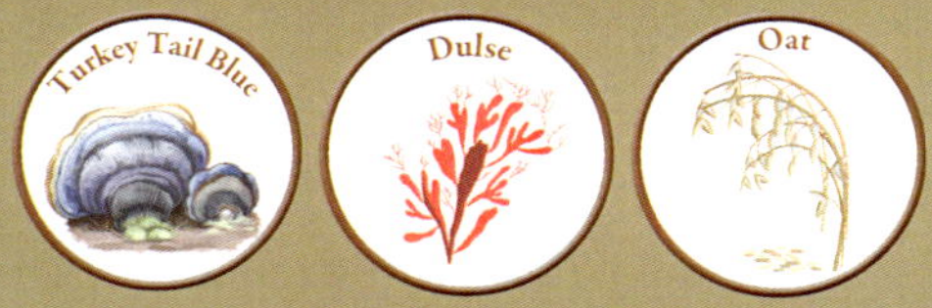

Beta-glucans
Present in mushroom, algae, and plant cell walls; broken down by glucanase

Improves lipid metabolism, balances blood sugar, protects the cardiovascular system

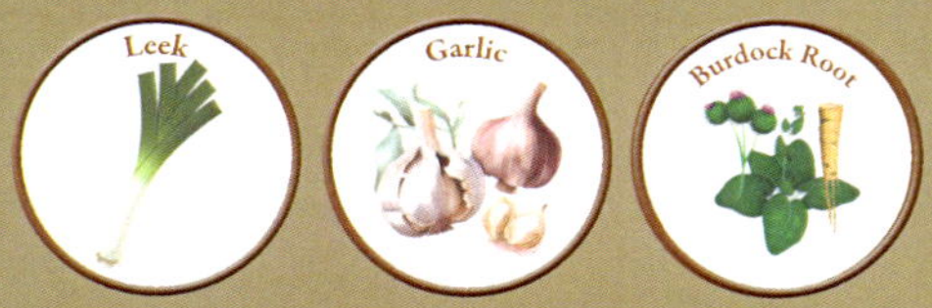

Fructo-oligosaccharides (FOS), *Manufactured in vacuoles of plant tissue; broken down by inulinase*

Prebiotic (primary probiotic food source), hydrates the stool and facilitates bowel movements

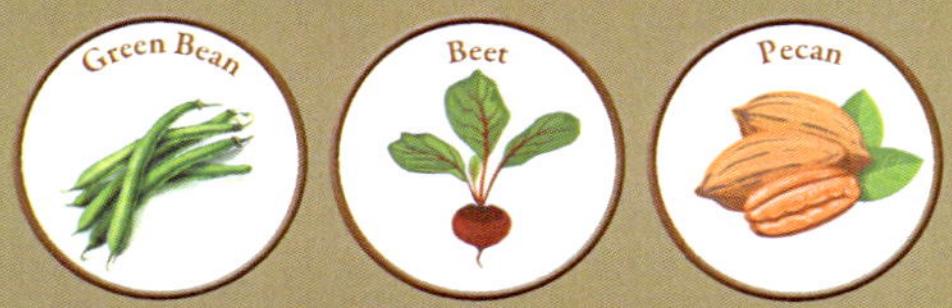

Hemicellulose
Main component of plant cell walls; broken down by hemicellulase

Reduces pathogenic bacteria and intestinal inflammation; antifungal, antiviral, anti-cancer

Lignin
Provides rigid structure to cell walls; broken down by microbial enzymes, such as laccase

Removes excess estrogen; anti-cancer; anti-bacterial; anti-viral; anti-parasite; anti-fungal (candida)

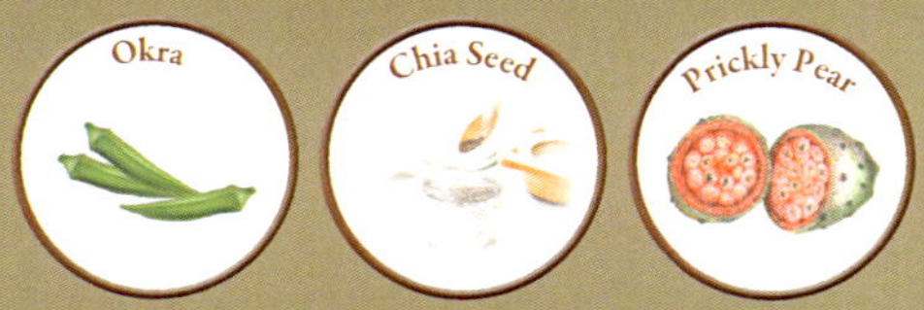

Mucilage
Gelatinous substances in plant seeds, bark, leaves, buds, cactus pads, and the cell walls of algae; broken down by pectinase

Soothes tissues, including the mouth, throat, esophagus, and lining of the intestines; wound healing

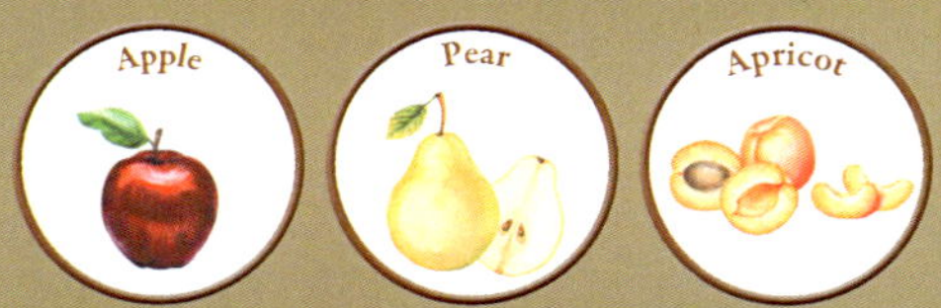

Pectin
Colloidal substance in plant tissue, especially the rinds of citrus fruit; broken down by pectinase

Improves lipid metabolism, relieves irritable bowl syndrome, binds with and eliminates toxins

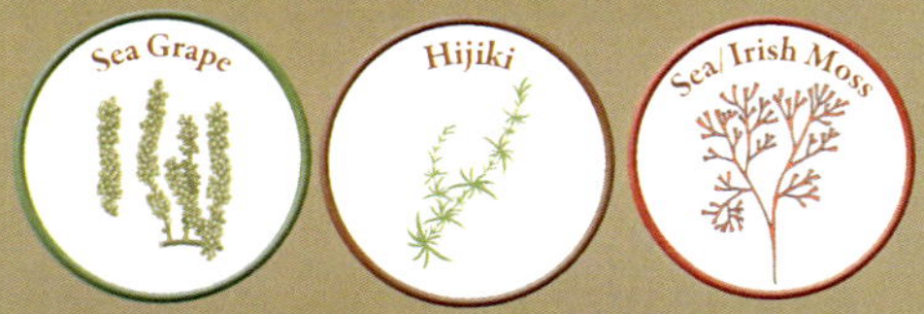

Sulfated Polysaccharides
Present in algae cell walls; broken down by phosphorylases and lyases

Neuro-protective, anti-oxidant, reduces inflammation, anti-viral, supports the immune system

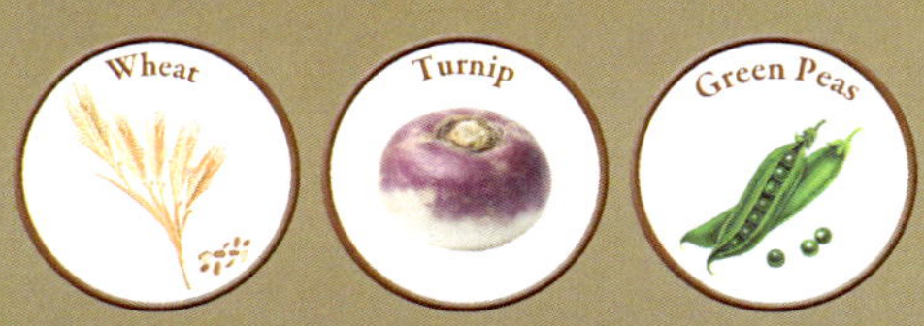

Cellulose
With lignin, forms important structural component of plant and algae cell walls; broken down by cellulase and alpha galactosidase (produced by probiotic microbes)

Binds with water, expands, and becomes bulk fiber that activates peristalsis* - reduces stagnation of fecal matter, aids in elimination, and strengthens the walls of the colon

*smooth, wave-like muscular movements that carry food through the intestinal tract

The Macro Nutrient Composition of Natural Foods
Protein, Lipids, and Carbohydrates

Food Combining for Optimal Digestion

Food combining practices for optimal digestion entail consuming:

- Simple carbohydrates (fruits) by themselves, ideally on an empty stomach (lemons and limes, however, digest well with protein)
- Mild starch and starchy complex carbohydrates with lipids (fats and/or oils), not with protein
- Non-starch complex carbohydrates with protein and lipids (fats and/or oils)

Ancestral foods were more robust in nutrients, fiber, and resistant starch (supports digestion and healthy level of blood sugar) than today's foods. For this reason, food combining may be more relevant now than in the past. Some people find the practice of food combining improves their digestion, eases their symptoms, and brings them to a higher state of health. Exploring how you feel when eating various combinations of foods may unveil what food combining practices are useful to adopt. Information on food combining is provided throughout the Macro Nutrient Composition of Natural Foods Chart.

Summary Table

Common food groups and their macro nutrient content, and digestion times based on a well-functioning digestive system with a healthy microbiome

COMMON FOOD GROUPS	MACRO NUTRIENTS	DIGESTION TIME (hours)
Animal Foods		
Seafood, meats, eggs	Protein (all essential amino acids) & fats	12
Milk products	Protein (all essential amino acids), fats, & simple carbohydrates	12
Animal fats	Lipids (fats)	12
Edible Plants, Algae, Mushrooms		
Fruits – acid, sub-acid, sweet, melons	Simple carbohydrates	2 or 3
Vegetables (non-starch), leafy greens, mushrooms	Complex carbohydrates (non-starch)	5
Vegetables and algae (mild starch)	Complex carbohydrates (mild starch, starch)	5
Grains	Complex carbohydrates (starch), protein	5
Legumes	Complex carbohydrates (starch), protein	12
Nuts, seeds	Protein, lipids (oils), (and varied complex carbohydrates)	12
Plant oils and fats	Lipids (oils and fats)	12

Continued...

The Macro Nutrient Composition of Natural Foods

Protein, Lipids, and Carbohydrates

Combinations of Foods May Hinder or Facilitate Digestion Based on Their Macro Nutrient Composition and pH

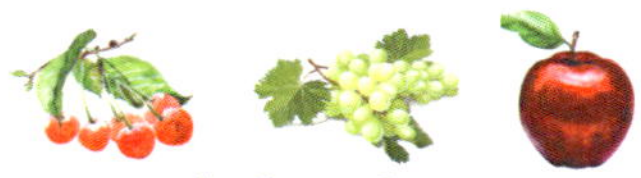

Simple Carbohydrates

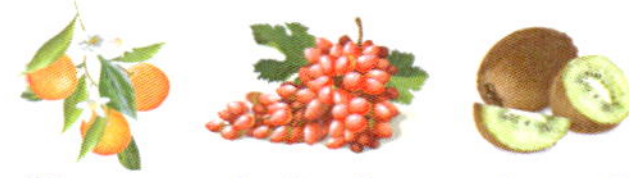

Fruits are comprised of simple carbohydrates. In addition to being nourishing, they are hydrating and cleansing. All fruits (acid, sub-acid, sweet, melons) are alkalinizing, easily digested, and detoxifying, especially when eaten only with other fruits of similar acidity and sweetness. Fruits contain biochemical compounds that neutralize and help remove waste and toxins from the body. These compounds include: vitamin C and bioflavonoids, limonene (may dissolve gallstones), and soluble fiber pectin which binds with heavy metals and other foreign substances and assists the body in eliminating them.

Soluble and insoluble fiber in whole fruits slow the digestive process and slow the rise in blood sugar. Additionally, when we eat fruits by themselves, we avoid introducing fructose into the digestion of complex carbohydrates or protein which may interfere with the efficient and complete digestion of all these foods. Low in fructose and high in acids, acid fruits, such as lemons and limes, are an exception. They combine well with seafoods and meats, helping to break down their protein and fats and facilitate their digestion.

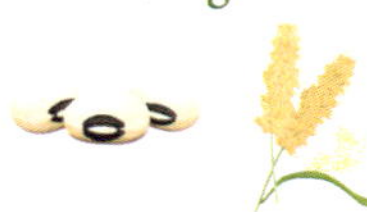

Complex Carbohydrates (Mild Starch and Starch)

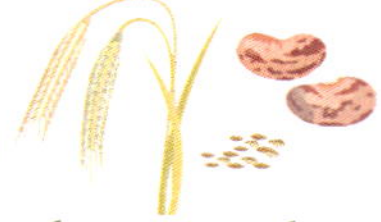

Mild starch and starchy vegetables, grains, and legumes digest well with a small amount of lipids (fats or oils) to facilitate the digestion of their fat-soluble vitamins A, D_2, E, and K_1. These starch-containing foods digest poorly with protein. This is because carbohydrates need a more alkaline environment for digestion than the acidic gastric juices that protein digestion requires.

Legumes have more protein than grains; and it is the combination of starch and protein that makes grains, and especially legumes, difficult to digest for many people. Soaking, sprouting, and fermenting these foods begins to break down the protein, lipids, and carbohydrates which facilitates digestion. Cooking grains and legumes after soaking and/or sprouting them may help to solve digestive issues associated with eating these foods. Consuming fermented foods may help too.

Blood Sugar and Insulin Resistance
Carbohydrate starches in grains and legumes can raise blood sugar and cause insulin resistance. Soaking, sprouting, and fermenting reduce these effects.

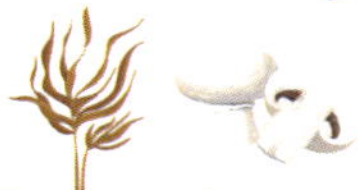

Non-Starch Carbohydrates, Protein, and Lipids

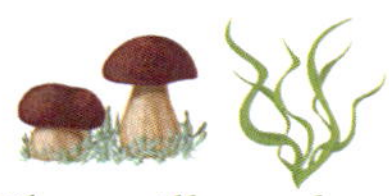

Algae, mushrooms, and plant foods, comprised of non-starch complex carbohydrates, digest well with animal protein and fat (animal protein and fat naturally occur together, side-by-side as in eggs or interwoven in seafood and meats). When milk products sit, the cream (fat) separates and rises to the top. Lipids (fats and oils) digest well with either the complex carbohydrates or protein.

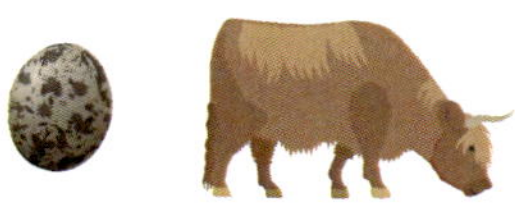

Animal Protein and Lipids (Fats)

HCL and Alkaline Phosphatase

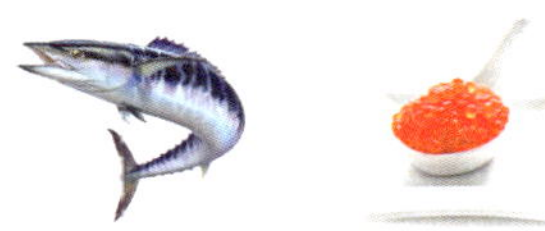

Hydrochloric acid (HCL) and alkaline phosphatase (AP) are needed to digest and assimilate animal protein and lipids (fats); and AP is important for maintaining a healthy microbiome and intestinal barrier integrity. People with Blood Type O generally produce the most HCL–*and Blood Type A the least*. Additionally, people with Blood Type O tend to have the greatest available amount of AP–*and Blood Type A the least*.

Even though Blood Type A may have lower amounts of HCL and AP, there are several kinds of seafoods, meats (including organ meats), eggs, and raw fermented milk products that contain high-quality animal protein with all the essential amino acids and associated nourishing fats that are beneficial for blood type A. Additionally, Peter J. D'Adamo, N.D. in his book, *Live Right for Your Type*, offers that "Fish and seafood represent a nutrient-rich source of protein for most Type A's. Because of this, fish is probably the best food source to build active tissue mass–especially for Type A non-secretors."[1]

Secretors and Non-Secretors
In people who are 'secretors,' blood type antigens occur in their secretions generally, including the blood and saliva; whereas, 'non-secretors' only secrete their blood type antigens in the blood.[2]

Continued...

The Macro Nutrient Composition of Natural Foods
Protein, Lipids, and Carbohydrates

Macro Nutrients In Animal Foods

Protein and Lipids (Fats)

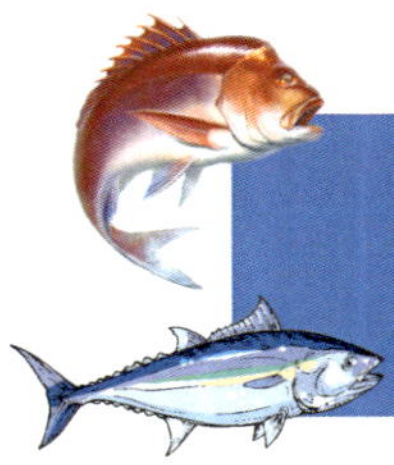

Seafoods

Meats

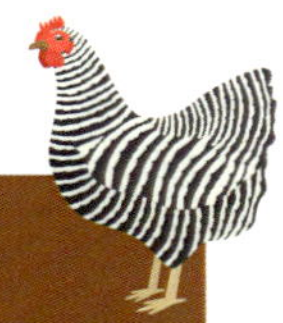

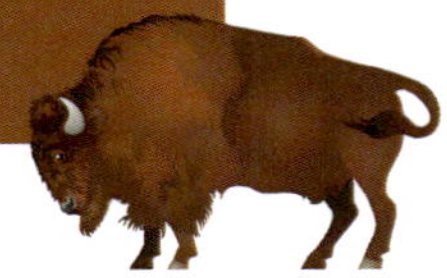

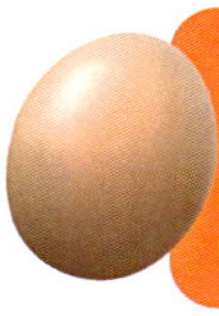

Land and Waterfowl Eggs

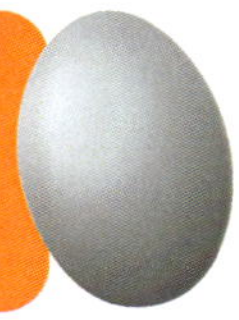

Animal foods contain no fiber

Digests in 12 hours

Combines well with lemon and lime, vegetables (non-starch), algae, mushrooms, spirulina

Protein, Lipids (Fats), and Simple Carbohydrates
(0% to 5% milk sugars)

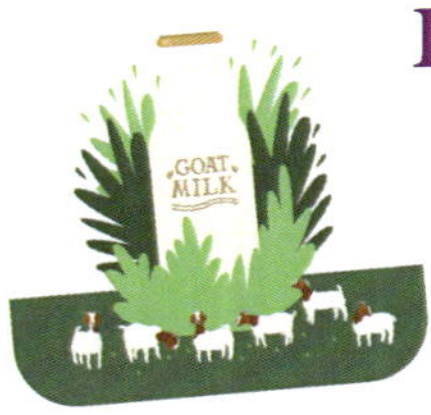

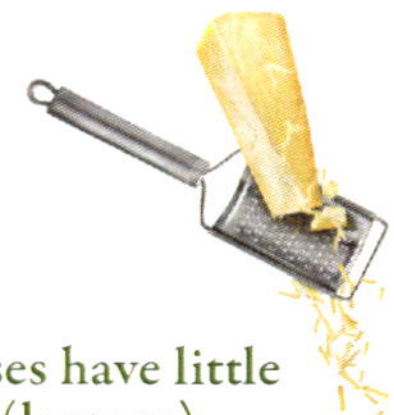

Milk Products

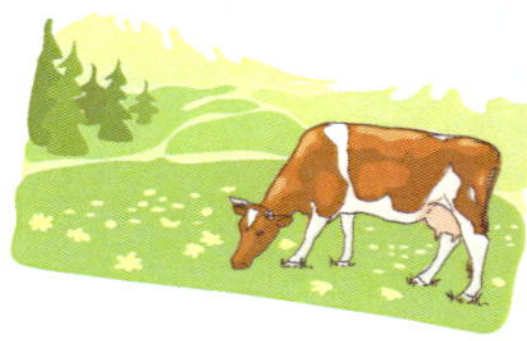

Hard, aged cheeses have little to no milk sugar (lactose); soft cheeses have more; and whole milk ~5% milk sugar.

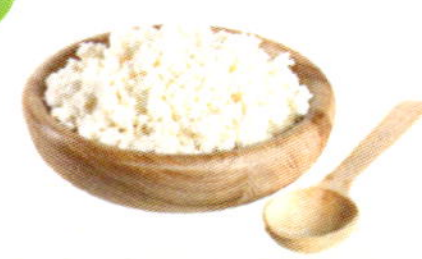

Animal foods contain no fiber

Digests in 12 hours

Combines well with vegetables (non-starch), algae, mushrooms, spirulina

Lipids (Fats)

Animal foods contain no fiber

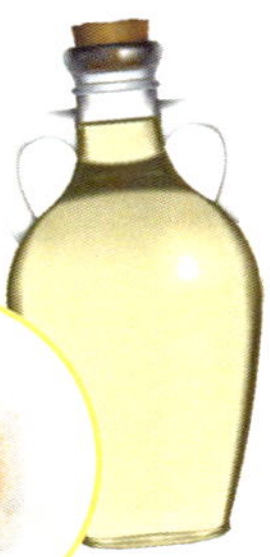

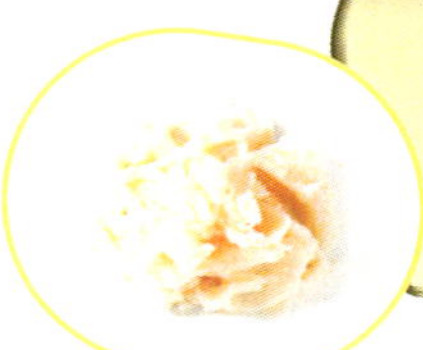

Animal Fat

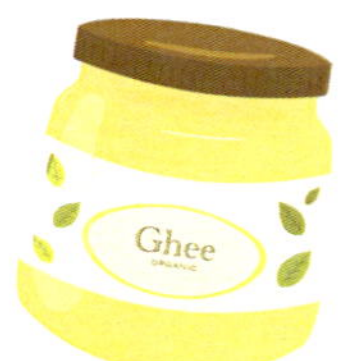

Digests in 12 hours

Combines well with any natural food (except fruit)

Continued...

The Macro Nutrient Composition of Natural Foods
Protein, Lipids, and Carbohydrates

Macro Nutrients In Plant Foods

Simple Carbohydrates
Acid Fruits

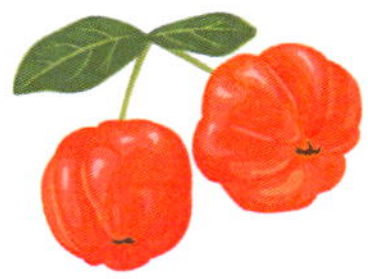
Acerola

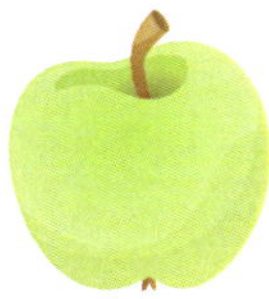
Apple (sour)

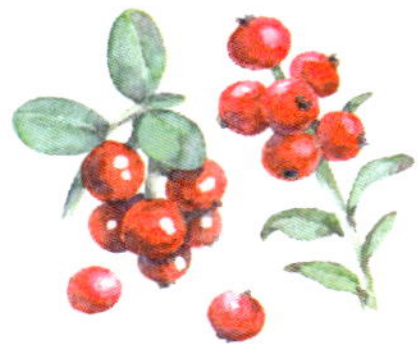
Cranberry

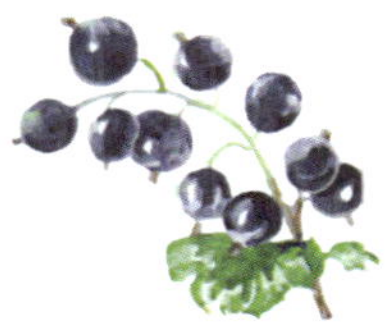
Currant

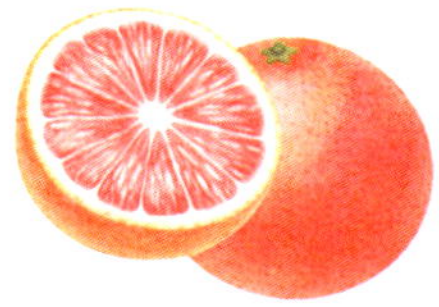
Grapefruit

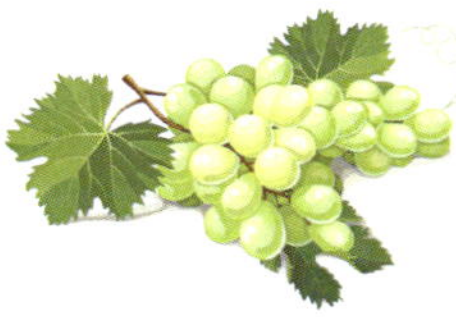
Grape (sour)

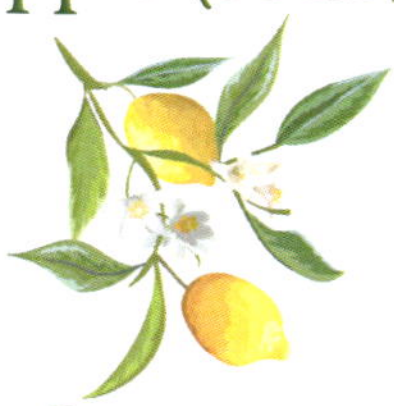
Lemon

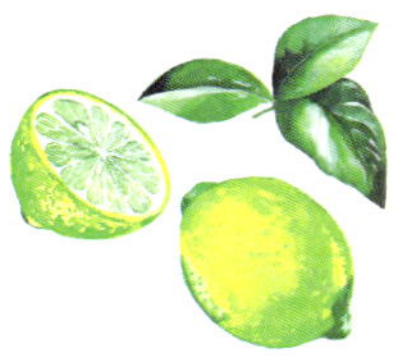
Lime

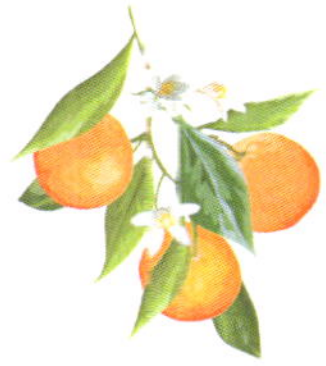
Orange

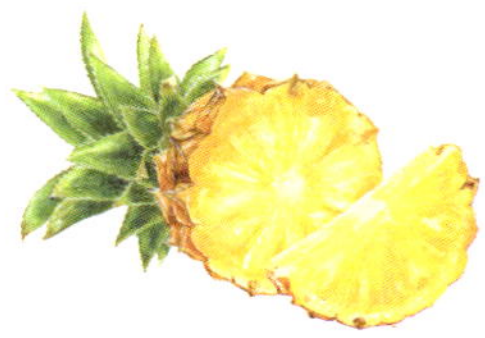
Pineapple

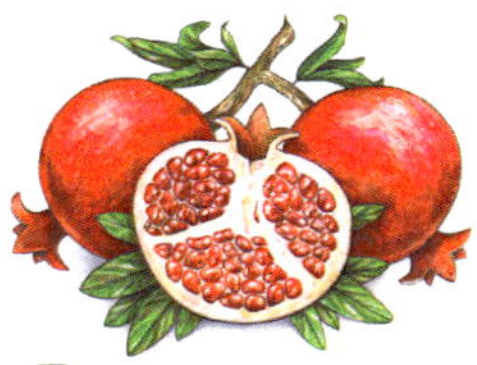
Pomegranate

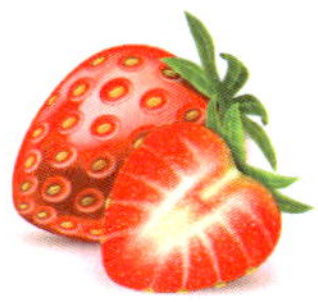
Strawberry

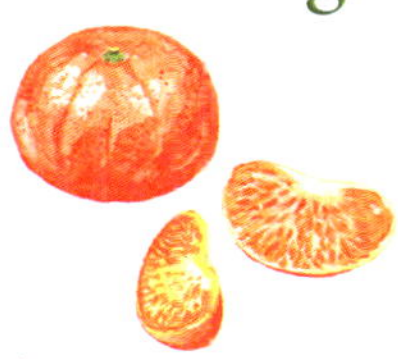
Tangerine

Digests in 2 hours

Combines well with other acid fruits, and maybe with sub-acid fruits

Simple Carbohydrates
Sub-Acid Fruits

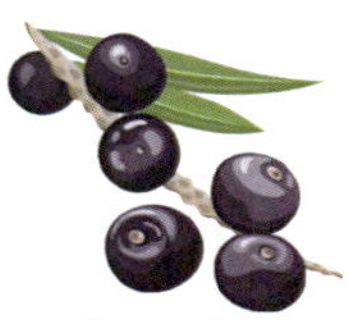
Acai

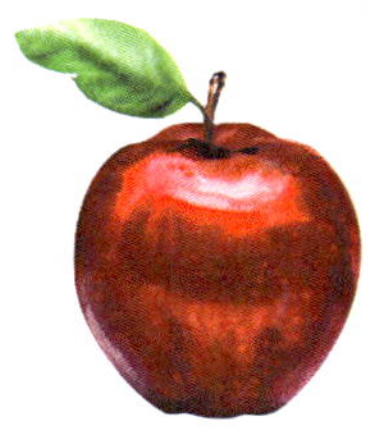
Apple

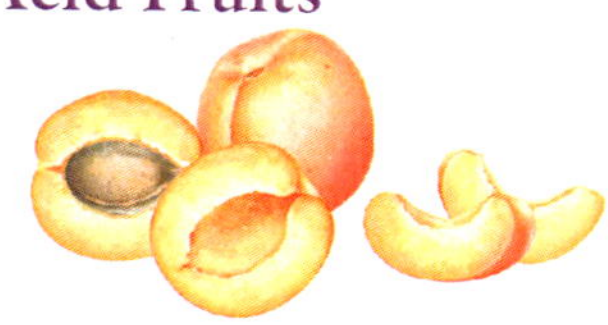
Apricot

Blackberry

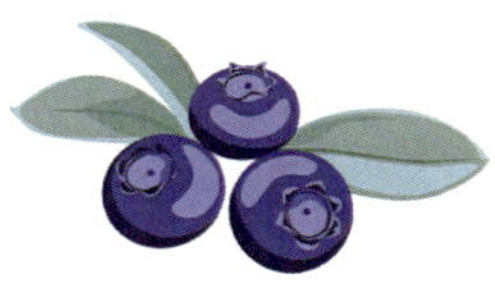
Blueberry

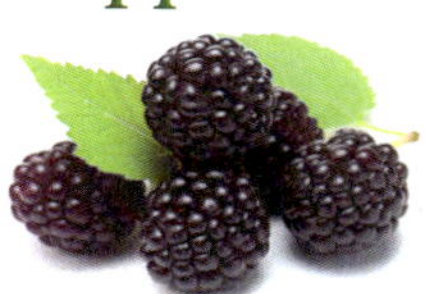
Boysenberry

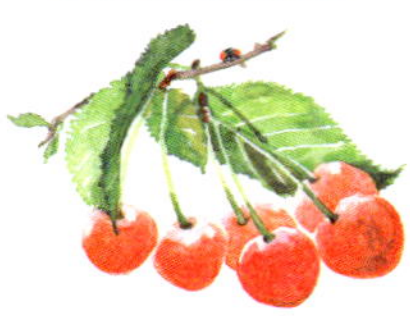
Cherry

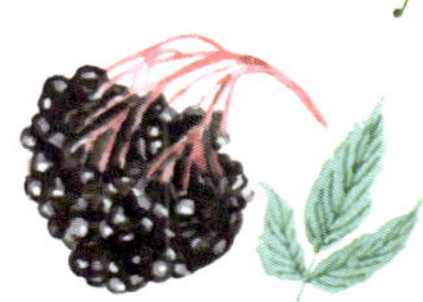
Elderberry

Digests in 2 hours

Combines well with other sub-acid fruits, and maybe either acid or sweet fruits but not both

Continued...

The Macro Nutrient Composition of Natural Foods

Protein, Lipids, and Carbohydrates

Macro Nutrients In Plant Foods

Simple Carbohydrates

Sub-Acid Fruits

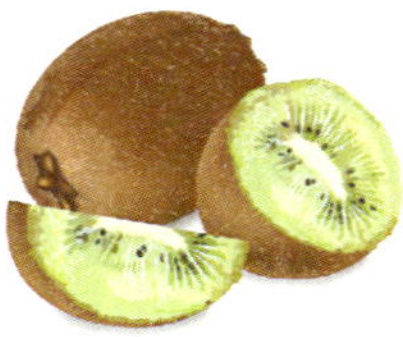

Kiwi

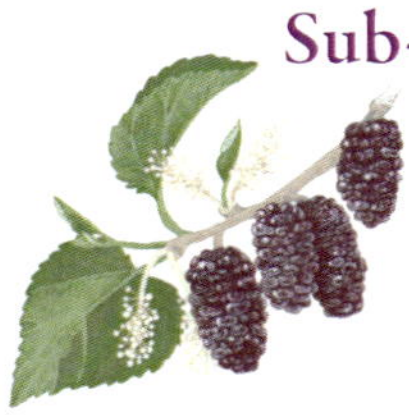

Mulberry

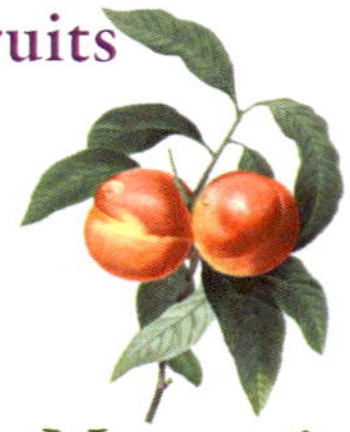

Nectarine

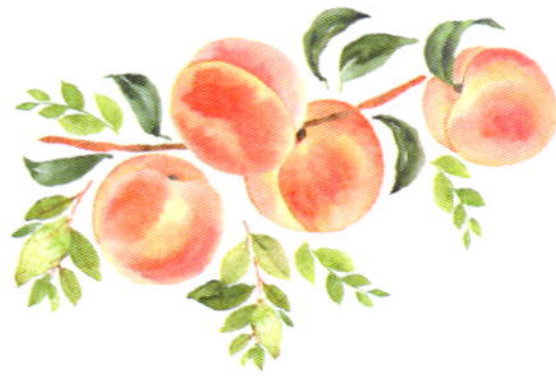

Peach

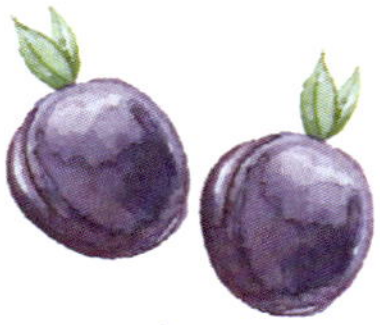

Plum

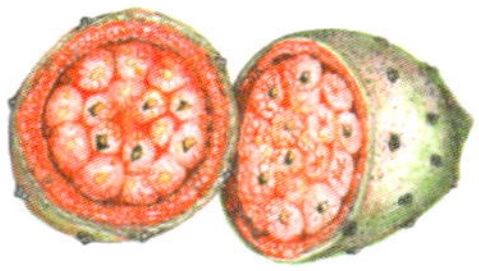

Prickly Pear

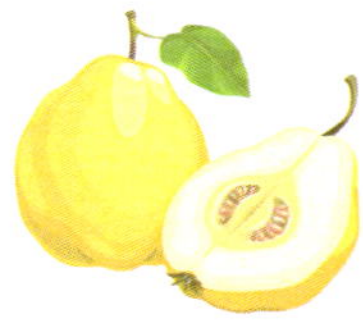

Quince

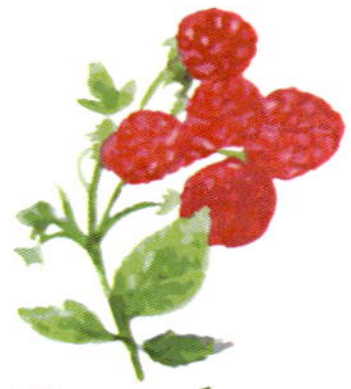

Raspberry

Digests in 2 hours

Combines well with other sub-acid fruits, and maybe either acid or sweet fruits but not both

Simple Carbohydrates

Sweet Fruits

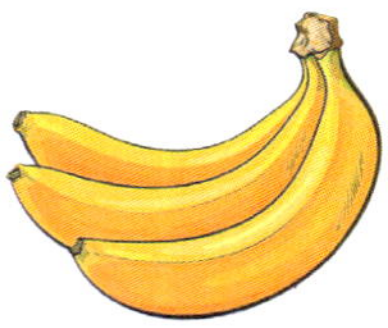

Banana

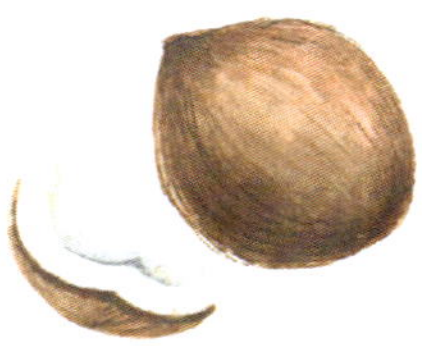

Coconut

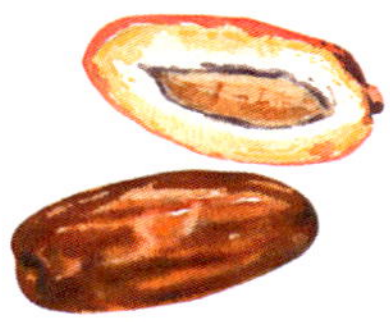

Date

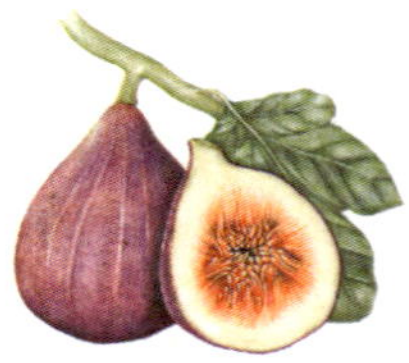

Fig

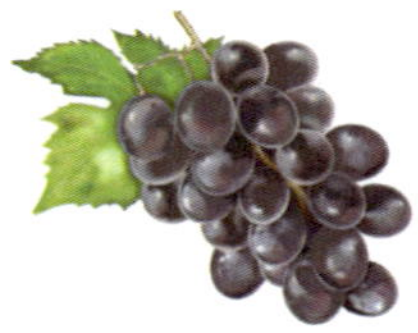

Grape

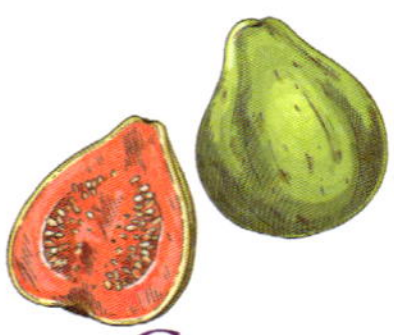

Guava

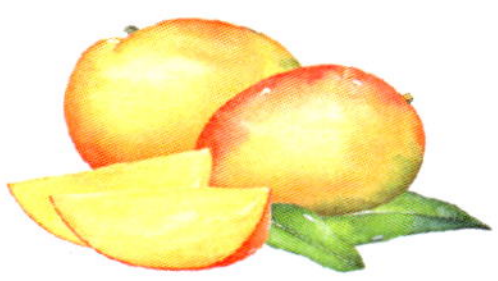

Mango

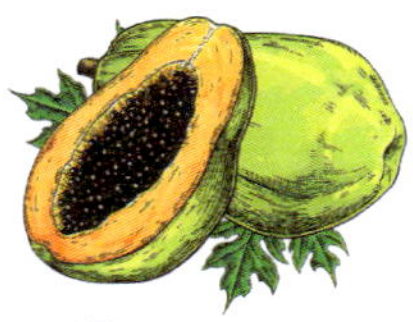

Papaya

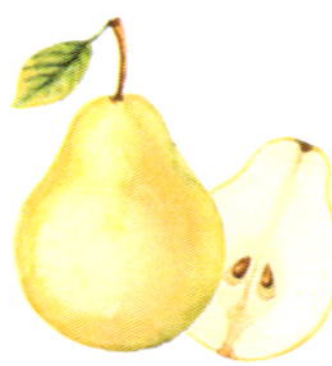

Pear

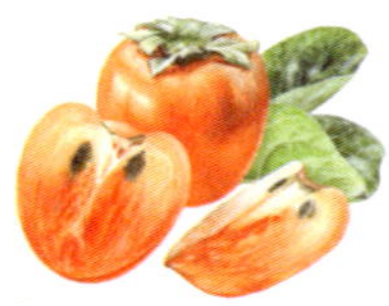

Persimmon

Digests in 3 hours

Combines well with other sweet fruits, and maybe with sub-acid fruits

Continued...

The Macro Nutrient Composition of Natural Foods

Protein, Lipids, and Carbohydrates

Macro Nutrients In Plant Foods

Simple Carbohydrates

Melons (sweet)

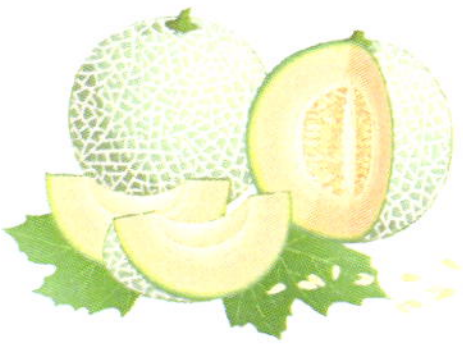
Cantaloupe

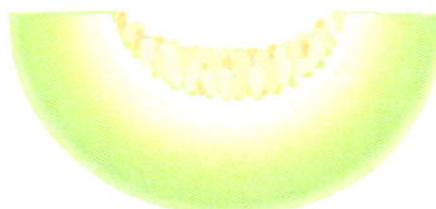

Honeydew

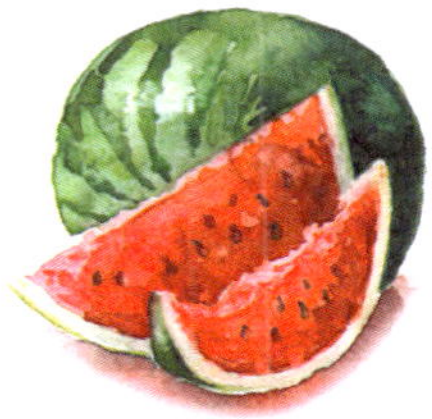
Watermelon

Digests in 2 hours — Combines well only with other melons

Complex Carbohydrates

(Non-Starch)

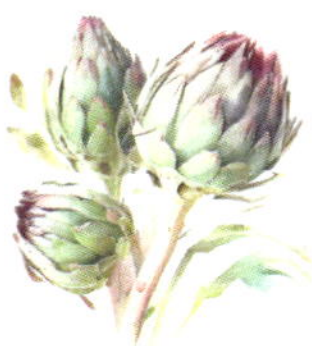
Artichoke

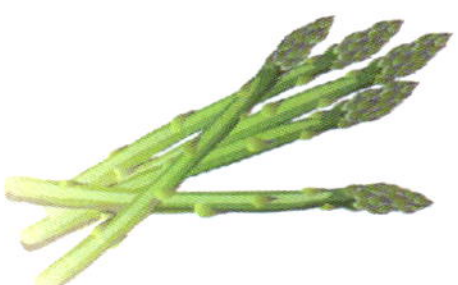
Asparagus

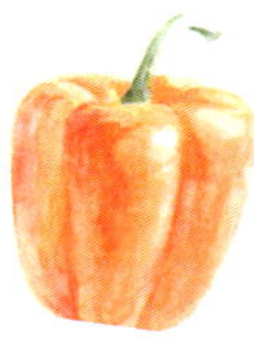
Bell Pepper

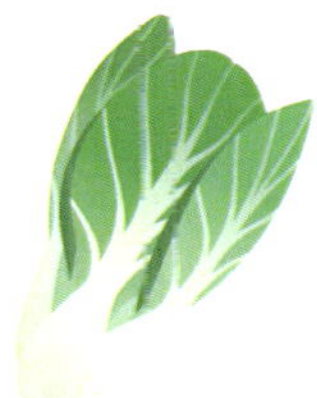
Bok Choy

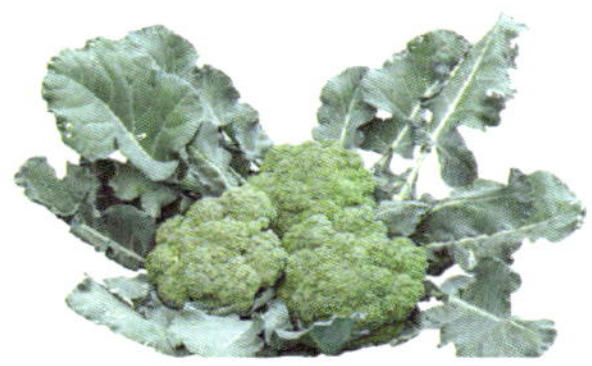
Broccoli

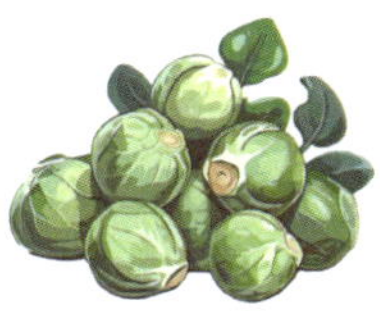
Brussels Sprouts

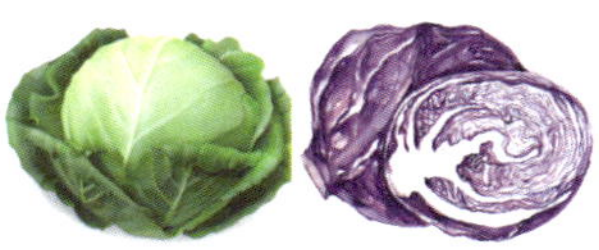
Cabbage (Green & Purple)

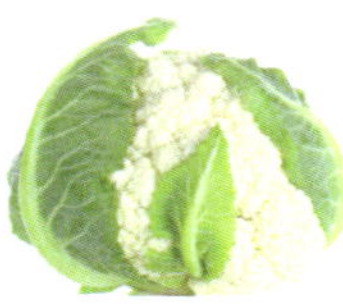
Cauliflower

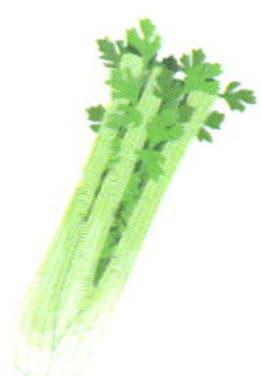
Celery

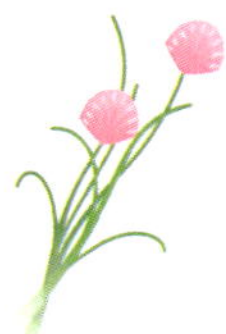
Chives

Digests in 5 hours — Combines well with any natural food (except fruit)

Continued...

The Macro Nutrient Composition of Natural Foods
Protein, Lipids, and Carbohydrates

Macro Nutrients In Plant and Algae Foods and mushrooms

Complex Carbohydrates
(Non-Starch, Mild Starch)

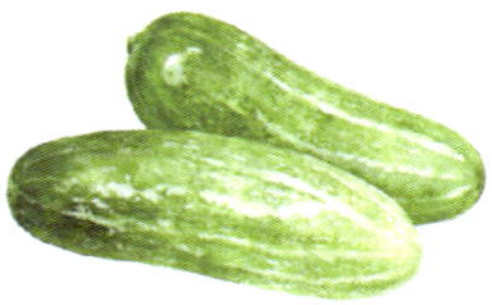
Cucumber

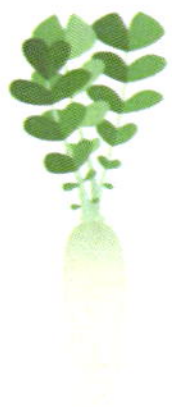
Diakon Radish

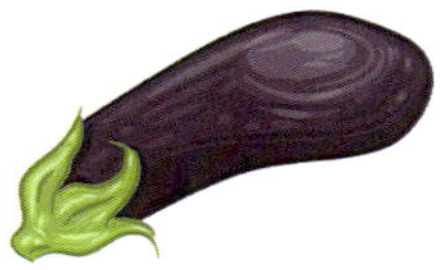
Eggplant

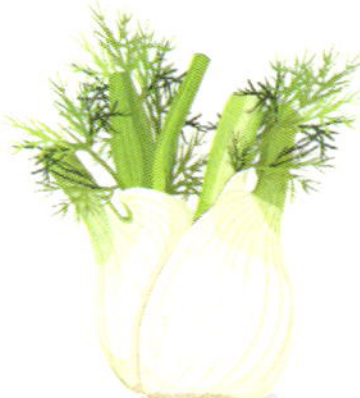
Fennel Bulb

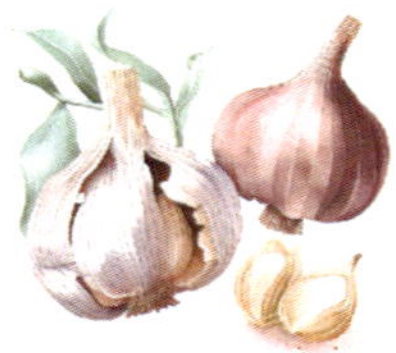
Garlic

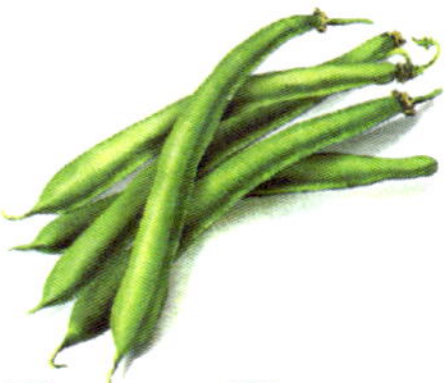
Green Bean

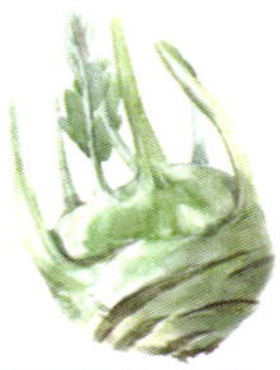
Kohlrabi

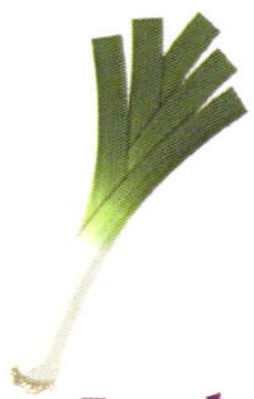
Leek

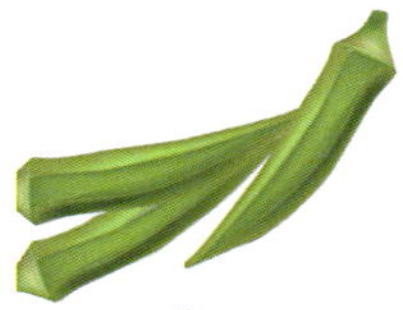
Okra

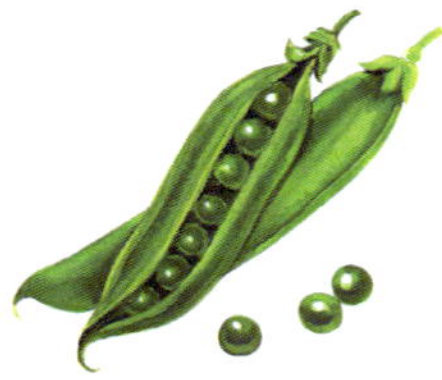
Peas (Fresh)

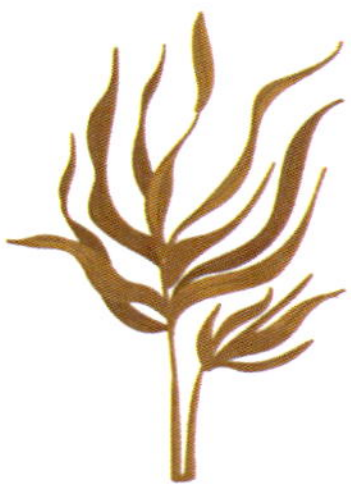
Arame

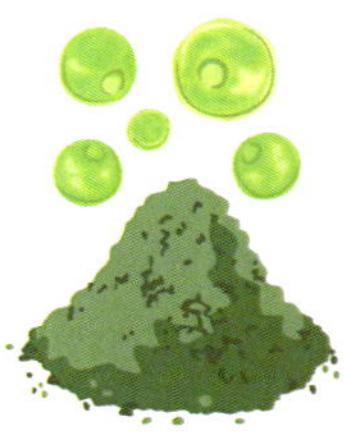
Chlorella

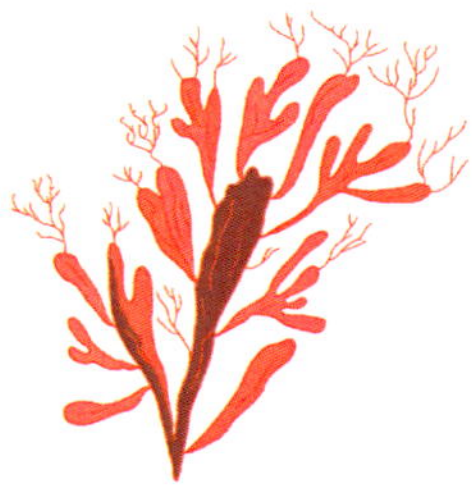
Dulse

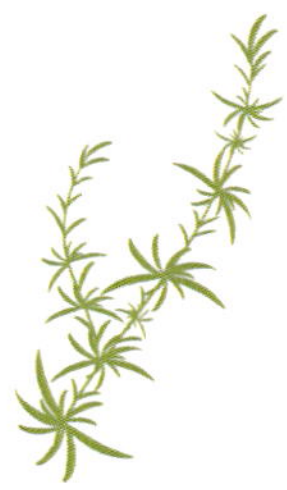
Hijiki

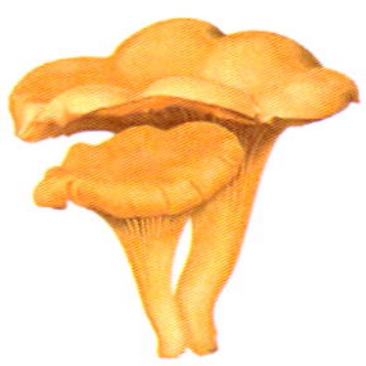
Chanterelle

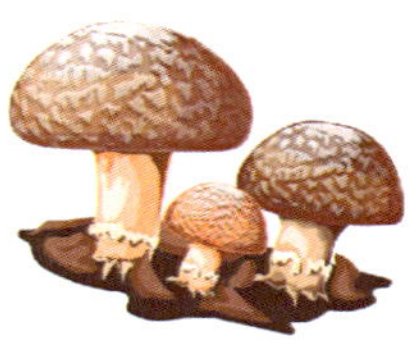
Shitake

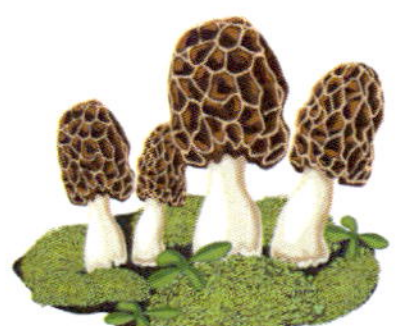
Morel

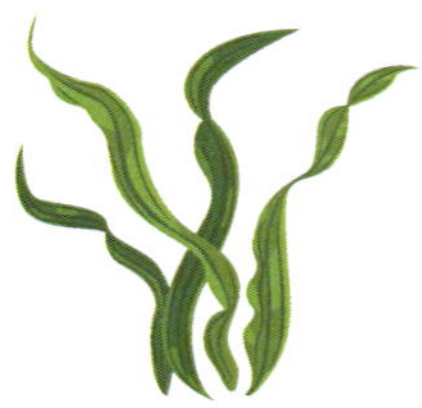
Spirulina

Digests in 5 hours   Combines well with any natural food (except fruit)

Continued...

The Macro Nutrient Composition of Natural Foods

Protein, Lipids, and Carbohydrates

Macro Nutrients In Plant Foods

Complex Carbohydrates

(Mild Starch)

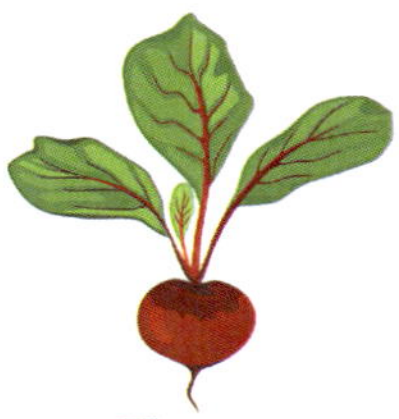

Beet

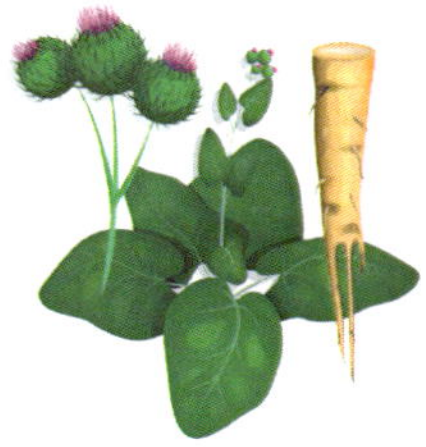

Burdock Root

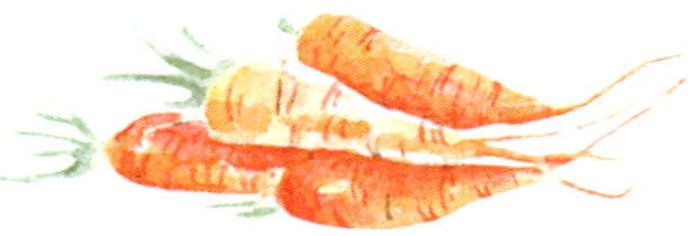

Carrot

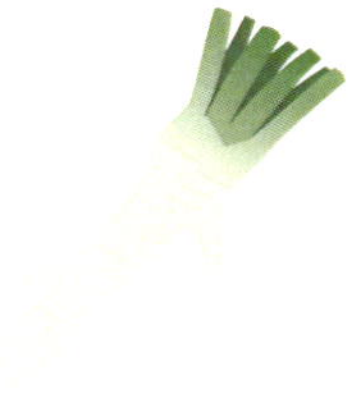

Horseradish

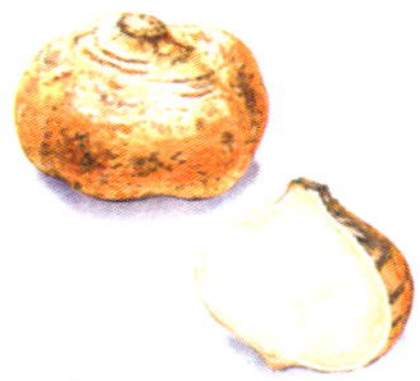

Jicama

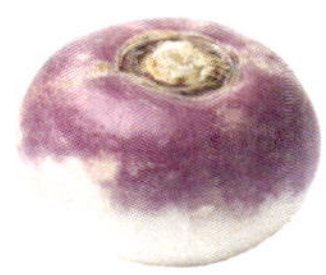

Turnip

Complex Carbohydrates

(Starch)

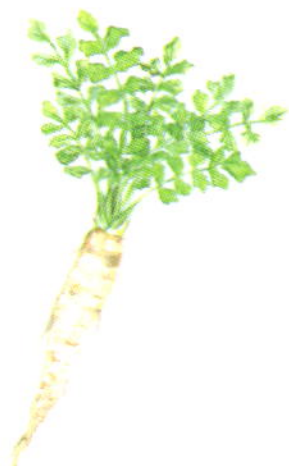

Parsnip

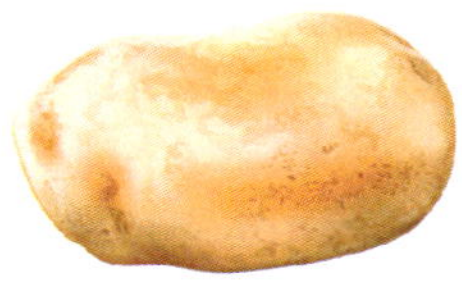

Potato

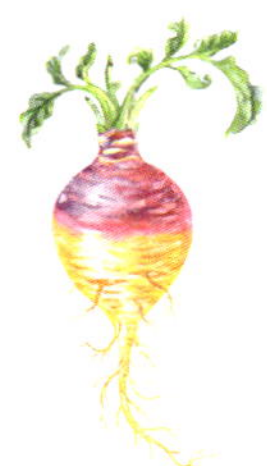

Rutabaga

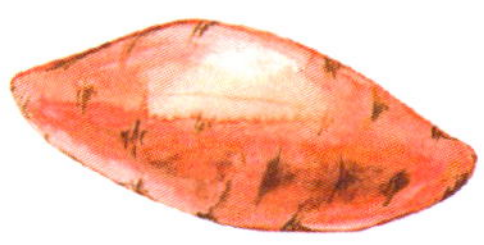

Sweet Potato

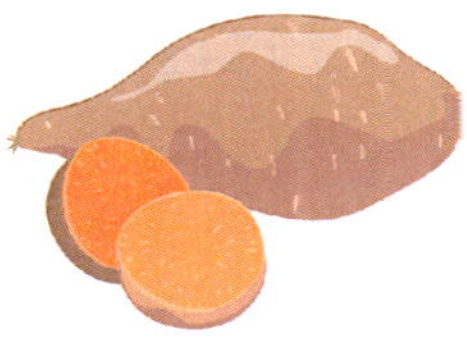

Yam

Digests in 5 hours

Combines well with vegetables (non-starch, mild starch, & starch), grains, and fats and oils

Continued...

The Macro Nutrient Composition of Natural Foods

Protein, Lipids, and Carbohydrates

Macro Nutrients In Plant Foods

Complex Carbohydrates and Protein
(Mild Starch, Starch)

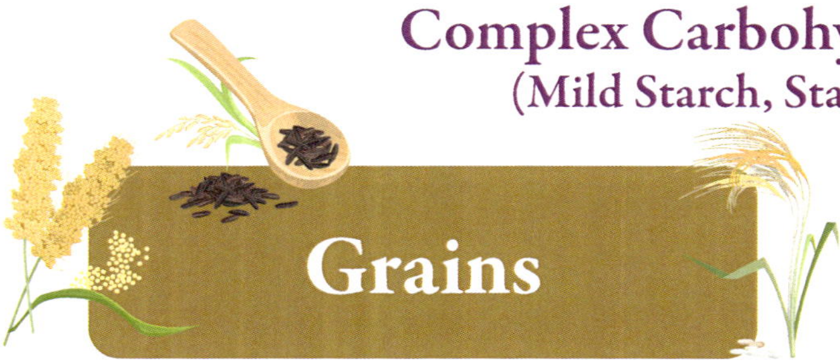

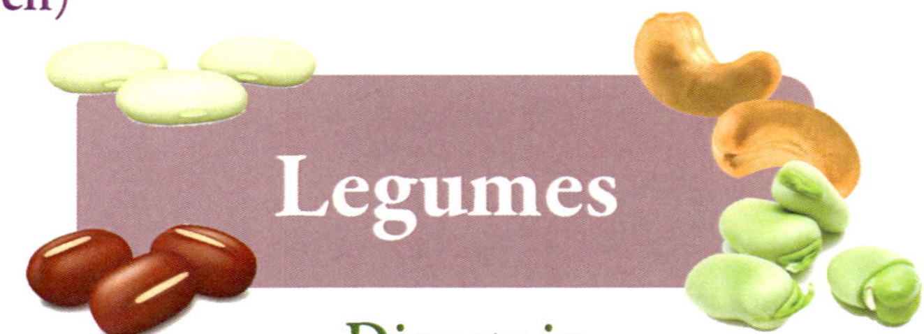

Digests in
5 hours - Grains

Digests in
12 hours - Legumes

Combines well with all vegetables, leafy greens, algae, spirulina, mushrooms, and fats and oils

Lipids (fats, oils extracted from fruits)

Some fruits, such as coconuts, olives, and avocados, are rich in lipids (fats and oils); the amount of protein and carbohydrates varies between them.

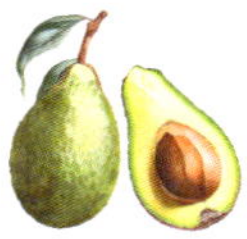

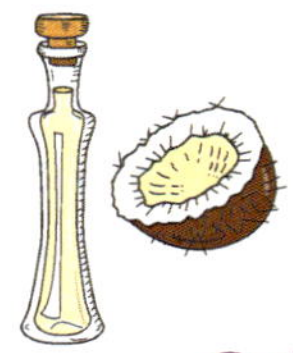

Coconut Oil

When extracted, coconut lipids can be fats or oils. Since coconut's lipids are predominantly saturated fatty acids, they are fats (solid) at room temperature. At higher temperatures they become oils (liquid).

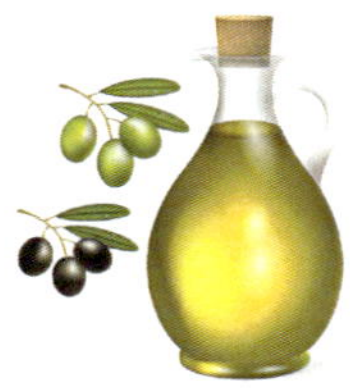

Olive Oil

Digests in 12 hours

Combines well with all vegetables, leafy greens, algae, spirulina, mushrooms,

Protein, Lipids, and Complex Carbohydrates
(10 to 50%)

Comprised mostly of monounsaturated and polyunsaturated fatty acids that are oils (liquids) at room temperature

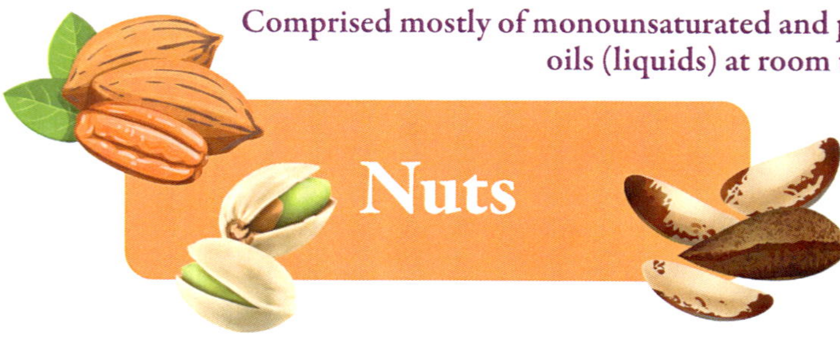

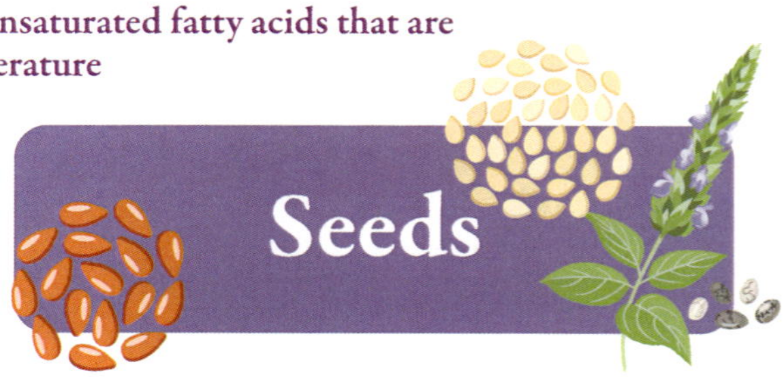

Digests in 12 hours

Combines well with vegetables (non-starch), leafy greens, algae, spirulina, mushrooms

Continued...

The Macro Nutrient Composition of Natural Foods
Protein, Lipids, and Carbohydrates

Macro Nutrients In Plant Foods

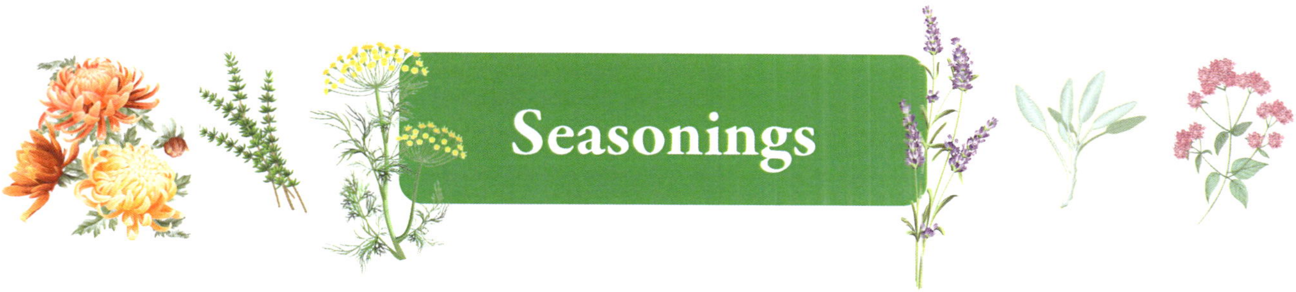

Seasonings

Complex Carbohydrates
(Non-Starch)

Bark

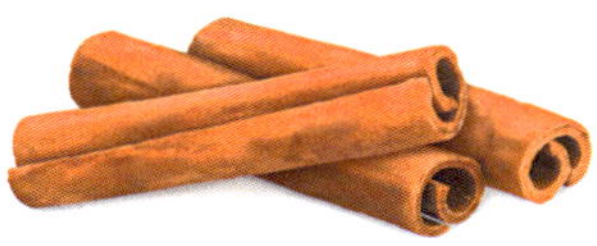
Cinnamon

Herbs

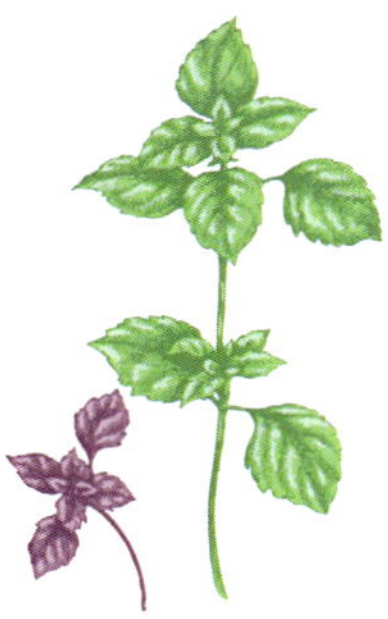
Basil

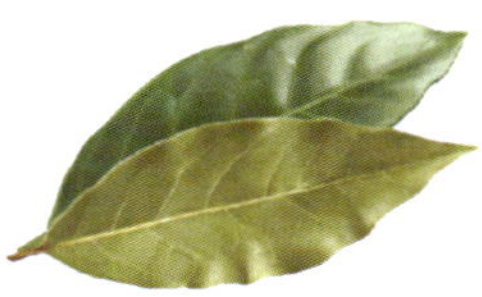
Bay Leaf

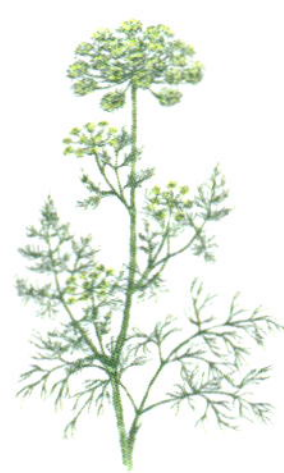
Dill

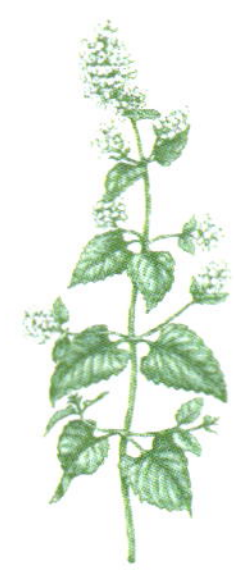
Lemon Balm/Melissa

Digests in 5 hours Generally combines well with all foods

Continued...

The Macro Nutrient Composition of Natural Foods
Protein, Lipids, and Carbohydrates

MACRO NUTRIENTS IN PLANT FOODS

Complex Carbohydrates
(Non-Starch)

Seasonings

Herbs

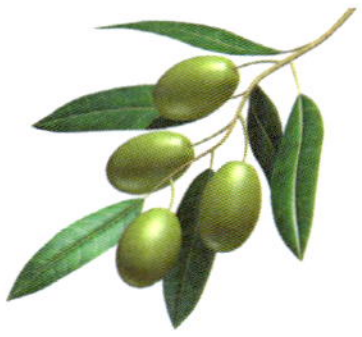
Olive Leaf

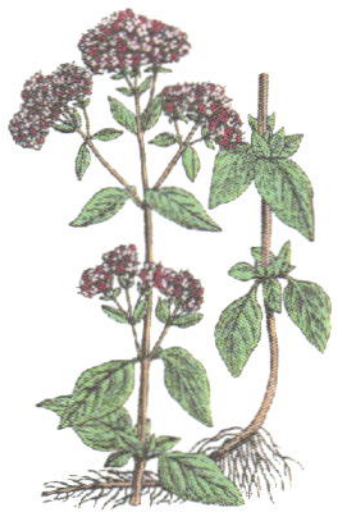
Oregano

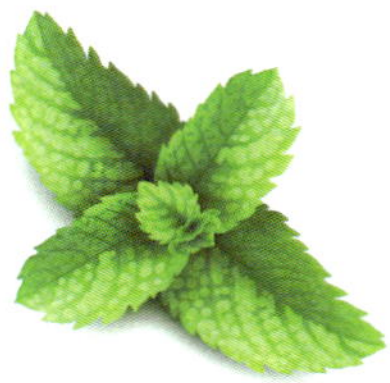
Peppermint

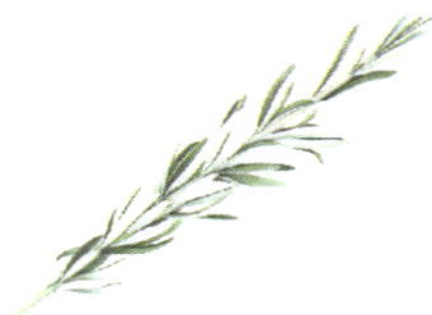
Rosemary

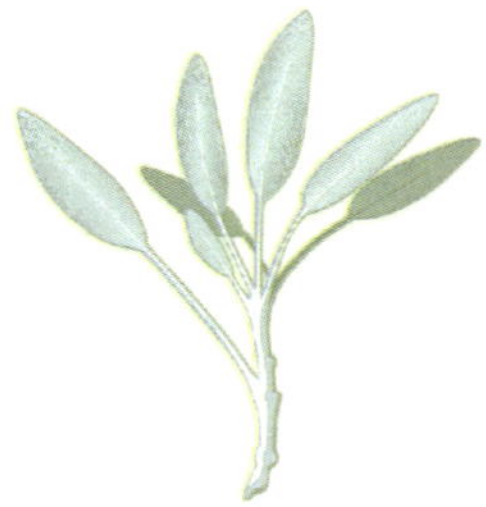
Sage

Flowers

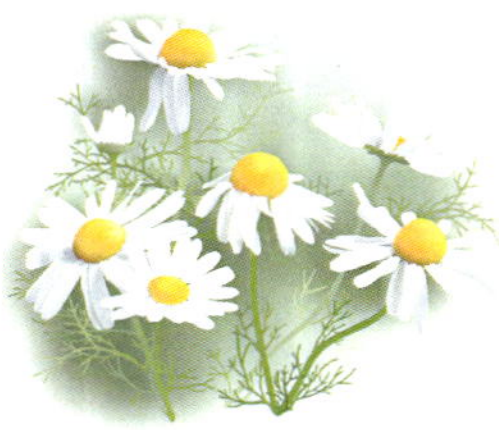
Chamomile

Chrysanthemum

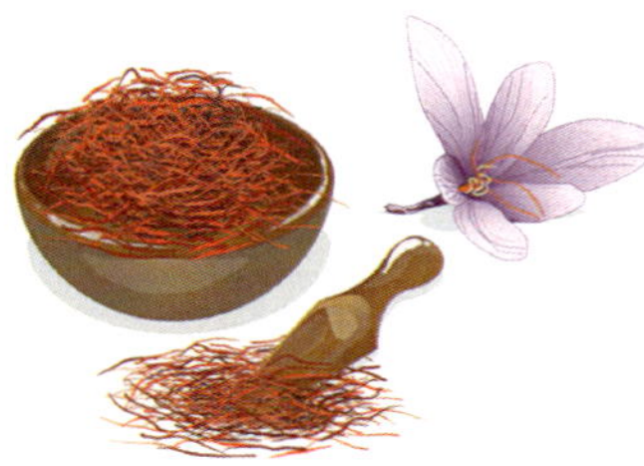
Saffron
Stigma "threads" that hold the pollen

Flower Buds

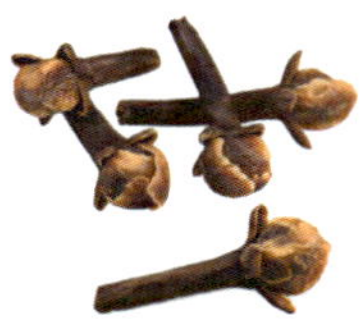
Cloves

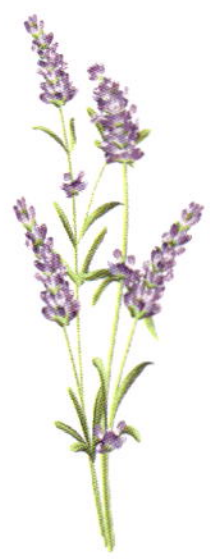
Lavender

Digests in 5 hours — Generally combines well with all foods

Continued...

The Macro Nutrient Composition of Natural Foods
Protein, Lipids, and Carbohydrates

Macro Nutrients In Plant Foods

Complex Carbohydrates (Non-Starch)

Seasonings

Piquant Fruits

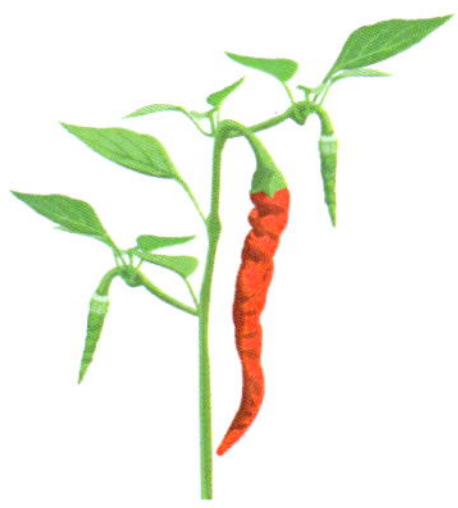

Cayenne Pepper

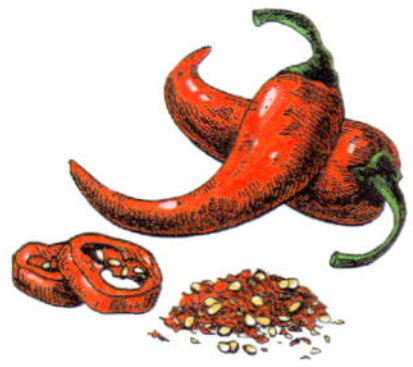

Chili Pepper

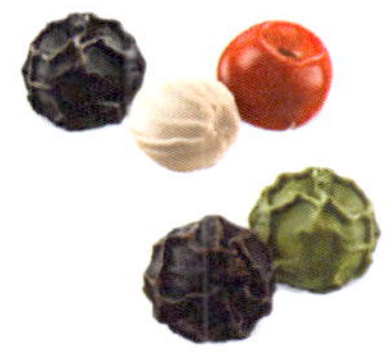

Peppercorn (non-starch)

Digests in 5 hours

Combines well with all foods

Complex Carbohydrates (Mild Starch, Starch)

Seasonings

Roots

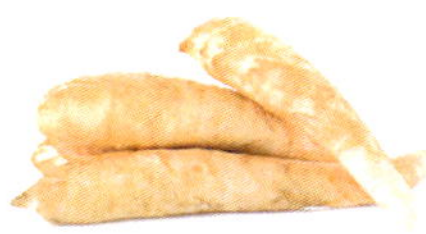

Arrowroot

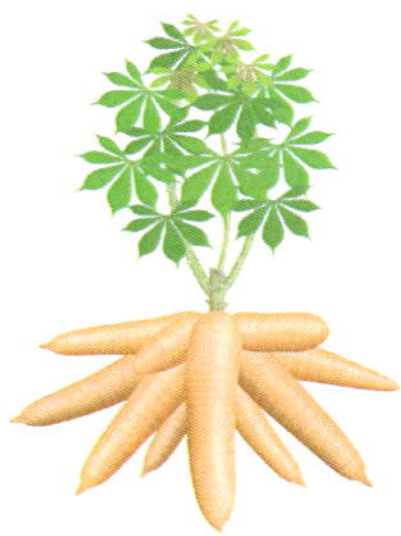

Cassava

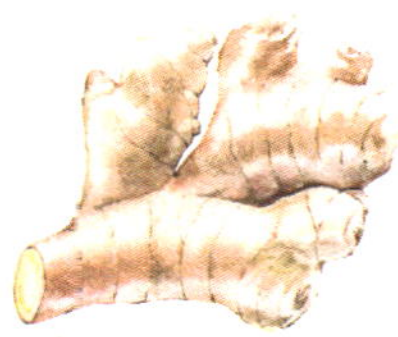

Ginger

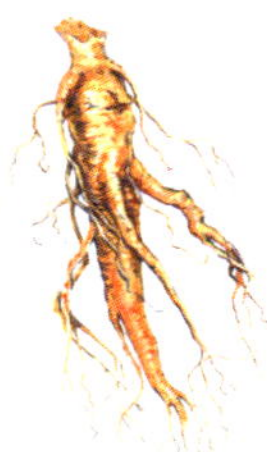

Ginseng

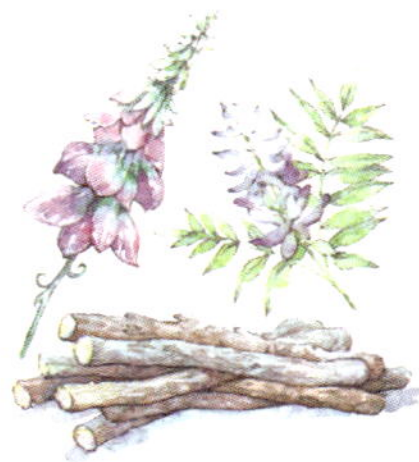

Licorice

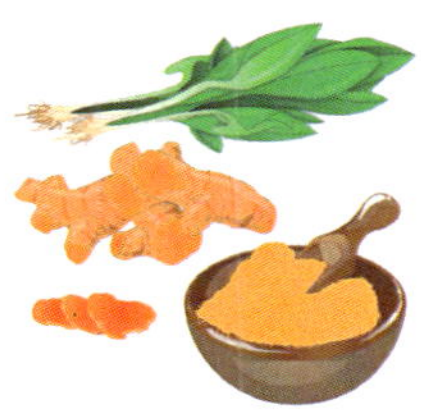

Turmeric

Digests in 5 hours

Combines well with vegetables (non-starch), leafy greens, algae, spirulina, mushrooms

Continued...

The Macro Nutrient Composition of Natural Foods

Protein, Lipids, and Carbohydrates

Macro Nutrients In Plant Foods

Protein and Lipids (Oils)

Seasonings

Seeds

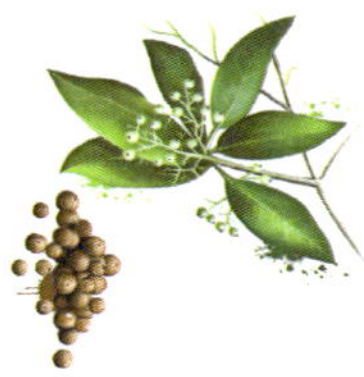

Allspice

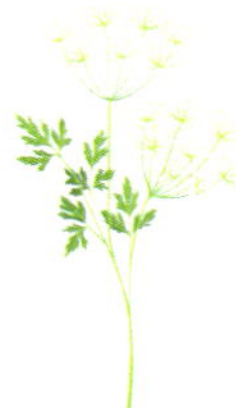

Anise

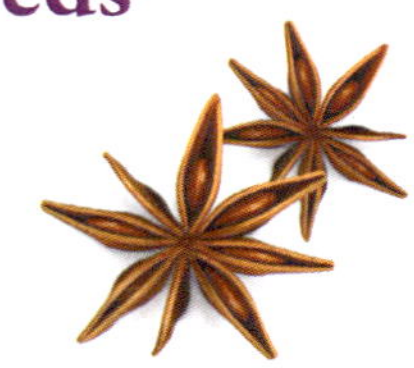

Star Anise

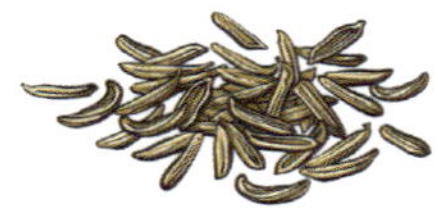

Caraway

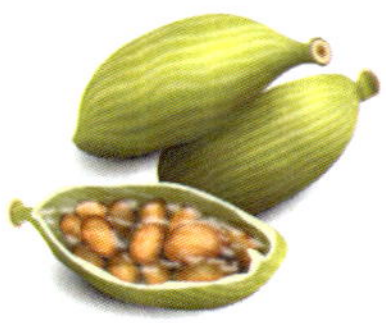

Cardamon

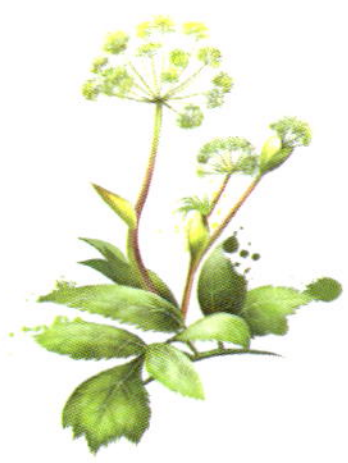

Celery

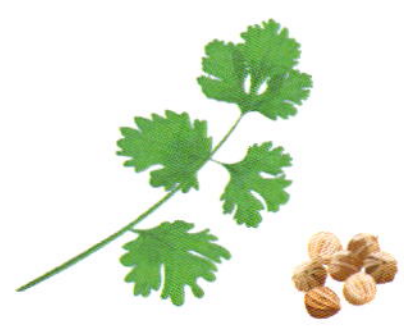

Coriander

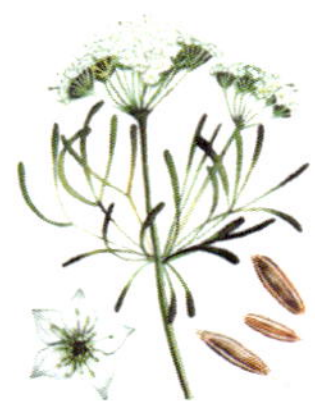

Cumin

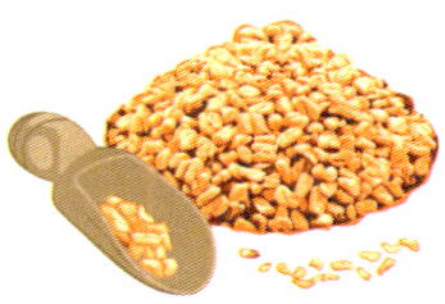

Fenugreek

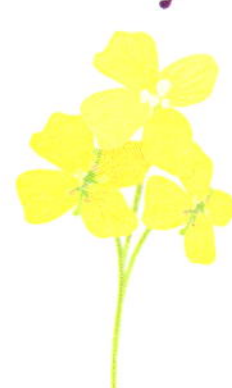

Mustard

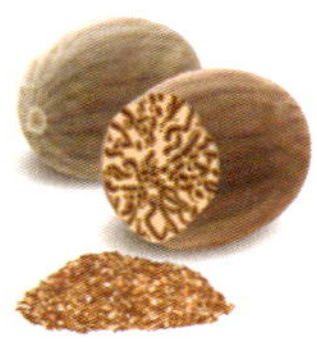

Nutmeg

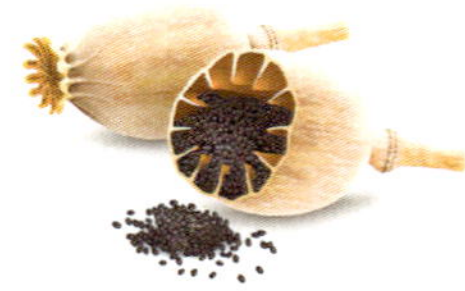

Poppy

Digests in 12 hours

Combines well with any natural food

Micro Nutrient Composition of Natural Foods–Sea Salts

Micro Nutrients In Mineral Foods

Salts from ancient seas, containing major and trace mineral nutrients

Celtic Sea Salt

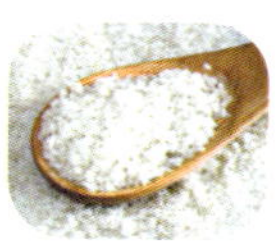

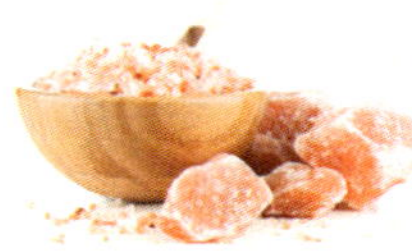

Pink Sea Salt

Seasonings

Combines well with any natural food

Vitamin Nutrients

VITAMINS		ROLES IN THE BODY
FAT-SOLUBLE VITAMINS	Lipids and bile are needed to digest, absorb, and assimilate fat-soluable vitamins into the lymph system, where they are circulated to nourish the cells and tissues throughout the body	The fat-soluble vitamins A, D_2, D_3, E, K_1, and K_2 are kept readily available (for when needed) in fat that is stored in the body; in high levels, the fat-soluable vitamins can be toxic (K_1, and K_2 have much less potential for toxicity)
Organ Meats  Butter 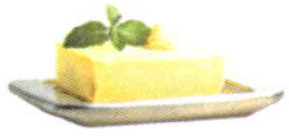	**VITAMIN A (retinol)** Animal foods contain the only source of active vitamin A *Less efficiently, using enzymes reserves, the body can convert provitamin A carotenoids from plant, algae, and mushroom foods into active, retinal vitamin A.*	Essential for cell growth, reproduction, gene expression, strong bones; bolsters white blood cells, macrophages, and lymphocytes; and protects the retina from oxidative stress
Cilantro 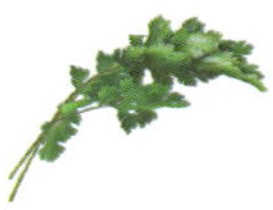 Escarole 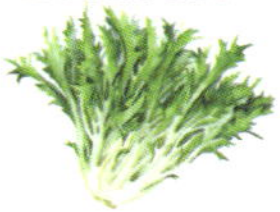	**VITAMIN D_2 (ergocalciferol)**	Supports skeletal, respiratory, and immune health; with folate, protects the skin from UV damage
Fish Roe 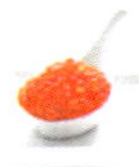 Salmon 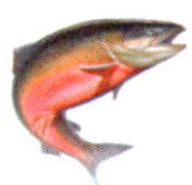	**VITAMIN D_3 (cholecalciferol)**	Necessary for bone development and regeneration, brain, nerve, and muscle function; cardiovascular protective
Sesame Seed 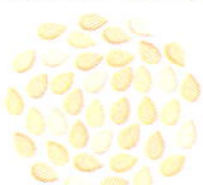 Hazelnut 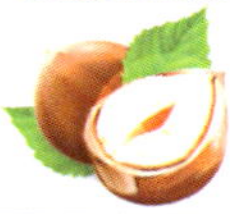	**VITAMIN E** *(alpha, beta, gamma, and delta tocopherols and tocotrienols – they work together, alpha tocopherol is the most active)*	Prevents oxidative damage to the cell membranes, protects vitamin A and increases its storage, vital for reproductive health, anti-coagulant
Kale 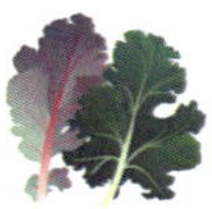 Watercress 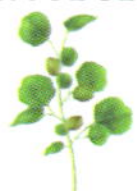	**VITAMIN K_1 (phylloquinone)**	Enhances cardiovascular health and elasticity; both vitamin K_1 and K_2 are essential for blood clotting (coagulation) as needed
Emu Oil 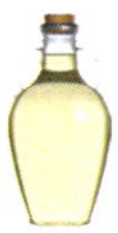 Sauerkraut 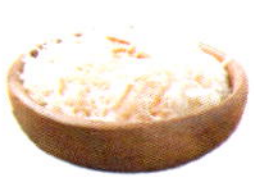	**VITAMIN K_2 (menaquinone)**	Important in forming strong bones, neuro and heart protective, K_2 MK-4 needed for brain function (memory); K_2 MK-7 reduces arterial calcification
WATER-SOLUBLE VITAMINS	Water-soluble vitamins are primarily absorbed in the small intestine. Then they are transported to the liver, then released into the bloodstream and delivered to the cells and tissues.	Widely available in natural foods, easily destroyed in heat (cooking); only a small quantity is stored in the body, any excess is excreted via the urine
VITAMIN B COMPLEX	B vitamins work synergistically, with key roles in energy production and relieving stress	
Spirulina 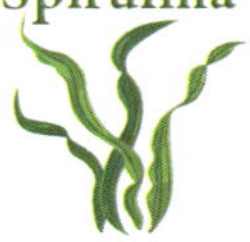 Pine Nuts 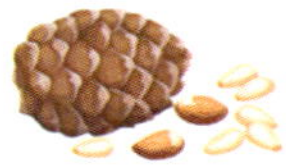	**VITAMIN B_1 (Thiamine)**	Critical role in synthesizing DNA, RNA, and the neurotransmitter acetylcholine which is important for cognition and memory
Trout 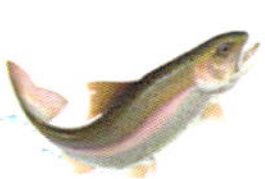 Kefir 	**VITAMIN B_2 (Riboflavin)**	Important in the synthesis of thyroid hormones, assists in the absorption of vitamin B6 and iron, and facilitates the metabolism of tryptophan

Continued...

Vitamin Nutrients

	VITAMINS	ROLES IN THE BODY
Meat Stock 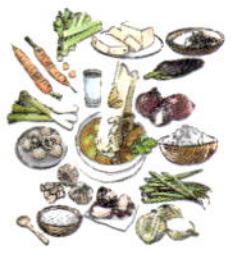 Chicken Egg 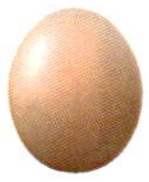	VITAMIN B_3 (Niacin and Niacinamide)	Central to adrenal function and the production of hydrochloric acid (HCL); involved in regulating glucose, metabolizing cholesterol, and repairing DNA
Shitake Mushroom 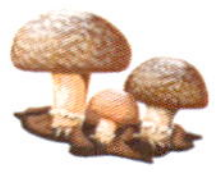 Offal 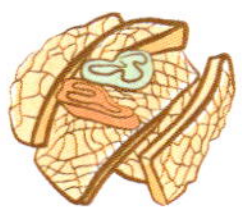	VITAMIN B_5 (Pantothenic Acid)	Supports the production of neurotransmitter acetylcholine, melatonin, adrenal hormones, and heme (the protein in hemoglobin that carries oxygen)
Tuna (Yellowfin) 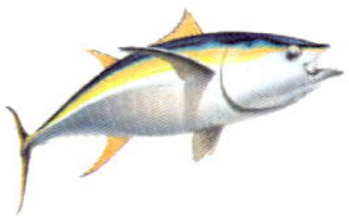 Sunflower Seeds 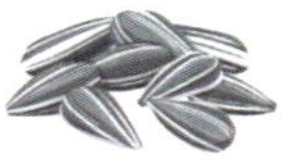	VITAMIN B_6 (Pyridoxal and Pyridoxamine) *(Pyridoxal and pyridoxamine are the two active, more bioavailable forms of vitamin B_6, of the six different B_6 forms)*	Needed for synthesizing hemoglobin and neurotransmitters and for achieving rapid eye movement (REM) sleep which enhances the immune system
Shrimp 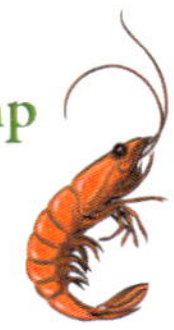 Barley 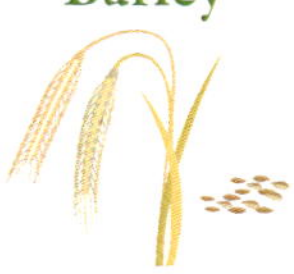	VITAMIN B_7 (Biotin) Can be synthesized by probiotic bacteria in the small intestines	Critical for the absorption and metabolism of fats and amino acids; strengthens hair and nails, and supports in gene expression
Black-eyed Pea 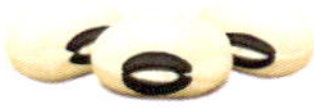 Cilantro 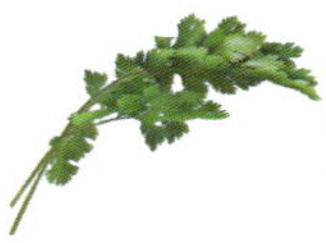	VITAMIN B_9 (Folate) Can be synthesized by probiotic bacteria in the small intestines	Functions closely with vitamin B_{12}, maintaining the nervous system; facilitates the synthesis of proteins, DNA, and RNA
Gizzards, Liver and Heart 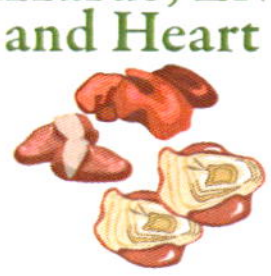 Crab 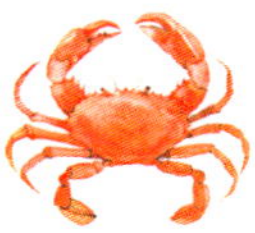	VITAMIN B_{12} (Cobalamin)	Necessary for the growth, function, and regeneration of the nervous system, including the protective myelin sheath; with folate, helps form red blood cells; required for the digestion and absorption of nutrients
Chick Pea 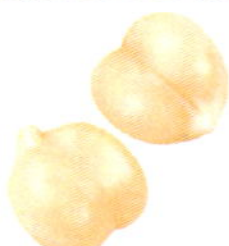 Green Bean 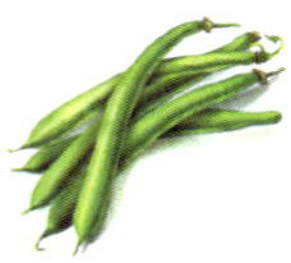	INOSITOL	Key component of every cell membranes (like choline), contributes to the metabolism of fats and cholesterol in the arteries and liver, and improves sleep
Organ Meats  Duck Egg 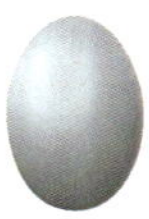	CHOLINE	Assists in the transmission of nerve impulses from the brain to the central nervous system; precursor of acetylcholine, lecithin, and phosphatidylcholine; essential for brain function; and helps maintain healthy cholesterol
Bell Pepper 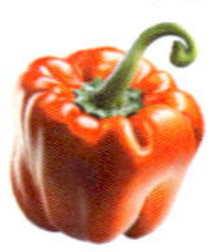 Kiwi 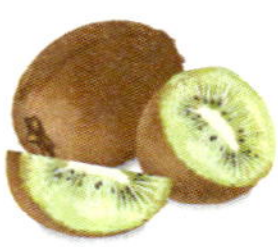	VITAMIN C (Ascorbic Acid)	Powerful anti-oxidant; anti-viral, anti-tumor, heals wounds; in conjunction with bioflavonoids, recharges enzymes; synthesizes collagen, tyrosine, neurotransmitters, and hormones

Nourishing and Protective Enzymes in Living Foods

Digestive enzymes (hydrolases) break down our foods. Specifically, the macro-nutrients, **protein**, **lipids** (fats and oils), and **carbohydrates**, are broken down into their micro-nutrients, principally amino acids; fatty acids and glycerol; glucose and other simple sugars. While hydrolases break down the macro-nutrients, metabolic enzymes capture the energy for use in our body's cells. Synthesizing enzymes (synthetases) then use the unbound micro-nutrients to construct and repair cells and tissues. As catalysts, remaining unaltered themselves, all of these enzymes start and accelerate these biochemical reactions by reducing the activation energy necessary for the reactions to take place.[1]

Without digestive, metabolic, and synthesizing enzymes,
essential biochemical reactions would not occur fast enough to sustain life.

Digestive Enzymes (Hydrolases)

In conjunction with organic compounds, including hydrochloric acid (HCL) in the stomach and secretin and bile in the small intestine, hydrolases facilitate digestion.

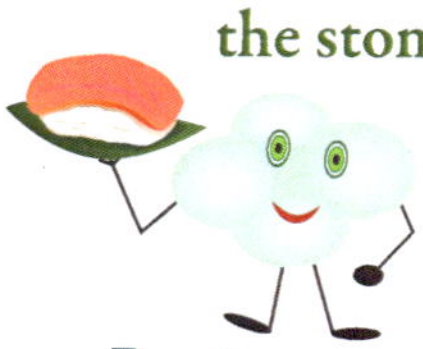

Protease

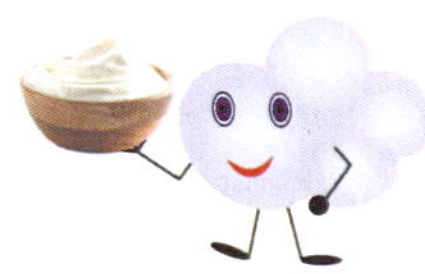

Lipase

Key Hydrolases Include:

- **Proteases – break down protein into amino acids**
- **Lipases – break down lipids (fats and oils) into their constituents: fatty acids, sterols (cholesterol), glycerol, and fatty alcohols[1]**
- **Amylases – break down carbohydrates into their constituents: glucose and other simple sugars**
- **Lactase – break down lactose (milk sugar) into lactic acid**

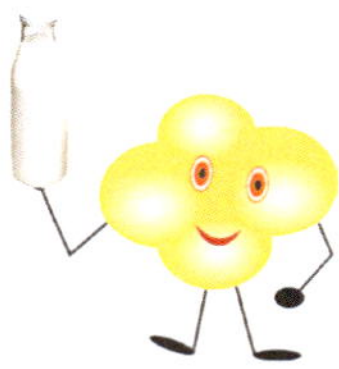

Lactase

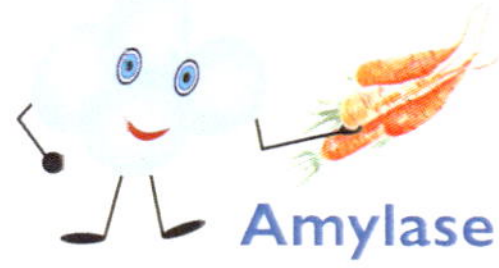

Amylase

The aroma of foods and movement of chewing activates the digestive "juices," preparing organs and glands for digestion and immune response. Chewing ". . . stimulates the parotid glands, behind the ears in the jaw, to release hormones that stimulate the thymus to produce T cells, which are the core of the protective immune system."[2] Since food can introduce foreign substances and microbes, the immune system is active throughout the digestive process, scavenging, neutralizing, and removing toxic, inflaming, and oxidizing compounds and pathogens.

Metabolic and Synthesizing Enzymes

Metabolic enzymes catalyze metabolic pathways to release energy and metabolites (such as, vitamins and DNA/RNA nucleotides) from protein, lipids, and carbohydrates for the activities of cells. Lipids are the most energy-dense (9 calories per gram) compared to protein and carbohydrates (4 calories per gram). The energy from these macro-nutrients is converted to adenosine triphosphate (ATP) for the synthesis of proteins and nucleic acids to repair cells and restore tissues. Other enzymes, like superoxide dismutase, act as strong anti-oxidants protecting the cells from free radicals that damage molecules, atoms, or ions.

Continued...

Nourishing and Protective Enzymes in Living Foods

Replenish your Enzymes with Soaked, Sprouted, and Fermented Foods

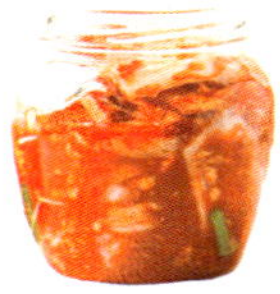

Kimchi

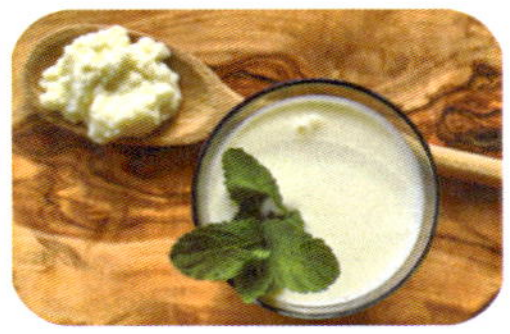

Kefir

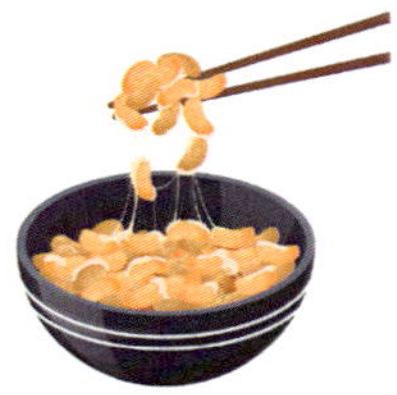

Natto

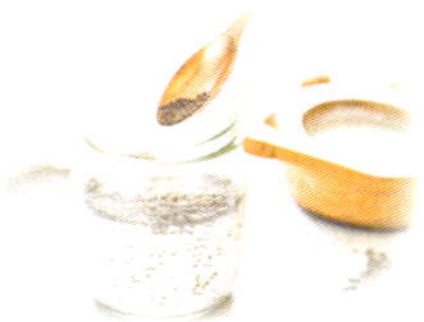

Soaked Seeds

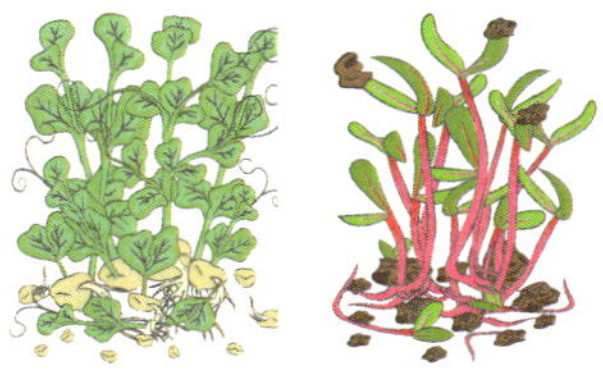

Microgreens (Sprouted)

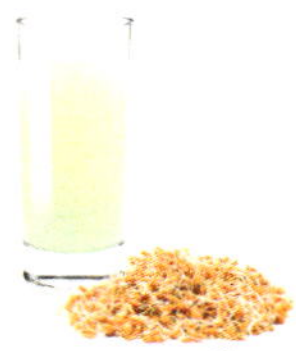

Rejuvelac

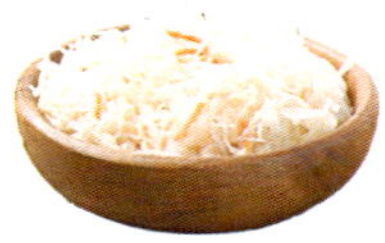

Sauerkraut

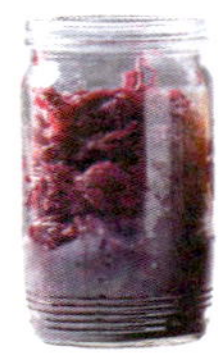

Vegetable

Our body can manufacture enzymes to a limited degree but cannot keep up with a lifetime need of enzymes. Fortunately, we can obtain plenty of enzymes from raw foods; they need to be kept at or below 117° F (47° C) because heat destroys enzymes. Germinating seeds (including nuts, grains, and legumes) through soaking or sprouting, offers an abundance of enzymes. Additionally, any food that has been healthfully fermented contains an abundance of enzymes generated by probiotic microbes. These probiotic microbes aid in the digestion, absorption, and assimilation of nutrients and work in concert with our immune system. We benefit tremendously when probiotic microbes find favorable habitat in our intestinal tract and make themselves a home.

There are no known traditional diets based exclusively on raw food. "Even in the tropics, where fires are not needed for warmth, the inhabitants build a fire every day to cook their foods. Some nutrients are made more available through cooking and cooking also neutralizes naturally occurring toxins in plant foods."[3] The traditional diets that built excellent human health over millennia included a variety of raw and cooked foods from the land and sea.

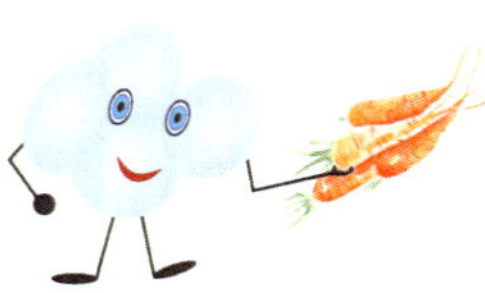

Amylase

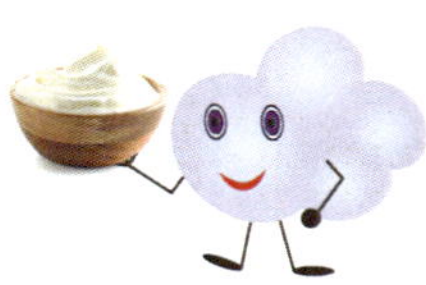

Lipase

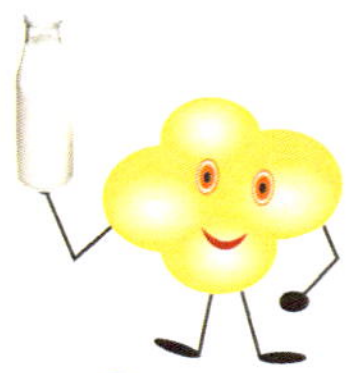

Lactase

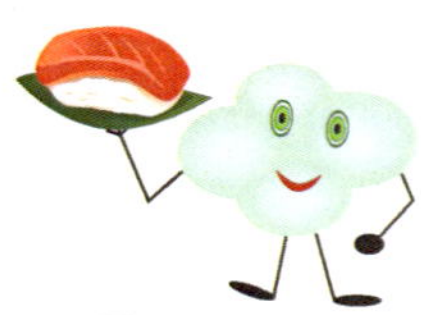

Protease

Continued...

Nourishing and Protective Enzymes in Living Foods

ENZYMES NECESSARY FOR DIGESTING PLANT, ALGAE, MUSHROOM, AND ANIMAL FOODS

HYDROLASES	DIGESTIVE, IMMUNE, AND RELATED ROLES IN THE BODY

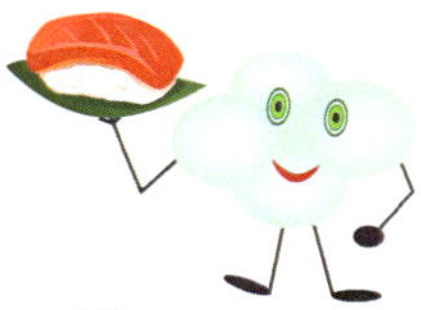

Protease

PROTEASES – Protein Digestion

Proteases are fundamental to the enzymatic process of breaking down protein, first into peptides (groups of amino acids) and then into individual amino acids. Playing key roles in protein digestion, too, are hydrochloric acid (HCL) and co-enzymes: betaine, bromelain, chymopapain, hyaluronidase, pancreatin, pepsin, plasmin, rennin, and trypsin.

Activates the optic nerve, eliciting melatonin production, facilitating sleep; initiates vitamin D_3 production in the skin, strengthening the bones; increases serotonin levels, improving concentration, memory, and homeostasis

Pineapple 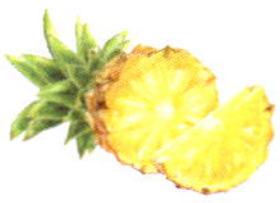 Kiwi 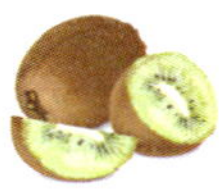 Papaya 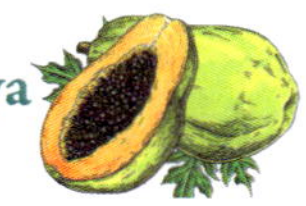

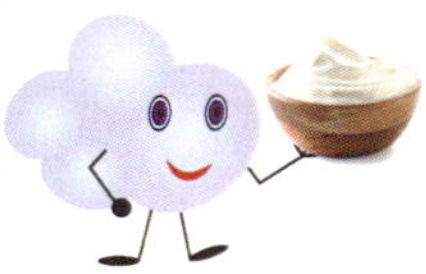

Lipase

LIPASES – Lipid Digestion

Lipases break down lipids (fats and oils). Lingual lipase is secreted in the saliva, gastric lipase in the stomach, and pancreatic lipase in the small intestine where bile emulsifies the lipids. Once the lipids are broken down small enough, they are first absorbed into the lymph system and then delivered to the blood stream where they are carried with other micro-nutrients to the cells where they are needed.

Supports healthy cholesterol levels and protect the cardiovascular system; helps relieve bloating, heartburn, irritable bowel syndrome, celiac disease, and cystic fibrosis.

Avocado 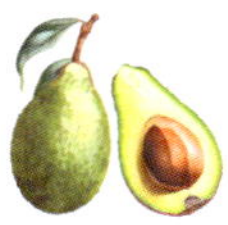 Walnut 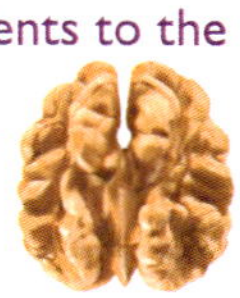 Coconut 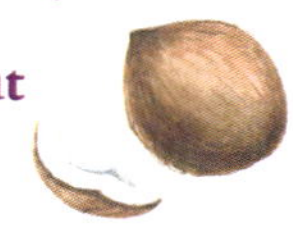

AMYLASES AND LACTASE – Carbohydrate Digestion

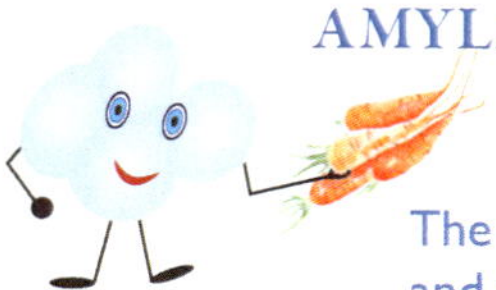

Amylase

Amylases break down plant foods, algae, mushrooms, and spirulina (cyanobacteria).

The amylases break the polysaccharides into disaccharides and then monosaccharides (simple sugars, including glucose). Insulin (secreted from the pancreas) and hormones (from the adrenal glands and thyroid) regulate glucose levels in the blood.

Amylase co-enzymes include: diastase, glucoamylase, hemicellulose, maltase, pancreatin, pectinase, phytase, and papain.

Provides energy; slow the absorption of glucose, lowering blood sugar; relieves diarrhea caused by undigested carbohydrates; anti-inflammatory; and anti-tumor

Mango 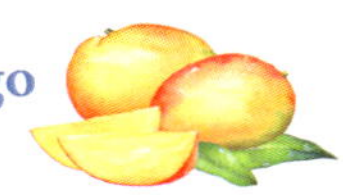 Banana 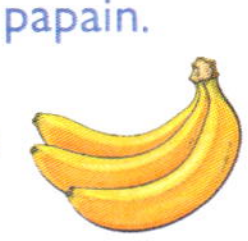 Sweet Potato 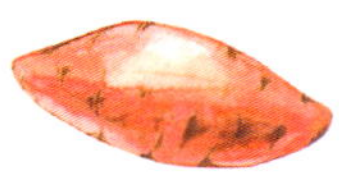

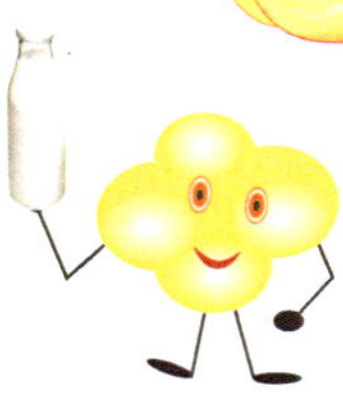

Lactase

LACTASE digests the lactose in raw milk

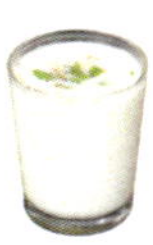 Buttermilk 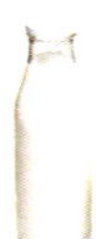 Kefir 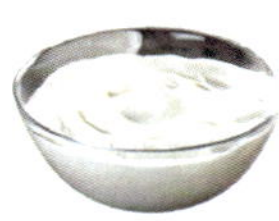 Yogurt

Essential for the complete digestion of raw milk products, breaking down the milk sugar (lactose) into galactose and glucose; supports mineral absorption

References
[1]Lewis T. & Stone W. L. (2024, January). Biochemistry, Proteins Enzymes. *StatPearls*. Treasure Island, FL: StatPearls Publishing. https://www.ncbi.nlm.nih.gov/books/NBK554481.
[2]Umpleby, A. M. & Russell-Jones, D. L. (1996, October). The hormonal control of protein metabolism. *Baillieres Clinical Endocrinology Metabolism. 10*(4):551–70. https://pubmed.ncbi.nlm.nih.gov/9022951.
[3]Fallon Morell, S. (2001). *Nourishing Traditions* (p. 47). Washington, D.C.: NewTrends Publishing, Inc.

Vital Photons and Molecules

Sunlight supports life with light, heat, and energy. Like us, mycelia (mushrooms) of the *Fungi* Kingdom need oxygen (O_2). They combine it with glucose to release energy. Mycelia also need carbon dioxide (CO_2), water (H_2O), and minerals to grow their mushrooms(fruiting bodies), whether inhabiting an area of full sun or a dark forest. Mycelia release CO_2 when they respire. Photosynthesizing algae and plants of the *Plantae* and *Chromista* Kingdoms use sunlight, CO_2, H_2O, and minerals to produce carbohydrates in the form of new algae and plant material. As a byproduct, algae and plants release O_2. Notably, in the *Bacteria* Kingdom, aerobic b acteria require O_2; whereas, anaerobic bacteria need CO_2 and only grow in places where O_2 is limited or absent. Cyanobacteria use CO_2, dissolved in marine, estuarine, and fresh water, for photosynthesis. Producing chlorophyll through photosynthesis, algae, plants, and cyanobacteria are the primary producers in food webs. Nitrogen is used throughout the kingdoms of life for making nucleic acids (DNA and RNA) and proteins. Water is essential for all forms of life.

VITAL PHOTONS AND MOLECULES	ROLE IN THE BODY
 SUNLIGHT	Activates the optic nerve, eliciting melatonin production, facilitating sleep; initiates vitamin D_3 production in the skin, strengthening the bones; increases serotonin levels, improving concentration, memory, and homeostasis
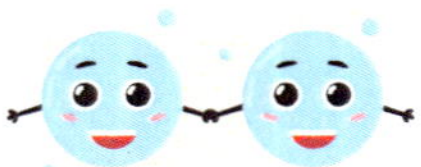 O_2 OXYGEN *(O_2 – two oxygen atoms)*	Critical for mitochondrial respiration, oxidative phosphorylation (production of energy), and brain, heart, and retinal function
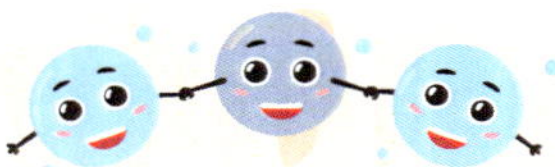 CO_2 CARBON DIOXIDE *(CO_2 – one carbon atom and two oxygen atoms)*	Drives respiration, facilitates the affinity of hemoglobin for oxygen, and helps regulate blood pH
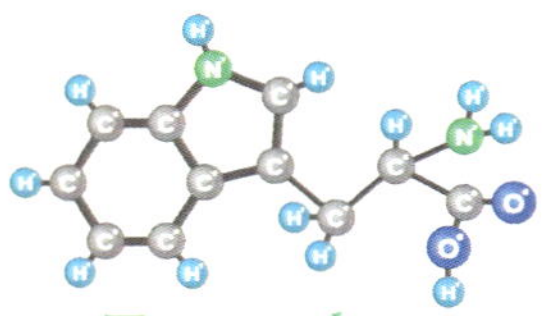 Tryptophan NITROGEN *(The amino acid tryptophan contains two nitrogen atoms)*	Required for producing DNA, RNA, proteins, creatine, peptide hormones, and several neurotransmitters Our body uses nitrogen in forming amino acids to build protein. Every amino acid has at least one nitrogen atom in its molecular structure. Nitrogen cannot be stored and must be obtained by consuming natural foods. The air we breathe contains ~78% nitrogen gas, ~21% oxygen and ~1% argon, carbon dioxide and other gases; however, our body cannot use nitrogen as a gas. We are dependent on nitrogen-fixing rhizobacteria, mycorrhizal fungi, and blue green algae that make the nitrogen available to plants and mushrooms that are then eaten by animals.
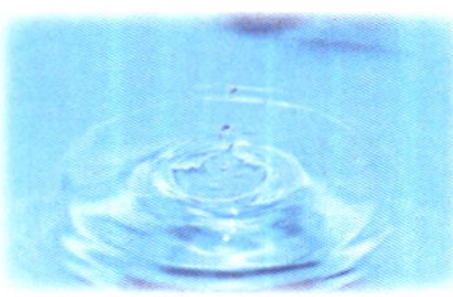 WATER *(H_2O – two hydrogen molecules and one oxygen molecule)*	Moistens tissues, transports oxygen and nutrients, helps maintains body temperature, cleanses, and detoxifies

Major Mineral Nutrients

MAJOR MINERALS

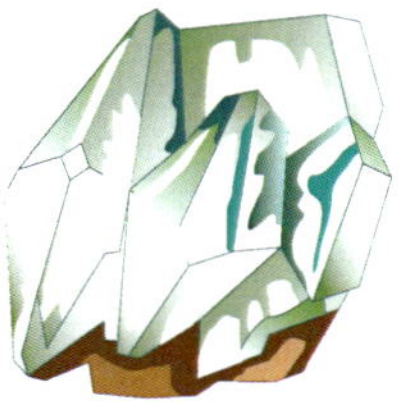

The seven minerals required in amounts greater than 100 mg per day are: calcium, chloride, magnesium, potassium, phosphorus, sodium, and sulfur. These major minerals (aside from sulfur) function as electrolytes. They are electrically charged and essential for producing energy, sending nerve impulses, contracting and relaxing muscles, keeping the tissues hydrated, and balancing pH.

INORGANIC MINERAL NUTRIENTS			ROLE IN THE BODY
CALCIUM *Most abundant mineral in the body*	Cheese (hard) 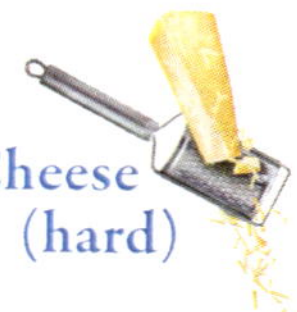	Collards 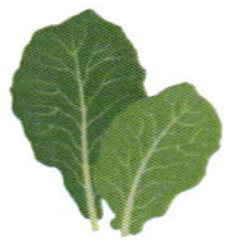	Required for building and maintaining strong bones, heart function and regulating blood pressure, the secretion of insulin and other hormones, and the absorption of vitamin B12.
CHLORIDE	Nori 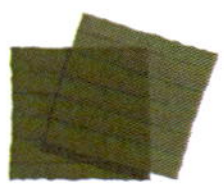	Scallops 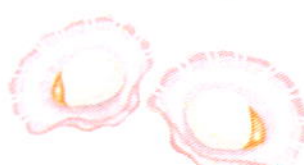	As an extracellular electrolyte like sodium, helps with balancing fluid, pH, and electrical charge from outside the cells; in the form of hydrochloric acid (HCL), aids in digestion
MAGNESIUM	Almonds 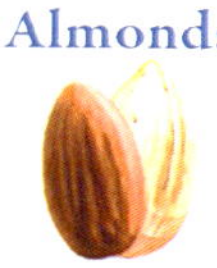	Buckwheat 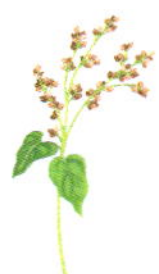	Predominant mineral in the cells; maintains healthy heart rhythm, necessary for bone formation, increases muscle strength and endurance, relaxes the nervous system and improves sleep
PHOSPHORUS *Second most abundant mineral in the body after calcium*	Pumpkin 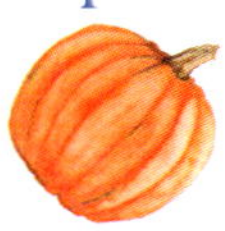	Sesame Seeds 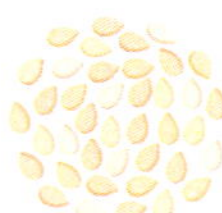	Facilitates calcium absorption and essential for bone formation and regeneration, phospholipids are the main component of cell membranes, significant to DNA and RNA synthesis, helps balance pH
POTASSIUM	Dulse 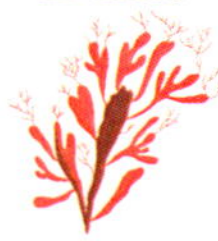	Honeydew Melon 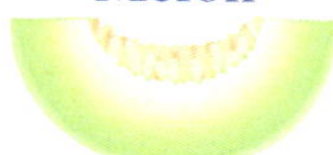	As an intracellular electrolyte, maintains fluid, pH, and electrical charge from inside the cells; helps facilitate the transmission of electrical signals (energy) through the nervous system and muscle contraction
SODIUM	Celery 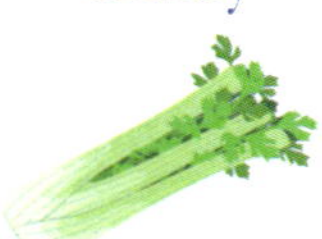	Wakame 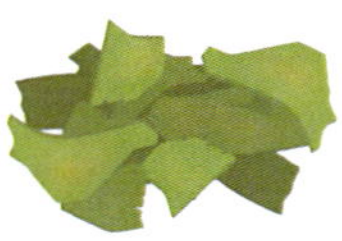	As an extracellular electrolyte like chloride, helps to maintain fluid, pH, and electrical charge from outside the cells; supports the cardiovascular system; regulates blood pressure; improves the elasticity of the subcutaneous (underneath) layer of skin
SULFUR	Chicken Egg 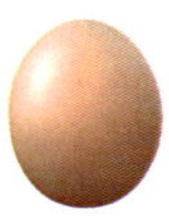	Onion (white) 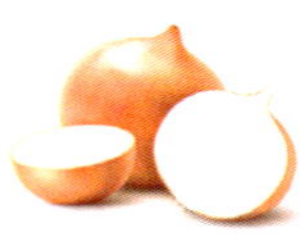	Helps solidify the protein in cartilage, strengthening joints, hair, skin, and nails; acts as a key component of insulin (regulating blood sugar), glutathione (detoxifying the body), and methyl sulfonyl methane (MSM) (relieving pain)

Continued...

Trace Mineral Nutrients

TRACE MINERALS
(12 Examples)

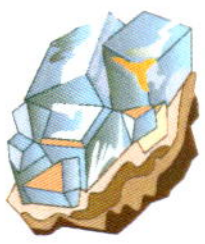

Trace minerals are required in amounts less than 100 mg per day. They are key activators of enzymes. For instance, zinc (along with the major mineral magnesium) is required by alkaline phosphatase for breaking down protein in the digestive process. Trace minerals are also fundamental to the structure of blood (iron in hemoglobin) and tissues (boron, copper, manganese, and silicon in bone).

INORGANIC MINERAL NUTRIENTS			ROLE IN THE BODY
BORON	Apricots 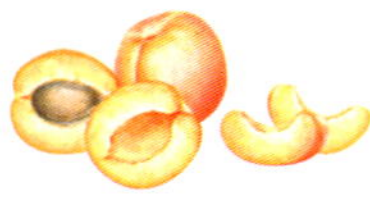	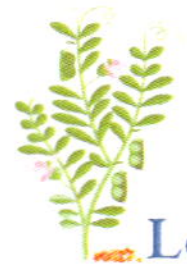 Lentils	Essential for bone and cartilage formation, anti-inflammatory, improves brain function (memory)
CHROMIUM	Offal 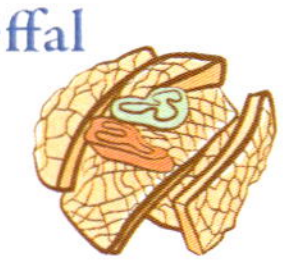	Rye 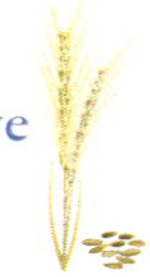	Increases the excretion of insulin from the pancreas, moving glucose from the blood into the cells for energy
COBALT	Oyster 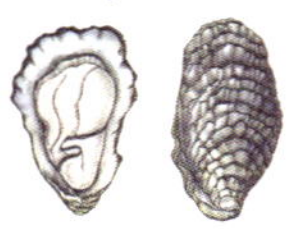	Fig 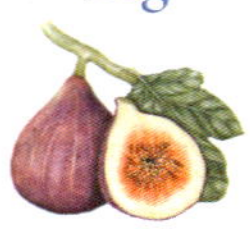	The core component of Vitamin B_{12} (methyl cobalamin), essential for red blood cell formation, and supports healthy nerve tissue
COPPER	Crab 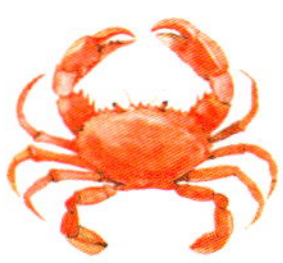	Pecans 	Needed for collagen production and the formation of red blood cells, bones, and connective tissue; supports eye health
IODINE *Thyroid hormone T4 (thyroxine) has four iodine molecules and T3 (triiodothyronine) has three*	Kelp 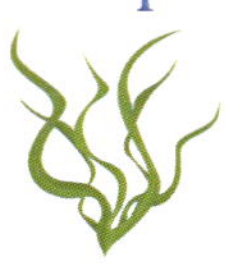	Muscles 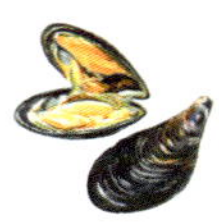	Prevents infection, critical for the production of thyroid hormones; important for metabolism and maintaining body temperature
IRON *Partner nutrients include: Vitamins A, B_2 (Riboflavin) and C and minerals copper and zinc*	Gizzards, Liver, and Heart 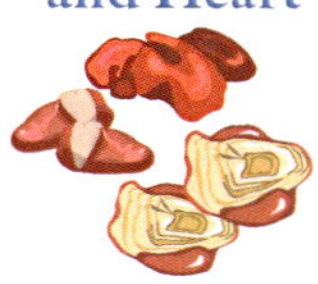	Wild Rice 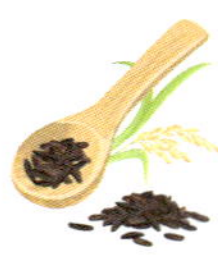	Used for brain function (concentration), the development of red blood cells and hemoglobin, and DNA and RNA synthesis

Continued...

Trace Mineral Nutrients

INORGANIC MINERAL NUTRIENTS			ROLE IN THE BODY
MANGANESE	Barley 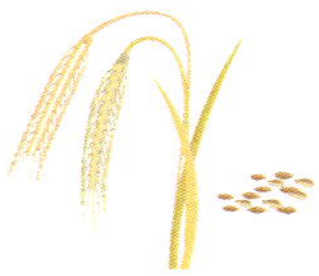	Beet Greens 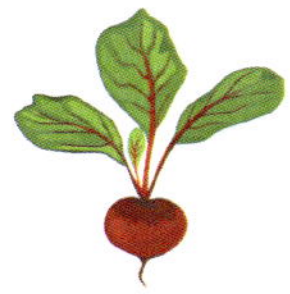	Prevents infection, critical for the production of thyroid hormones, important for metabolism and maintaining body temperature
MOLYBDENUM	Split Peas 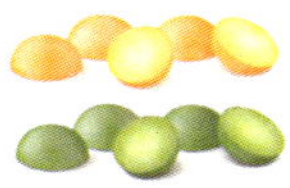	Cauliflower 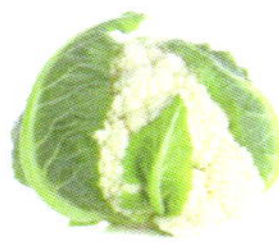	Metabolizes the sulfur-containing amino acids: methionine, cysteine, cystine, and taurine; supports detoxification
SELENIUM	Brazil Nut 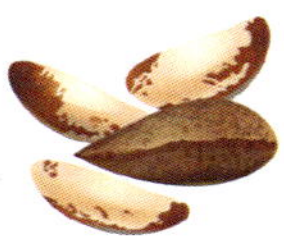	Herring 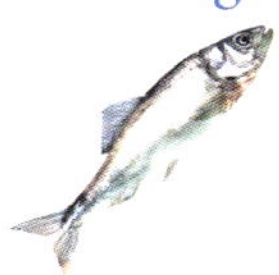	Important for DNA repair and converting T4 (thyroxine) to the more biologically active T3 (triiodothyronine); anti-oxidant
SILICON *The third most abundant mineral in the body*	Green Beans 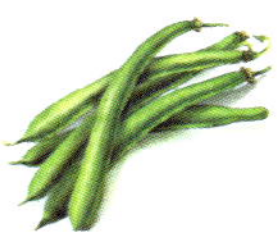	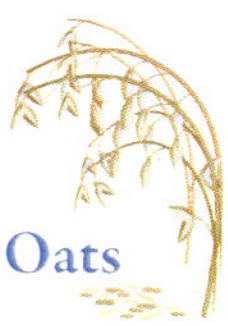 Oats	Strengthens bone and cartilage, increases the elasticity of connective tissue, and supports the thymus gland
VANADIUM	Parsley 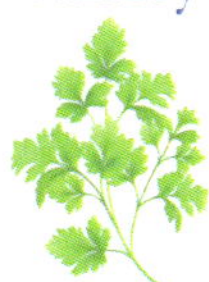	Quail Egg 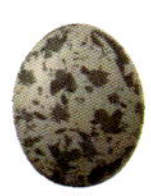	Helps metabolize glucose, increasing insulin sensitivity; helps metabolize fats; and protects the cardiovascular system
ZINC	Oyster 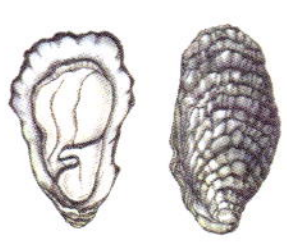	Ginger 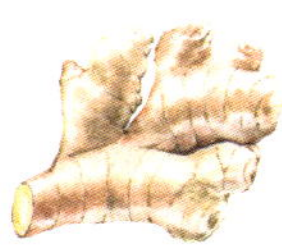	Fights infection, improves thyroid function, helps heal wounds, needed for night vision, and enables the sense of taste and smell

PART V

Study Of

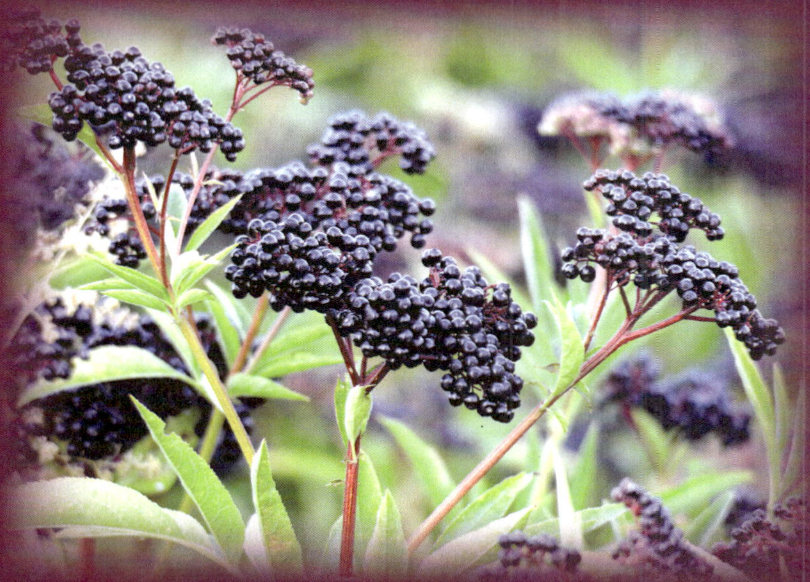

The Energy and Wound Healing Vitamin

The Youth Mineral

A Well-Being Hormone

A Regenerative Organ

Study of the Energy and Wound Healing Vitamin – Vitamin C

Produces Energy, Fights Infection, Heals Wounds

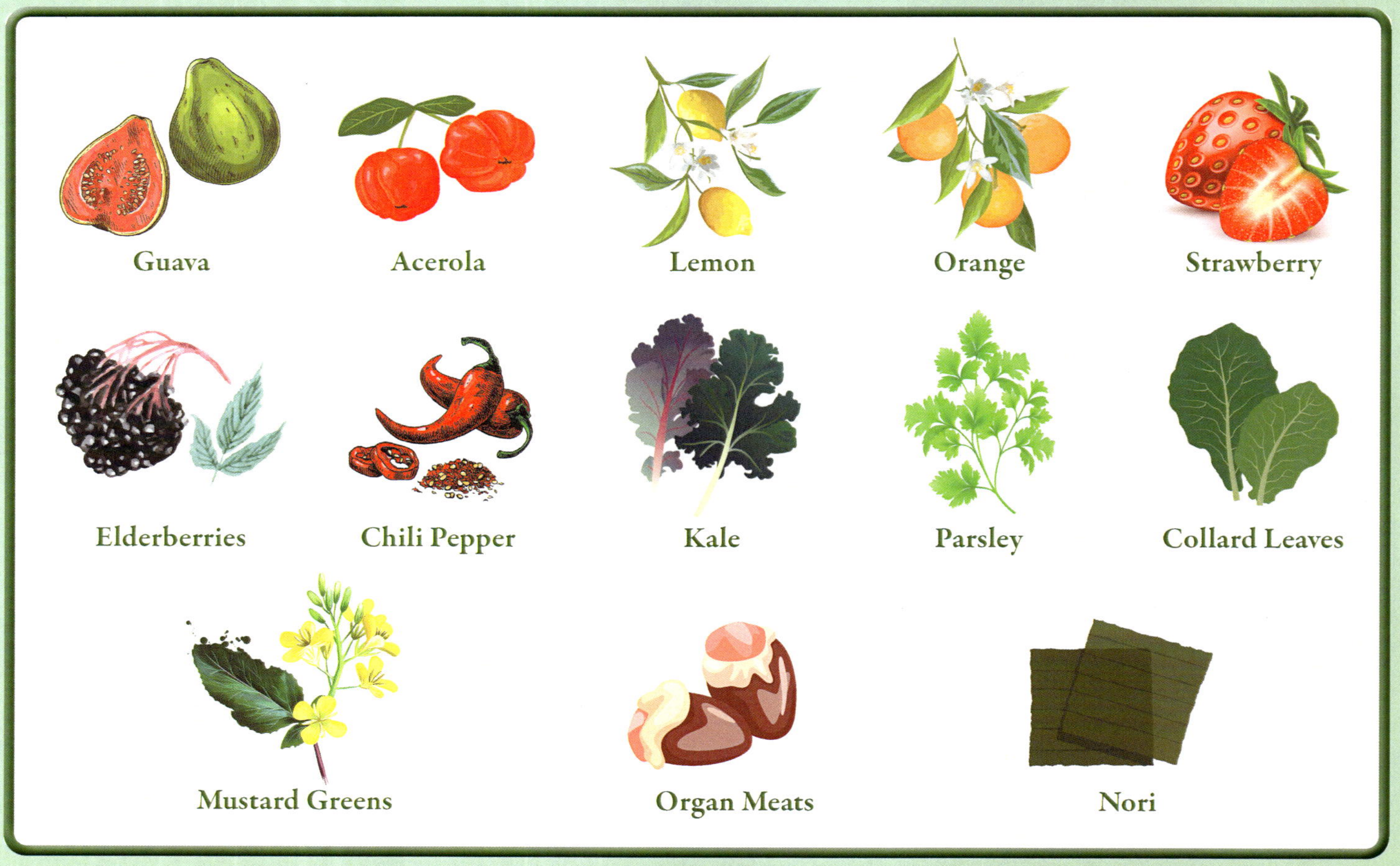

Vitamin C (ascorbic acid) and co-occurring bioflavonoids are cardinal to many foundational processes in the body. We need a frequent supply of them and higher amounts than most other nutrients. Our bodies do not manufacture vitamin C or bioflavonoids; and, being water-soluble, they cannot be stored. Any extra is excreted. Loose stools can be an indication of having consumed more than is needed. Another consideration is that vitamin C and bioflavonoids degrade when exposed to heat or light.

Handily, fruits and vegetables (especially the rinds, skin, and pulp) and leafy greens contain an abundance of vitamin C and bioflavonoids. When fully ripe, fruits and vegetables are at the peak of their vitality; and freshly harvested, such as hand-picked from a home garden, their flavor is superior. As an anti-oxidant, vitamin C slows down the degradation of other nutrients exposed to oxygen in the air. We obtain the most nutritional benefit from raw fruits, vegetables, and leafy greens when we consume them soon after chopping, blending, or juicing them.

Continued...

Study of the Energy and Wound Healing Vitamin – Vitamin C

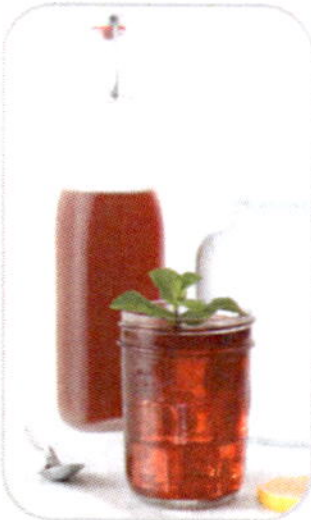

Hibiscus Tea

Working in Concert, Vitamin C and Bioflavonoids

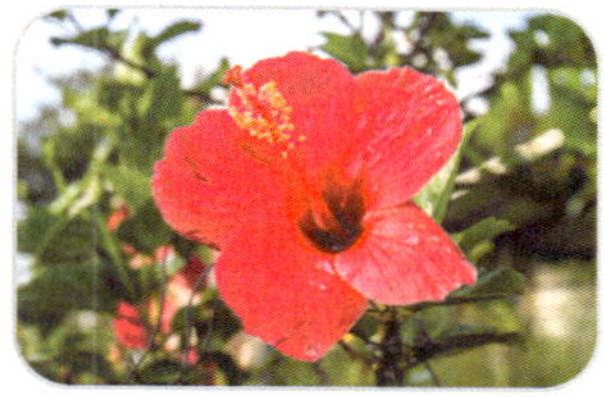

Hibiscus Flower

- Facilitate energy production and aid in adrenal function
- Destroy pathogenic microbes and build white blood cells
- Anti-cancer[1]and support the immune system
- Act as powerful anti-oxidants and anti-inflammatory
- Enhance the bioavailability and absorption of iron
- Prevent bleeding gums and nose bleeds
- Protect the eyes from the formation of cataracts
- Essential for the formation of collagen in connective tissue
- Protect the skin from UV damage
- Strengthen the walls of arteries, veins, and capillaries
- Aid in repairing damage caused by inflamed tissue
- Reduce bruising, relieve swelling, and heal wounds

Individual bioflavonoids offer specific health benefits and enhance the absorption and assimilation of vitamin C. For instance, the bioflavonoid citrin increases energy production in mitochondria. Eriodyctiol has anti-oxidant and anti-inflammatory properties. Heperidin supports blood circulation and heart function. Naringenin is anti-fungal and anti-cancer.[2] Quercetin safeguards vitamin C from oxidation. Rutin maintains blood vessel elasticity and reduces hypertension. In nature, thousands of bioflavonoids evolved in plants to protect them from disease and dissuade herbivores from eating them. Many of these compounds are nutritive and healing.

References

[1]Lee, Y. (2023, November 30). Role of vitamin C in targeting cancer stem cells and cellular plasticity. *Cancers. 15*(23):5657. https://www.ncbi.nlm.nih.gov/pmc/articles/PMC10705783.

[2]Duda-Madej, A., Stecko, J., Sobieraj, J., Szymańska, N., & Kozłowska, J. (2022, November 15). Naringenin and its derivatives-health-promoting phytobiotic against resistant bacteria and fungi in humans. *Antibiotics. 11*(11):1628 https://www.ncbi.nlm.nih.gov/pmc/articles/PMC9686724.

Study of the Youth Mineral – Sodium

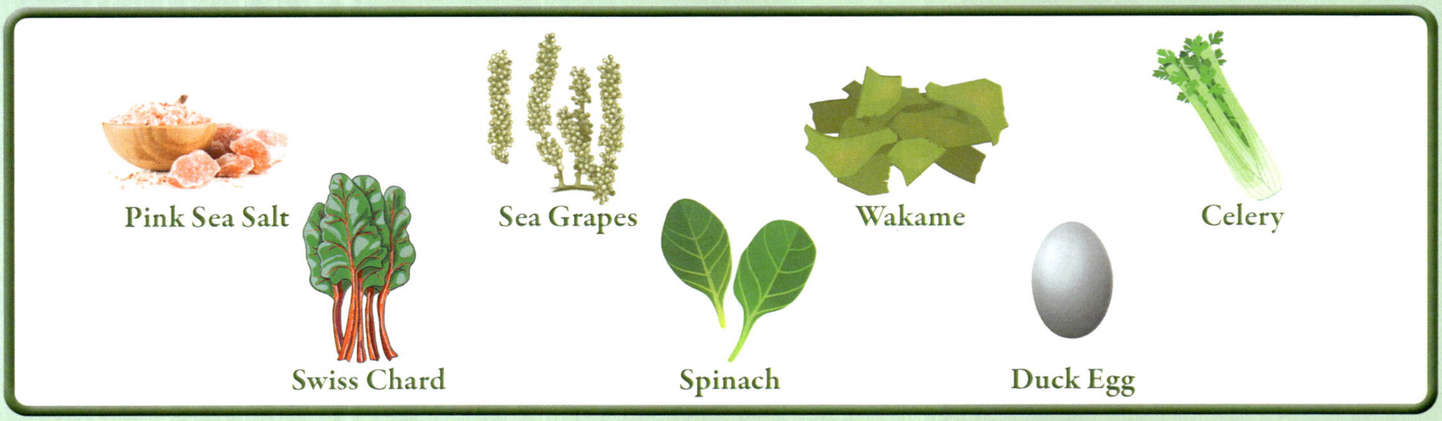

Naturally-occurring sodium, in sea salt and other natural foods, supports all the systems of the body. Sodium is one of the major minerals, along with chloride, potassium, calcium, magnesium, phosphorus, and sulfur. Our bodies require these minerals in amounts greater than 100 mg per day.[1] Most of our sodium is in our blood plasma and extracellular fluids, a significant amount is in our bones, and a small amount is in our organs and cells. As electrolytes, sodium and potassium send nerve impulses that signal the contraction and relaxation of muscles. Sodium and chloride ion (electrical charge) concentrations are lower inside the cells than outside, in contrast to potassium ions which concentrate inside the cells. Based on ionic polarity, sodium, chloride, and potassium balance the volume of fluid inside and outside the cells and regulate blood pressure.

In her book, *Health Is Your Birthright: How to Create the Health You Deserve,* Ellen Tart-Jensen highlights that Bernard Jensen, D.C., N.D. called sodium the youth element because of its importance in maintaining limber and pliable joints. Tart-Jensen describes how sodium nourishes the lymph and helps hold fluids in areas where they are needed, including: around the eyes, sinus cavities, mouth, lungs, and around the joints. She details how sodium normalizes the glandular secretions in the endocrine system, lubricates cellular membranes, and maintains proper blood pH.[2] Sodium also aids in the transport of carbon dioxide, supporting the respiratory system.

We can help maintain internal homeostasis by staying hydrated and replenishing our minerals. Sodium may be lost through dehydration, sweating, diarrhea, and kidney disease. Pamela W. Smith in her book, *What You Must Know About Vitamins, Minerals, Herbs and So Much More,* outlines symptoms of sodium deficiency (hyponatremia), including: decreased elasticity of subcutaneous tissue, diminished reflexes, impaired adrenal function, neurological disorders, and tiredness. On the other hand, fever and vomiting are among the causes of excess sodium (hypernatremia) which may result in edema, high blood pressure, seizures, thirst, and weakness.[3] Notably, table salt is detrimental to our health due to the extreme heat and industrial purification processes used to refine it from rock salt. The added anti-caking chemicals are also a concern, such as: dextrose, sodium fluoride, ferrous fumarate, calcium aluminosilicate, and sodium ferrocyanide/prussiate of soda.

Sea salt and organic foods that naturally contain sodium were a part of all the traditional diets that Weston A. Price, D.D.S. studied in the 1930s. The indigenous people he researched, who enjoyed excellent health and high immunity to disease, obtained sodium from sea salt, algae, animal, and plant foods. The isolated indigenous groups he studied included: the people of the Outer Hebrides off the coast of Scotland; Alaska and the Far North Eskimos and Indians; Polynesian, Melanesian, and Micronesian South Sea islanders; Australian aborigines; New Zealand Māori; and the North and South American coastal tribes.[4] "Lacking a local source, sea salt was one of a few items the people of the alpine valley Lötschental in Switzerland brought into their village."[5] Natural foods containing sodium and other nourishing minerals, including sea salt, are widely available and life-sustaining.

References

[1]Murrey, M. (2005). *The Encyclopedia of Natural Foods* (p. 115). New York, NY: Atria Books, .

[2]Tart-Jensen, E. (2006). *Health Is Your Birthright: How to Create the Health You Deserve* (pp. 20, 228). Berkeley, CA: Celestial Arts.

[3]Smith, P. W. (2020). *What You Must Know About Vitamins, Minerals, Herbs And So Much More* (2nd ed., pp. 87–89). Garden City Park, NY: Square One Publishers.

[4]Nienhiser, J. (2000). *Characteristics of traditional diets.* Washington, D.C.: Weston A. Price Foundation. https://www.westonaprice.org/health-topics/abcs-of-nutrition/characteristics-of-traditional-diets/.

[5]Price, W.A. (2019). *Nutrition and Physical Degeneration* (8th ed., p. 22). Lemon Grove, CA: Price Pottenger.

Study of a Hormone

Serotonin Promotes Well-Being

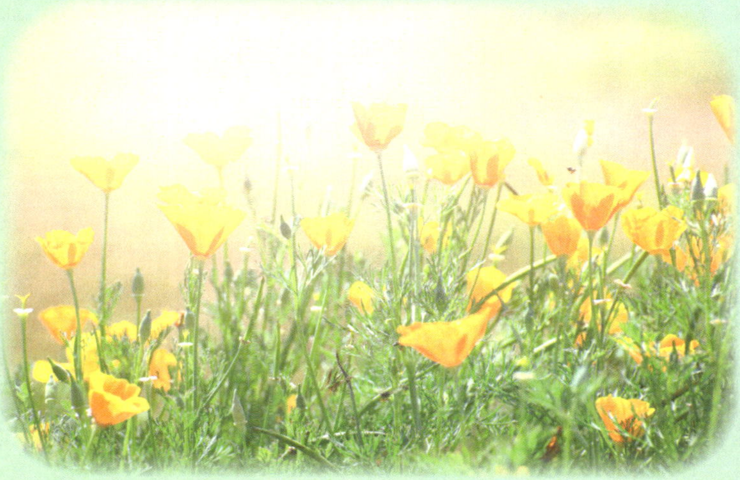

Serotonin is a compound made in our brain that is vital for maintaining a healthy appetite, sound sleep, and feelings of well-being.[1] It signals satiety as we are finishing our meals and is used by the body to make melatonin, the hormone that governs the sleep-wake cycle. Stress, lack of sunlight, and insufficient physical activity can lower serotonin levels. On the other hand, relaxation, sunlight each day, and regular exercise increases serotonin levels. Consuming foods rich in tryptophan can increase serotonin and melotonin levels.[2,3] Example foods that are high in tryptophan are displayed below.

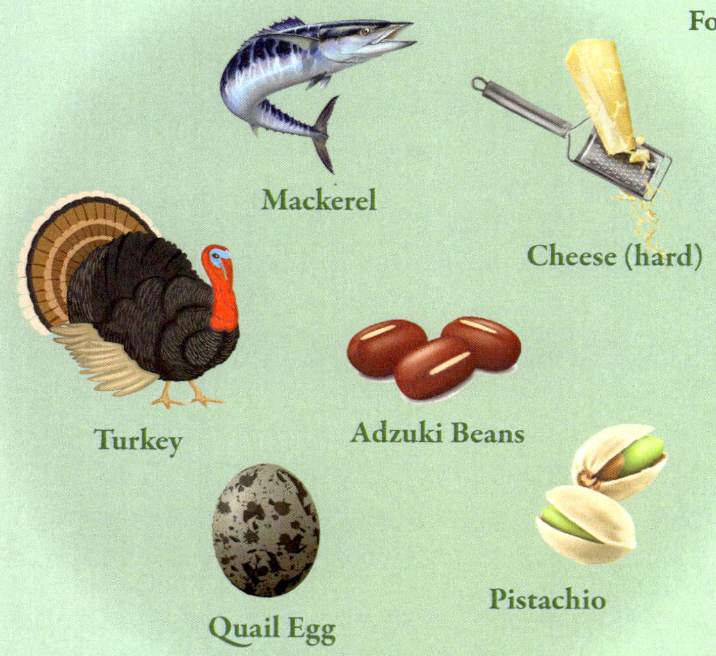

Foundational to the biochemical messaging of our nervous system, serotonin-producing neurons comprise a large complex system in the human brain. In their *Annual Review of Medicine* article titled, "The Expanded Biology of Serotonin," the authors stated that virtually every cell in the brain is close to a serotonergic fiber, and many brain functions are associated with serotonin.[4] Most serotonin is released in the digestive system where the intestinal microbiota influences its pathways and concentration. Serotonin supports peristalsis (the involuntary waves of muscle contractions that move food through the gastrointestinal tract) and the assimilation and absorption of nutrients. While traveling on the brain-gut axis, and to each of our organs, serotonin supports calmness within the body.

References

[1,3]Smith, P. W. (2020). *What You Must Know About Vitamins, Minerals, Herbs, and So Much More* (2nd ed., pp. 179, 180). Garden City Park, NY: Square One Publishers.

[2]Murray, M. & Pizzorno, J. (2005). *The Encyclopedia of Healing Foods* (p. 63). New York, NY: Atria Books.

[4]Berger, M. Gray, J. A., & Roth, B. L. (2018, March 22). The expanded biology of serotonin. *Annual Review of Medicine.* https://www.ncbi.nlm.nih.gov/pmc/articles/PMC5864293/#:~:text=In%20the%20central%20nervous%20system,system%20in%20the%20human%20brain.,1,2 and Bryan L. Roth3.

Study of a Regenerative Organ – Bone

"Despite its inert appearance, bone is a highly dynamic organ that is continuously resorbed by osteoclasts and neoformed [newly formed] by osteoblasts."[1]

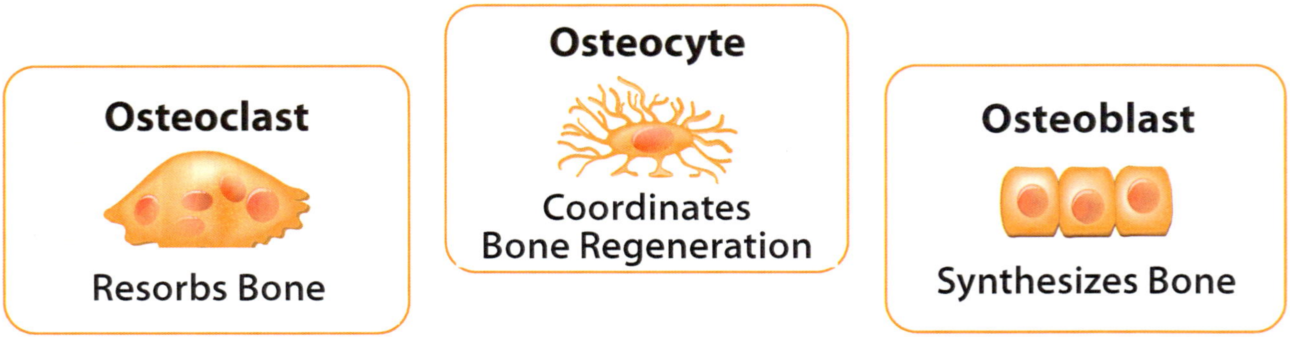

Bone is illuminative of life. It is self-organizing, complex, and regenerative. Most of our skeletal structure takes many years to mature, initially made of cartilage and then gradually replaced by bone. Considering the slow development of bone (ossification), the skeletal system becomes fully formed about the time we are age twenty-five. Bone regeneration (remodeling), on the other hand, is a life-long process.

The body is continually repairing bone from daily wear and tear. For example, microtears occur in bone and muscle when doing strengthening and weight-bearing activities. Knocks against the body cause tiny bone fractures. When our diet lacks sufficient calcium or phosphorous, the body takes these minerals from the bone to meet more urgent needs elsewhere. Once added to the diet, the bone can replenish these minerals. However, borrowing minerals from the bones without resupplying them, over time, can result in loosening teeth and shrinking skeletal structure.[2] Bone malnourishment can be passed on to the next generation and cause narrowing of the facial structure, including the dental arch; crowded for space, the teeth come in crooked.[3]

Continued...

Study of a Regenerative Organ – Bone

Traditionally-prepared whole natural foods provide the nutrients needed to build and maintain healthy bones.

Essential Nutrients Include

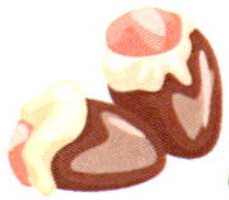

Organ Meats

Vitamin A — Required for the growth and development of bones

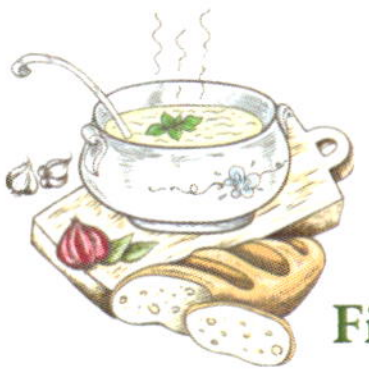

Fish Bone Broth

Collagen — Principal component of bone and cartilage

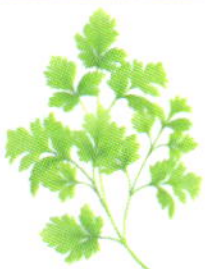

Parsley

Vitamin C

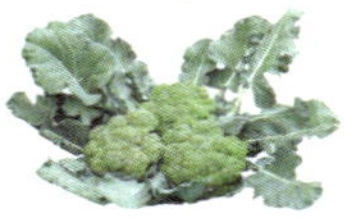

Broccoli

Vitamin K_1

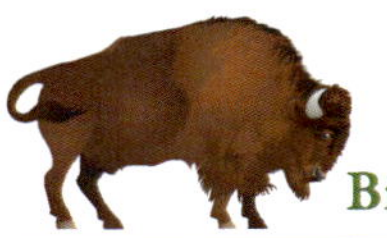

Bison

Zinc

Facilitates the formation of collagen

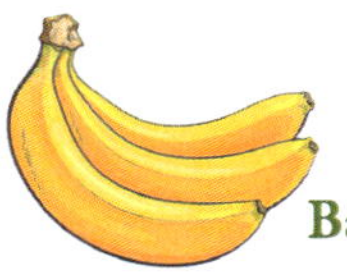

Banana

Silicon — Used in collagen synthesis and making bones sturdy

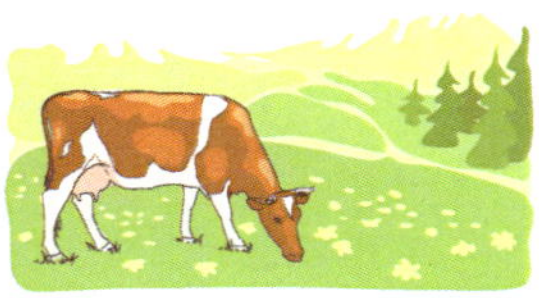

Raw Milk Products

Calcium

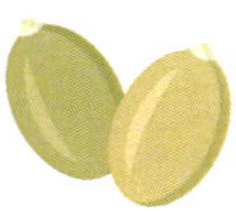

Pumpkin Seed

Phosphorus

Principal mineral components of bone

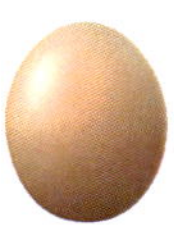

Chicken Egg

Vitamin K_2

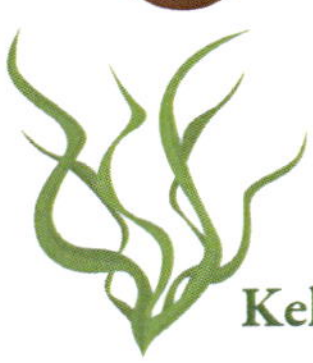

Kelp

Magnesium

Needed for bone formation and density

Continued...

Study of a Regenerative Organ – Bone

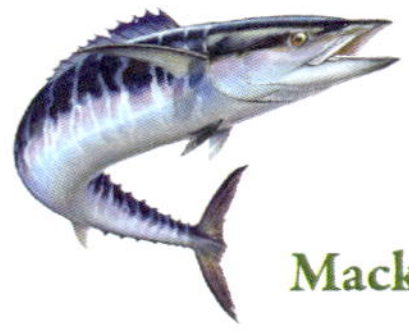
Mackerel

Vitamin D_3

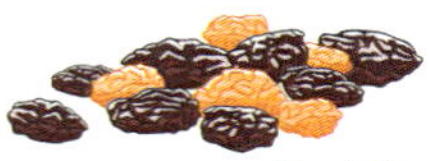
Raisins

Boron

Aid in mineral absorption; support estrogen production

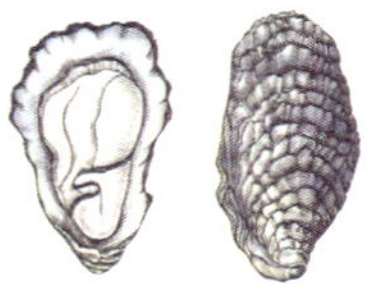
Oysters

Copper

Pecan

Manganese

Necessary for bone mineral deposition

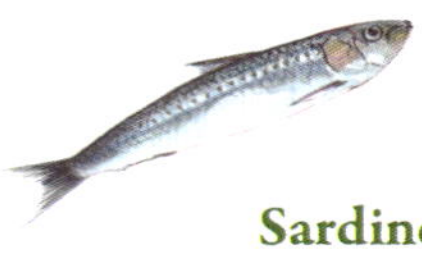
Sardine

Fatty Acids

Critical energy source for bone-building osteoblasts[4]

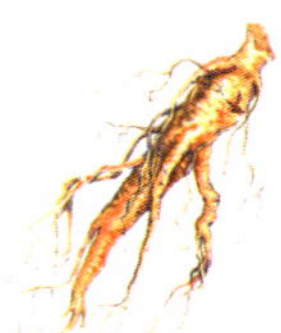
Ginseng

Estrogen

Protect bone from unnecessary resorption

Bone is built in a hierarchical structure; wherein, calcium phosphate crystals are arranged around helices of collagen. The structure occurs from the nanoscale upward in nested, helix-like patterns for twelve or more levels.[5] Osteocytes orchestrate the construction of bone, coordinating groups of osteoclasts and osteoblasts. The osteoclasts resorb worn and damaged bone cells by secreting acid phosphatase that unglues calcium phosphate. The osteoblasts secrete alkaline phosphatase and collagen to construct the organic bone matrix; then they deposit hydroxyapatite (mostly calcium phosphate) to mineralize and harden the bone. The inner bone has elastin and is porous and spongy, protected by a denser outer bone shell. The development of bone incorporates blood vessels that are transformed into bone marrow.[6]

Continued...

Study of a Regenerative Organ – Bone

Osteocytes are one of the longest living types of cells in the body. They affect phosphate reabsorption in the kidneys, insulin secretion in the pancreas, and skeletal muscle function.[7] Occupying lacunae (small spaces in the bone matrix), osteocytes are mechano-sensors, adapting bone responses to mechanical loading. They receive hormonal signals from hormones locally, such as prostaglandins, and more broadly from the endocrine system, including: parathyroid hormone, calcitonin, vitamin D_3, glucocorticoids, androgens, and estrogens. The estrogens protect bone by inhibiting unnecessary osteoclast resorption of bone.[8]

Overall, our skeletal structure protects our organs and other soft tissue. It is also integrated with other systems in the body. For instance, as part of the endocrine system, bone produces hormones, including osteocalcin which is involved in energy metabolism.[9] Bone marrow manufactures oxygen-carrying red blood cells and platelets that support the respiratory and cardiovascular systems, and marrow-producing white blood cells supply the lymph and immune system. Our skeletomuscular system works in conjunction with the nervous system, enabling our capacity for movement.

References

[1]Breeland, G., Sinkler, M. A, & Menezes, R. G. (2024, May 1). *Embryology, bone ossification*. StatPearls Publishing. https://www.ncbi.nlm.nih.gov/books/NBK539718.

[2, 3]Price, W. A. (2019). *Nutrition and Physical Degeneration* (8th ed., pp. 344, 75). Lemon Grove, CA: Price-Pottinger.

[4]Nandy, A., Helderman, R. C. M., Thapa, S., et al. (2023, November 24). Lipolysis supports bone formation by providing osteoblasts with endogenous fatty acid substrates to maintain bioenergetic status. *Bone Research. 11*(62). https://www.nature.com/articles/s41413-023-00297-2#Fun.

[5]Reznikov, N., Bilton, M., Lari, L., Stevens, M. M., & Kröger, R. (2018, May 4). Fractal-like hierarchical organization of bone begins at the nanoscale. *Journal of Science. 360*(6388). https://www.science.org/doi/10.1126/science.aao2189.

[6]Florencio-Silva, R., Sasso, G. R., Sasso-Cerri, E., Simões, M. J., & Cerri, P. S. (2015, July 13). Biology of bone tissue: structure, function, and factors that influence bone cells. *Biomed Research International*. https://www.ncbi.nlm.nih.gov/pmc/articles/PMC4515490.

[7]Robling, A. G. & Bonewald, L. F. (2020, February). The osteocyte: new insights. *Annual Review of Physiology. 82*:485–506. https://www.annualreviews.org/content/journals/10.1146/annurev-physiol-021119-034332.

[8]Dallas, S. L., Prideaux, M., & Bonewald, L. F. (2013, April 26). The osteocyte: an endocrine cell ... and more. *Endocrine Reviews. 34*(5):658– 690. https://www.ncbi.nlm.nih.gov/pmc/articles/PMC3785641.

[9]Zhou, R., Guo, Q., Xiao, Y., et al. (2021, May 20). Endocrine role of bone in the regulation of energy metabolism. *Bone Research. 9*(25). https://www.nature.com/articles/s41413-021-00142-4#citeas.

PART VI

Natural Foods Support the 11 Systems of the Body

In concert, the 11 Systems synchronize to carry out the functions of the body and maintain homeostasis.

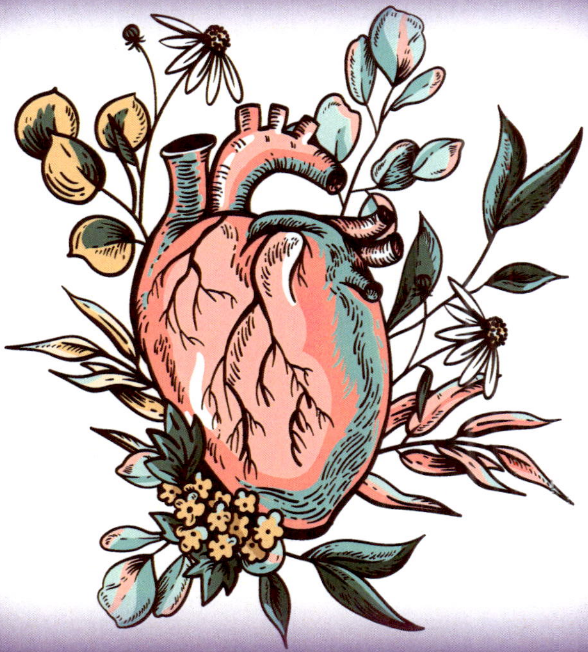

Cardiovascular
Digestive
Endocrine
Immune
Integumentary
Muscular
Nervous
Reproductive
Respiratory
Skeletal
Urinary

Cardiovascular System

Freshly oxygenated blood from the heart acquires nutrients, electrolytes, enzymes, and hormones and delivers these constituents through the arteries to nourish the organs and tissues. Capillaries in the tissues connect to tiny arterioles and venules where nutrients and metabolites diffuse into the cells. Then, the veins, traveling closer to the surface of our skin, bring the blood back to the heart to be reoxygenated.

Beneficial Foods

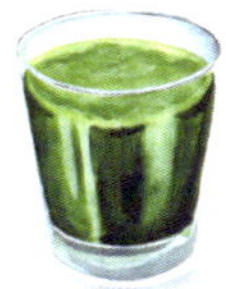

Chlorophyll enhances the oxygen-carrying capacity of hemoglobin in the blood

---

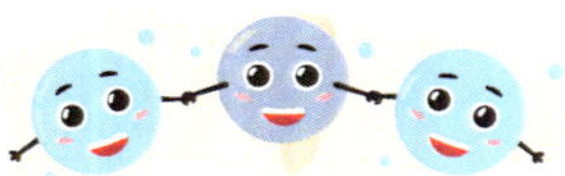

CO_2

The required amount of CO_2 in the blood constricts the blood vessels and hemoglobin, releasing oxygen into the tissues[1]

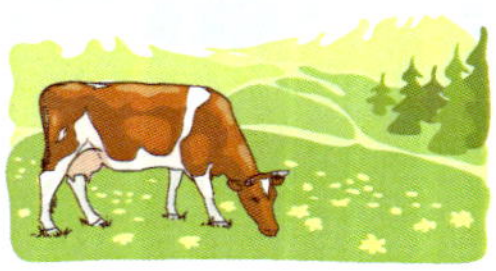

Raw Cow's Milk

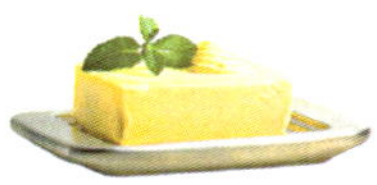

Raw Butter

Conjugated linoleic acid (CLA) protects against atherosclerosis;[1] saturated fats (non-oxidizing, heat stable) and fat-soluble vitamins A, D_3, E, and K_2 protect against atherosclerosis[2]

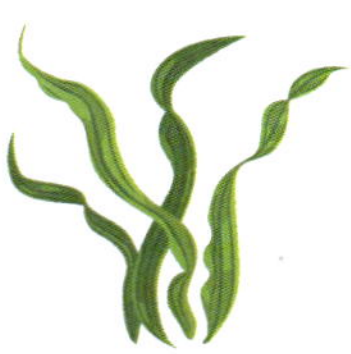

Spirulina

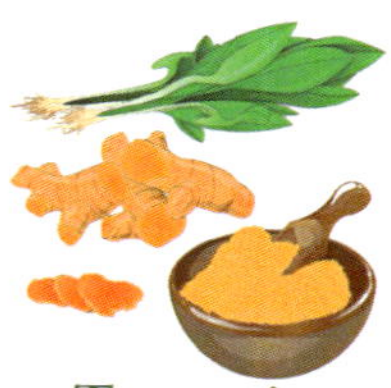

Turmeric

Reduces the oxidation of lipids[3] and inhibits platelet clumping in the body[4]

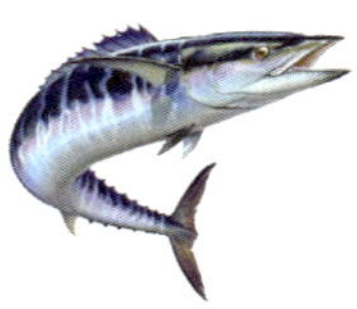

Mackerel

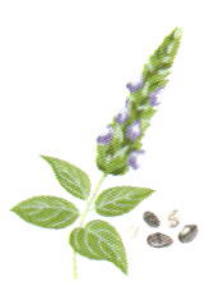

Chia Seed

Omega-3 fatty acids keep blood vessels supple

Continued...

Cardiovascular System

Beneficial Foods

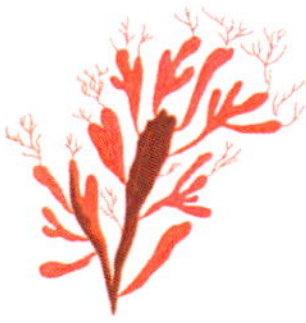
Dulse

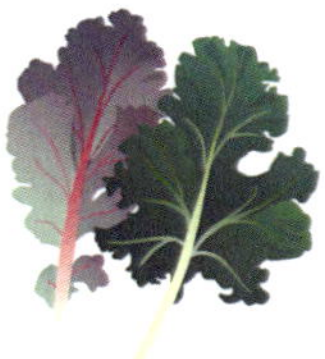
Kale

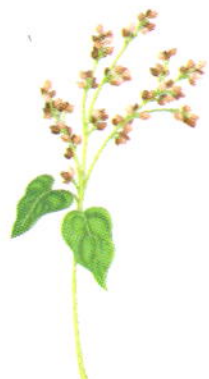
Buckwheat

Magnesium supports a healthy heartbeat and reduces inflammation

---

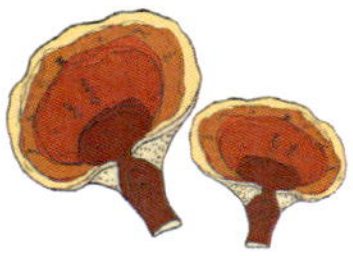
Reishi Mushroom

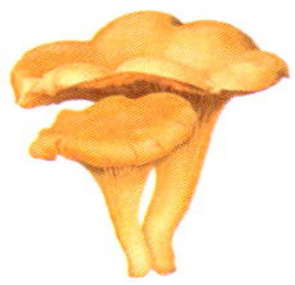
Chanterelle Mushroom

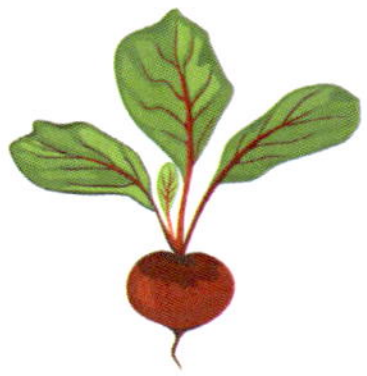
Beet

Triterpenoids in reishi and chanterelle mushrooms protect the heart; and betanin and nitrate and nitrite in beets improve blood flow

---

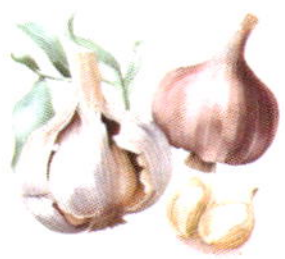
Garlic

Allicin and other sulfur containing compounds support the blood vessels making them more supple and strong

---

Grape seed extract

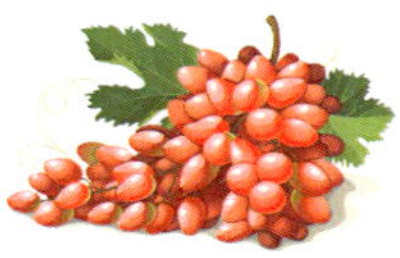
Grape (red)

Proanthocyanidins strengthen the walls of the blood vessels and veins, improve the flow of blood and lymph fluid, and reduce swelling in the legs and feet

Resveratrol protects the heart from inflammation-induced oxidative damage[5]

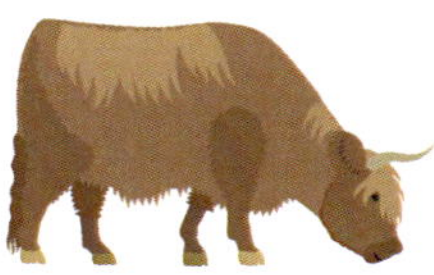
Cow

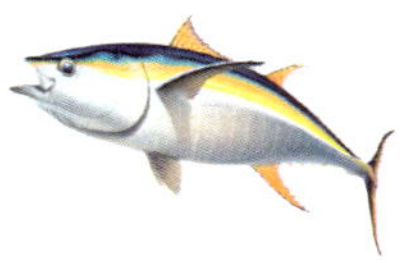
Tuna (yellowfin)

Coenzyme Q10 (ubiquinone) is an anti-oxidant that protects the heart and supports the mitochondria in energy production

References

[1]McKeown, P. (2015). *The Oxygen Advantage* (p. 29). New York, NY: HarperCollins Publishers.

[2]Wannamethee, S. G., Jefferis, B. J., Lennon, L., Papacosta, O., Whincup, P. H., & Hingorani, A. D. (2018, January 6). Serum conjugated linoleic acid and risk of incident heart failure in older men: The British regional heart study. *Journal of the American Heart Association*. 7:e006653. https://doi.org/10.1161/JAHA.117.006653.

[3]Dinicolantonio, J. & Land, S. (2020). *The Immunity Fix* (p. 152). Kansas City, MO: http://drjamesdinic.com.

[4]Hussain, Y., Abdullah, Khan, F., Alsharif, K. F., Alzahrani, K. J., Saso, L., & Khan, H. (2022, December 8). Regulatory effects of curcumin on platelets: An update and future directions. *Biomedicines. 10*(12):3180. https://www.ncbi.nlm.nih.gov/pmc/articles/PMC9775400.

[5]Gal, R., Deres, L., Toth, K., Halmosi, R., & Habon, T. (2021, September 21). The effect of resveratrol on the cardiovascular system from molecular mechanisms to clinical results. *International Journal of Molecular Science*. https://www.ncbi.nlm.nih.gov/pmc/articles/PMC8466271.

Digestive System

With saliva and chewing, food becomes masticated and is sent down the throat (pharynx) and esophagus to the stomach where digestive enzymes break it down into chyme. Peristaltic muscular contractions move the chyme into the small intestine for further digestion. Nutrients are absorbed into the blood and lymph for assimilation by cells and tissues. The pancreas, liver, and gall bladder play key roles in digestion. In the large intestine (colon), nutrients and water are absorbed and waste products are moved to the rectum and anus for elimination.

Beneficial Foods

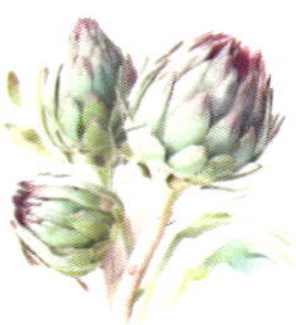
Artichokes

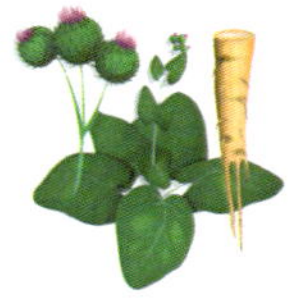
Burdock Root

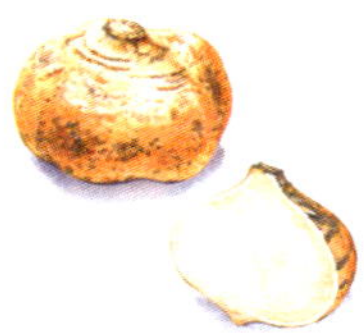
Jicama

Inulin nourishes probiotics in the microbiome

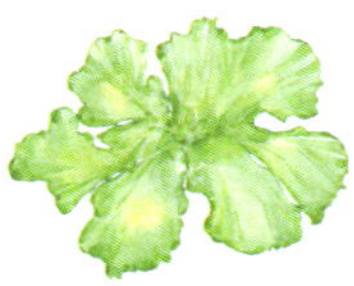
Sea Lettuce

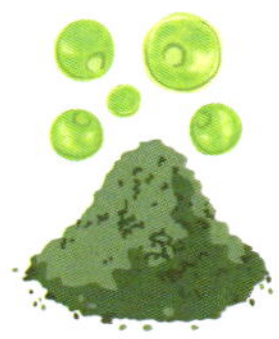
Chlorella

Oligosaccharides nourish probiotics in the microbiome

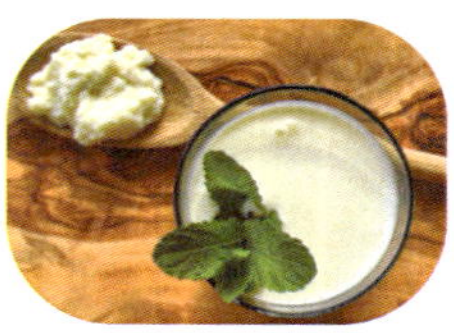
Kefir

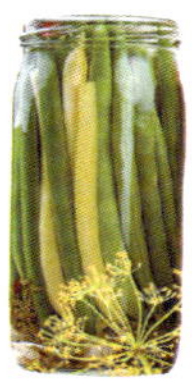
Vegetables (wild fermentation)

The probiotics in fermented foods replenish and support the microbiome

---

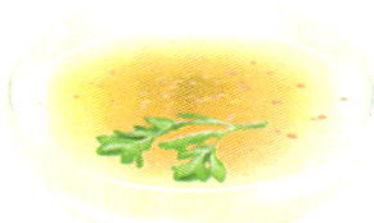
Bone Broth

Collagen repairs damage to the lining of the intestines

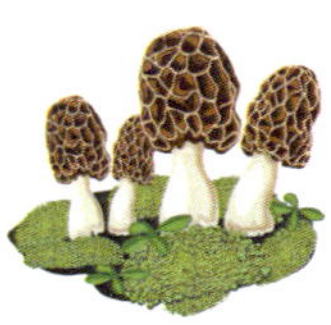
Morel Mushroom

Soluble polysaccharides are prebiotic and improve digestion by nourishing probiotic bacteria[1]

Continued...

Digestive System

Beneficial Foods

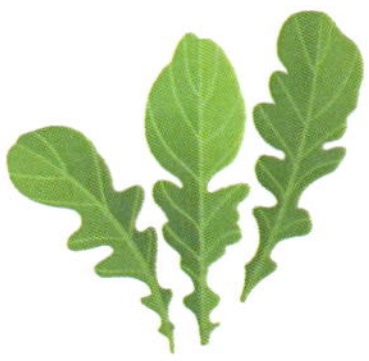

Arugula

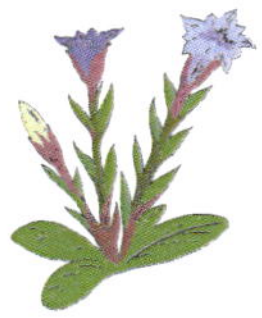

Gentian

Bitters promote the secretion of digestive enzymes and bile and tone the entire digestive system

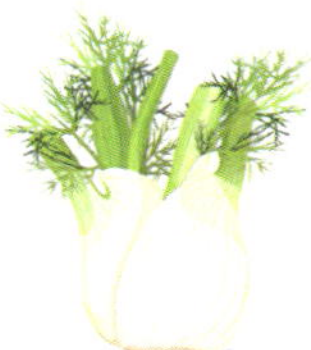

Fennel Bulb

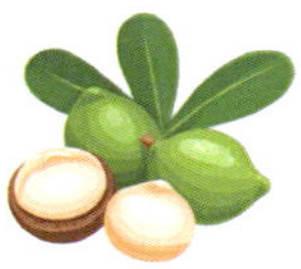

Macadamia

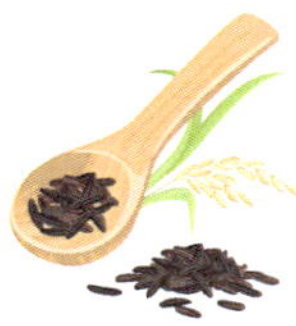

Wild Rice

Soluble and insoluble fiber is prebiotic, supporting the microbiome and provides bulk that aids in digestion

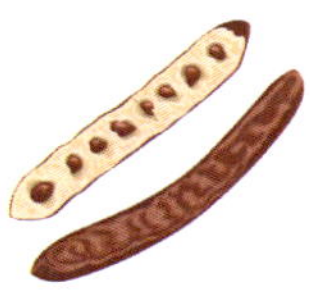

Carob Pod and Bean

Phenolic acids, such as quercetin, cinnamic, and coumaric protect the mucosal lining of the digestive tract

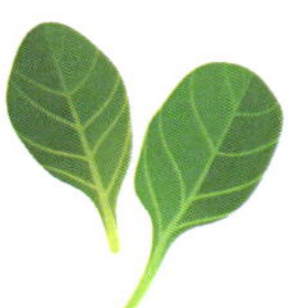

Spinach

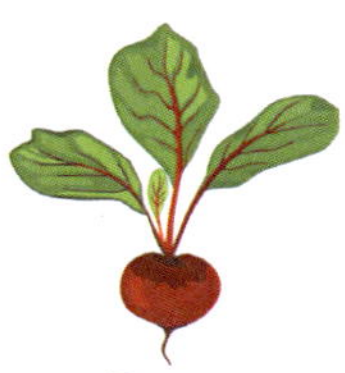

Beets

Supports digestion; aids the liver in processing fat and detoxifying the body, reducing homocysteine in the blood (which can damage the arteries)

References

[1]Li, Y., Chen, H., & Zhang, X. (2023, March 17). Cultivation, nutritional value, bioactive compounds of morels, and their health benefits: A systematic review. *Frontiers in Nutrition*. 10:1159029. https://www.ncbi.nlm.nih.gov/pmc/articles/PMC10063854.

[2]Murray, M. & Pizzorno, J. (2005). *The Encyclopedia of Healing Foods* (p. 389). New York, NY: Atria Books.

Endocrine System

The glands of the endocrine system produce and release hormones into the blood, lymph, and interstitial fluids that support the functions of the body, including: growth and development, reproduction, metabolism, and sleep. The hypothalamus gland in the brain secretes neurotransmitters and neurohormones that promote homeostasis. Receiving signals from the organs, the hypothalamus informs the pituitary gland in synchronizing hormonal activity. The endocrine system encompasses the: pineal, thymus, thyroid, parathyroid, and adrenal glands; heart; bones; skin; stomach; small and large intestines; pancreas; liver; kidneys; ovaries; testes.

Beneficial Foods

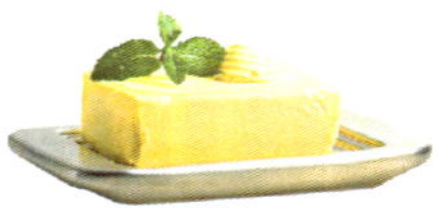

Butter

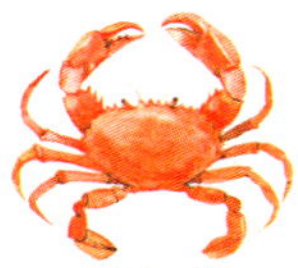

Crab

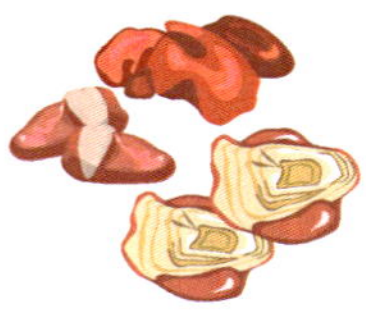

Gizzards,
Liver, & Heart

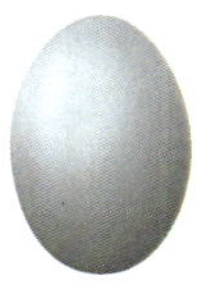

Duck Egg

Cholesterol is the precursor to vitamin D3 and all steroid hormones, including: cortisol, glucocorticoids (regulates blood glucose levels), mineralocorticoids (balances cellular electrolytes and water): and dehydroepiandrosterone (DHEA) which is used to make estrogen (estradiol, estriol, and estrone), progesterone, and testosterone.[1]

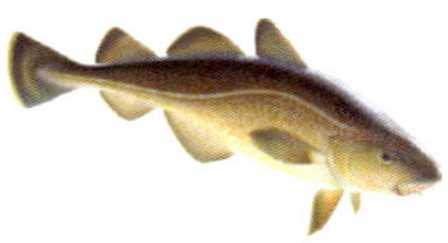

Cod

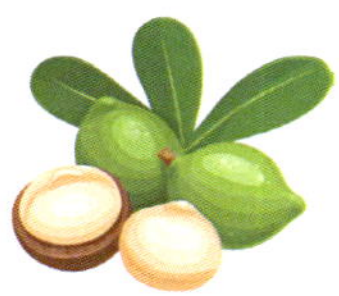

Macadamia Nut

Omega-3 fatty acids aid in the production of hormones and promote healthy metabolism

---

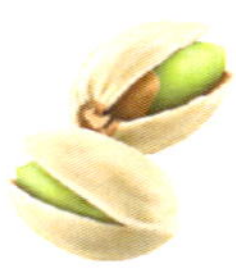

Pistachio

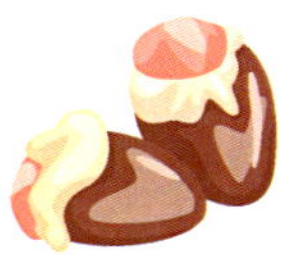

Organ Meats
Vitamin B6
(pyridoxine)

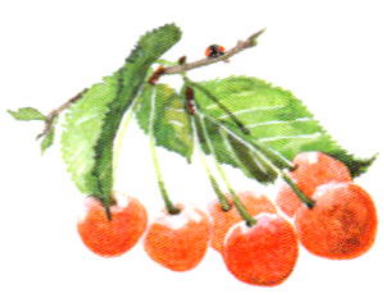

Cherry

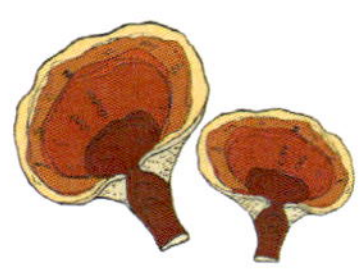

Reishi Mushroom
Melatonin

Vitamin B6 (pyridoxine) and Melatonin are used by the pituitary gland to make human growth hormone (somatostatin), which is needed for healthy cell growth and repair and restful, restorative sleep

Continued...

Endocrine System

Beneficial Foods

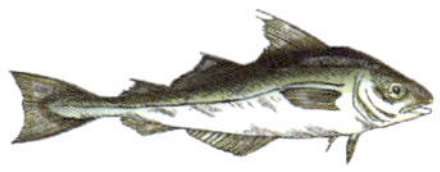

Haddock
(iodine)

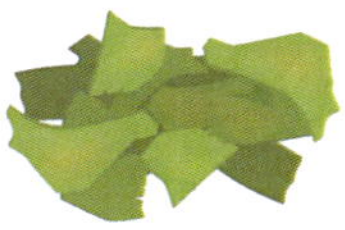

Wakame
(iodine)

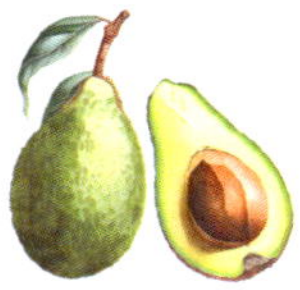

Avocado
Tyrosine (amino acid)

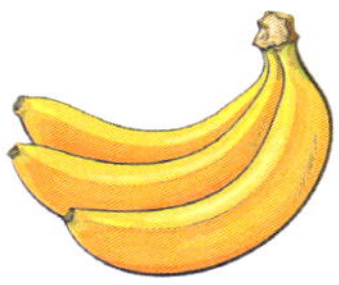

Banana
Tyrosine (amino acid)

Iodine and Tyrosine (amino acid) are used by the thyroid gland to make thyroglobulin as the precursor to producing the thyroid hormones T3 (triiodothyronine) and T4 (thyroxine) which are crucial for brain development and regulating the rate of metabolism

---

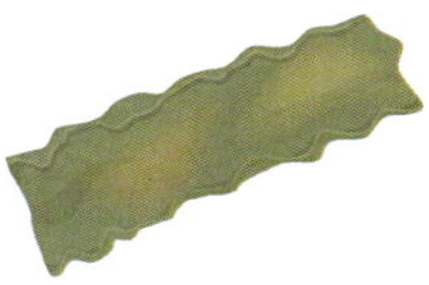

Kombu

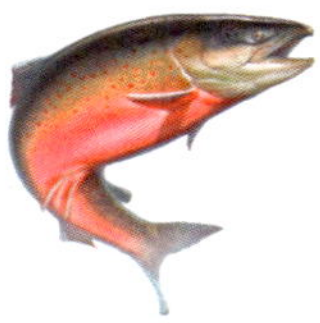

Salmon

Magnesium protects the pancreas, increases insulin sensitivity, and healthy glucose levels in the blood

---

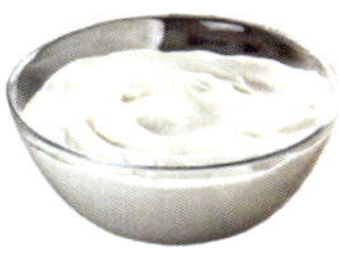

Yogurt

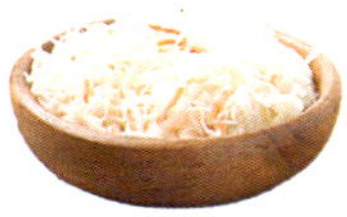

Sauerkraut

Probiotic fermented foods assist the body in regulating hormones, such as insulin, ghrelin, and leptin to support healthy blood sugar levels, appetite, and satiety; also help balance steroid hormones (for example, estrogen and glucocorticoids) supports bone remodeling[1]

References

[1]Hu, J., Zhang, Z., Shen, W. J., & Azhar, S. (2010, June 1). Cellular cholesterol delivery, intracellular processing and utilization for biosynthesis of steroid hormones. *Nutrition & Metabolism* (London). *1*(7):47. https://www.ncbi.nlm.nih.gov/pmc/articles/PMC2890697.

[2]Zhang, L., Zhang, R., & Li, L. (2023, April 25). Effects of probiotic supplementation on exercise and the underlying mechanisms. *Foods*. *12*(9), 1787. https://doi.org/10.3390/foods12091787.

Immune System

Slow-flowing lymph fluid defends against pathogens and delivers lipids and fat-soluble vitamins to the blood for delivery to cells and tissues. The contractions of surrounding muscles in daily movement compress the lymph vessels, bathing the tissues with interstitial lymph fluid. As a result, waste products, bacteria destroyed by lymphocytes, and worn cells are filtered out. The immune system encompasses the: tonsils; tear glands; adenoids in the back of the nasal passage; thymus gland; spleen; Peyer patches in the small intestine; liver; appendix; bone marrow; and lymph vessels, nodes, and ducts.

Beneficial Foods

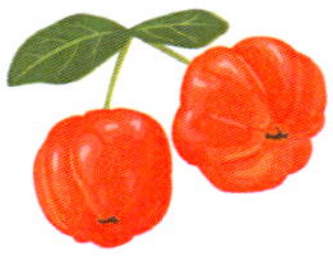
Acerola

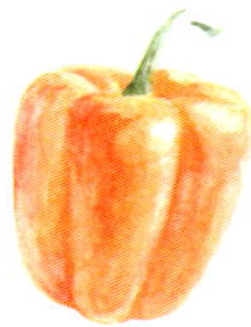
Bell Pepper

Vitamin C, polyphenols, and carotenes protect the thymus gland[1]

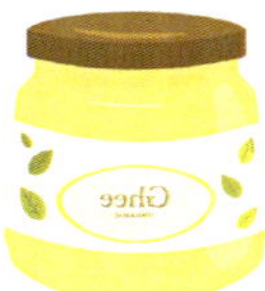
Ghee

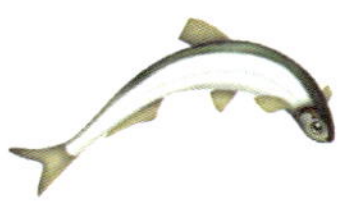
Anchovies

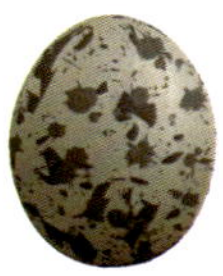
Quail Egg

Fats facilitate the absorption of fat-soluble vitamins A, D_2, D_3, E, K_1, K_2 into the lymph system and protect the body from disease;[2] omega-3 fatty acids reduce inflammation; and docosahexaenoic acid (DHA) strengthens the immune system[3]

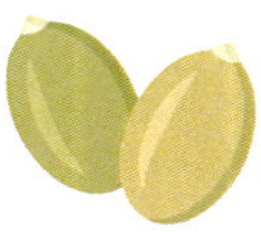
Pumpkin Seed

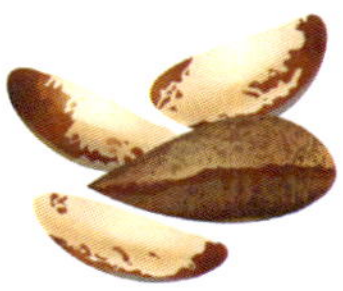
Brazil Nut

Magnesium and zinc are essential the proper functioning of the immune system

---

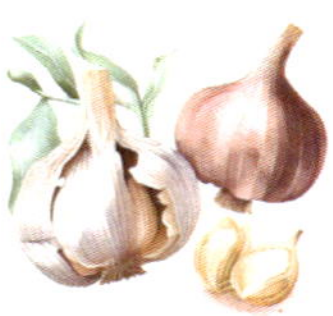
Garlic

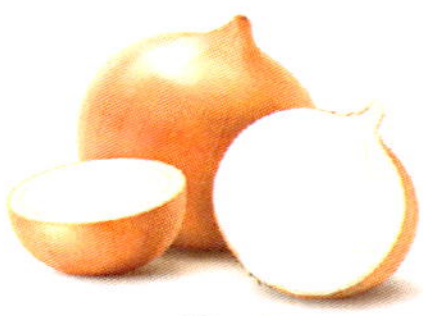
Onion

Allicin provides anti-microbial protection; quercetin is anti-oxidant and anti-inflammatory

---

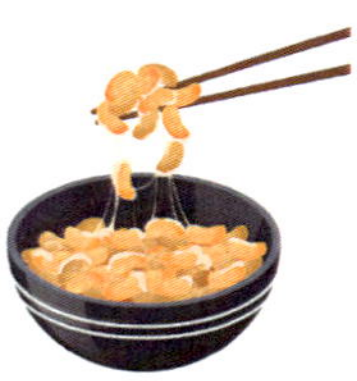
Natto

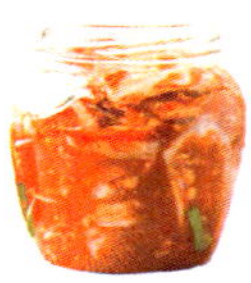
Kimchi

Probiotics create a healthy microbiome, fight pathogens, and enhance the immune system

Continued...

Immune System

Beneficial Foods

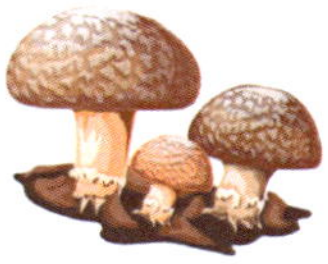
Shitake Mushroom

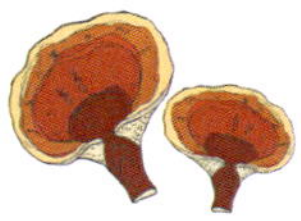
Reishi Mushroom

Beta-glucans, terpenes, ergosterols, and other bioactive compounds reduces inflammation and strengthen the immune system

---

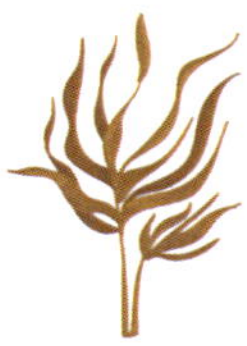
Arame

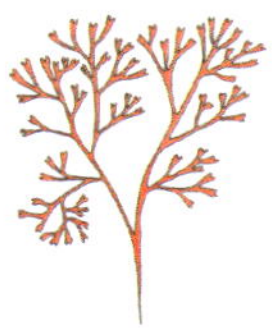
Sea/Irish Moss

Phenolic compounds and mineral nutrients, including iodine, prevent infection, help remove toxins, and support the immune response

---

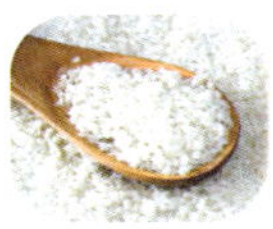
Celtic Sea Salt

Chloride is used by the body to make hydrochloric acid and hypochlorous acid to fight infection; taurine and chloramine calm excessive inflammatory response[4]

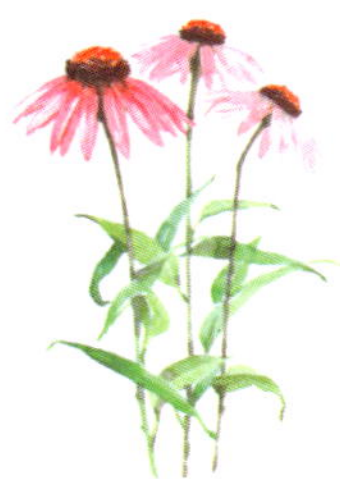
Echinacea

Echinocoside and other caffeic acids are anti-oxidant, anti-inflammatory, and wound healing

References

[1]Murray, M. & Pizzorno, J. (2005). *The Encyclopedia of Healing Foods* (p. 737). New York, NY: Atria Books.

[2]McGuire, M. & Beerman, K. (2018). *Nutritional Sciences* (3rd ed., p. 461). Boston, MA: Sengage Learning.

[3,4]Dinicolantonio, J. & Land, S. (2020). *The Immunity Fix* (pp. 143, 81, 224–225). Kansas City, MO: http://drjamesdinic.com.

Continued...

Immune System

Natural Foods with Anti-Microbial Properties

Plants and fungi (mushrooms) have evolved strong defenses against harmful bacteria, viruses, micro-fungi, and parasites. The foods listed, below, have traditionally been used to fight infection and strengthen immunity.

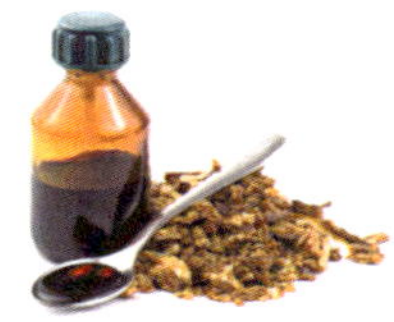

Bee Propolis
Pinocembrin

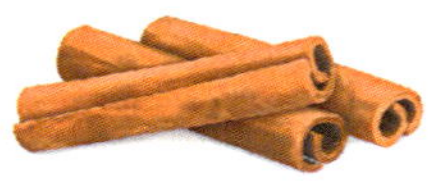

Cinnamon
Cinnamaldehyde

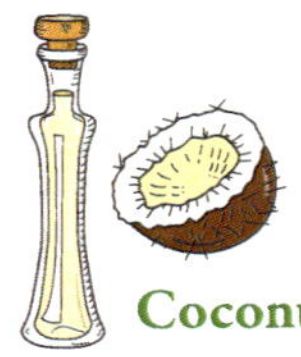

Coconut
Lauric Acid

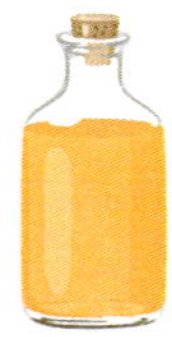

Cod Liver Oil
Omega-3 fatty acids:
eicosapentaenoic acid (EPA) and docosahexaenoic acid (DHA)

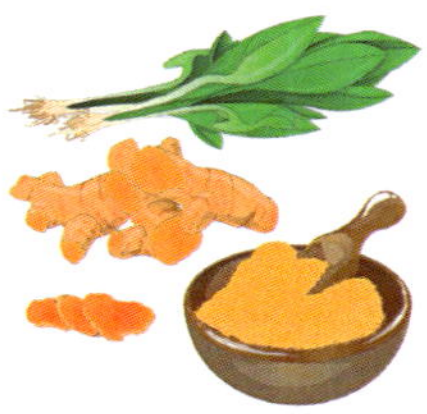

Turmeric
Curcumin

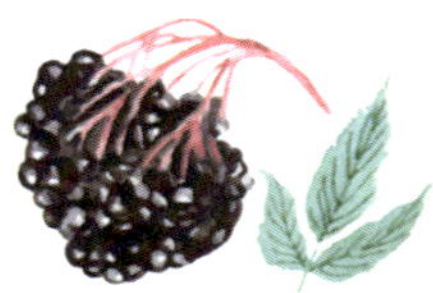

Elderberry
Anthocyanin

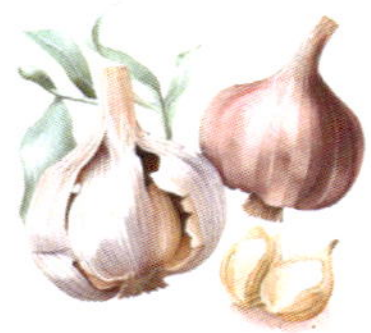

Garlic
Allicin

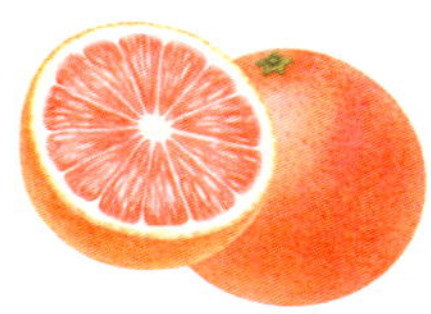

Grapefruit (seed extract)
Procyanidins

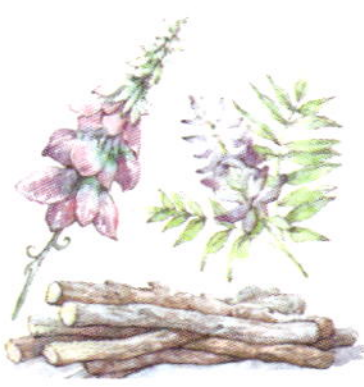

Licorice
Triterpenoids

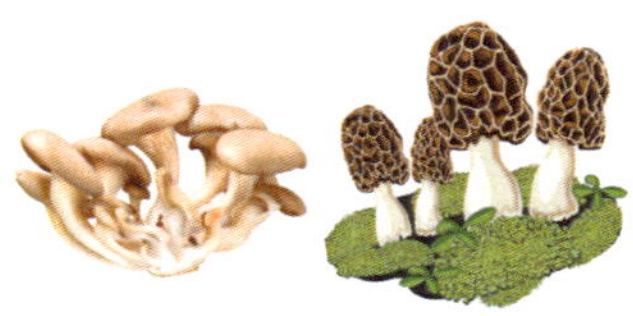

Mushrooms
Anthraquinone

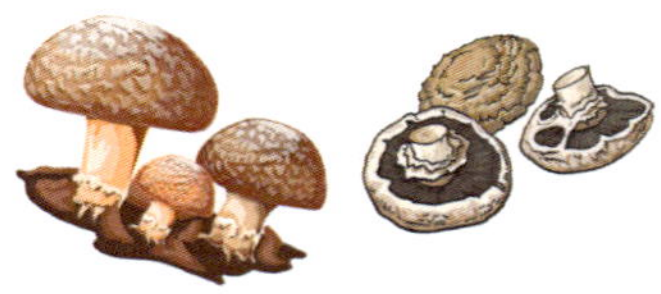

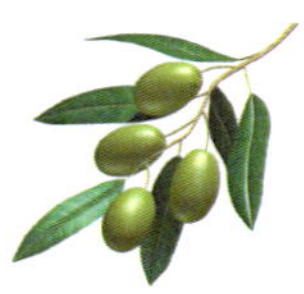

Olive (leaf extract)
Secoiridoids

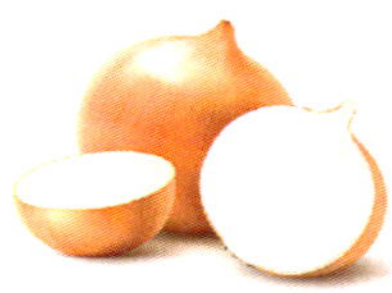

White Onion
Quercetin

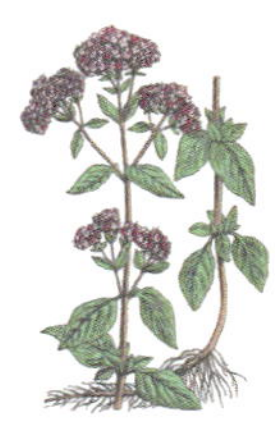

Oregano (oil extract)
Carvacrol

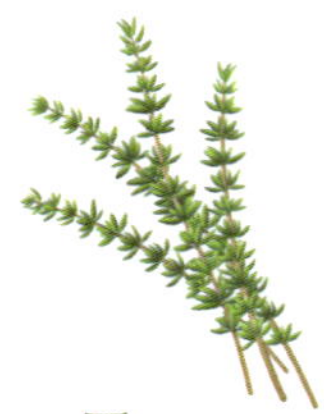

Thyme (oil extract)
Thymol

Integumentary System

The integumentary system is comprised of the skin, hair, and nails, furnishing a resilient protective covering for the body. Within the skin, hair follicles, and beneath the nail plates are vascular and nerve networks. The skin enables touch and makes the hormone-like vitamin, vitamin D_3, using a cholesterol metabolite and UV B rays of sunshine. Integral to the endocrine system, the skin's sweat glands cleanse and cool while the sebaceous glands lubricate. The outer layer of the skin, hair, and nail plates are primarily made of keratin. The under layers of skin are subcutaneous connective tissue, including collagen, and a fat store of energy that is insulating, shock absorbing, and cushioning.

Beneficial Foods

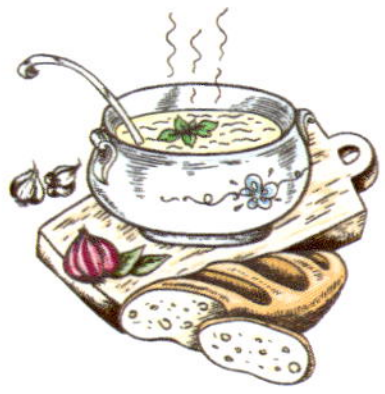
Fish Broth

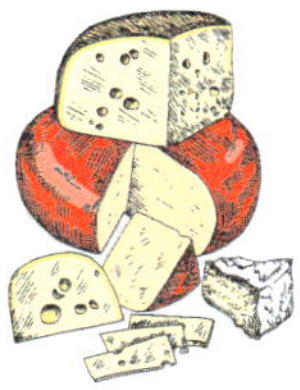
Cheese (soft)

Threonine, cysteine, methionine (amino acids) are used in making connective tissue (collagen and elastin) for maintaining the skin

---

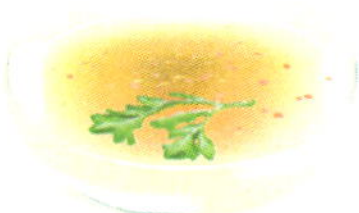
Bone Broth

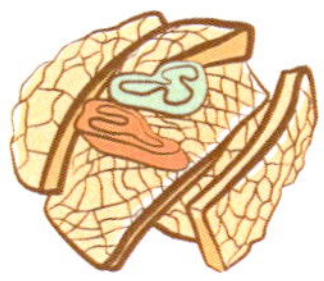
Offal

Collagen is used to construct connective tissue and maintain skin elasticity

---

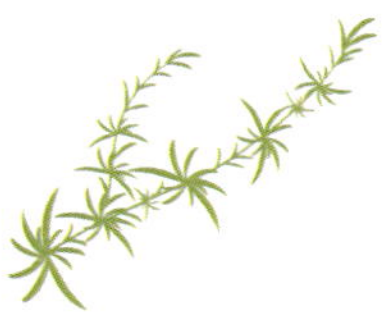
Hijiki

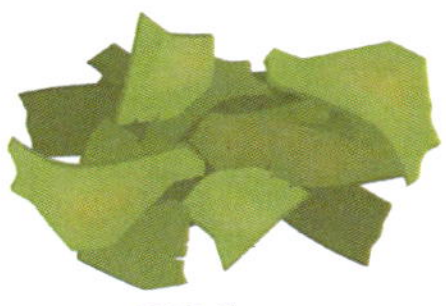
Wakame

Mucilage and alginic acid soothe and enhance the elasticity of the skin

---

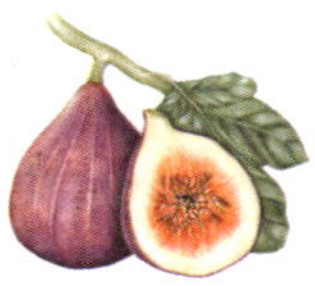
Fig

Plum

Rutin and vitamin C are used in making collagen

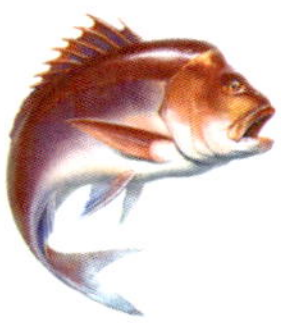
Red Snapper

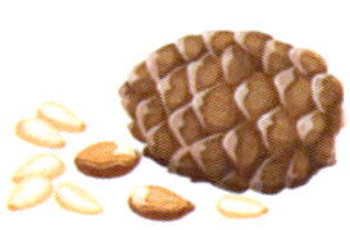
Pine Nut

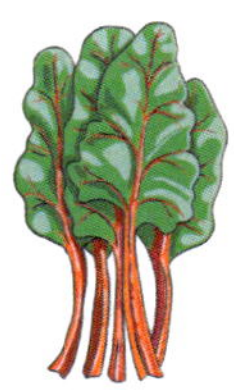
Swiss Chard

Omega-3 fatty acids nourish the skin and promote the growth of hair and nails

Continued...

Integumentary System

Beneficial Foods

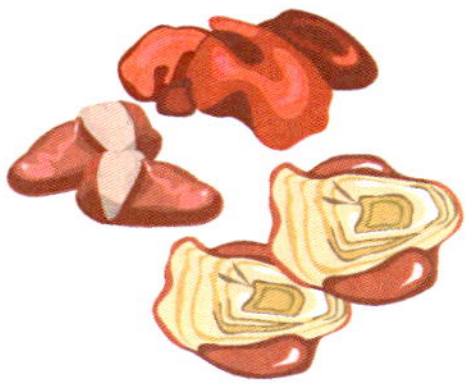

Gizzards, Liver, and Heart

Beef Tallow/Suet

Biotin (vitamin B_7) is needed for developing and maintaining healthy skin, hair, and nails

---

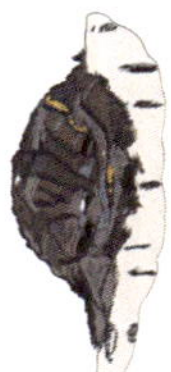

Chaga Mushroom

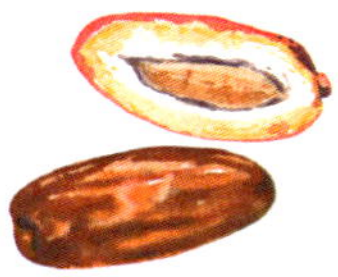

Date

Melanin provides the natural coloring (pigment) of the skin and hair and protects the skin from ultraviolet radiation damage

---

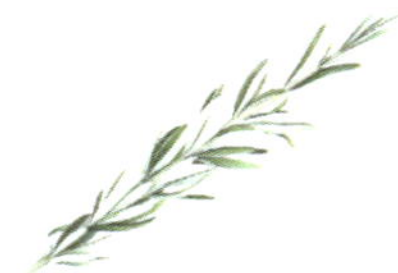

Rosemary

Has astringent properties, cleansing and closing pores in the skin, and promotes healthy hair and nails

---

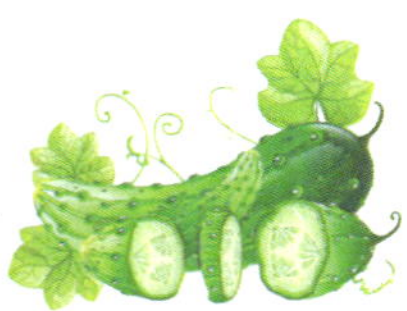

Cucumber

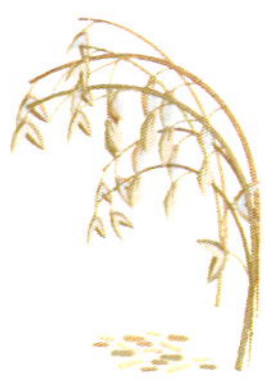

Oat

Silicon hydrates and strengthens connective tissue

Grape fleshy parts and seed extract

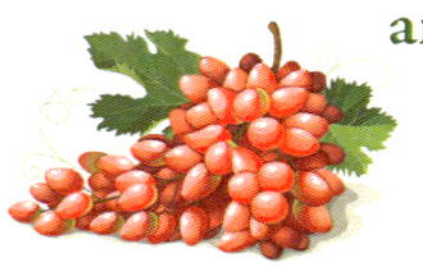

Grape (red)

Proanthocyanidins and resveratrol enhances collagen production, bone strength, and wound healing

Muscular System

Bands of muscles (bundled myofibers) layer the human body. They are controlled by the nervous systems and work in pairs, flexors and extensors. The skeletal muscles are attached to the bones by the tendons. Smooth muscles are located in the organs, including the fine muscles of the sensory organs such as the eyes. Blood supplies the muscles with oxygen and energy.

Beneficial Foods

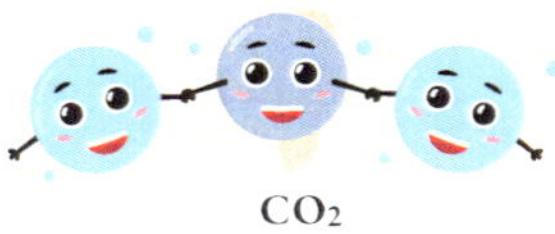 Carbon Dioxide	Facilitates oxygen reaching the blood and muscles
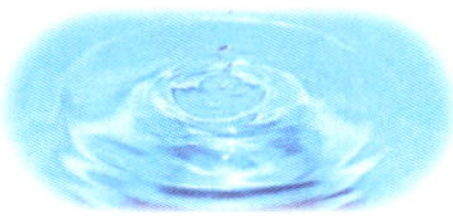 Water	Hydration enhances muscle performance and recovery and reduces soreness and tension
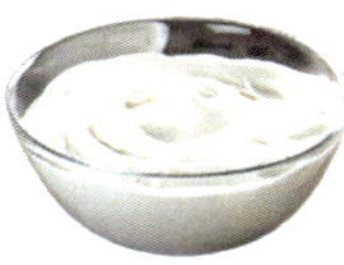 Yogurt	Whey, in conjunction with weight-bearing activities, increases energy (glycogen) while stabilizing blood sugar, promotes the synthesis of glutathione (anti-oxidant and essential for immune function); and helps burn fat and build lean muscle tissue
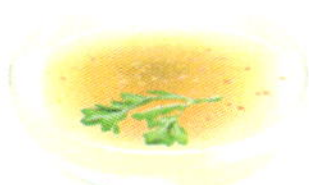 Bone Broth 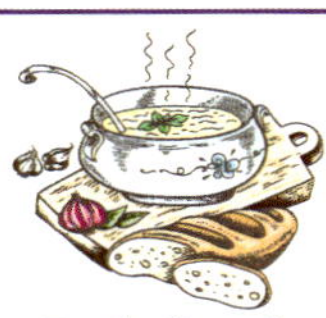 Fish Stock	Collagen in gelatinous bone broth "strengthens the tendons that connect muscle to the bones and the ligaments that connect bones together;"[1] and the amino acid alanine helps build muscle and endurance.[2]
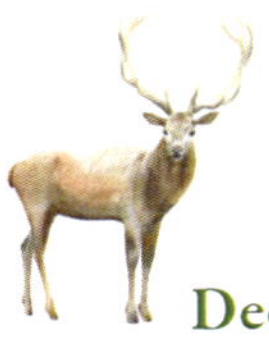 Deer 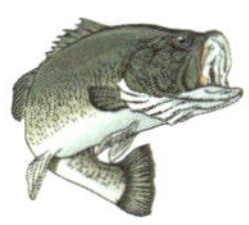 Bass 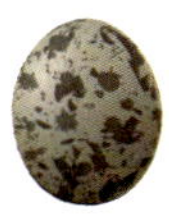 Quail Egg	Protein and fat are used to build muscle tissue and the amino acid lysine is significant for strengthening skeletal muscles
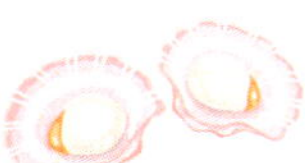 Scallop 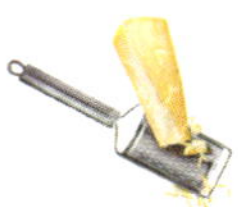 Cheese (hard) 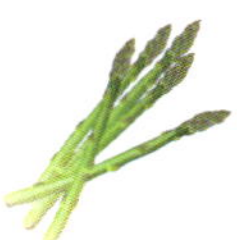 Asparagus 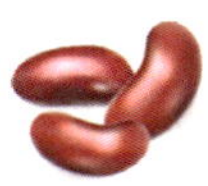 Kidney Beans	Leucine and lysine (amino acids) promote muscle metabolism and improve athletic performance
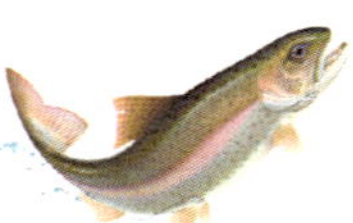 Trout 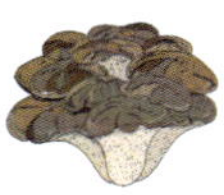 Maitake Mushroom 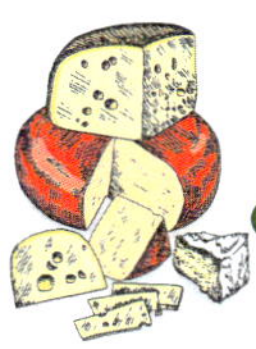 Cheese (soft)	Vitamin D_3 nourishes the musculoskeletal framework

References

[1]McKeown, P. (2015). *The Oxygen Advantage* (p. 29). New York, NY: HarperCollins Publishers.

[2,3]Fallon Morell, S. & Daniel, K. T. (2014). *Nourishing Broth* (p. 13, 38). New York, NY: Grand Central Life&Style.

Nervous System

The nervous system is an intricate communication network encompassing the brain, spinal cord, and peripheral nerves connecting with the organs and tissues. Embedded in insulated fatty connective tissue (myelin sheath), neurons project fibers that enable them to pass messages (neurotransmitters) between them via electrical waves and synapses, measured in millivolts.

Beneficial Foods

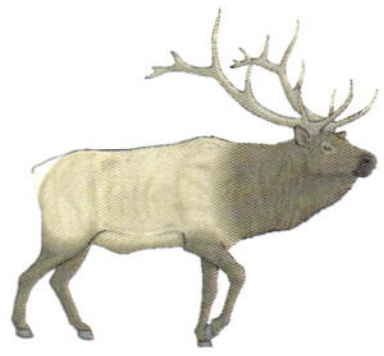
Elk

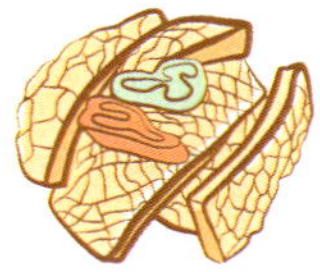
Offal

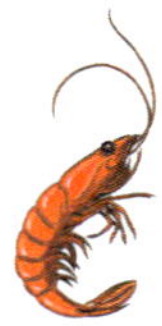
Shrimp

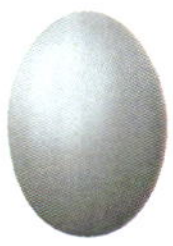
Duck Egg

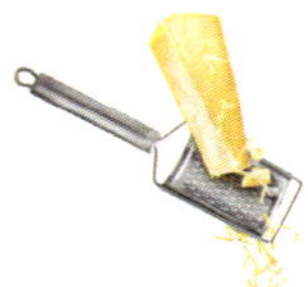
Cheese (hard)

Vitamin B12 (cobalamin) (water-soluble) and vitamins A, D3, K2 (fat-soluble) are essential for proper development and function of the brain and nervous system.[1]

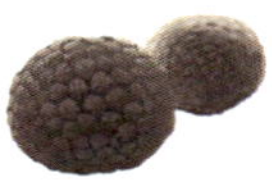
Truffle Mushroom

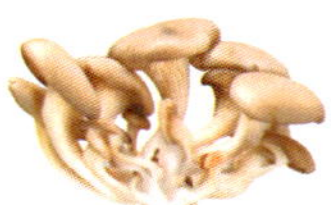
Oyster Mushroom

Lion's Mane Mushroom

Bioactive compounds that are neuro-protective, regenerate nerve tissue, facilitate the synthesis of neurotransmitters,[2] improve sleep [3]

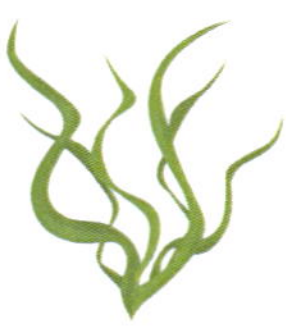
Kelp

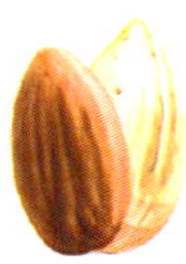
Almonds

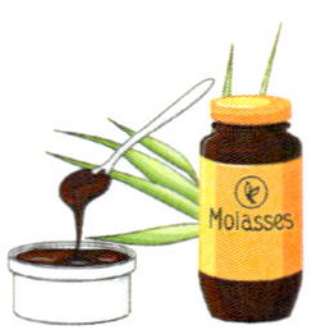

Molassas

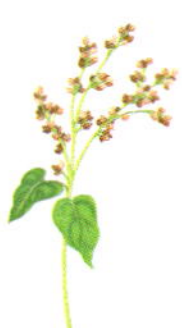
Buckwheat

Magnesium initiates gamma-aminobutyric acid (GABA) receptors in the brain, soothing the central nervous system and fostering optimal sleep; as an electrolyte, maintains a healthy electrical charge in the cells of muscles and nerves

Continued...

Nervous System

Beneficial Foods

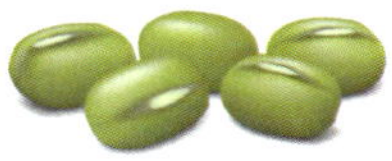

Mung Bean

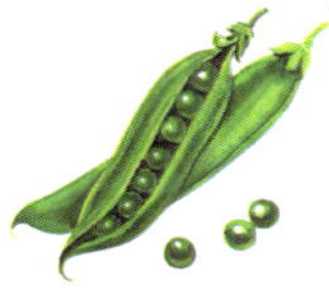

Green Peas

Vitamin B_9 (folate) and vitamin B_{12} (cobalamin) are critical to development of the nervous system[4]

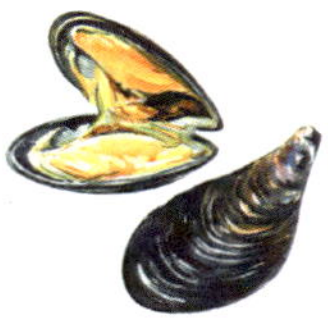

Mussels

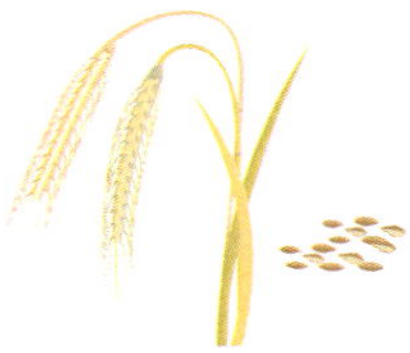

Barley

Manganese is essential for brain and nervous system function

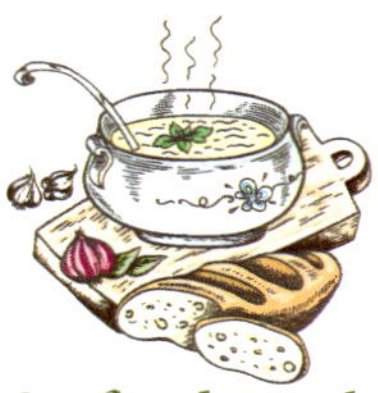

Seafood Broth

Glutamine in gelatin-rich broths is used by the body to manufacture gamma amino butyric acid (GABA) which has a calming effect, reduces anxiety, and aids in mental clarity.[5]

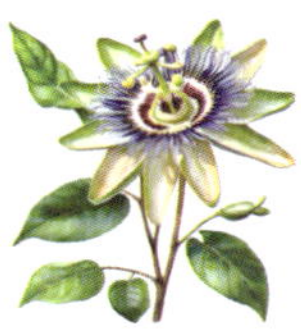

Passionflower Herb

Flavinoids and phenolic compounds have a calming effect and support the nervous system[6]

References

[1]Fallon Morell, S. (2001). *Nourishing Traditions* (2nd ed., pp. 38, 16). Washington, D.C.: NewTrends Publishing Inc.

[2]Lee, H., Nam, K., Zahra, Z., & Farooqi, M. Q. U.. (2020, June 17). Potentials of truffles in nutritional and medicinal applications: a review. *Fungal Biology and Biotechnology. 17*(7):9. https://www.ncbi.nlm.nih.gov/pmc/articles/PMC7301458.

[3]Rai, S. N. R., Mishra, D., Singh, P., Vamanu, E., & Singh, M. P. (2021, May). Therapeutic applications of mushrooms and their biomolecules along with a glimpse of in silico approach in neurodegenerative diseases. *Biomedicine & Pharmacotherapy. 137*, 111377.

[4]Murray, M. & Pizzorno, J. (2005). *The Encyclopedia of Healing Foods* (p. 109). New York, NY: Atria Books.

[5]Fallon Morell, S. & Daniels, K. T. (2014). *Nourishing Broth* (pp. 122–124). New York, NY: Grand Central LifeStyle.

[6]Hearm, S. (2015, September 13). *Passiflora incarnata. The Naturopathic Herbalist.* https://thenaturopathicherbalist.com/2015/09/13/passiflora-incarnata.

Reproductive System

The reproductive organs and glands are an integral part of the endocrine system. They support the major stages of life, including: puberty; fertility; potentially conception, pregnancy, and raising children; menstruation and menopause, postmenopause, andropause, and postandropause. The adrenal glands produce dehydroepiandrosterone (DHEA) which is a precursor of the reproductive hormones: estrogen (estradiol, estriol, and estrone), progesterone, and testosterone. These reproductive hormones support other systems of the body, for example, protecting the integrity of the bones.

Beneficial Foods

"Traditional cultures make provisions for the health of future generations by providing special nutrient-rich animal foods for parents-to-be, pregnant women and growing children. . ."[1] In her book, *Nourishing Traditions*, Sally Fallon Morell states that isolated traditional societies consumed high quality animal protein and fat with "activator" fat-soluble vitamins A, D_3, and K_2, in foods like shellfish, fish eggs, the blubber of sea animals, and organ meats because these natural foods provide optimal fertility, growth, and development in children.[2]

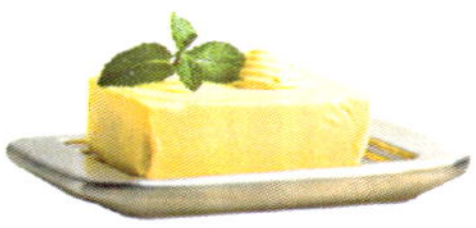

Butter

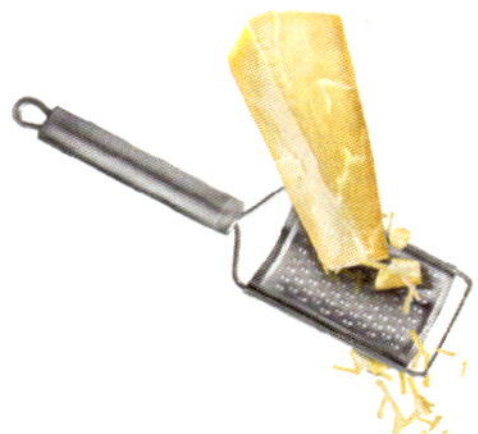

Cheese (hard)

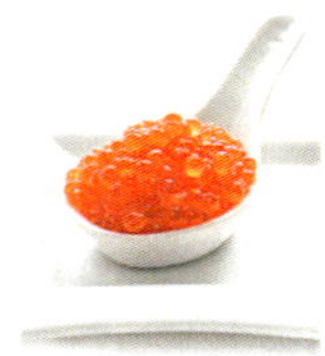

Fish Eggs

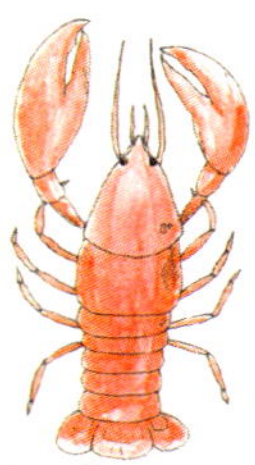

Lobster

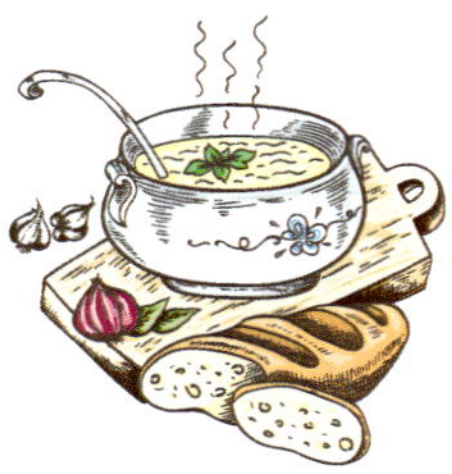

Fish Stock

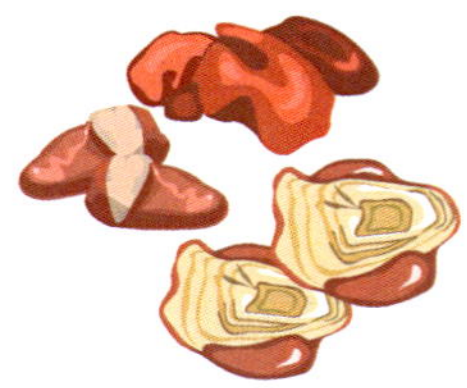

Gizzards, Liver and Heart

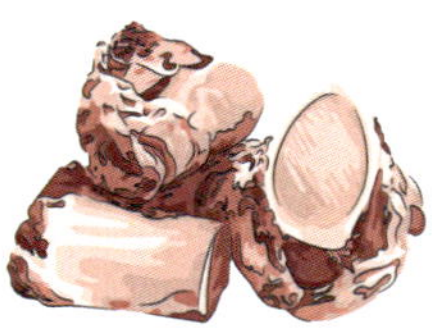

Bone Marrow

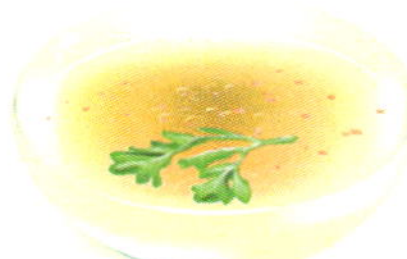

Bone Broth

Continued...

Reproductive System

Beneficial Foods

Key nutrients required for healthy reproduction, growth, and development include:

- Water-soluble vitamins: Fava Bean, Lamb folate (vitamin B_9); Red Chili Pepper and Guava (vitamin C)
- Trace minerals: Bone Marrow and Nori (iron); Pecans and Spinach (manganese); Buckwheat and Green Beans (vanadium); Mussels and Quail (zinc)
- Amino acids: Broccoli and Quail Egg (arginine); Bison and Goat Milk (histidine)

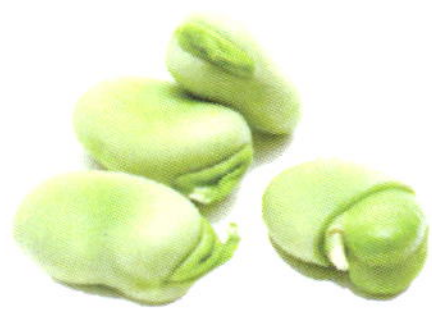
Fava Bean

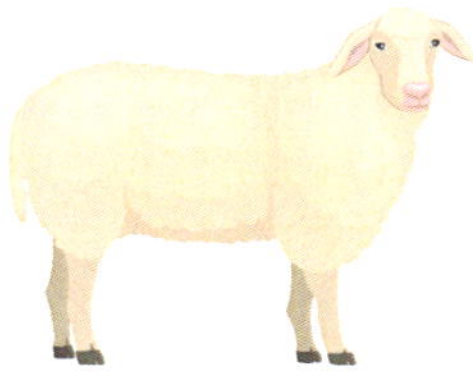
Lamb

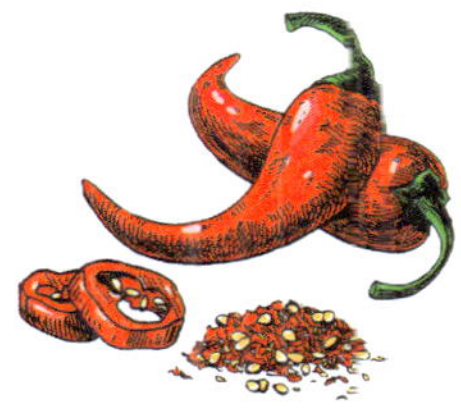
Red Chili Pepper

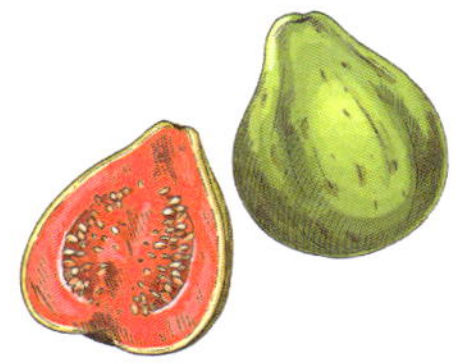
Guava

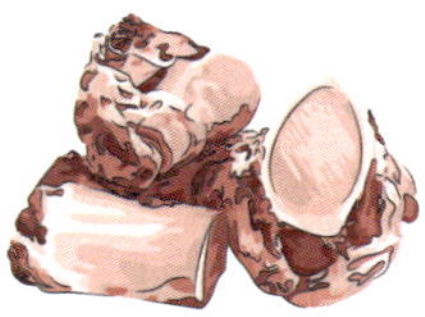
Bone Marrow

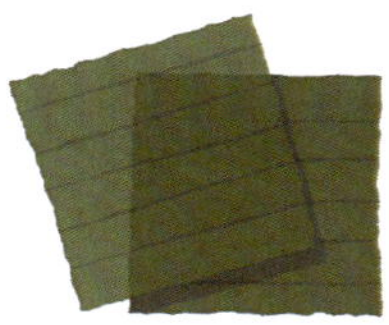
Nori

Pecans

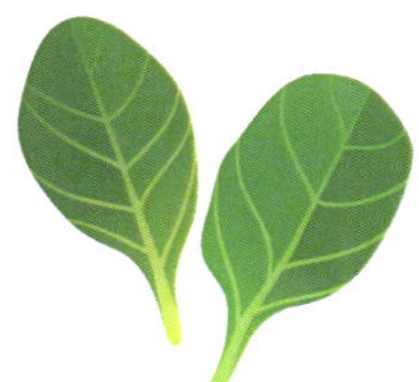
Spinach

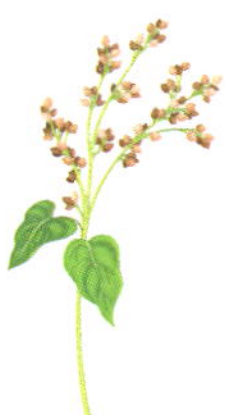
Buckwheat

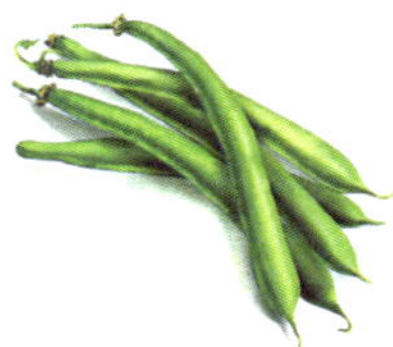
Green Beans

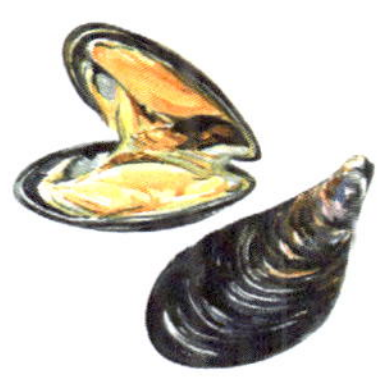
Mussels

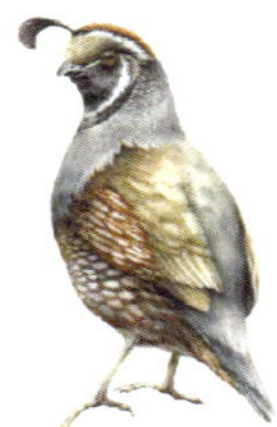
Quail

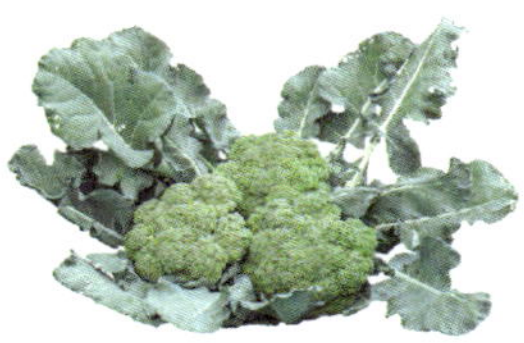
Broccoli

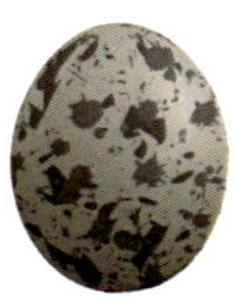
Quail Egg

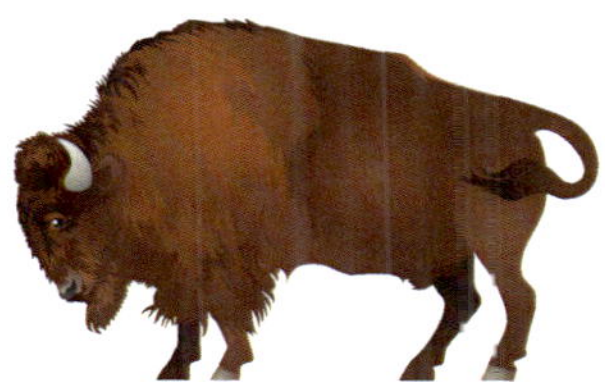
Bison

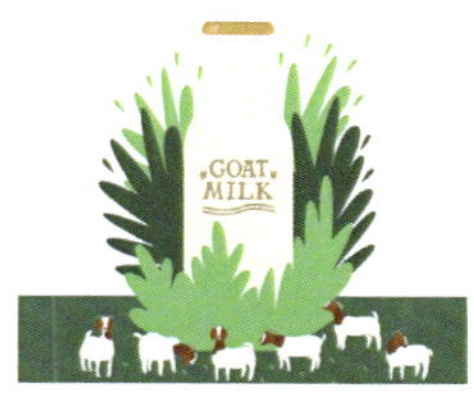

Goat Milk

Continued...

Reproductive System

Beneficial Foods

Bioactive compounds including hormones in these seeds, roots, and herbs calm the nerves, balance reproductive hormones, and support the immune system.[3]

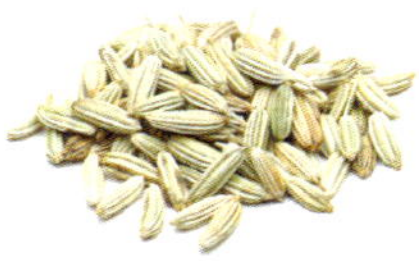

Fennel Seed

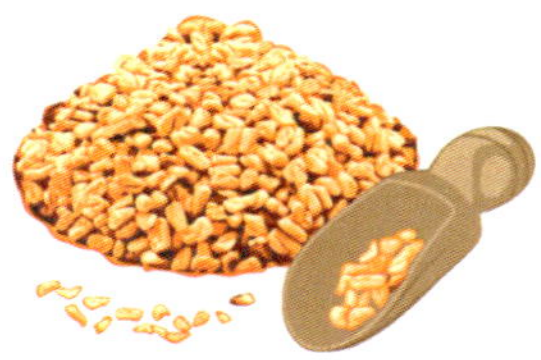

Fenugreek Seed

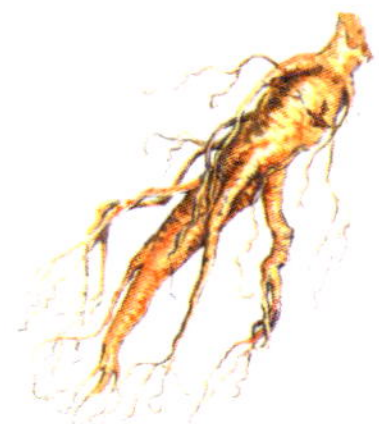

Ginseng

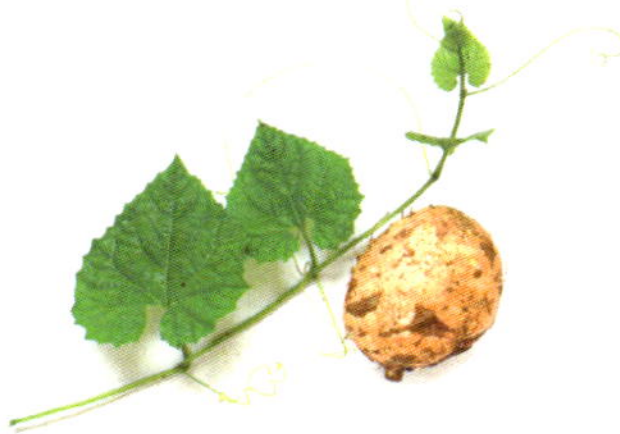

Wild Yam

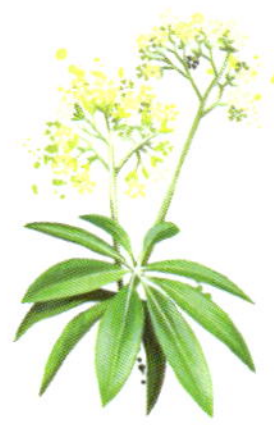

Saw Palmetto

References

[1]WAPF. (1999). *Timeless principles of healthy traditional diets*. Washington, D.C.: The Weston A. Price Foundation. https://www.westonaprice.org/health-topics/abcs-of-nutrition/principles-of-healthy-diets-2.

[2]Fallon Morell, S. (2001). *Nourishing Traditions* (2nd ed., p. 16). Washington, D.C.: NewTrends Publishing Inc.

[3]ABC. (2021). *Herbalgram*. American Botanical Council. https://abc.herbalgram.org/site/SPageServer.

Respiratory System

In breathing, the diaphragm muscles bring air into the respiratory tract through the nasal passages, mouth, throat (pharynx), windpipe (trachea), and into the lungs. Deep in the lungs, the oxygen, essential to life, is absorbed by the bronchi, bronchioles, and alveoli, diffuses into the blood, and is carried to every cell in the body. Carbon dioxide facilitates oxygen reaching the blood and muscles and has a key role in maintaining the blood pH; excess carbon dioxide is released with exhalation.[1]

Beneficial Foods

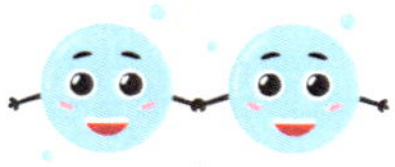

O_2

Oxygen is crucial for the life and growth of every cell in the body[1]

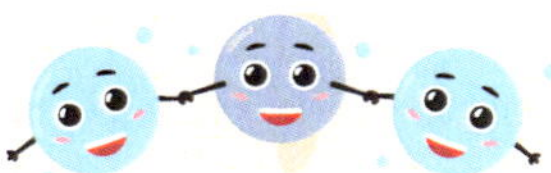

CO_2

Carbon dioxide largely determines how much oxygen is released into the cells and tissues[2]

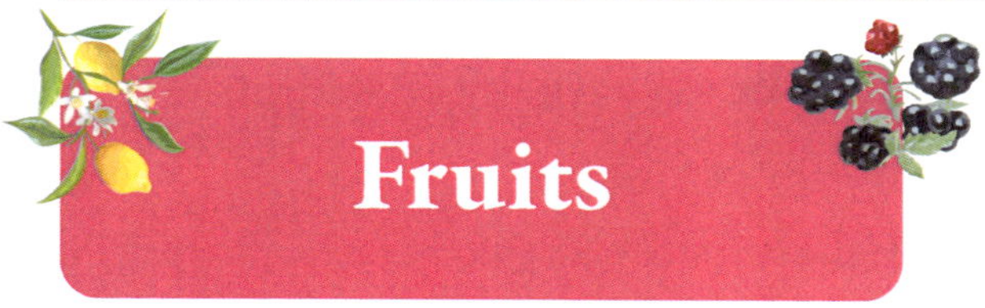

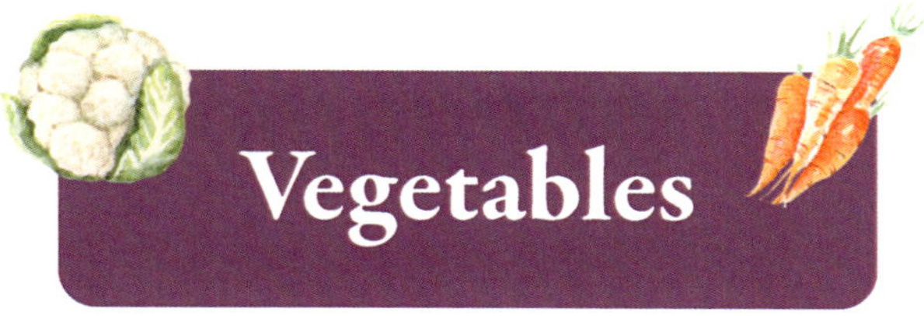

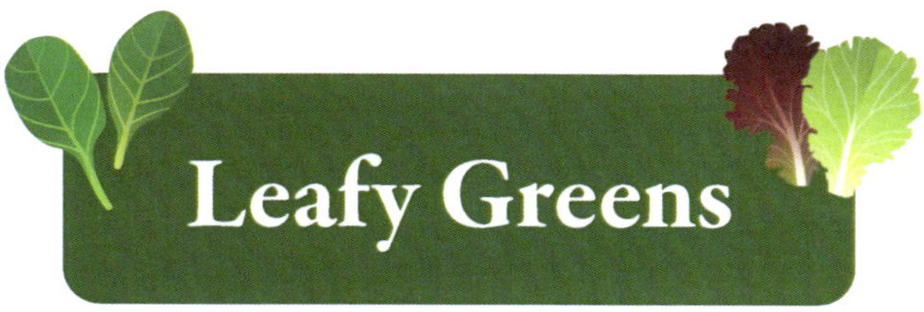

Phytonutrients, such as lycopene, beta carotene, indoles, and lutein, nourish the respiratory system and protect the lungs and bronchial from infection[3]

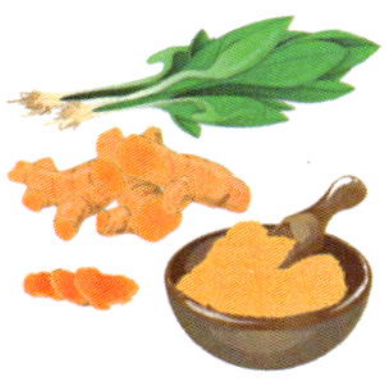

Turmeric

Curcumin provides relief from asthma, acute respiratory distress, lung injury, and pulmonary fibrosis[3]

Continued...

Respiratory System

Beneficial Foods

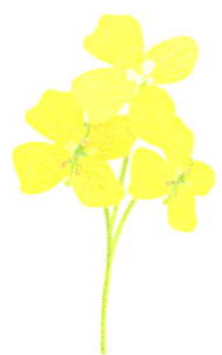

Mustard

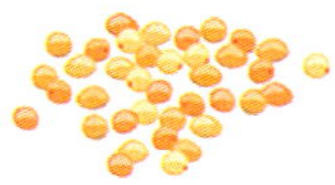

Mustard Seed

Glucosinolates help reduce cough and chest congestion[4]

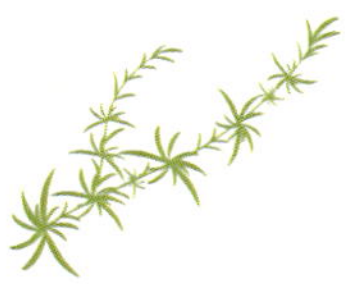

Hijiki

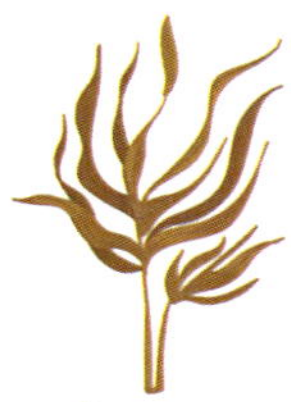

Arame

Fucoxanthan, flavinoids, and carotenoids strengthen the blood vessels and capillaries, increasing the oxygen capacity of the lungs

---

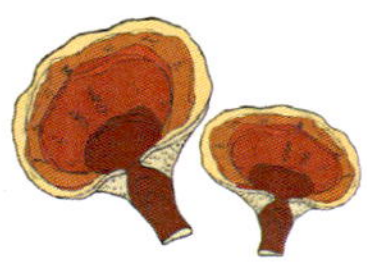

Reishi Mushrooms

Triterpenoids and other bioactive compounds improve the absorption of oxygen in the cells and tissues

---

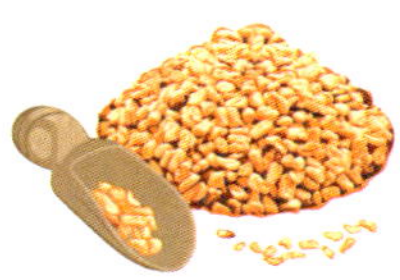

Fenugreek Seeds

Volatile oils and mucilage soothe, clear the airway, and improve lung function

References

[1]Trayhurn, P. (2019, February 12). Oxygen-a critical, but Overlooked, nutrient. *Frontiers in Nutrition*. https://www.ncbi.nlm.nih.gov/pmc/articles/PMC6379287.

[2]McKeown, P. (2015). *The Oxygen Advantage* (pp. 22 – 25). New York, NY: HarperCollins Publishers.

[3]Link, R. (2020). Best foods for your lungs. *Ancient Nutrition*. https://draxe.com/nutrition/best-foods-for-your-lungs.

[4]Fallon Morell, S. (2001). *Nourishing Traditions* (2nd ed., p. 104). Washington, D.C.: NewTrends Publishing Inc.

Skeletal System

In the central core of the body is the axial skeleton, encompassing the skull, spine, sternum, ribs, and breastbone. The paired appendicular bones include the shoulders, limbs, and hips. Bone is made mostly of minerals, especially calcium phosphate, collagen, and water. It continually rebuilds itself. Strong, lightweight, and durable, bone enables ease of movement. In the bone marrow, fresh blood cells (red, white, and platelets) are produced and added to the blood stream. The ligaments and cartilage, comprised largely of collagen, connect to the bones and act as cushioning and shock absorbers.

Beneficial Foods

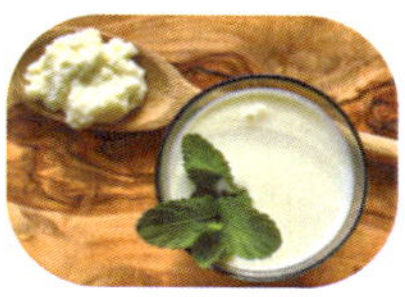
Kefir

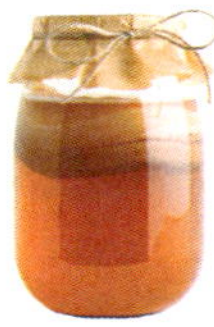
Kombucha

Probiotics enhance vitamin D_3 and calcium absorption, increasing bone density[1]

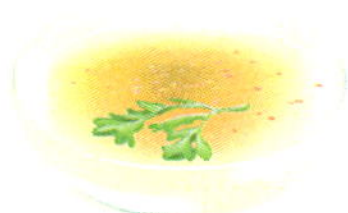
Bone Broth

"Collagen is what holds us together, creates the framework for our bones, forms the basis of strong tendons and joints, surrounds our organs, lines the intestinal tract, interlaces our fatty tissue and undergirds our skin."[2]

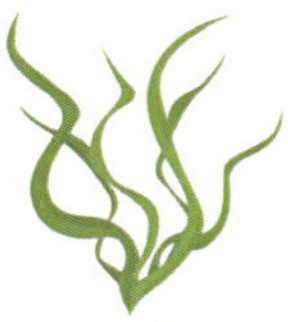
Kelp

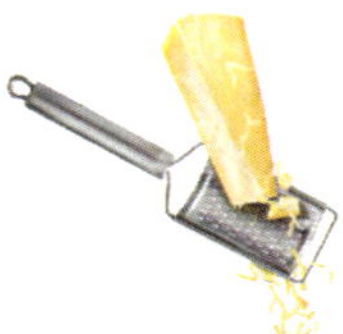
Cheese (hard)

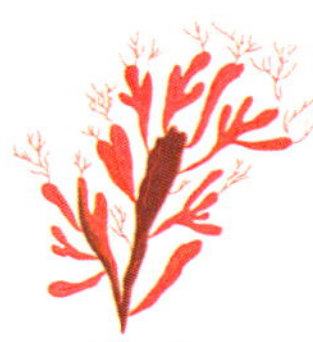
Dulse

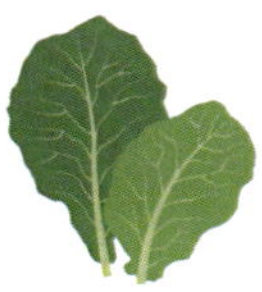
Collard Greens
Calcium

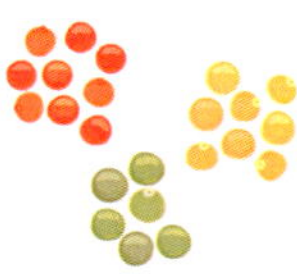
Lentils

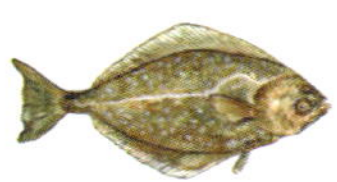
Halibut

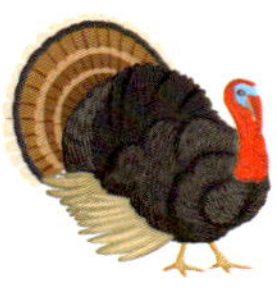
Turkey
Phosphorus

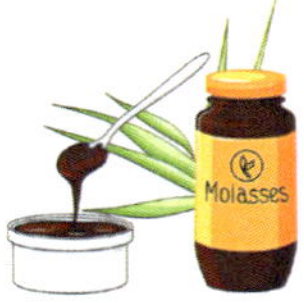

Molasses

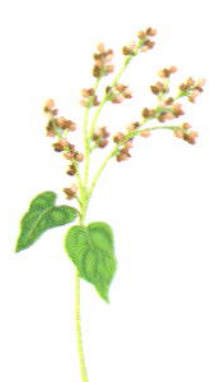
Buckwheat
Magnesium

Calcium, phosphorus, and magnesium provide the minerals needed for healthy bones and teeth; magnesium helps regulate the metabolism of calcium and vitamin D_3 [3]

Continued...

Skeletal System

Beneficial Foods

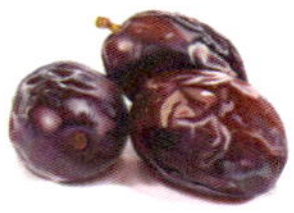
Prunes

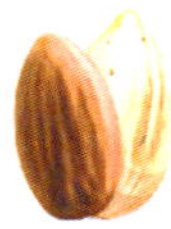
Almonds

Boron is required to activate estrogen and vitamin D_3 in constructing and maintaining bone structure[4]

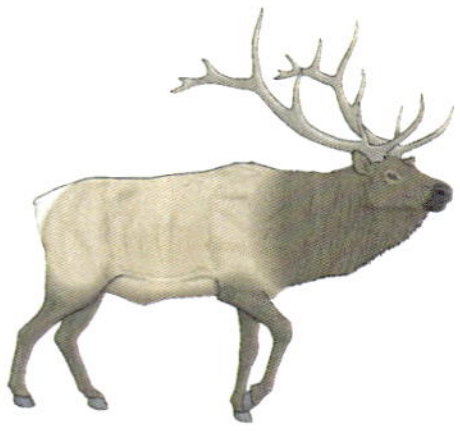
Elk

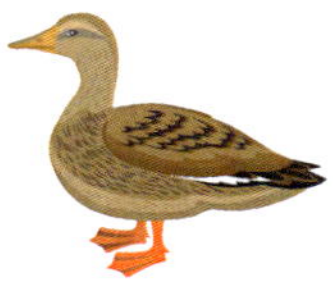
Duck

"Vitamin K_2 helps us put calcium and phosphorus in the bones and teeth where they belong, and prevents their deposition in the arteries and other soft tissues, where they do not belong"[5]

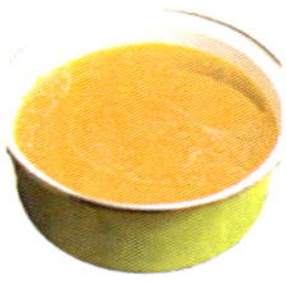
Goose Fat

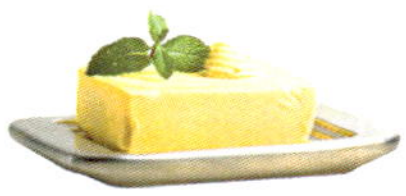
Butter

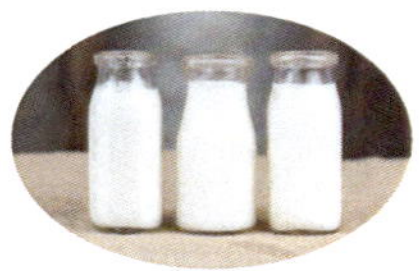
Buttermilk

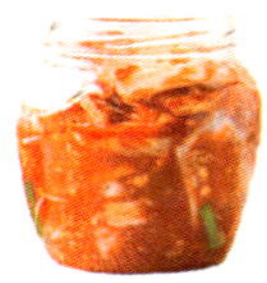
Kimchi

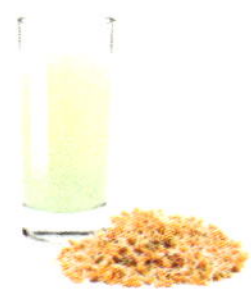
Rejuvlac

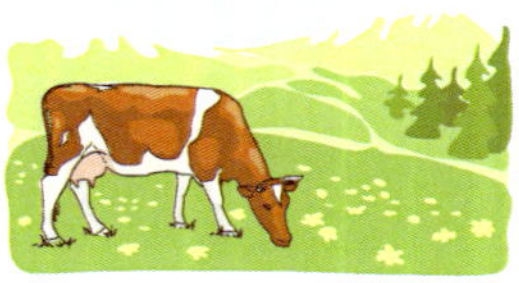
Milk (cow)

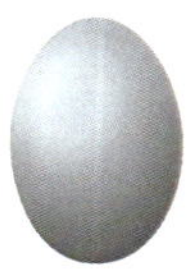
Duck Egg

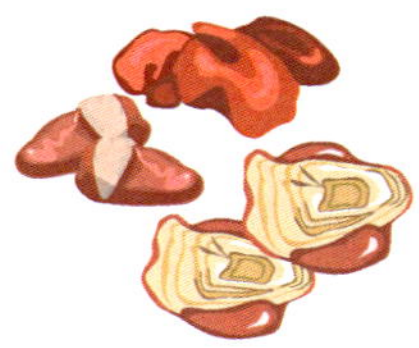
Gizzards, Liver, and Heart

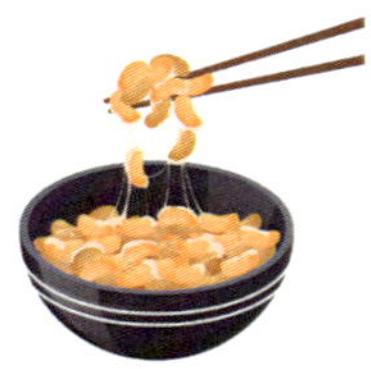
Natto

References

[1]Zhang, L., Zhang, R., & Li, L. (2023, April 25). Effects of probiotic supplementation on exercise and the underlying mechanisms. *Journal of Foods*. *12*(9), 1787. https://doi.org/10.3390/foods12091787.

[2, 5]WAPF. (2021). *Eleven Dietary Wise Traditions Principles* (pp. 52, 16). Washington, D.C.: Weston A. Price Foundation. westonaprice.org.

[3]Low Dog, T. (2020). *Fortify Your Life* (p. 180). Washington, D.C.: National Geographic.

[4]Murray, M. & Pizzorno, J. (2005). *The Encyclopedia of Healing Foods* (p. 755). New York, NY: Atria Books.

Urinary System

The kidneys are paired organs situated behind the abdominal cavity. They conduct many key functions in the body, including helping to maintain the volume, pH, salinity, and composition of the blood, lymph, and other fluids of the body. The kidneys filter and cleanse the waste to be eliminated as urine. The urinary system also involves the: ureters; bladder; urethra; and in men, the prostrate.

Beneficial Foods

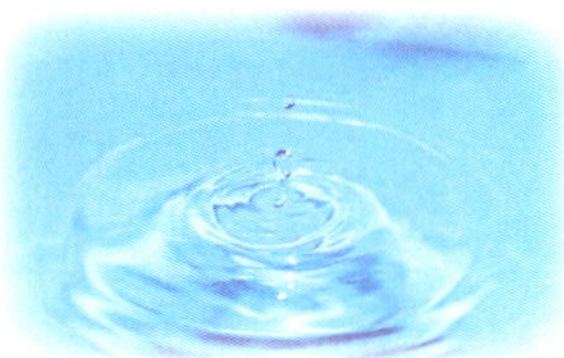

Water

Cleanses the urinary system

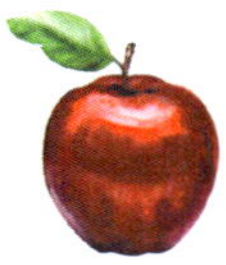

Apple

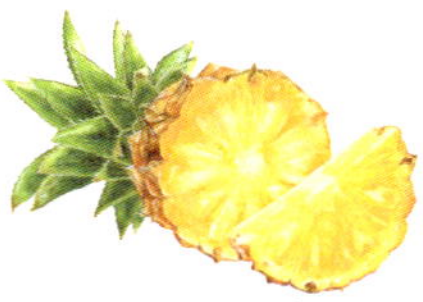

Pineapple

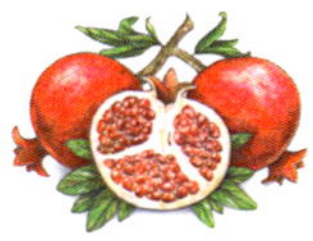

Pomegranate

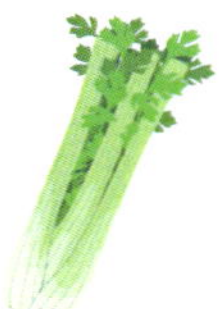

Celery

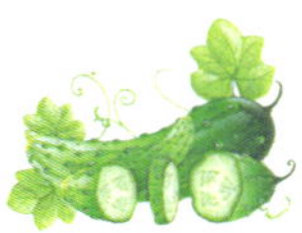

Cucumber

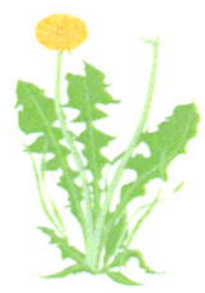

Dandelion

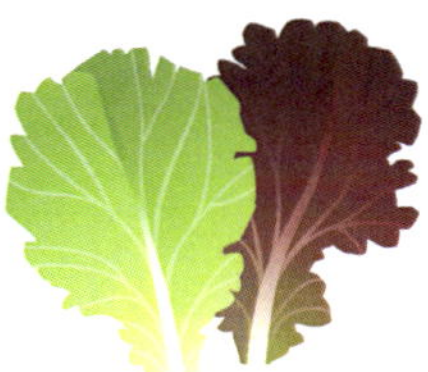

Lettuces

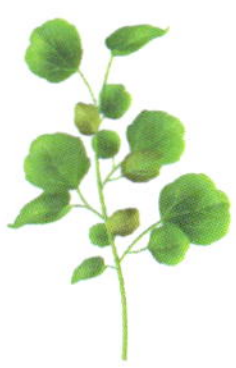

Watercress

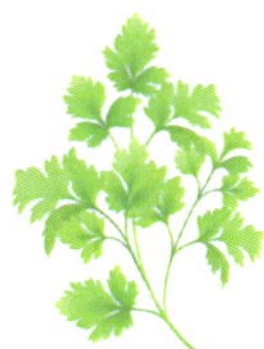

Parsley

Fresh raw fruits (acid or subacid) and vegetables, eaten whole or juiced, nourish and cleanse the urinary system

---

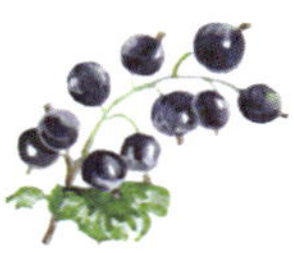

Currant

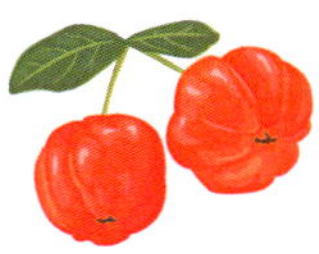

Acerola

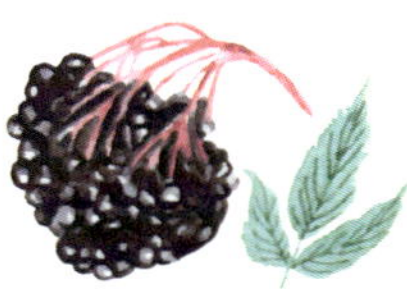

Elderberry

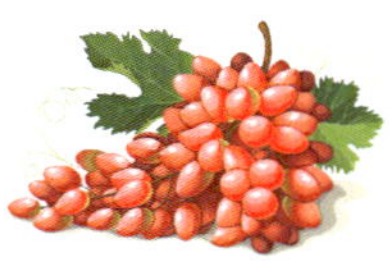

Grape (red)

Resveratrol, antioxidants, and vitamin C are anti-bacterial, anti-viral, and strengthen the immune system; proanthocyanins inhibit the adhesion of pathogenic bacteria, such as *Escherichia coli*, to the mucosal wall of the urinary tract[1]

Continued...

Urinary System

Beneficial Foods

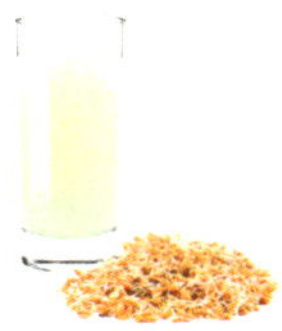

Rejuvelac

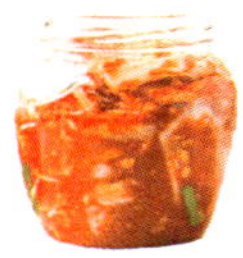

Kimchi

Probiotics maintains a healthy microbiome, fight infection, and support the immune system

---

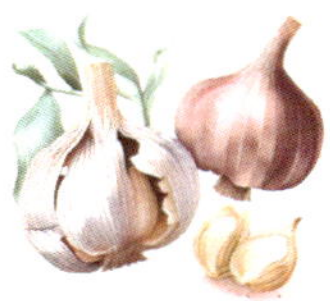

Garlic

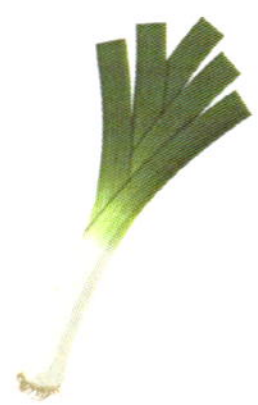

Leek

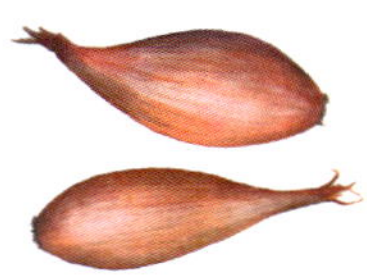

Shallot

Sulfur compounds, including allicin, are antioxidant; anti-inflammatory; and increase glutathione, which enhances detoxification and protects against infection

---

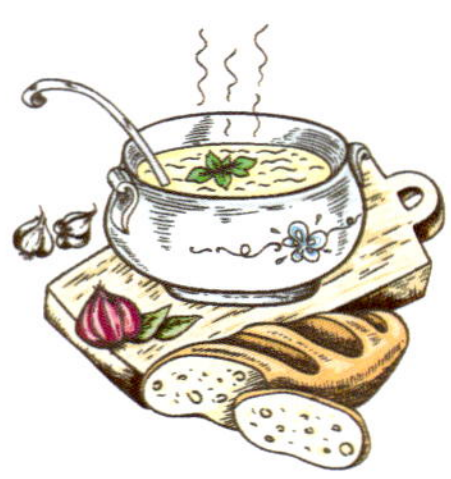

Seafood Bone Broth

Gelatinous collagen heals tissue membrane, including the bladder; eases inflammation; and supports the immune system

References

[1]Murray, M. & Pizzorno, J. (2005). *The Encyclopedia of Healing Foods* (p. 269). New York, NY: Atria Books.

Part VII

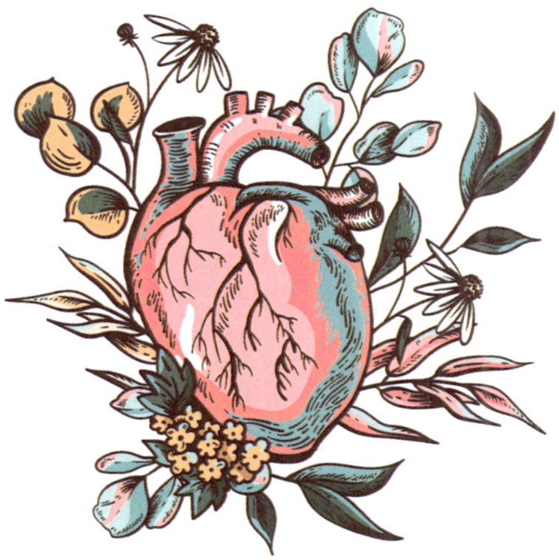

Medical Vintage Card

Illustrator Belusuab, Dreamstime

Human Health and Homeostasis

While disease takes many forms, health is the state of vitality

Attributes of Human Health

Examples for each of the eleven systems of the body

Cardiovascular

Steady heartbeat, continuous blood flow, resonance in the chest

Digestive

Symbiotic microbiome; complete digestion; efficient nutrient absorption and assimilation

Endocrine

Hormones in balance; metabolism and internal temperature fully support body functions

Integumentary

Skin supple with turgor and warm to touch, indicating healthy blood circulation; hair strong with luster; nail cuticles lay flat

Immune

Self-protective, wards off pathogens, restorative

Muscular

Full range of motion, symmetry in movement when walking and running, excellent eye/hand coordination

Nervous

Brain manages physiological pathways holistically; keen sense of touch, hearing, sight, smell, and taste; sound sleep, waking up refreshed

Reproductive

Balanced hormones; well-nourished to support fertility and child-rearing

Respiratory

Quiet, easy breath, through the nose with clear airway; oxygen supports the heart and physical activity; carbon dioxide efficiently facilitates oxygen delivery to the blood and helps maintain optimal blood pH.[1]

Skeletal

Straight teeth and dense, strong bones; body alignment (posture), without strain, that supports the natural curvature of the neck and spine when the body is still or in motion

Urinary

Body hydrated; waste and toxins effectively eliminated

Homeostasis and The Endocannabinoid System

In its overarching role, the endocannabinoid system (ECS) integrates the systems of the body to continually maintain an optimal internal state (homeostasis); wherein, the body can function in a changing environment. For example, the ECS coordinates the cardiovascular, integumentary, and nervous systems in regulating body temperature–when too hot, the body sweats and expands small blood vessels to bring heated blood to the surface of the skin where it can cool; when too cold, the body shivers, producing warmth. Via lipids within the tissues, organs, and fluids, the ECS functions in an elaborate network of endocannabinoids (neurotransmitters) that bind to cannabinoid receptors synthesized and degraded, as needed, in the brain, central nervous system, and immune cells. Modulating the frontal cerebral cortex, hypothalamic-pituitary-adrenocortical axis, and central nervous system the ECS manages inflammation and stress. Fundamentally, the ECS supports the regeneration of cells and tissues essential to homeostasis and our overall well-being.

The Body Depends on Natural Foods to Regenerate

"... proper nutrition changes the course of disease at its source. Food alone can accomplish this feat."[2] *-Bernard Jensen, D.C.*

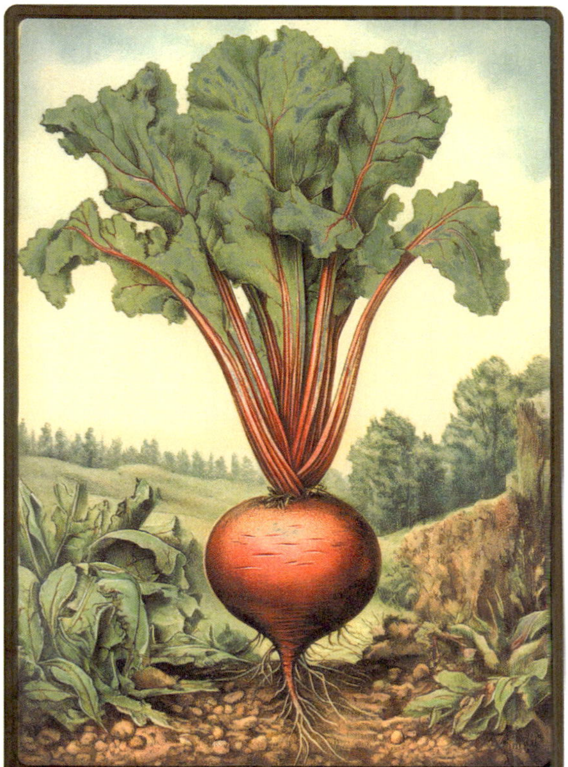

Illustrator Karen Foley, Dreamstime

Beet and Beet Greens

Natural foods – pristine from the land and sea – **build and maintain human health**

Natural foods provide the nourishment required to produce superb health and high immunity to disease. Foods containing omega-3 fatty acids are particularly beneficial for the endocannabinoid system. In his research, Weston A. Price, D.D.S. found that each of the indigenous groups he studied, living on the natural foods they harvested from the land and sea, had sturdy bone structure; skulls with ample room for the hypothalamus, pineal, and pituitary glands; and straight teeth.[5] In his comparative analysis of members of the indigenous groups who left their isolated communities and adopted the diet of modern commerce, Dr. Price consistently found innumerable deformities, including narrowed skulls and dental arches, crooked teeth, and dental decay. He described the "... displacing diet of modern commerce as mankind's most universal disease. . ."[6] As Dr. Price further demonstrated, nutritional deficiencies and the resulting afflictions can be passed on from one generation to the next, just as robust health is passed on from one generation to the next.[7]

***'Like feeds like'** – organic, gelatinous bone broth, for example, furnishes the essential assemblage of nutrients needed to regenerate our bone and cartilage*[3]

A hundred years ago, people who were unexposed to modern commerce were largely free of dental decay and osteoarthritis. Today, as Sally Fallon Morell points out in her book *Nourishing Broth*, "The problem is not old age, but the fact that cartilage is breaking down faster than it is built up."[4]

Our Native Microbiome

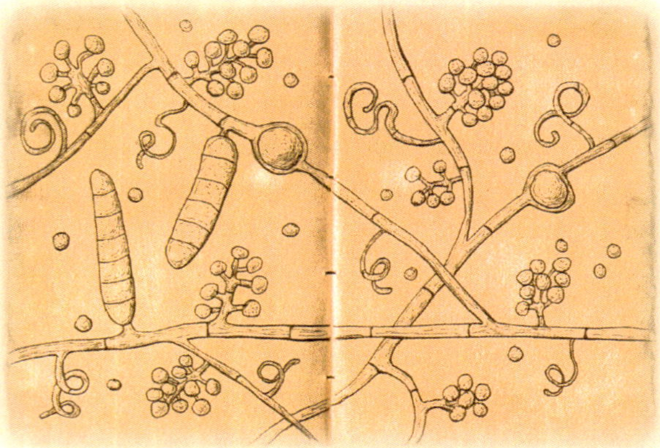

Illustrator Kateryna Kon, Dreamstime

"Lactic bacteria/intestinal bio-cultures are so important that they must be considered agents that protect life and are essential companions to human beings."[8] -Silas K. Everett

Probiotic bacteria and micro-fungi chimera (strains) vary throughout the digestive tract (mouth, throat, esophagus, stomach, small and large intestines, anus) based on our internal micro-habitats, which they influence and adapt to over time. Lactic acid bacteria are acid-producing and 'acid-loving,' thriving in the environment they produce. In our microbiome, lactic acid bacteria:

- aid in the breakdown, absorption, and assimilation of natural foods
- produce B vitamins and vitamin K_2, and lactase (which they use to breakdown of the lactose in milk into glucose and galactose)

- solubilize mineral nutrients, making them more bioavailable
- help alleviate diarrhea and constipation
- protect the mucosal lining of the intestinal tract, instituting a barrier that keeps food particles from slipping out ('leaky gut')
- facilitate peristalsis (muscle contractions), which moves the mass of digesting food (bolus) through the intestinal tract, and accelerate the evacuation of excrement from the large intestine (bowel).
- produce natural anti-biotics, including: acidophilin, reutericin, plantaricin, and bulgarican
- destroy pathogens, including *Candida albicans* yeast and Epstein-Barr[9]
- symbiotically interact with cells of our lymphoid tissue (including lymphocytes, macrophages, and T cells) within the intestinal tract, which comprises the body's largest immunological organ
- prevent the invasion of *Salmonella typhimurium* (salmonella infection) and *Helicobacter pylori* (diarrhea) and activate immune production of interferon and interleukin (anti-tumor)
- support the immunological activity of the spleen, thymus, and other organs of the immune system
- reduce inflammation and influence the internal environment to promote homeostasis

Healthy Tissue Isn't a Home for Pathogens

Disease-causing micro-organisms require an environment quite different from healthy, vital tissue. Instead, they thrive on weakened, depleted substrates. Once established, invading microbes make way for more detrimental pathogens. Candida (*Candida albicans*) fungal yeast, for example, proliferates on nutritionally-depleted tissue and make way for more dangerous micro-organisms to penetrate our organs. Putrefactive yeasts, molds, parasites, and bacteria produce ammonia, hydrogen sulfide, amines, and other harmful compounds that can bring on allergies, bronchitis, asthma, pneumonia, cancer, and other ailments.

On the other hand, probiotic bacteria create a robust internal environment. They produce lactic acid with the pH level (acidity) that is needed for digestion and anti-septic conditions inhospitable to pathogens. Probiotics also destroy pathogens with the anti-microbial compounds they excrete. When probiotics are getting established, they may cause temporary die-off symptoms as our body gets rid of pathogens. The elimination of pathogens is followed by an improvement in the health of each cell, tissue, organ, and system of the body. Since our cells and tissues are always self-repairing, especially when we sleep, we can change our biochemistry by consuming natural foods and engaging in health-giving activities that favor our native microbiome and promote healing.

Helping the Body Replenish and Heal

The practice of naturopathic medicine is founded on the following principles:

- *First do not harm*
- *The healing power of nature*
- *Identify and alleviate the causes of disease*
- *Treat the whole person*
- *Prevention*
- *The physician as teacher*

Illustrator Somesun, Dreamstime

Ways to facilitate the body's innate healing process may include: intermittent fasting,[10] consuming nourishing natural foods; drinking fresh vegetable juices; applying cleansing (detoxing) natural substances, such as algae and clays; having uplifting experiences and reducing stress with yoga, meditation, swimming, dance, and walks in nature; rebuilding the microbiome; and using medicinal herbs and mushrooms to strengthen the immune systems. Encompassing many fields of study and practice, natural health professionals help support the body's self healing process.

References

[1]McKeown, P. (2015). *The Oxygen Advantage* (p. 29). New York, NY: HarperCollins Publishers.

[2]Jensen, B. (1993). *Foods That Heal.* Avery Publishing Group, Inc.: Garden City Park, NY

[3,4]Fallon Morell, S. & Daniels, K. T. (2014). *Nourishing Broth* (pp. 20, 59). New York, NY: Grand Central LifeStyle.

[5]Fallon Morell, S. (2008). *Nourishing traditional diets: The key to vibrant health* [Film]. White Plains, MD: New Trends Publishing.

[6,7]Price, W.A. (2019). *Nutrition and Physical Degeneration* (8th ed., pp. 1, 419). Lemon Grove, CA: Price-Pottenger.

[8]Silas K. Everett, Ph.D., collaborating with Dr. Edouard Brochu (1986, August 10)

[9]Mazziotta, C., Tognon, M., Martini, F., Torreggiani, E., & Rotondo, J. C. (2023). Probiotics mechanism of action on immune cells and beneficial effects on human health. *Journal of Cells.* 12(1):184. https://pmc.ncbi.nlm.nih.gov/articles/PMC9818925.

[10]Fung, J., Mayer, E., & Ramos, M. (2020). *Live in the Fasting Lane.* New York, NY: HarperCollins Publishers. https://www.thefastingmethod.com.

PART VIII

NATURAL LIVING

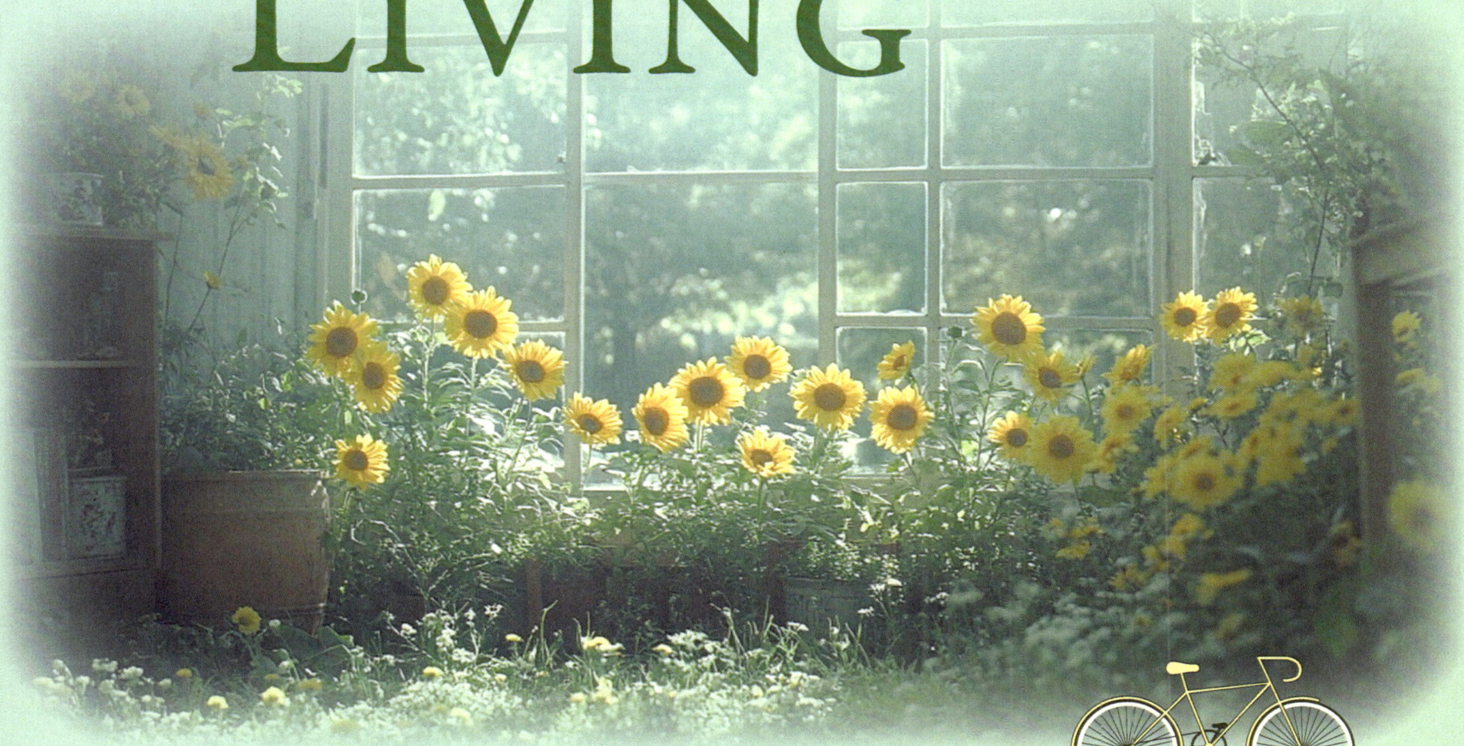

Soothing and Relaxing
Physical Activities
Rejuvenation

Natural Living

Soothing and Relaxing

Fresh Air, Sunshine, and Beneficial Ions

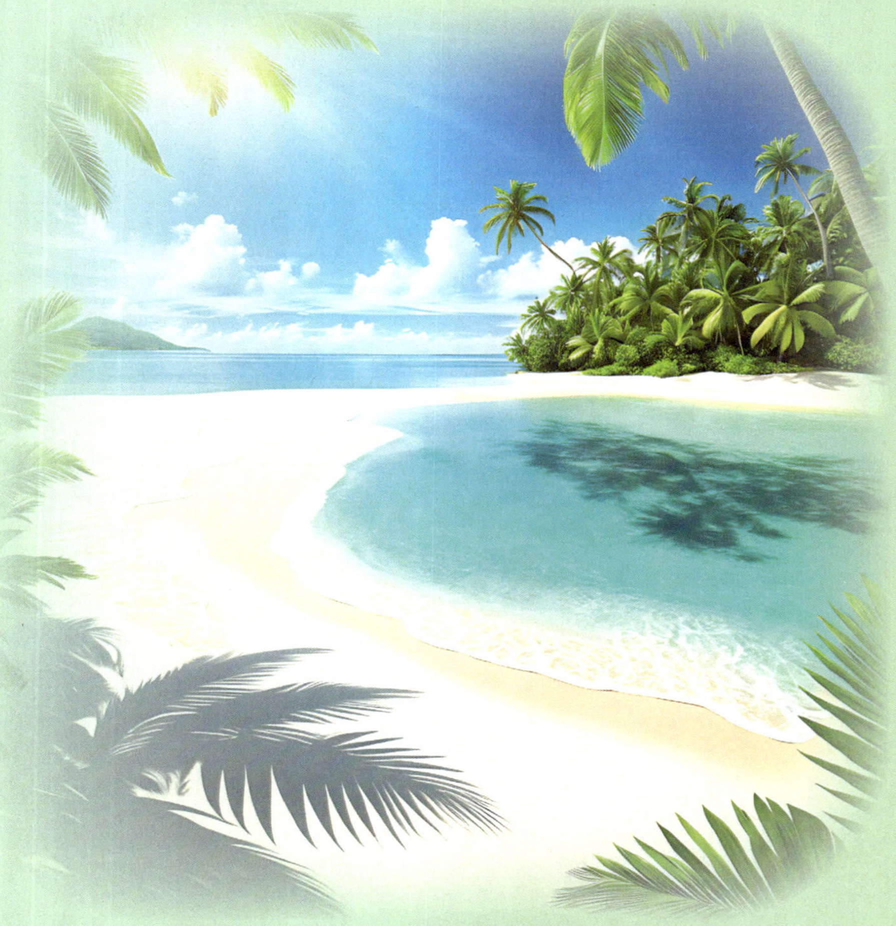

Plants are the only true air fresheners. They filter the air, removing pollutants, and release oxygen.

(ref. plants also improve water and soil quality, pages 60, 85)

Fresh air, clean water, sunlight, shade, and negative ions are primary for our health. Negative ions concentrate along beaches, by waterfalls, in forests, and on mountains. When oxygen molecules have an extra electron they are negatively charged ions that clean the air–by attaching to positively charged electrons in bacteria, viruses, dust, pollen, mold spores, and pollutants floating in the air. This causes these particles to clump together and, with enough weight, to drop to the ground.[1] In addition to clearing the air, negative ions support the flow of oxygen to the brain, facilitate cell metabolism, and foster a state of tranquility.

References

[1]Kaur, S. (2019, September 5). *The healing properties of the beach: negative ions for health*. Pura Veda Gurukulam. https://www.puraveda.org/post/the-healing-properties-of-the-beach-negative-ions-for-health.

1

Soothing and Relaxing

The Science of Healthy Breathing

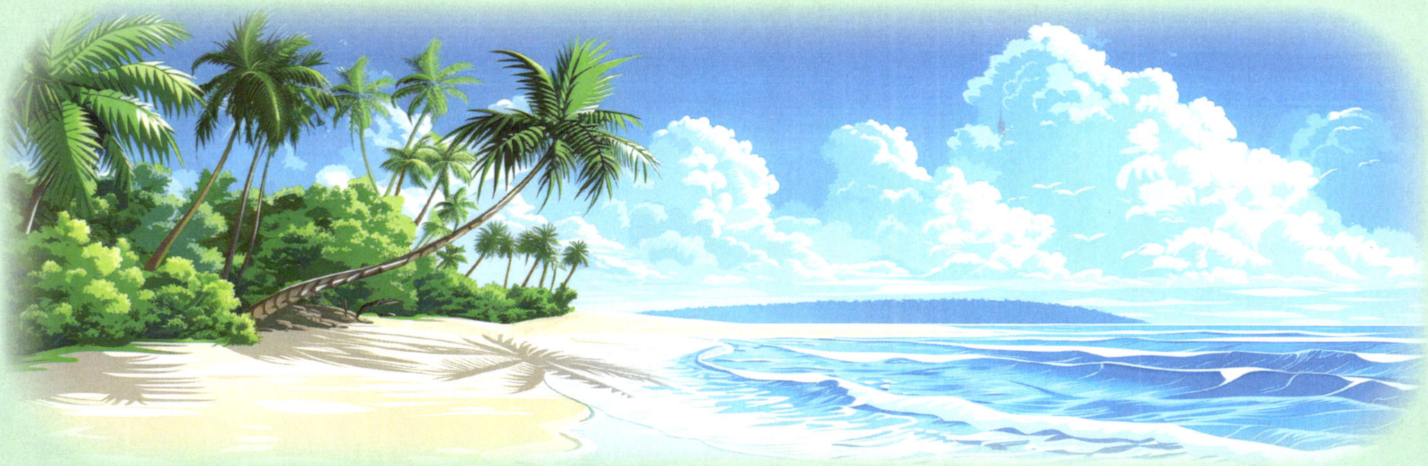

Natural breathing integrates the respiratory system with the other systems of the body. In his book, *The Oxygen Advantage*, Patrick McKeown describes healthy breathing as: slow, gentle, calm, regular, silent, relatively unnoticeable, and occurring through the nose. Placidly bringing the breath into the diaphragm assists the lymph system in carrying away waste.[1] McKeown studied the breathing techniques of Konstantin Pavlovich Buteyko, M.D. (1923-2003) who is world-renowned for having taught his patients how to restore their health with their breath.[2] James Nestor, in his book, *Breath*, illuminates ancient and contemporary breathing practices, including yoga traditions, that increase longevity.[3]

The natural way to breath is through our nose. McKeown describes how when we inhale, our nose slows down the airstream, warms and humidifies the incoming air, removes pathogenic bacteria, and furnishes a reservoir of nitric oxide to maintain good health.[4] Carbon dioxide facilitates the release of oxygen from red blood cells into our organs and tissues. First documented by physiologist Christian Bohr in 1904, this crucial role of carbon dioxide is known as the Bohr Effect.[5] More carbon dioxide in the bloodstream means more efficient delivery of oxygen to where it is needed in the body, and nasal breathing facilitates this important function. McKeown emphasizes that while many of us have

Continued...

Natural Living

Soothing and Relaxing

The Science of Healthy Breathing

forgotten the innate way of breathing, anyone can relearn how to nose breathe. Mouth breathing results from poor diets, environmental toxicity, overheated homes, and lack of fitness. This can lead to carbon dioxide deficiency, poor oxygenation, weakened respiratory system; and mental and physical ailments.

Nasal breathing can be adopted anytime and improves overall health and the capacity for aerobic exercise. It involves the inhalation of a smaller volume of air and provides more time between breaths. This gives the lungs a chance to hold onto the carbon dioxide and deliver more oxygen to the cells before the next breath. Nasal breathing also lowers blood pressure and heart rate, increases blood flow to the brain and the rest of the body, and builds muscle tone and endurance.[6]

References

[1,4,6]McKeown, P. (2015). *The Oxygen Advantage* (pp. 73, 56 – 57, 2). New York, NY: HarperCollins Publishers.

[2]McKeown, P. (2024). *Transform Your Health with the Buteyko Breathing Method.* Buteyko Clinic International. https://buteykoclinic.com.

[3]Nestor, J. (2020). *Breath* (p. 212). New York, NY: Riverhead Books.

[5]Somnifix. (2022). *The Bohr effect: the key to unlocking new levels of physical endurance.* https://somnifix.com/blogs/snews/bohr-effect-and-fitness.

NATURAL LIVING

Soothing and Relaxing
REFRESHING WATER

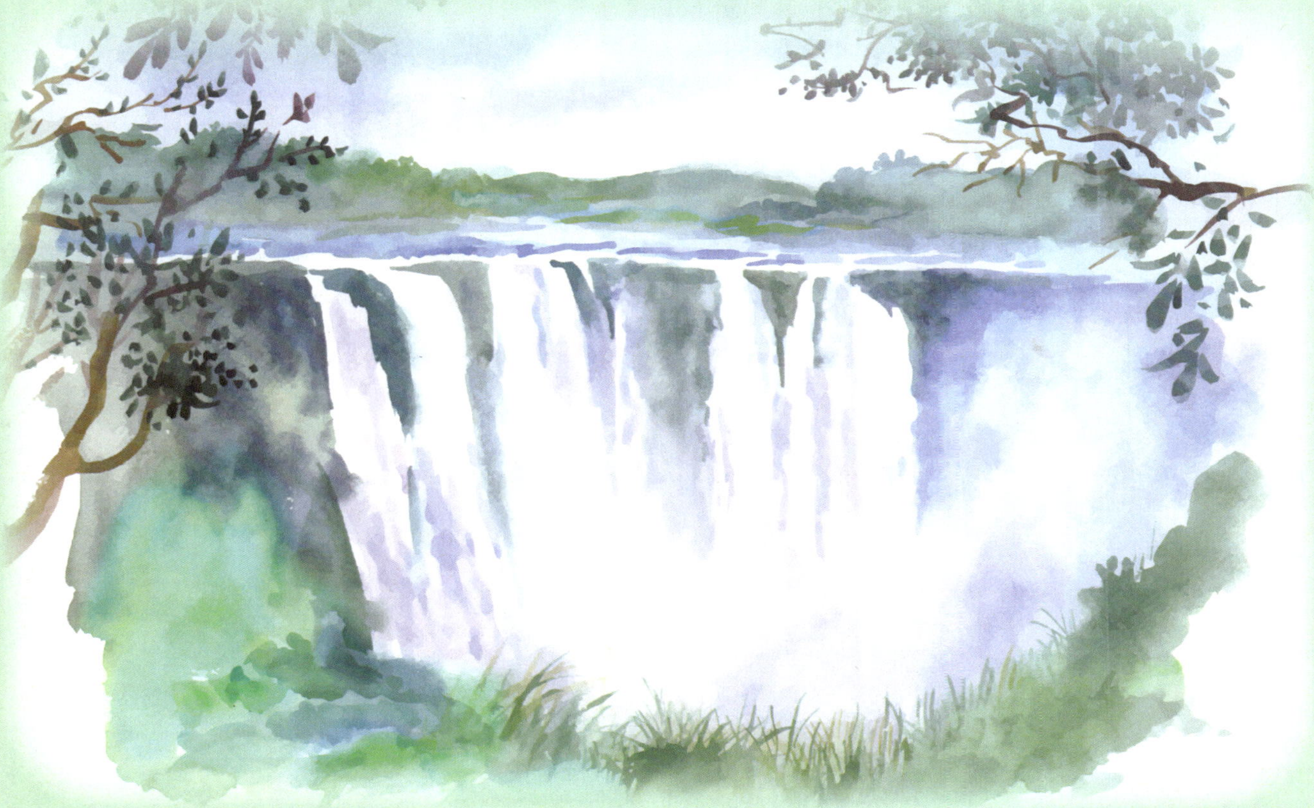

Breathing in moisture from the air by a waterfall or river is refreshing. We need more water in a dry climate and when we are active. Drinking plenty of water everyday keeps us hydrated. Glass is one of the best, non-toxic vessels for holding water.

Our body uses water for:

- transporting oxygen and nutrients
- regulating body temperature and blood pressure
- repairing and cushioning joints
- balancing minerals
- digesting food, forming stool, and removing waste from the body

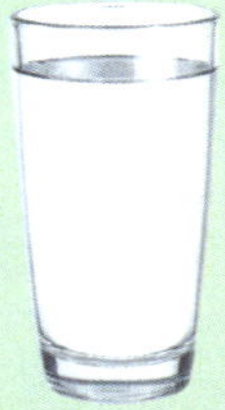

The body needs fresh clean water to carry out its functions

Infused Water Imparts Aroma, Flavor, and Health Benefits
Fresh herbs, such as mint, basil, lemon balm, and rosemary and/or sliced cucumbers can be added.

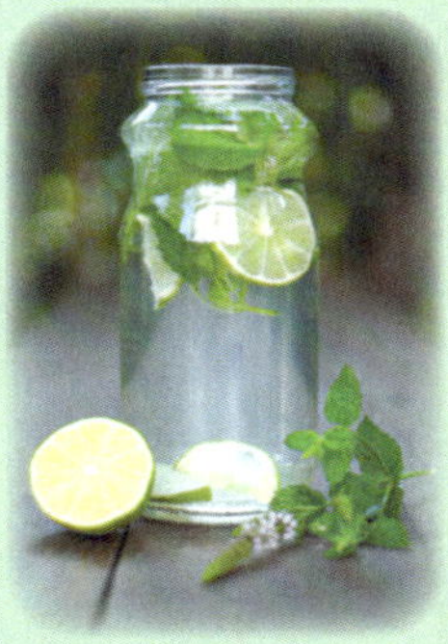

Acid Fruits and Tooth Enamel
Acidic foods, such as lemons, limes, and apple cider vinegar, while cleansing and aiding digestion, also dissolve tooth enamel. A remedy is to swish the mouth with baking soda or sea salt mixed in water, which washes away the acids and balances the pH.

During a meal, sipping a little water helps wash the food down; otherwise, waiting to drink water ½ an hour before and one hour after eating is a way to avoid diluting gastric, hydrochloric, and other digestive juices needed for digestion. Additionally, finishing drinking water and other beverages a couple of hours or more before going to sleep can minimize waking up during the night to urinate; uninterrupted sleep cycles throughout the night promote well-being.

NATURAL LIVING

Soothing and Relaxing

Restful Sleep

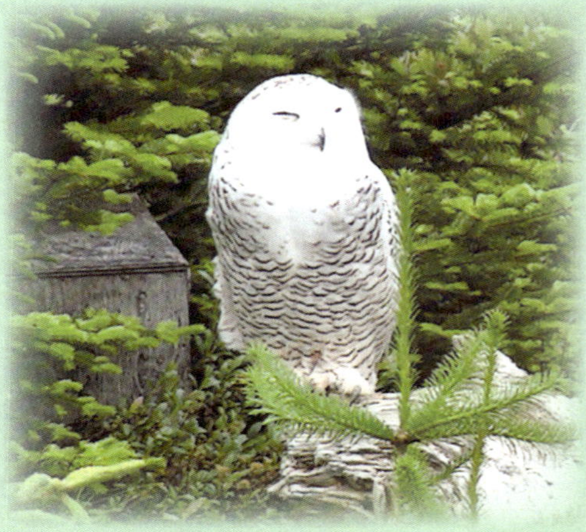

Deep, restful sleep each night is important for good health, healing, and longevity. Turning in when tired at night, especially at sundown, allows our sleep cycle to attune to our inner rhythms which coincide with the sun's 24-hour cycle. Circadian rhythms regulate our physiological processes, including the autonomic nervous system, body temperature, and hormone levels. During sleep, the body mends and repairs itself. Dr. James DiNicolantonio and Siim Land, in their book, *The Immunity Fix: Strengthen Your Immune System, Fight Off Infections, Reverse Chronic Disease and Live a Healthier Life*, point out that during sleep our body improves T-cell function and eliminates intracellular pathogens. They explain that "Sleeping is important for the adaptive immune system, which works like an immunological memory, helping the body remember how to respond effectively to infectious agents and how to fight them."[1]

There are several ways to support the nervous system and prepare for a good night's sleep. Here are some sleep-friendly practices:

- turn in to sleep and wake up around the same time each night and day
- consume foods with natural sodium, magnesium, and L-tryptophan to support the nervous system
- finish drinking caffeine, including, matcha green tea or eating chocolate, early in the day
- exercise after the nervous system has warmed up, and finish exercising a few hours before sleep
- spend time in nature, such as, walking in a forest, tending a garden, watching the sunset
- place green plants in your home for more oxygen and to freshen the air
- take a warm bath with ancient sea salt to relax tight or aching muscles
- wind down from the day listening to music
- before bed, avoid artificial blue light, such as TV and computer screens
- sleep in a quiet, cool room, with no cell phone due to harmful Wi-Fi radiation[2] (use a battery-run alarm clock)

The blackness of night (absence of light) enables the eyes to completely relax, since any amount of light stimulates the eyes. A padded eye mask worn at night helps provide darkness that supports sleep.[3]

References

[1]DiNicolantonio, J. & Land, S. (2020). *The Immunity Fix: Strengthen Your Immune System, Fight Off Infections, Reverse Chronic Disease and Live a Healthier Life* (pp. 202, 292). Monee, IL: http://drjamesdinic.com.

[2]Pall, M. L. (2018, July). Wi-Fi is an important threat to human health. *Journal of Environmental Research, 164*, 405–416. https://pubmed.ncbi.nlm.nih.gov/29573716.

[3]Bates, W.H. (1981). *The Bates Method for Better Eyesight Without Glasses* (p. 194). New York NY: Henry Holt and Co.

Soothing and Relaxing

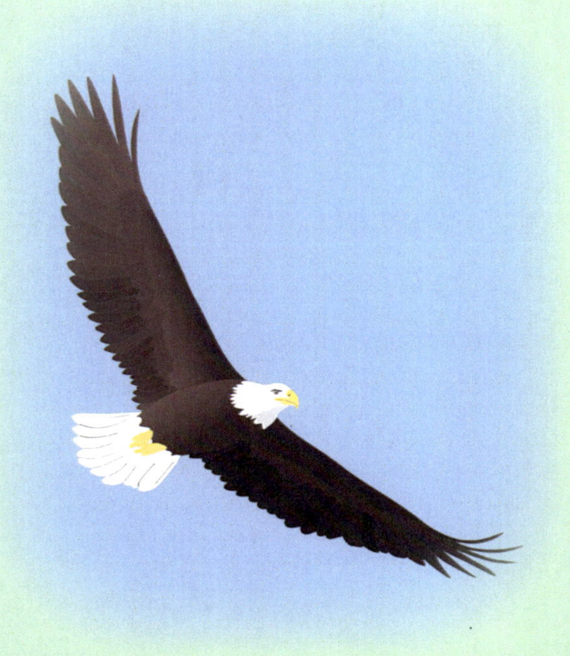

Eagles have the best vision in the animal Kingdom

(ref. https://www.lasikbyoclivision.com/90-animals-ranked-by-eyesight/)

Natural Vision

Ophthalmologist Dr. William H. Bates, M.D. (1860-1931) discovered the principles of natural vision, examining thousands of people and different species of animals with a retinoscope. From the knowledge he gained, he developed a system of eye education and taught people how to improve their eyesight naturally. His system became known as The Bates Method and is taught by practitioners around the world. In his book, *The Bates Method for Better Eyesight Without Glasses*, Dr. Bates explains that chronic eye strain is the cause of errors of refraction (the deviation of light waves as they enter the eye), including blurriness and near and far-sightedness. Poor eyesight can be corrected by relieving tension and relearning to see, applying Dr. Bates system of activities regularly.

Centralizing sight with the fovea centralis of the eye focuses and improves vision (rather than diffusing sight).[1] This aids digestion, assimilation, and elimination.[2] Gently blinking lubricates the eyes. Noticing color, variation, contrast, and spatial and depth perception improves vision. Dr. Bates explains that "The act of seeing is passive.[3] Things are seen, just as they are felt or heard or tasted, . . without effort or volition on the part of the subject."[3]

Dr. Bates illustrated that all sense perceptions are based on movement. Hearing involves sound waves which vibrate the eardrum. Molecules flowing through the nose allow us to smell. Taste involves molecules moving over the taste buds on the tongue. With the sense of touch, moving over an object enables us to feel it. Dr. Bates summed this up by stating, "We sense changes which are based on movement." He taught patients that swinging the arms and legs alternately across the body (while standing) helps the coordination of the two hemispheres of the brain. Thus, Dr. Bates emphasized that natural vision occurs when there is movement. He states that in complete darkness (seeing only black) without any stimulation of light, gives our eyes full rest. Dr. Bates recommends 'palming;' wherein, he had his patients cover their eyes with the palms of both hands.[4]

Continued...

Natural Living

Soothing and Relaxing

Natural Vision

Human vision may have been keener in ancient times than it is today. Westin A. Price, D.D.S. illustrates in this book, *Nutrition and Physical Degeneration*, that a prehistoric cave painting of Pleiades shows the the constellation as having ten stars; whereas, most of us only see a cluster of seven stars–which is now known as 'The Seven Sisters.' We need a telescope to see the additional stars. If astronomers are correct in determining that the stars were ***not brighter*** at the time of the cave painting, then it appears the artist must have been able to see all ten stars.[5]

Iridology

The iris of the eye is the most complex tissue of the body meeting the outside world. It is an extension of the brain, with hundreds of thousands of nerve endings, microscopic blood vessels, muscles, and other tissues. The iris is connected to every organ and tissue of the body through the brain and nervous system. Nerve fibers in the iris respond to changes in the body's tissues; therefore, it is possible to see the condition of every part of the body in the iris. This is the science and practice of Iridology.[6] For over fifty years, Bernard Jensen, D.C. developed and refined one of the most comprehensive iris charts used in the field of Iridology; wherein, Jensen mapped each of the organs reflected as reflexes in the iris of the eye.[7]

Colorful Phytonutrients Nourish the Eyes

Chris Kresser, M.S., L.Ac. points out some of the key nutrients that maintain eye health. For example, Dr. Kresser states that pigmented phytonutrients, lutein (green) and zeaxanthin (yellow) help maintain the structure and function of the macula of the eye. The nutrient astaxanthin (deep orange) in certain species of seafoods nourishes the retinal ganglion cells. Vitamin C helps regulate intraocular pressure and Vitamin E lipids protect the retina. The omega-3 fatty acid docosahexaenoic acid (DHA) is essential for the photoreceptor cells and guards against glaucoma. Vitamin A (retinol) from animal sources is a critical component of the protein rhodopsin, which is needed for vision. Vitamin D receptors are found in several structures in the eye, including the retina, retinal pigment epithelium, and the vascular layer known as the choroid. Herbs and nutrients to research that may help protect the eyes and support vision include: bilberry (*Phytonutrient anthocyanin*), ginkgo (*Ginkgo biloba*), Co-enzyme Q10, alpha-lipoic acid (ALA), and curcumin (orange).[8]

References

[1,2,3,4,5]Bates, W.H. (1981). *The Bates Method for Better Eyesight Without Glasses* (pp. 54, 62, 46, 63, 194). New York, NY: Henry Holt and Co.

[5]Price, W.A. (2019). *Nutrition and Physical Degeneration* (8th ed., p. 452). Lemon Grove, CA: Price-Pottenger.

[6,7]Jensen, B. (1980). *Iridology Simplified.* (5th ed., p. 3). New York, NY: Penguin Publishing.

[8]Kresser, C. (2019, April 11). *Your Guild to Eye Health.* https://chriskresser.com/your-guide-to-eye-health.

Natural Living

Soothing and Relaxing

Reducing, Releasing, and Alleviating Stress

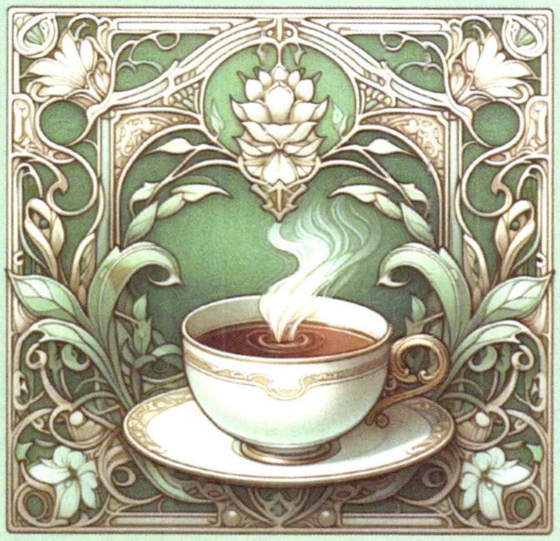

Stress is not something to put off dealing with until later, emphasizes Dr. Chris Kresser, Co-Director of the California Center for Functional Medicine. He states that if we could only do one thing to help ourselves, it would be stress management, not supplements or changing our diet.[1] In modern society, new types and levels of stress are being introduced from Wi-Fi radiation[2] and pervasive toxicity in the environment, causing inflammation and distressing the microbiome.

In his book, Essentials of Managing Stress, Brian L. Seaward expresses that "There is a huge health crisis in the world today . . . " and he discusses the physiology of stress.[3] When under duress, the body releases stress hormones that can lead to chronic adrenal fatigue and depress the immune function. The 'fight or flight response; Seward explains, elevates the heart rate and blood pressure, increases serum glucose, mobilizes free fatty acids as an energy source, decreases gastric flow, and increases perspiration. The nervous system releases catecholamines, epinephrine, and norepinephrine for blood redistribution and muscle contraction. Cortisol, vasopressin, aldosterone, and other glucocorticoids infiltrate the bloodstream.[4] If the fight or flight response becomes chronic, it is exhausting, emotionally and physiologically. A longer term effect could result in the detrimental shortening of telomeres (which are at the end of each DNA strand, protecting chromosomes from deterioration).[5]

Physical activity, needed for all the systems of the body to function properly, can free us from a significant amount of stress. Cardio-respiratory efficiency and endurance improve with regular exercise, building a stronger heart, improving blood flow, lowering systolic blood pressure, and making healthier blood lipids. Benefits of physical activity also increase: bone density, muscle mass (resistance training), range of motion, flexibility, and mental clarity. Broths and herbal teas can be hydrating and calming.

References

[1]Kresser, C. (2022, October 18) *RHR: high cortisol and brain fog*. https://chriskresser.com/high-cortisol-and-brain-fog.

[2]Pall, M. L. (2018, July). Wi-Fi is an important threat to human health. *Journal of Environmental Research, 164*, 405–416. https://pubmed.ncbi.nlm.nih.gov/29573716.

[3, 4, 5]Seaward, B. L. (2021). *Essentials of Managing Stress* (5th ed., pp. xiii, 11, 43). Burlington, MA: Jones & Bartlett Learning.

NATURAL LIVING

Physical Activities

Movement is Life – Matthew A. Holten, D.C.
Jack Harless, D.C.

WALKING FORWARD AND BACKWARD

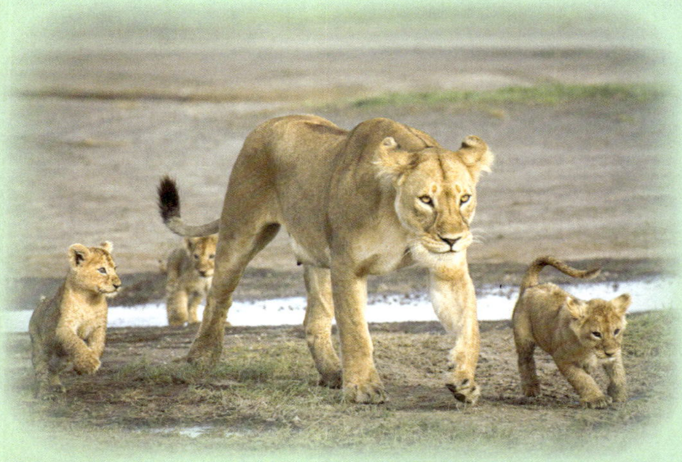

One of our most natural movements is walking. At any pace, walking improves our well-being and lubricates the joints. A leisurely walk through nature engages the senses and can enhance visual, olfactory, and auditory acuity. The scents from evergreen trees and shrubs, including pine, fir, and cedar (the resin in their bark and needles), as well as wildflowers, are nourishing and healing. Striding up a hill, or adding more energy into each step on level ground, can provide benefits. On an energetic walk, the body burns more energy and the heart beats faster, delivering the needed oxygen to the muscles, brain, and other organs. Walking helps maintain the cardiovascular system, relieves tension and anxiety, and facilitates a positive outlook.

Walking backward safely offers the advantage of exercising lesser-used muscles and improves balance and adds variety to a routine. Walking backward can give the muscles that propel us forward relief. Strengthening the muscles used in walking backward protects the joints and can help heal knee injuries. Walking backward takes away the heel-strike, puts less pressure on the joints, and changes the pelvic alignment, easing off back pain.

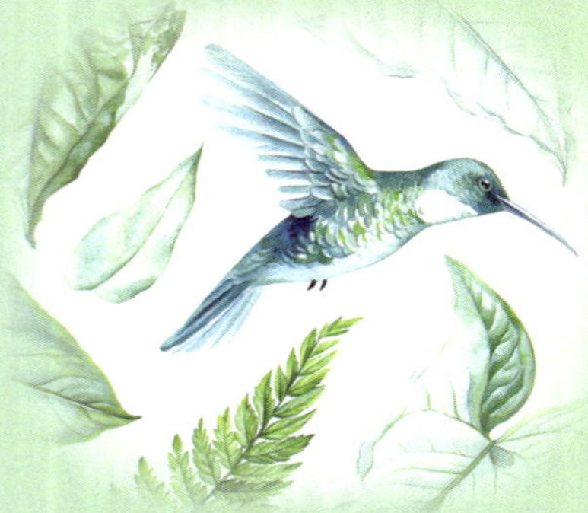

Hummingbirds are the only bird species that hover and fly both forward and backward

Dancing Supports Brain Health

Waltz

The complexity of ballroom dance involves a high degree of mind-body coordination while syncing with music and a partner. This activates multiple parts of the brain, creating new neural pathways, strengthening existing connections, and promoting neuroplasticity which facilitates mental and physical agility.

Natural Living

Physical Activities

Hatha Yoga for Balance, Flexibility, and Strength

Iyengar Hatha yoga, developed by of B.K.S. Iyengar, encompasses classic poses (asanas) and breathing techniques (pranayama) from the traditions of India that he devised to revitalize and tone all the internal systems the body. In his book, *Yoga: The Path to Holistic Health*, Iyengar emphasizes that the benefits of attentively engaging the mind and body in doing the asanas carries over into everyday life.[1]

The asanas stretch the fascia connected to the bones, keeping the fascia elastic, and creating room for the joints to move smoothly, easing the flow of blood and lymph throughout the body. Bob Anderson, in his book, *Stretching*, explains how doing stretches, as with yoga, prepares you for more vigorous types of physical activity, enhances coordination, and allows more freedom of motion.[2] Maxine Tobias, in her book, *Complete Stretching*, states that stretching is quieting, keeps us in touch with ourselves, and builds confidence.[3]

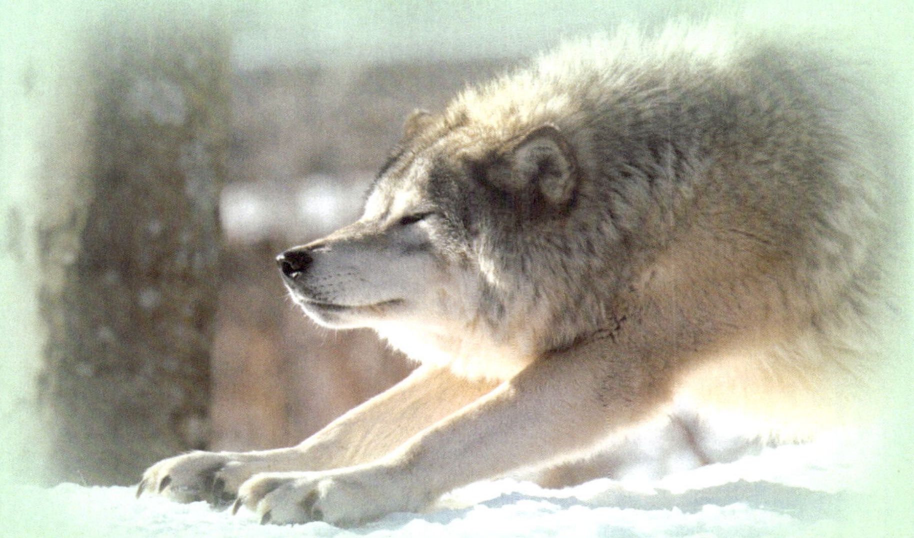

In the different asanas, yoga takes us to the edge of our physical limits without straining, gradually expanding our range of motion. It is more effective to do yoga frequently for short periods of time than to do it once in a great while for long periods. Some people like to dedicate a special place and time to do yoga. When the room temperature is warm, we tend to be more flexible than when it is cold.

Restorative yoga involves fully supporting the body with props, such as bolsters, blankets, blocks, or belts. The props make the asanas effortless; letting go, the props and gravity do the work, supporting and healing the muscles and organs. Restorative asanas are generally held for a longer time than other asanas, releasing physical and emotional tension. An eye pillow is often used while doing restorative asanas, keeping out the light and bringing serenity.

References

[1]Iyengar, B.K.S. (2001). *Yoga: The Path to Holistic Health* (p. 11). New York, NY: Dorling Kindersley.

[2]Anderson, B. (1980). *Stretching* (p. 11). Bolinas, CA: Shelter Publications, Inc.

[3]Tobias, M. & Sullivan, J. P. (1994). *Complete Stretching: A New Exercise Program for Health and Vitality* (p. 13). New York, NY: Alfred A. Knopf, Inc.

Physical Activities

Gliding Through Your Pilates Routine

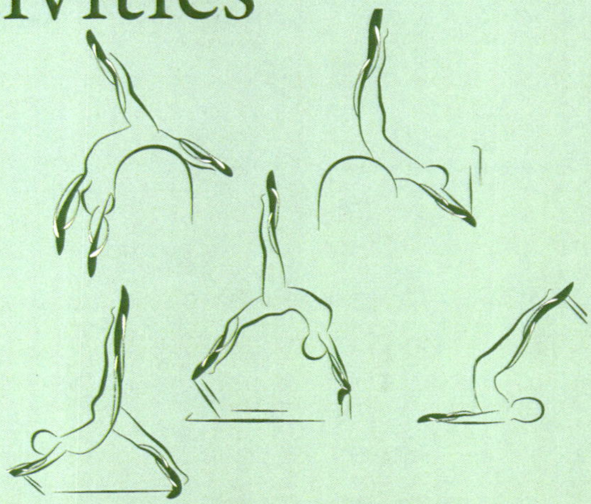

When doing Pilates, unlike yoga, we are in continual motion, like dance, swimming, and Tai Chi. Pilates is different from yoga in that you slowly and smoothly move continuously from one pose to another; whereas, in yoga you hold the poses (asanas). As a cardio exercise, Pilates aerobically raises your heart rate; whereas, yoga is mostly anaerobic, involving lifting your own body weight. On a similar note, Pilates and yoga poses are alike in that they are performed on a floor mat; and, the techniques of Pilates and yoga are both founded on the optimal functioning of the human anatomy and physiology.

Alycea Ungaro, Director of Pilates Center of New York–Tribeca Bodyworks, offers a complete Pilates workout in her book, *Pilates: Body In Motion*.[1] While attending the New York School of Ballet, she studied under Romana Kryzanowska who was Joseph Hubertus Pilates's successor.[1] Joseph H. Pilates (1880–1967) developed this form of exercise to increase concentration, strength, flexibility, and stamina. As a diver, skier, and gymnast, he drew from his experience as an athlete in creating the Pilates system. He emphasized inhaling when preparing for movement and exhaling when executing movement. The flow of the movement is one of the main principles of Pilates, improving balance and coordination.
As you glide from one pose to another, Ungaro explains, mat-work becomes seamless from the first exercise to the last. Joseph H. Pilates intended for the Pilates method to be performed at the rhythm of each person's heart.[1]

In our center, core muscles (such as the adominal, back and gluteal muscles) stabilize the body. Pilates is designed to exercise muscles in opposing ways which helps achieve balance and symmetry in the body. Opening the chest is important for enhancing posture, restoring alignment, and making space for breathing. Pilates focuses on the natural curvature of the spine to accomplish proper alignment. Challenging oneself to increase proficiency entails exertion to the threshold one's ability (referred to as your "edge" in yoga). This increases flexibility and endurance. It is valuable to dress comfortably and avoid eating for 45 minutes before your practice. In only ten minutes per day of Pilates or yoga, people can see a difference in their health and well-being.[1]

References

[1]Ungaro, A. (2002). *Pilates: Body In Motion* (pp. 22, 24). New York, NY: DK Publishing, Inc..

NATURAL LIVING

Physical Activities

ROLLING INTO GOOD HEALTH

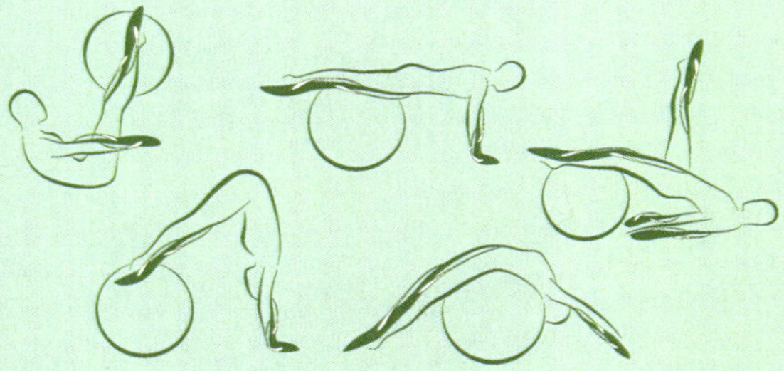

Aquilino Cosani made the first inflatable fit ball in 1963 to for developing gymnastic skills. He called it the 'Pezzi Ball.' Physical therapists across Europe then adopted the Pezzi Ball to rehabilitate people with neurological conditions, including cerebral palsy and spinal injuries.[1] In the United States, Yamuna Zake designed a ball rolling method for longevity.[2] She uses fit balls of varying sizes to tone, strengthen, and realign the entire body, creating space for freer movement of the bones, muscles, blood, and lymph.[3]

Zake explains that with pressure from the fit ball, bone tissue, even when ossified and brittle, becomes more supple; and it will initiate a release of the tendons to all muscles that have attachments anywhere else on the bone. Each muscle has a natural memory of its function. Zake applies pressure at a muscle's origin and waits for the muscle to respond. She explains that this communicates to the muscle that there is greater space for it to expand into, awakening it to relax and elongate muscle fibers to fill the space. Once elongated, the muscle, taking up its full length, may decompress and relieve the tension on bones, joints, and nerves, potentially restoring full function.[4]

Ball rolling is a mild form of weight-bearing exercise. "The weight of your body sinking into the ball applies pressure directly into the bone to stimulate bone-building. The pressure brings increased circulation to bone, tendons, and muscles simultaneously."[5] Zake teaches people to find the places in their body that need attention and how to fix these places on their own. Observing the breath, she states, is the quickest, most effective way to identify where the restriction is to then begin to address it.

Zake uses small specialized balls for hard-to-reach places, such as between the shoulder blades. Her methods of ball rolling benefits individual fascia, organs, muscles, tendons, ligaments, and bones, including the arm and leg abductors, hip rotators, and the entire spine.[6] Since 1979, Zake has trained and certified hundreds of instructors. Through her workshops, she taught thousands of people around the world. Attending Zake's school, people gain an understanding of human anatomy and learn strategies for problem solving common musculoskeletal issues. Her students learn how to use different size fit balls to elongate muscles multidimensionally, create space, and improve circulation and range of motion. Zake demonstrates how to use fit balls to guide strained parts of the body back to their natural position, releasing tension, alleviating pain, and supporting the parasympathetic nervous system.[7]

References

[1]Heffernan, C. (2016, January 4). *A brief history of the Swiss ball.* https://physicalculturestudy.com/2016/01/04/a-brief-history-of-the-swiss-ball.

[2]Zake, Y. (2003). *Yamuna.* Retrieved on December 30, 2024: https://www.yamunausa.com.

[3, 4, 5]Zake, Y. & Golden, S. (2003). *The Ultimate Body Rolling Workout* (pp. 3, 10, 13). New York, NY: Broadway Books. https://www.yamunausa.com.

[6, 7]Suzuki, S. (2013, October 20). The Theory and Technique of Yamuna Body Rolling. *Journal of Physical Therapy Science, 25*(9): 1197–1200. https://pubmed.ncbi.nlm.nih.gov/24259945.

Natural Living

Physical Activities

Resistance Exercise and Impact Training

Resistance and impact training promote cardiovascular and musculoskeletal health. Examples of resistance exercises that use bodyweight are: pull-ups, push-ups, squats, leg raises, and plank pose. Other resistance training includes:

- exercise bands – resists when stretched
- weights – free weights engage the secondary muscles (stabilizers) as well as major muscles
- impact activities – dancing, running, and jumping have cardiovascular and musculoskeletal benefits

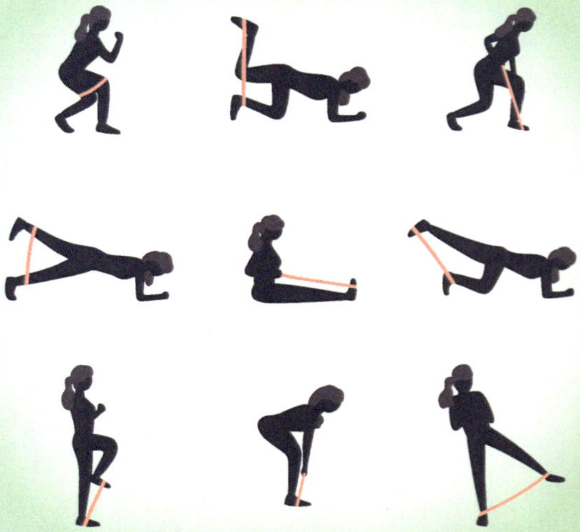

Resistance Bands

Resistance bands are light and easy to take anywhere. Made of elastic rubber, each band's thickness, width, and length is suitable for different exercises. Light-weight bands are recommended for beginning users. Typically, the bands are from 1 to 2½ meters (~3 to 8 feet) in length. They can be used as they are or be wrapped around a door knob or a tree for traction. Resistance bands aid in healing. Physical therapists facilitate recovery, using the bands to stabilize and regenerate injured areas of the body. Professional athletes engage the bands for stretching before and after rigorous workouts. Stretching and strengthening is accomplished by pulling the band with joint-friendly movements. The bands gently give and provide a counter-pull that challenges the muscles and makes them stronger. Band exercises can include: lateral lift, lat pull, rowing, leg extension, triceps stretcher, bicep curl, and squat.

Continued...

Physical Activities

Lifting weights

Professional fitness trainers highlight how muscle mass increases when you lift more weight and do fewer repetitions per set; strengthens and tones when you use less weight and do more repetitions per set; and boosts endurance when you use less weight and do even more repetitions per set. During resistance workouts, muscle fibers tear down. When the body repairs them, they are made stronger. It is important to allow muscles time to recuperate, rest, and rebuild between workouts. Muscle is metabolically active tissue, burning calories while we are at rest.

Impact Training

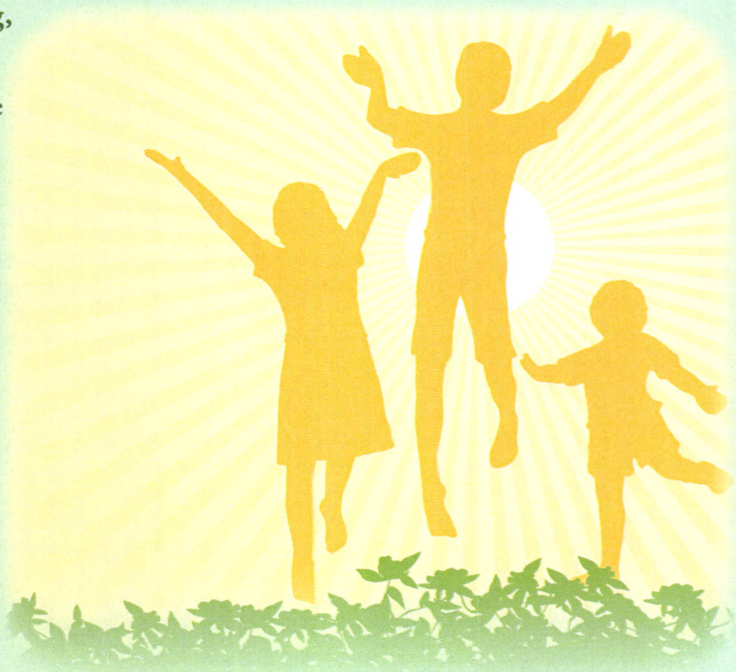

Landing on one or both feet, such as with dancing, hiking in the hills or mountains (especially when going downhill), running, and jumping, can cause various amounts of impact to the body. Medium to high impact sports can significantly increase the density and strength of the bones and build and tone muscle. If our bones, cartilage, tendons, and muscles are healthy and strong this can have a positive effect and build strength. Bouncing on a flexible medium, such as, a mini trampoline, is low impact like walking, gardening, bicycling, swimming, and Tai Chi. These activities generally lack the impact needed to strengthen bones; although, these activities are excellent for cardiovascular health, strengthening muscles, greater coordination and mobility, and supporting the flow of lymph which enhances the immune system. It is important to be mindful of the level of impact, to avoid putting too much pressure on vulnerable bones which could weaken instead of strengthen them. Osteopathic physicians and fitness coaches can help individuals assess optimal impact exercises. Resistance activities, weight training, and impact sports are important for well-being, especially for protecting bone health.

Physical Activities

Staying Active in the Water

Swimming, like dancing, Tai Chi, gymnastics, and Pilates, engages the whole body in movement

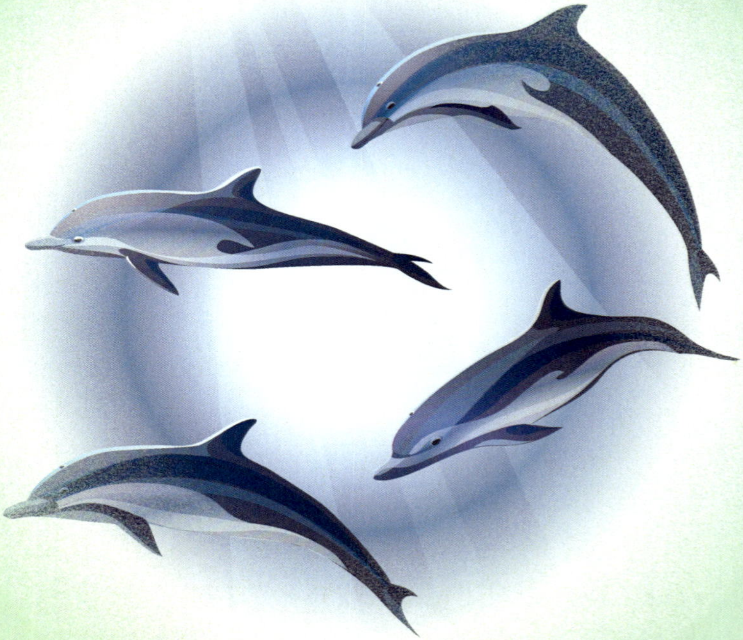

Water is an ideal medium for staying active and fit. Physical therapists Lynda Huey and Robert Forster, authors of *The Complete Waterpower Workout Book*, highlight that water furnishes support (buoyancy), three-dimensional resistance, and a fresh, clean feeling. Providing a cushion for weight-bearing joints, water is largely a low-impact and injury-free environment. Because water is denser than air, your muscles work harder. Simply by moving through the water, you accomplish weight-training. This works because water matches the energy you put into it; the harder you push or pull, the more resistance you get. Those who may not have exercised for months or years can enter the water and begin exercising immediately. People of all ages and abilities can do the same exercises and each will be challenged at their own level. Water is remarkable in how it responds to you.[1]

Water as a medium facilitates strong body alignment, including the anti-gravity muscles: trapezius, rhomboids, gluteal, hamstrings, and erector spinae which, in water, hold you effortlessly in postural alignment. Back-and-forth movements of the arms and legs are beneficial because muscles work in synchronized pairs, while one contracts, the opposing one relaxes, such as the quadriceps/hamstrings, biceps/triceps, and abductors/adductors. Any exercise in the water naturally works both muscles of the pair. Water is a low-gravity, safe, and relaxing environment.

Continued...

Physical Activities

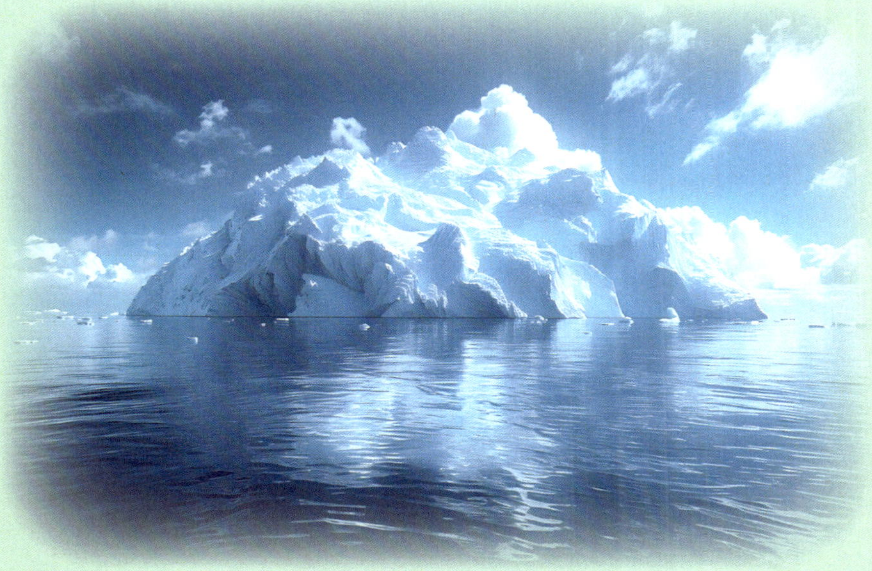

Healing Ice

When frozen, water is a healing agent that can help us recover from a physical injury. Authors Huey and Forester describe how 'PRICE' is a checklist used by Olympic athletes for treating an injury. The 'P' is for protection, including immobilizing or bracing the injured part of the body. 'R' is for resting the affect area until movement is pain-free. The 'I' is for ice, surrounding an injury with ice compresses the capillaries around the injury, preventing or diminishing swelling and bleeding. Ice is often applied for ten to twenty minutes, the frequency depends on the degree and type of injury. 'C' is for compression, immediately applying pressure to an injured area is sometimes recommended, such as with an Ace bandage or compression sleeve. Compression helps prevent swelling and the leaking of excess fluids into the tissues. Lastly, the 'E' is for elevation, keeping the injured part of the body above the heart; this helps the body drain fluids that may accumulate in the tissues surrounding the injury, keeping swelling to a minimum.[1]

For rehabilitation after PRICE, Huey and Forester offer water therapy recommendations for recuperating in the pool, introducing gentle range of motion exercises that support the healing process. They explain that ice reduces pain and diminishes muscle spasms, as does exercise in the water.[2]

References
[1,2]Huey, L. & Forester, R. (1993). *The Complete Waterpower Workout Book* (pp. 3–4). New York, NY: Random House.

Natural Living

Physical Activities
Tai Chi

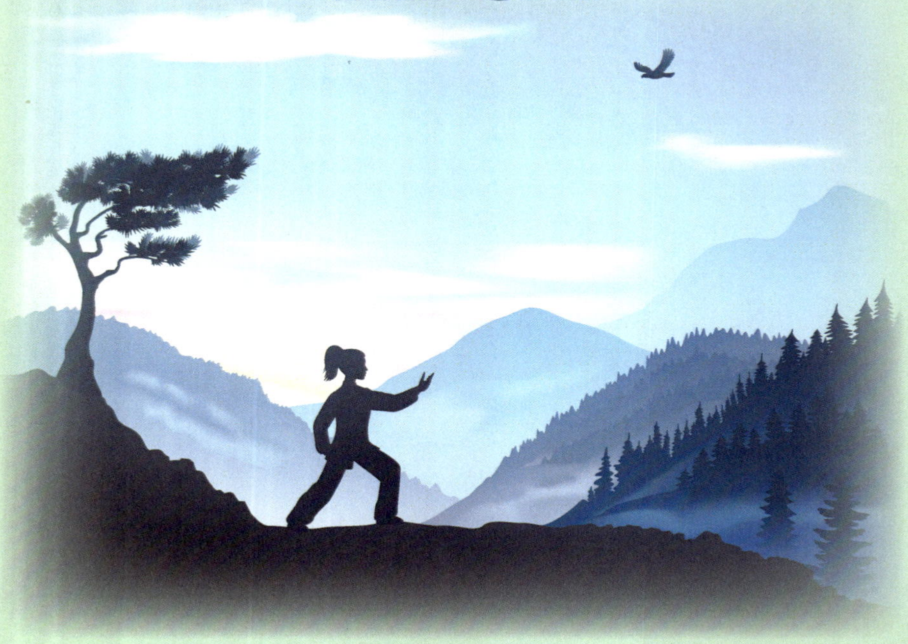

The ancient Chinese martial art of Tai Chi is short for Tai Ji Quan; and is based on the philosophy of Taoism, which fosters an awareness of the Qi universal life energy that flows through and sustains all things in nature. Tai chi was developed to attain physical and mental fitness and for self-defense, including skills in deflecting an incoming force and redirecting this energy. The movements are performed in a continuous flow, sometimes sinking into the joints, making deliberate circular motions, or fluidly when springing into action. Tai Chi is meditative and involves moving slowly and steadily. It requires great discipline and balance. Many health benefits are derived from Tai Chi, enhancing mental and physical coordination; flexibility in the muscles, tendons, and ligaments; improving circulation; lowering heart rate and blood pressure; reducing stress; and massaging the internal organs. Many of the postures and movements of Tai Chi were inspired by the agility and poise in the stances and movements of animals. Building on the techniques of those that came before him, physician Huá Tuó (华佗 - 141-208 A.D.) created the Wu Qin Xi (五禽戏) form of Tai Chi. Integrating the breath, he devised new postures and movements, like: a crouching tiger (虎), the complete stillness of a crane (鹤), and graceful deer (鹿).[1]

References
[1] Buhmann, E. (2020, September 29). *Animals and Heroes*. Tai Chi Notebook. https://taichinotebook.com/2020/09/29/animals-and-heroes.

Natural Living

Rejuvenation

Healing the Digestive System and Related Ailments with the GAPS Diet

Neurologist and nutritionist Natasha Campbell-McBride, M.D. a leader in the field of healing with natural foods, brought to light the connections between the functions of the digestive system and the brain. In developing the GAPS Diet, Dr. McBride drew on her work, helping hundreds of children and adults recover from neurological and psychiatric conditions, including: autistic spectrum disorders, attention deficit hyperactivity disorder (ADHD/ADD), schizophrenia, dyslexia, dyspraxia, depression, obsessive–compulsive disorder, bi-polar disorder, and other neuro-psychological and psychiatric problems.[1]

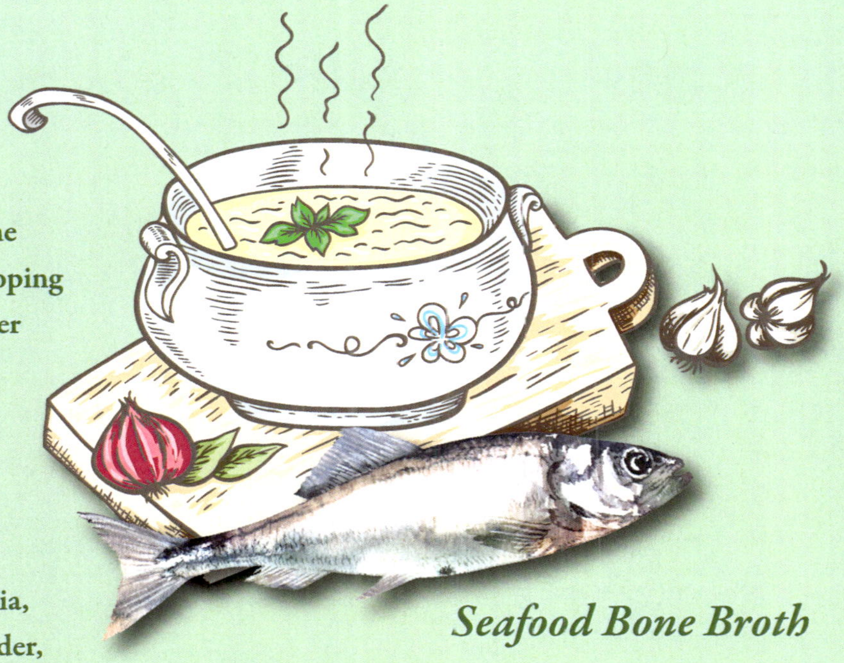

Seafood Bone Broth

Dysbiosis is the disruption of the microbiome, leading to nutritional deficiencies, proliferation of pathogenic micro-organisms, and increased permeability of the mucosal membrane of the intestinal tract (leaky gut). Elson M. Hass, M.D., in this book, *The New Detox Diet*, explains that when there is increased permeability in the wall of the digestive tract, larger than normal molecules pass through the wall of the intestines. This can cause allergic reactions and abnormal immune responses. Associated complaints may include: headaches; inflammation; swollen joints; excess mucus, acidity, and other flu or cold-like symptoms; and accumulation of oxidized fats and cholesterol in the arteries.[2]

In her book, *Gut and Psychology Syndrome*, Dr. Campbell-McBride illustrates how the microbiome facilitates the digestion, absorption, and assimilation of nutrients; metabolism; and neurotransmitter production and transport. Dr. Campbell-McBride designed the GAPS Diet Nutritional Protocol to reduce inflammation, heal the mucosa of the digestive tract, and encourage healthy probiotic diversity.

Continued...

Natural Living

Adhering to the protocol, people have found relief from physical ailments including: Crohn's disease, irritable bowel syndrome, gastritis, colitis, celiac disease, rheumatoid arthritis, diabetes type one, multiple sclerosis, asthma, allergies, eczema, chronic fatigue syndrome, fibromyalgia, chronic infections, and endocrine disorders. With targeted supplementation, detoxification, and lifestyle changes described in Dr. Campbell-McBride's program, people have restored their digestive system, brain function, and overall health.[3]

Oxalic acid presents a problem for many people. It occurs in a many common plant foods; for example, ocalic acid is high in spinach, sweet potatoes, and green tea. When oxalic acid combines with calcium, it forms calcium oxalate crystals, where it can cause muscle and joint pain and more serious inflammatory conditions. Diet can make a positive difference. The essential amino acid lysine plays an important role in dissolving oxalate crystals and preventing their formation.[4] Meats, fish, eggs, and milk products are high in lysine; however, legumes and grains contain trypsin inhibitors which block the absorption of lysine.[4] Consuming fatty acids can be part of the solution. Eicosatetraenoic acid (EPA), docosahexaenoic acid (DHA), and arachidonic acid (AA), help clear oxalates from the kidneys.[5]

Traditionally-prepared, home-cooked meals are the foundation of the GAPS Diet. Monica Corrado, author of *The Complete Cooking Techniques for the GAPS Diet*, provides easy-to-follow instructions for making bone broth and meat stock.[6] She explains that bone broth is simmered at a low temperature for many hours, long enough to allow the connective tissues to dissolve and the minerals to be drawn into the broth. This is why bone broth is an exceptionally nourishing and healing food, helping the body rebuild bone, cartilage, tendons, and the integumentary system (hair, skin, and nails).

In her article, 'The Dark Side of Bone Broth,' Corrado points out that long cook times result in a tremendous amount of glutamic acid, which for "... many people—including the vast number of children in our country with nervous system disorders such as ADD, ADHD, and Autism Spectrum Disorders..."[7] (associated with a leaky gut).

Caution: *people who have compromised digestion and immune system may be sensitive to glutamic acid, a main component of bone broth. They may do better with fish and meat stocks. Avoiding bone broth may be important until having addressed this issue, for instance, through working with a certified GAPS Diet practitioner.*[7]

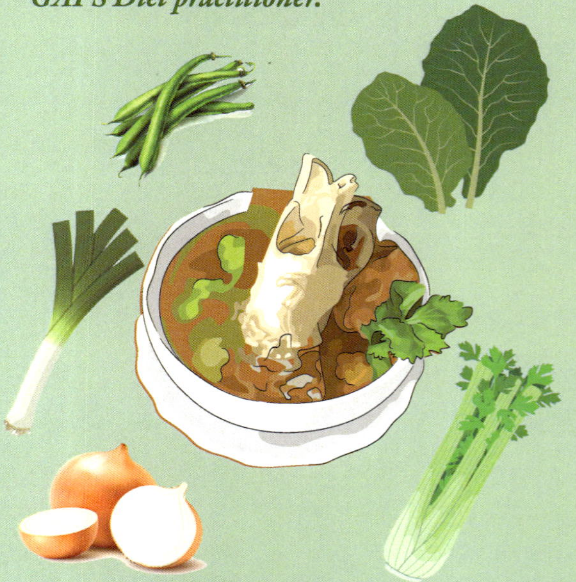

Meat Stock

Continued...

Natural Living

High amounts of glutamic acid can trigger additional neurological symptoms including: brain fog, migraine headaches, or even seizures. Corrado offers that many of the benefits of bone broth can be obtained without high amounts of glutamic acid by consuming meat stock instead. She explains, "It's cooked slow and low and not long. The short cook time means glutamic acid levels will be low—and therefore, not problematic."[7] Once people heal their digestive tract and immune system, they can once again benefit from bone broth. GAPS practitioners are trained by Dr. Campbell-McBride to help people rebuild their digestive health so they can handle the full breadth of health-giving foods.

References

[1]Campbell-McBride, N. (2024) *Natural digestive healing.* https://www.gapsdiet.com.

[2]Haas, E. M. (2004). *The New Detox Diet* (pp. 14–15). *Berkeley*, CA: Celestial Arts.

[3]Boynton, H., & Brackett, M. (2014). *The Heal Your Gut Cookbook* (pp. ix–x). White River Junction, VT: Chelsea Green Publishing.

[4]Tendler, J. M. & Arch. M. (2023, summer). *Journal of Wise Traditions* (p. 26). Washington, D.C.: The Weston A. Price Foundation.

[5]Rodgers, A. L. & Siener, R. (2020, April 12). The Efficacy of Polyunsaturated Fatty Acids as Protectors against Calcium Oxalate Renal Stone Formation: A Review. *Nutrients Journal. 12*(4): 1069. https://www.mdpi.com/2072-6643/12/4/1069.

[6]Corrado, M. (2019,). *The Complete Cooking Techniques for GAPSTM Diet*. Fort Collins, CO: Selene River Press.

[7]Corrado, M. (2015, August 27). *The dark side of bone broth*. Fort Collins, CO: Selene River Press. https://www.seleneriverpress.com/the-dark-side-of-bone-broth.

Natural Living

Rejuvenation

Cleansing and Healing with Fresh Juices

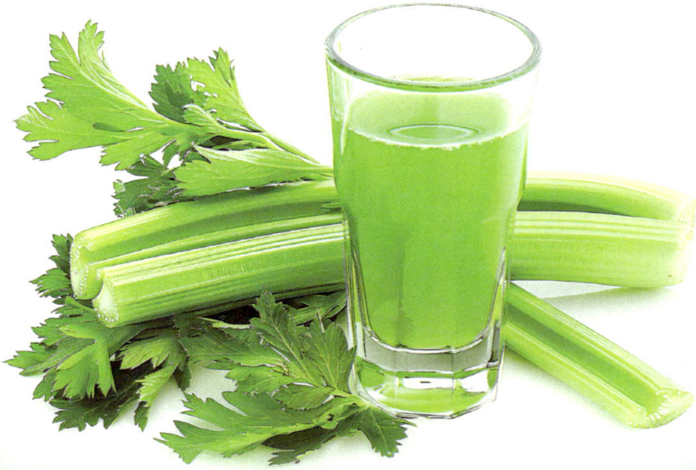

Vegetable and fruit juices furnish a wealth of nutrients that are readily absorbed and assimilated. When we suffer from malnutrition, the body is weakened and has a lessened ability to properly digest, absorb, and assimilate nutrients, guard against pathogens, eliminate toxins, heal worn out cells and wounds, and build new healthy cells and tissues. Pathogenic micro-organisms produce toxic byproducts that alter our biochemistry. They can target specific organs and/or impact the body systemically. Juicing and intermittent fasting[1] are ways of bringing about a higher state of health by enabling the body to: 1) neutralize and eliminate toxins, 2) create an environment that supports a healthy microbiome, and 3) optimize nutrition to nourish and renew the body.

Cleansing clears the way for healing. Elson M. Hass, M.D., in this book, *The New Detox Diet*, details the many avenues the body has for eliminating toxins and foreign substances, summarized, below:[2]

- gastrointestinal (GI) – liver, gall bladder, colon, and the whole GI tract
- urinary – kidneys, bladder, and urethra
- respiratory – lungs, bronchial tubes, throat, sinuses, and nose
- lymphatic – lymph channels and lymph nodes
- skin – sweat and sebaceous glands and tears
- head – nose, eyes, and ears

> Nutrients in fruits and vegetables are concentrated in and just beneath the skins and rinds.

Fresh, raw vegetable and fruit juices, with the fiber removed, helps the body cleanse and revitalize, supplying an abundance of bioavailable vitamins, minerals, phytonutrients, and enzymes. Drinking juice from colorful vegetables and fruits is a way to correct a suite of nutritional deficiencies. Michael T. Murray, N.D., in his book, *The Complete Book of Juicing*, describes

Continued...

how vegetable and fruit juices containing antioxidants, including manganese, carotenes, bioflavonoids, and vitamin C, increase the body's enzyme tissue levels of catalase, superoxide dismutase, and glutathione peroxidase. These enzymes are superlative in protecting the body from free radicals (unstable oxygen molecules).[3] Dr. Murray describes how plant foods incorporate minerals from the soil into their own tissues and complex them, making them more bioavailable to the body.[4]

Known as the Juiceman, Jay Kordich, made juicing into a lifestyle. He stated, "Every day I nurture the trillions of cells in my body with fresh juices and raw foods."[5] Pulp-free, juice contains concentrated nutrients and replenishes the body's need for enzymes. On the other hand, Kordich points out in his book, *The Juiceman's Power of Juicing*, that fruits, like pears and apples, have pectin which is best absorbed by eating the fruit whole rather than juiced (which could damage the pectin).[6] Additionally, the fiber in fruit slows down the digestion of the natural sugars (fructose) in fruit, which helps maintain low blood sugar levels. Nevertheless, juicing (or blending) may be a good option for fruit in certain circumstances. For instance, while the richest nutrients are concentrated in the skins of fruits (such as, purple-pigmented resveratrol and anthocyanin), their skins may be too tough to chew. In this case, juicing fruits makes it possible for us to more fully access these valuable phytonutrients.

Organic Vegetables and Fruits

Consuming only organic (pesticide free), regeneratively-grown produce is extremely important, especially when juicing, because juicing concentrates not only the nutrients but also any pesticides and/or herbicides. It may be beneficial to rinse produce in filtered water and an organic biodegradable wash (such as, baking soda dissolved in water).

References

[1]Fung, J., Mayer, E. & Ramos, M. (2020). *Life in the Fasting Lane*. New York, NY: Harper Collins Publishers.

[2]Haas, E. M. (2004). *The New Detox Diet* (p. 28). Berkeley, CA: Celestial Arts.

[3,4]Murray, M. T. (1998). *The Complete Book of Juicing* (pp. 16, 28). New York, NY: Three Rivers Press.

[5,6]Kordich, J. (1992). *The Juiceman's Power of Juicing* (pp. 27–28). New York, NY: William Morrow and Company, Inc.

Natural Living

Rejuvenation

Detoxing with Activated Charcoal

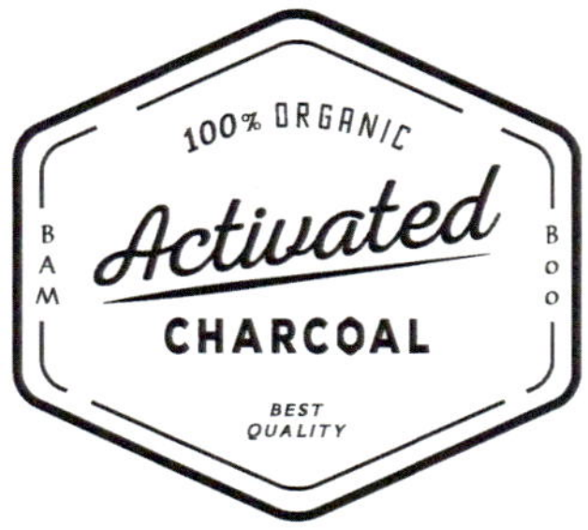

Naturally activated charcoal is a lightweight black carbon residue made from burned coconut husks, bamboo, peat, or other organic matter. At high temperatures, the gases expand in the charcoal making it very porous. When ingested, the charcoal absorbs toxins and facilitates the body in eliminating them. Research scientists in the Division of Emergency Medicine/Clinical Toxicology, Regional Poison Center, and Medical Intensive Care Unit at the Department of Internal Medicine, University of California Davis Medical Center Sacramento, California, published an article in the *Western Journal of Medicine*, stating that, "Activated charcoal may be the single most effective treatment in many types of poisoning."[1]

High quality charcoal, such as made from coconut, can be used as part of a detox and cleansing program, for example, HealthForce SuperFoods' Intestinal Drawing Formula with a blend of flax seeds, activated coconut charcoal, slippery elm bark, carob pod, nopal cactus leaf, marshmallow root, kelp leaf.[2] It has been used to improve pH balance in the mouth; reduce cavities, gum disease, and bad breath; and help eliminate pesticides, mold, and heavy metals from the body. Activated charcoal, like healing clay and psyllium husks, help with elimination in the colon (bowel); however, too much activated charcoal, healing clay, or psyllium husks can interfere with the absorption of nutrients and cause dehydration. (Too much psyllium husk can cause constipation and even block the intestinal tract.) These substances should only be used on a temporary basis and in consultation with experienced natural health professionals.

References

[1]Derlet, R. & Albertson, T. (1986). Activated charcoal--past, present and future. *Western Journal of Medicine. 145*(4):493 – 496. https://www.ncbi.nlm.nih.gov/pmc/articles/PMC1306980.

[2] HealthForce SuperFoods, (2025). *Intestinal Drawing Formula*. HealthForce Superfoods. https://healthforcesuperfoods.com.

Natural Living

Rejuvenation
Healing Clay

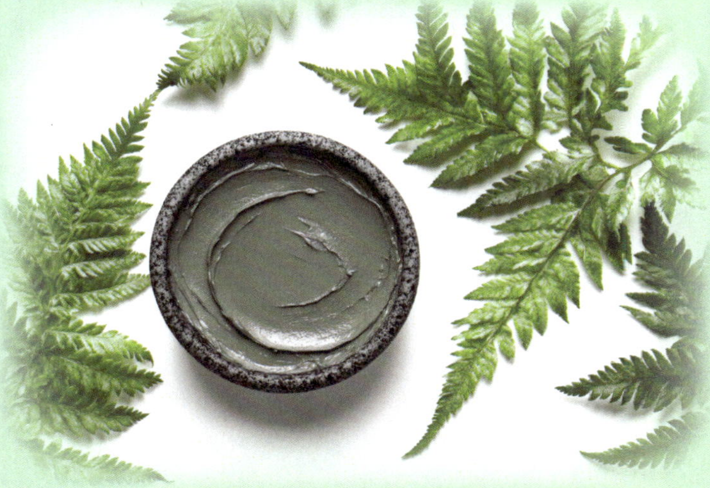

Many animals use muds and clays to restore their health. In their book, *Our Earth Our Cure*, Raymond Dextreit and Michel Abehsera, note that the curative properties of clay were discovered in Siberian forests when wild pigs, roe-deer, red deer, and other wildlife were observed wallowing in mud. They point out that gangrene hooves of horses and foot-and-mouth diseases (aphthous fever) in cows has been cured with applications of clay; and clay has been used to treat tree wounds. Clay contains minerals and serves as a natural fertilizer. "Added to organic debris, clay increases the production of humus and also the amount of carbon fixation in the soil."[1]

Dextreit and Abehsera highlight the natural healing principle that ". . . treating the general condition is more primary than relieving a specific manifestation, for 'a local disease is usually the consequence of a general disorder.'" The manifested trouble can even be seen as a 'beneficial crisis,' leading to diagnosis and treatment of a latent abnormality of the organism as a whole.[2] They explain that clay acts directly to alleviate minor ailments, such as diarrhea or constipation, through its local application; while at the same time, it acts on the whole organism, eliminating unhealthy cells and activating the rebuilding of healthy cells.[3]

In Switzerland and Germany, doctors effectively treated people who had tuberculosis with clay. In France, clay was used to treat burns.[4] Clay is highly absorptive and has the capacity to pull toxins out of the body, including pathogenic microbes and parasites. Clay's negatively charged molecules bind with positively-charged toxins and heavy metals, making it easier for the body to remove them. Colloidal properties in clay are greasy and act as a cleansing agent, facilitating the elimination of noxious substances. The diastases, oxidase, and other enzymes in clay fix free oxygen, protecting the body from oxidative damage. In the presence of clay, some of the most problematic pesticides have been removed from the body.[5]

To improve health, high quality clay, free of contaminants, should be selected and used with the consultation of an experienced natural clay practitioner. Dextreit and Michel Abehsera state

Continued...

Natural Living

Rejuvenation

Healing Clay

that when applied in poultices and compresses, ". . . clay provides numerous benefits. It can heal sores and ulcers and aid in the rebuilding healthy tissues and cells, and even of fractured bones and vertebrae."[6] In addition to being used externally, clay has been ingested in small amounts, dissolved in water or, as in Mexico, India, Sudan, and South America, kneaded into balls, dried, and then consumed.[7] As a magnetic component of the Earth, clay may transmit energy that helps strengthen and rebuild an organism's vital potential for self-healing.[8] Words of caution, clay can interfere with the absorption of nutrients; therefore, it should only be used when not eating meals. The more that clay is exposed to the sun, air, and rainwater, the more active it becomes, enhancing its restorative capacity.[9]

References

[1,2,3,4,6,7,8,9]Dextreit, R. & Abehsera, M. (1990). *Our Earth Our Cure* (pp. 196, 2–3, 12, 14, 12, 14, 13, 15). New York, NY: First Carol Publishing Group Edition.

[5]Moosavi, M. (2017, September). Bentonite clay as a natural remedy: A brief review. *Iran Journal of Public Health*. *46*(9):1176 – 1183. https://www.ncbi.nlm.nih.gov/pmc/articles/PMC5632318.

Natural Living

Rejuvenation

Seaweeds (marine algae), Seawater, Sea breeze for Health

In her book, ***Seaweed: Nature's Secret to Balancing Your Metabolism, Preventing Disease, and Revitalizing Body and Mind***, Valerie Gennari Cooksley explains the holistic practices of 'thalassotherapy' (related to the sea) with seaweeds (marine algae) and 'climatotherapy,' which encompasses spending time in a place where the temperature, altitude, humidity, and air quality improve health. Warm seawater: increases circulation; cleanses the skin, improves complexion and mobility of joints; helps heal muscle and bone injuries; eases nervous tension; and relieves arthritic pain and rheumatism. Inhaling sea air can reduce respiratory ailments and restore the lungs. Thalasso and climato spas offer seaweed wraps, masks, mudpacks, sand baths, pastes, scrubs, and soaks with seaweed, seawater, and marine coastal mud.[2] Additionally, breathing in sea breezes supports overall health.

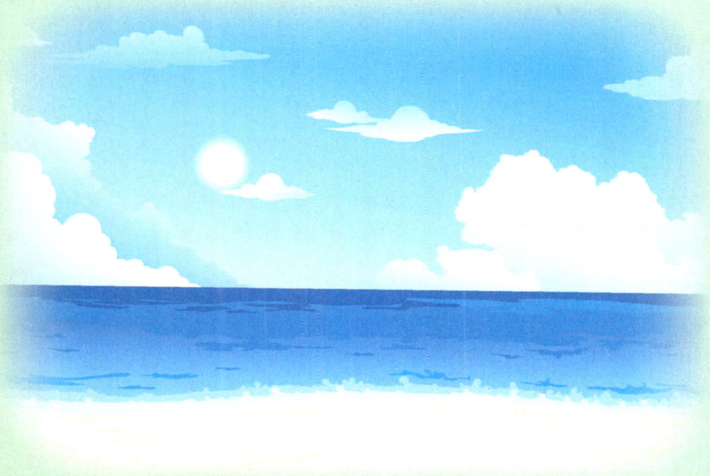

Caution: Seaweed is significantly higher in minerals than other natural foods. Absorbing minerals through the skin or air via marine products could cause mineral levels in the body to become too high, especially for those who are iodine sensitive or who have hypertension, kidney disease, or congestive heart issues. Consulting with a physician about one's own condition would be wise before applying topical seaweed.

'Balneotherapy' involves immersing in sea soaks and brine baths containing seawater and seaweed. Skin brushing beforehand enhances the benefits of the soaking, promoting skin tone, increasing blood and lymph flow, and energizing the nerve system.[3] 'Pelotherapy,' the regenerative use of sea mud in various colors, can be mixed with seaweed and herbs to draw out toxins, exfoliate, reduce inflammation, and soothe the autonomic nervous system.

References

[1,2,3]Cooksley, V. G. (2018). *Seaweed: Nature's Secret to Balancing Your Metabolism, Preventing Disease, and Revitalizing Body and Mind* (pp. 126, 124–126, 129–131, 143). The Woodlands, TX: Floramed Publishing.

Natural Living

Rejuvenation

Connecting with the Earth for Nourishment and Negative Ions

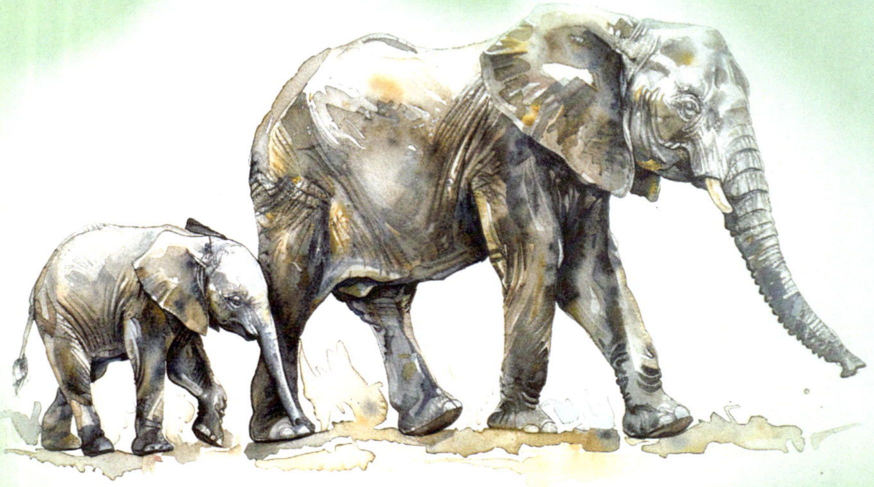

Walking barefoot on the nourishing earth–including through a pristine meadow; forest; or organic, regenerative garden–can bring us into contact with beneficial probiotic micro-organisms and negatively-charged ions. Joseph Mercola, D.O. explains that the reservoir of negatively-charged ions on the Earth's surface is maintained and influenced by several environmental factors, including solar and ionospheric winds and thunderstorms. Dr. Mercola describes the benefits of negative ions; for instance, they may help our cells and tissues heal from damage due to Wi-Fi radiation, cell phones, and computers; support better sleep; and promote homeostasis and a sense of well being.[1,2]

References

[1]Mercola, J. (2017). *Fat for Fuel* (pp. 238–239). Carlsbad, CA: Hay House, Inc.

[2]Pall, M. L. (2018, July). Wi-Fi is an important threat to human health. *Journal of Environmental Research, 164*, 405–416. https://pubmed.ncbi.nlm.nih.gov/29573716.

PART IX

PLANNING

Nourishing Meals

Tastes of Foods
Acid and Alkaline-Forming
Contracting and Loosening
Ideas for Meal Planning

Tastes of Foods and their Healthful Properties

The distinct tastes of sweet, salty, sour, bitter, and pungent in natural foods have long been recognized by Chinese and India's Ayurvedic traditions. In Ayurveda, the astringent taste is a sixth taste. In addition to these basic tastes, there are thousands of flavors, aromas, and textures in natural foods. Innovating dishes with new combinations of tastes and flavors offer endless, delectable possibilities.

The six fundamental tastes are associated with health-giving properties. These distinct tastes are best consumed in small amounts. When consumed in excess, these properties are no longer beneficial; for instance, too much sweet may cause indigestion and/or high blood sugar; too much sour may cause acidity and/or weakness; too much saltiness may cause thirst and/or hypertension; too much pungency may cause dehydration and/or tissue depletion; too much bitter may cause indisgestion, heartburn, and/or insomnia; and too much astringency may cause dryness and/or indigestion.

Each natural food has its own blend of tastes. One or two tastes are often predominate, such as sweet and sour in apples, and bitter and astringent in artichokes. Being mindful of these six tastes can reveal what kind and how much of these taste nutrients we need to support our health.

The six tastes presented here were inspired by Chinese and Ayurvedic traditions (astringent from Ayrveda).

FOODS	TASTES	HEALTH BENEFITS
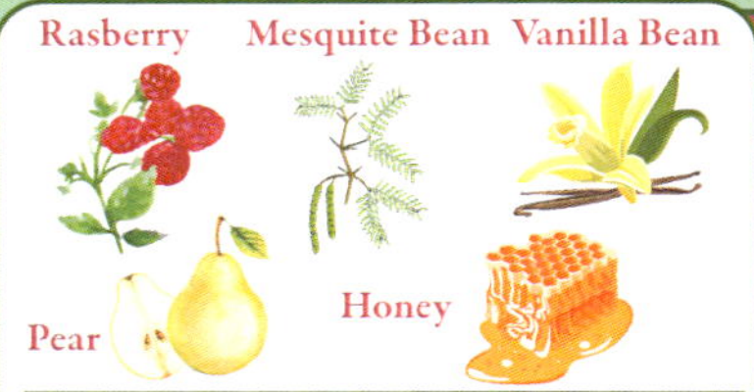 Rasberry, Mesquite Bean, Vanilla Bean, Pear, Honey	**SWEET** glucose fructose mannose	Enhances absorption; tones organs; lessens bleeding; reduces excess moisture (diuretic); and helps to bind stool and alleviate diarrhea
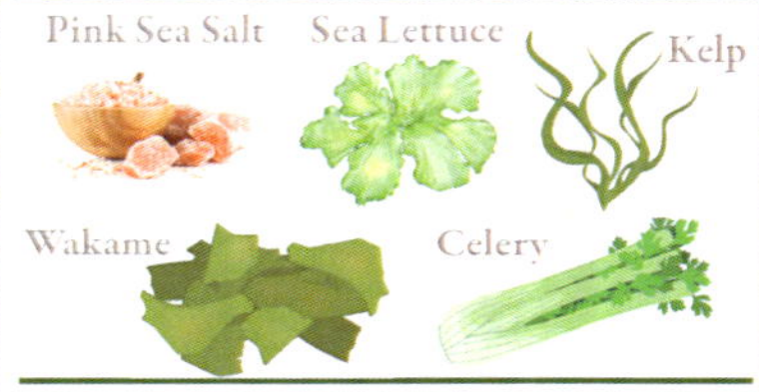 Pink Sea Salt, Sea Lettuce, Kelp, Wakame, Celery	**SALTY** sodium chloride potassium chloride	Balances body fluids; softens and lubricates tissues; calms nerves; and has an alkalinizing, cleansing, and antiseptic effect
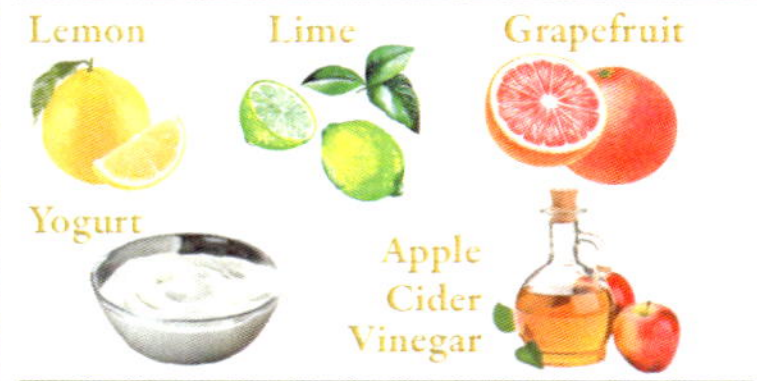 Lemon, Lime, Grapefruit, Yogurt, Apple Cider Vinegar	**SOUR** lactic malic and acetic acids	Stimulates digestion and metabolism; improves blood circulation; aids in eliminating waste. Soured (probiotic fermented) foods support the microbiome and immune system
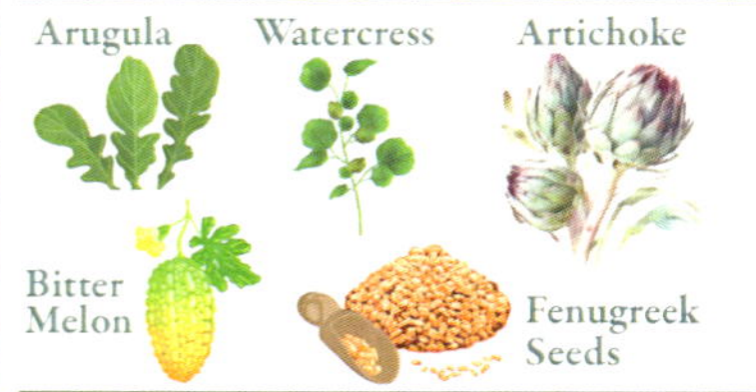 Arugula, Watercress, Artichoke, Bitter Melon, Fenugreek Seeds	**BITTER** flavonoids phenols catechins	Detoxifies; decreases inflammation, removes excess dampness and phlegm; aids in digestion and peristalsis (the movement of food through the digestive tract); and reduces blood sugar
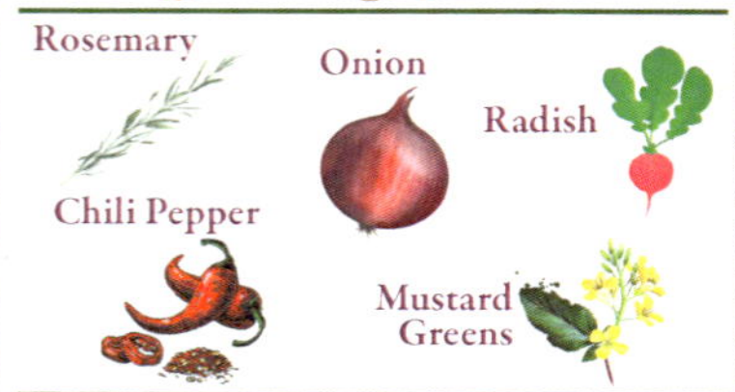 Rosemary, Onion, Radish, Chili Pepper, Mustard Greens	**PUNGENT** allicin capsaicin piperine	Supports digestion and metabolism; reduces swelling and nerve pain; stimulates the removal of stagnated waste in the lymph system
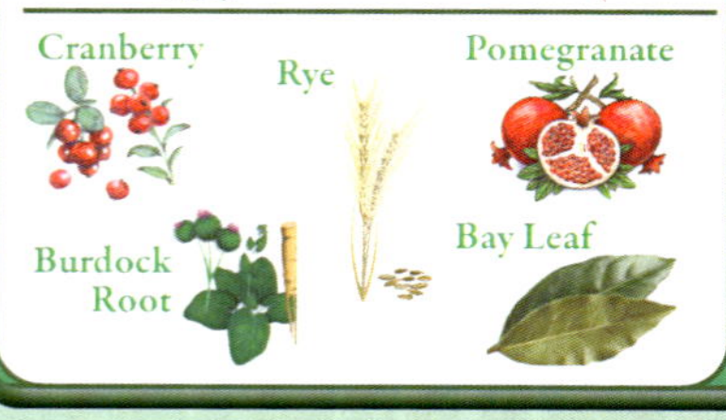 Cranberry, Rye, Pomegranate, Burdock Root, Bay Leaf	**ASTRINGENT** procyanidins saponins tannins	Enhances absorption; tones organs; strengthens prolapsed muscles; lessens bleeding; reduces excess moisture (diuretic); and helps to bind stool and alleviate diarrhea

Acid and Alkaline-Forming

The pH level of our cells and tissues is important for maintaining health. Acid-forming foods principally build and repair our cells and tissues while alkaline-forming foods hydrate, cleanse, and rejuvenate the cells and tissues. When our diet is too acidic, the acid-forming foods may be drying and/or contracting. When our diet is too alkaline, the alkaline-forming foods may water-log tissues and loosen stool.

Balancing the pH effects of foods is often key to regaining our health when we face an illness. Many chronic and degenerative diseases and constipation are associated with an over-acid condition (acidosis); whereas, *Candida* yeast overgrowth and other ailments occur when the body becomes too alkaline (alkalosis). Too much acidity or alkalinity may cause a biochemical environment that favors pathogenic microorganisms. With a holistic approach, naturopathic doctors and nutritionists, with expertise and experience in restoring pH, use lab tests and pH strips of the saliva, blood, and urine to recommend dietary and lifestyle changes to improve pH levels and, therefore, overall health.

Balancing pH is analytical and intuitive. We can adjust relative quantities of acid and alkaline-forming foods to achieve healthful results. Combining acid and alkaline-forming foods in meals and then giving attention to how we feel after eating can provide feedback for balancing pH. A meal that balances both might include:

- Seafood (acid-forming)
- Leafy greens, cooked non-starch vegetables, a salad with a dressing of herbs and lemon juice or apple cider vinegar (alkaline-forming)
- Olive oil (slightly acid-forming)
- Sea Salt (alkaline-forming)

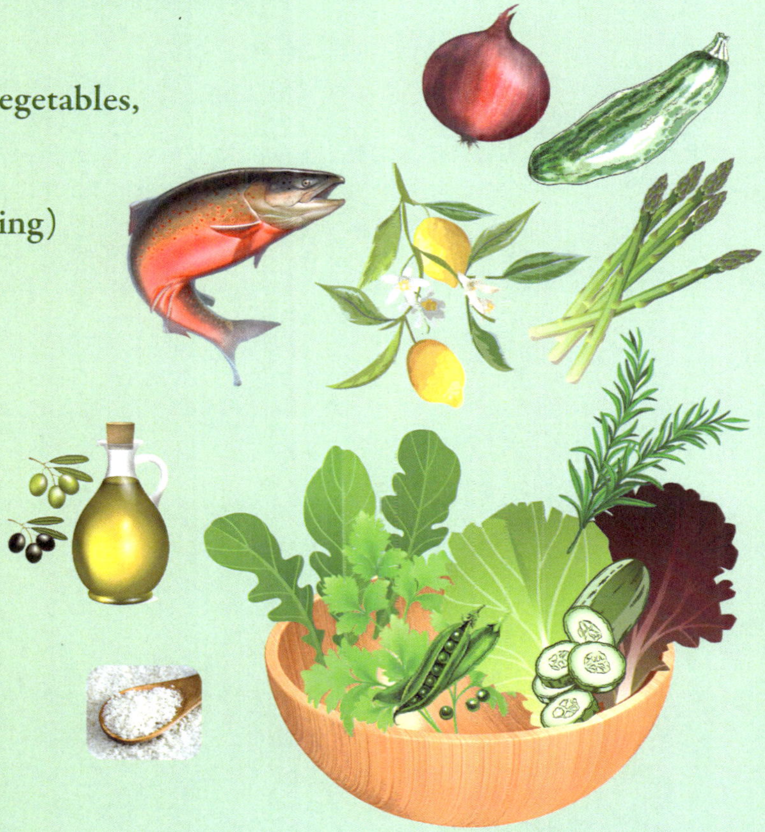

Continued...

Acid and Alkaline-Forming

Sea salt is a unique food. Not only is it our most comprehensive source of mineral nutrients, with anti-septic properties, sea salt is alkaline-forming and astringent. This unusual combination of being both alkaline-forming and astringent (contracting) is the opposite of other alkaline-forming foods, which have a loosening effect. Given these properties, sea salt simultaneously cleanses and strengthens the cells and tissues.

Hydrochloric acid (HCL) is required for digestion, particularly of acid-forming foods, including eggs, meats, and seafoods. For this purpose, the stomach has a very acidic pH of 0.8 to 1.5.[1] Without this degree of acidity, the body is unable to effectively break down acid-forming foods that are comprised largely of protein. Bitter leafy greens, including arugula, stimulate the production of HCL. Chloride, the main constituent of HCL, can be obtained by consuming sea salt (the main ingredient being sodium chloride), celery, lettuce, or other natural foods.

The major minerals in natural foods determine their pH effect on the body. Phosphorus, chloride, and sulfur have acidifying effects; whereas, calcium, sodium, potassium, and magnesium have alkalizing effects. Fruits and vegetables, for example, have more of the alkalizing minerals, therefore, they have more of an alkaline effect on the body. Notably, when we eat citrus fruits, their organic acids create a sour taste. Once they are digested, however, citrus fruits leave a mineral residue (alkaline ash). In fact, the more acidic the fruit (such as lemons and limes) the more alkaline the effect. The alkaline ash resulting from the digestion of citrus fruits tends to neutralize toxins and have an overall cleansing action on the body.

Acid and Alkaline-Forming diagram on next page

Reference

[1]Lipski, E. (2020). *Digestive Wellness.* (5th ed., p. 42) New York, NY: McCraw Hill.

Continued...

Acid and Alkaline-Forming

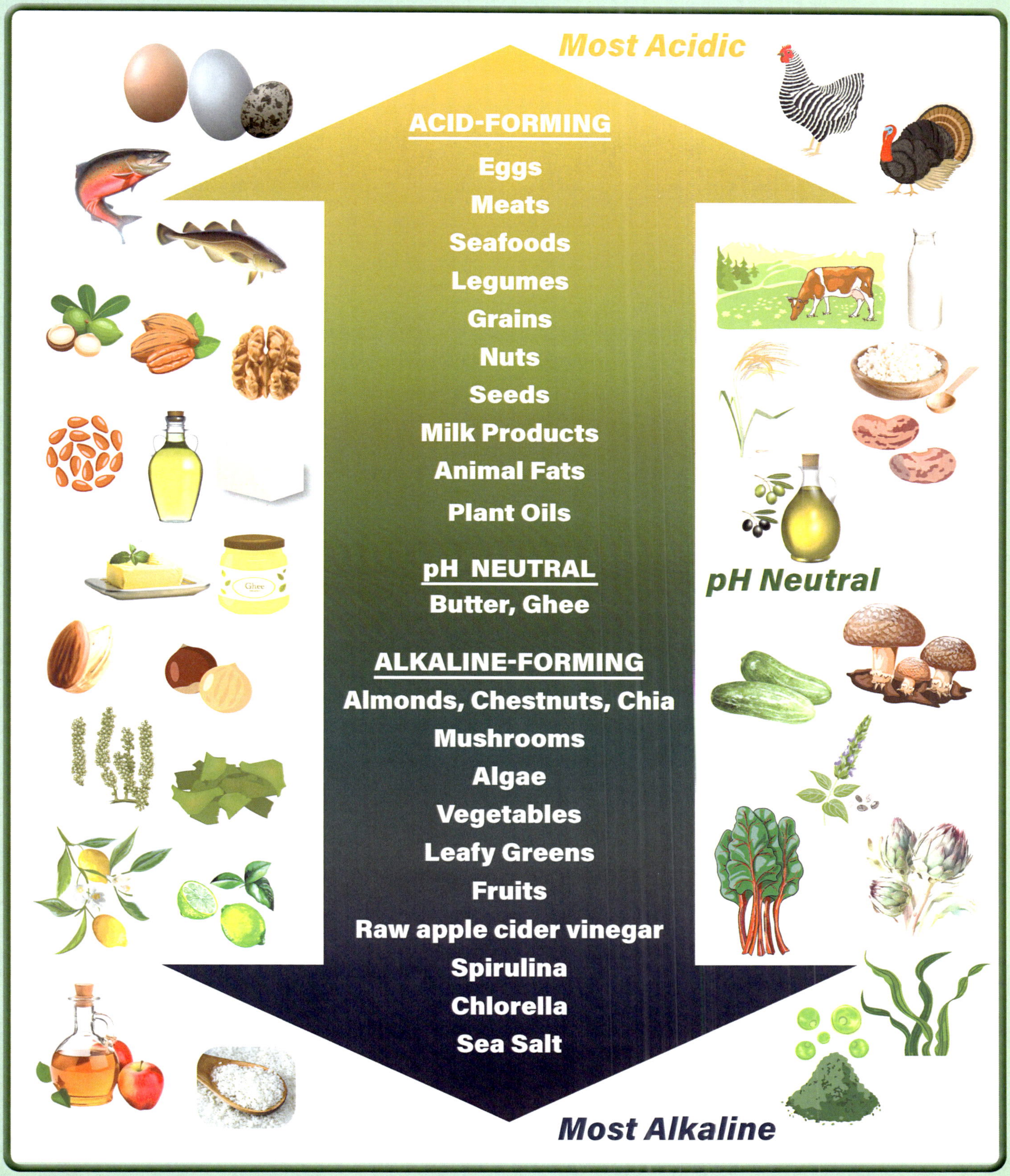

Contracting and Loosening Natural Foods

Relief from Constipation and Diarrhea

Generally, we can adjust our diet to form healthy stool that moves easily through the colon, rectum, and anus for elimination. Without drinking enough water and consuming enough hydrating foods, such as bone broth–with its 'water-loving' (hydrophilic), lubricating, and soothing (colloidal) properties–these contracting foods, such as:

Land and Water Fowl Eggs | **Meats** | **Legumes**

can cause the stool to be compacted and lead to constipation. In contrast, hydrating, loosening foods, such as: **Fruits** **especially**

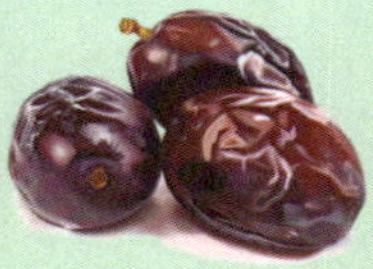

Plums, Prunes, and Dates may cause stool to become loose and result in diarrhea.

Acid-forming (and cooked) foods tend to be contracting/compacting while alkaline-forming (and raw) foods have expanding/loosening effects; sea salt is an exception, with contracting and alkaline-forming effects (ref. the Acid and Alkaline-Forming Chart, pages 245 - 247)**. Observing how foods effect our stool can reveal how to balance these foods.**

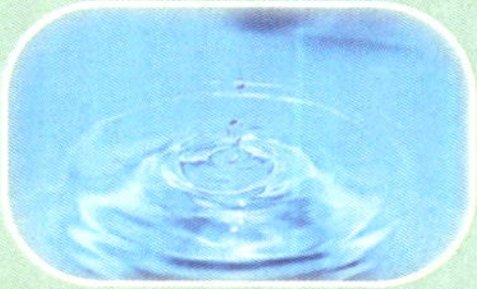

Water Is Essential

Hydration relieves constipation; and water is needed in the case of diarrhea too, because diarrhea is dehydrating. In general, drinking about ½ of our body weight in ounces of water every day can keep us hydrated and support the functions of the body. Typically, when our urine is a light yellow color this indicates we are adequately hydrated.

Constipation – Foods that May Offer Some Relief

Okra
(mucilage and mild laxative)

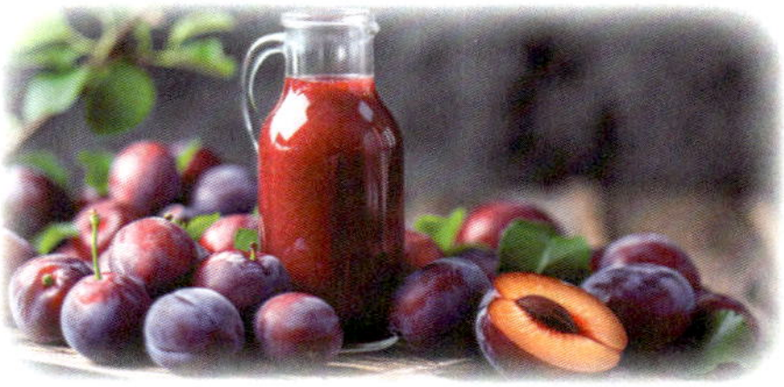

Plum and prune juice activate bowel movement

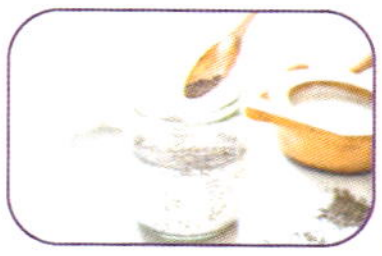

Chia, Flax, and Fenugreek Seeds
These foods are mild laxatives. They soften stool; their mucilage reduces irritation; and their fiber helps regulate bowels.
They should be soaked, rinsed, cooked or roasted, ground, and consumed with plenty of water.

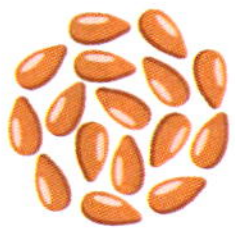

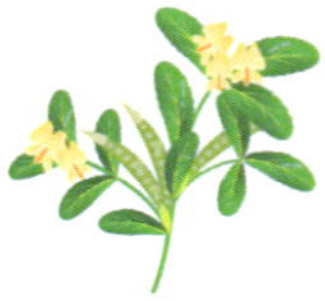

Continued...

Contracting and Loosening Natural Foods

Diarrhea - Foods that May Help Form Healthy Stool

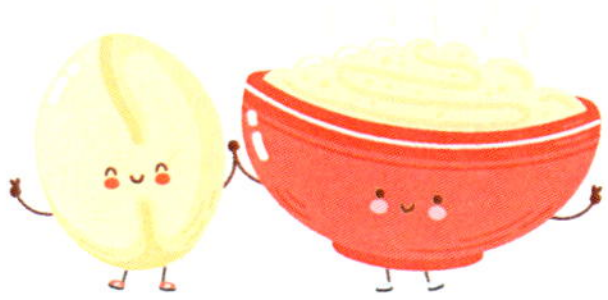

Oatmeal
(bland, soluble fiber)

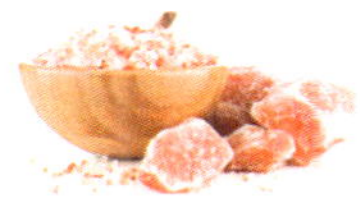

Celtic Sea Salt
(electrolytes)

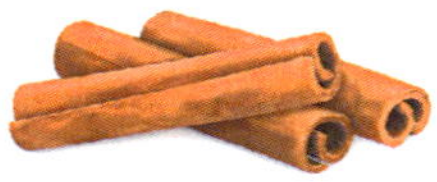

Cinnamon
(coumarin, cinnamic acid)

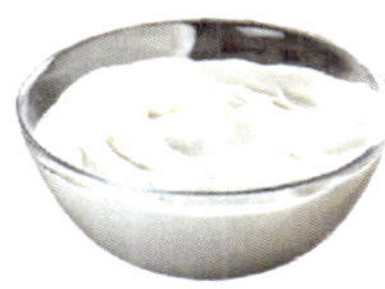

Raw milk Yogurt
(probiotics)

Fruits with pectin, such as

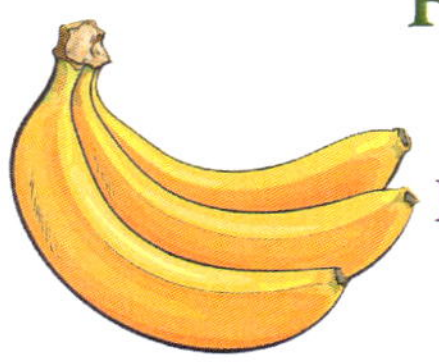

Banana and

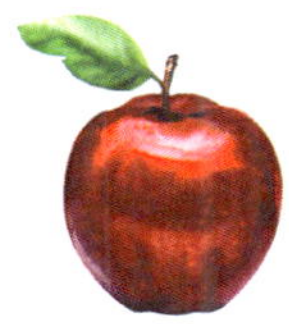

Apple
(apple sauce may be more easily digested)

Natural Foods and Herbs that May Be Beneficial for BOTH Constipation and Diarrhea

Soothe, Lubricate, and Heal Intestinal Tissue

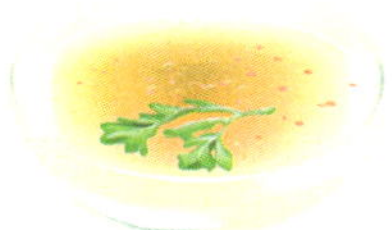

Bone Broth
(collagen used by the body to repair the intestinal lining)

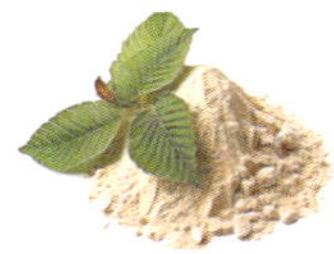

Slippery Elm Bark
(protective gel-like mucilage)

Probiotic Immune Support in Fermented Foods

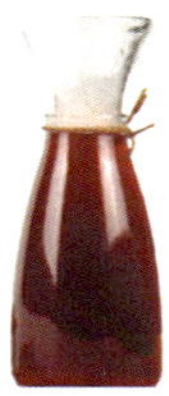

Beet Kvass and **Rejuvelac** solubilize mineral salts which make electrolytes available to the body, protect the intestinal mucosa,

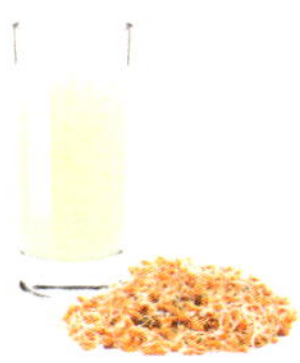

contribute to peristalsis (the smooth muscle contractions that move food through the digestive tract and keep it from stagnating), and facilitate bowel evacuation.

Intestinal Movement Formula

A blend of rhubarb root, peppermint leaf, aloe leaf, nopal cactus leaf, ginger root, *Chanca piedra* (whole herb extract); digestive enzymes (protease, alpha-galactosidase, amylase, cellulase, lipase, bromelain, papain), thyme leaf, and oregano leaf.

(ref. https://healthforcesuperfoods.com/product/intestinal-movement-formula)

Foot Rest to Facilitate Elimination

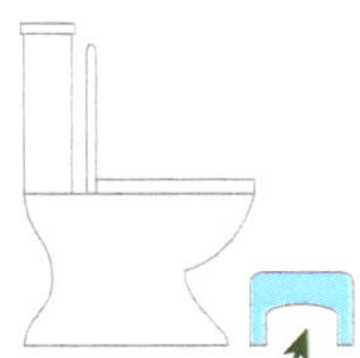

Foot Rest

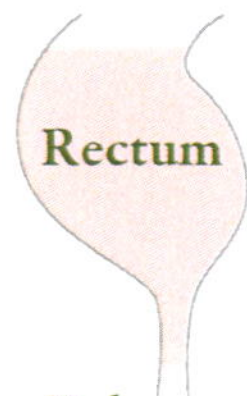

Relaxes and straightens the rectum

"As humans we are designed to squat in order to 'eliminate' properly."

PROPPR. (2022). *Getting into the 'PROPPR' position to poop on a pedestal toilet*. https://www.youtube.com/watch?v=RgkpFyulE1Q [Film].

PROPPR. (2025). The PROPPR. https://theproppr.com.

Note: Flush with the lid closed to avoid breathing in toxins eliminated that flushing releases into the air

Illustrator Yulia Gapeenko, Dreamstime

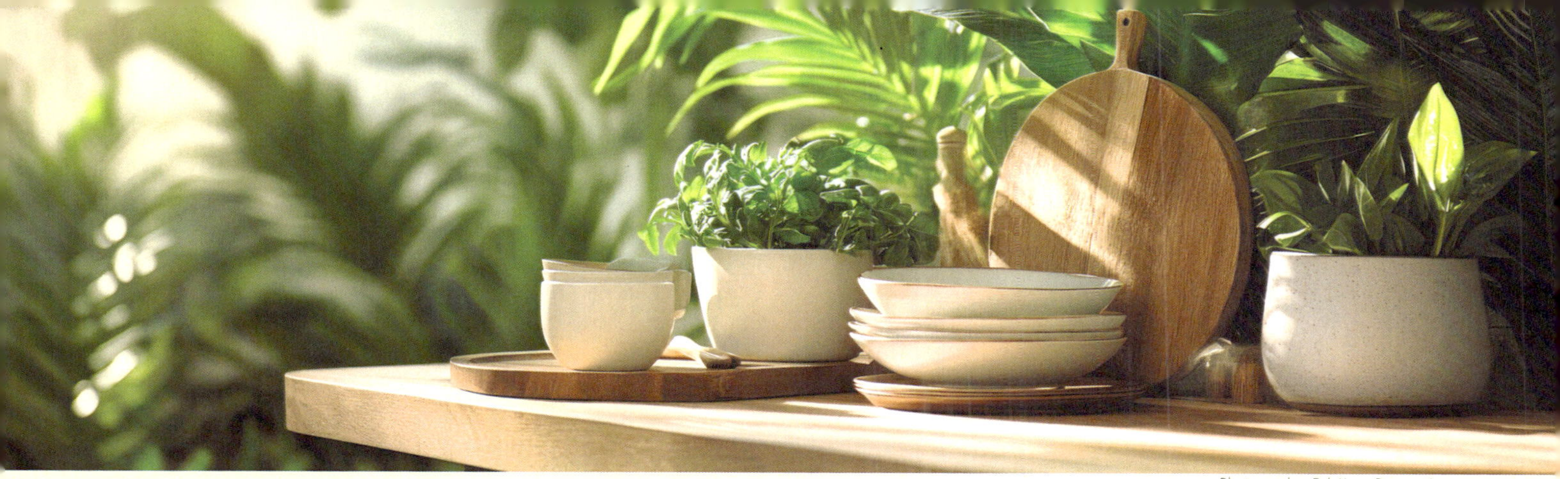

Photographer Eak Kem, Dreamstime

Planning Nourishing Meals

Nourish Yourself and Your Loved Ones with Natural Foods

Harvested in the wild or cultivated in our gardens and farms, natural foods come from nature, five kingdoms of life:

- *Animalia*–animal foods
- *Bacillati* (*Bacteria* Domain)–probiotic bacteria, spirulina
- *Chromista*–brown algae
- *Fungi*–mushrooms, probiotic micro-fungi
- *Plantae*–plant foods and green and red algae

Supplying and Organizing Your Kitchen

Create a place for your favorite recipes

Organize recipes in categories and place in a book or card file

List of staple foods

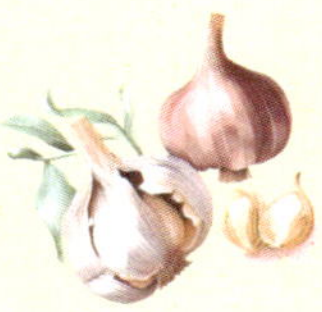
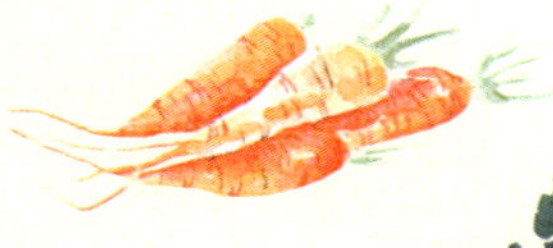
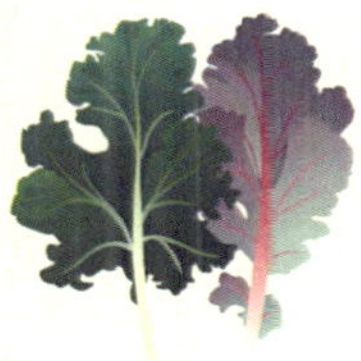
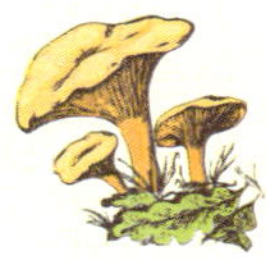

Seafood
Organ & muscle meat
Gelatin-rich bone broth
Eggs
Raw cream, butter, cheese, yogurt, kefir
Vegetables (a variety, including leafy greens and herbs)
Fruits
Seeds, nuts, grains, legumes
Mushrooms
Algae foods
Fermented foods
Sea salt

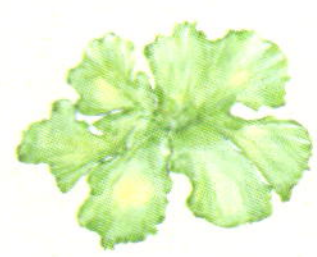
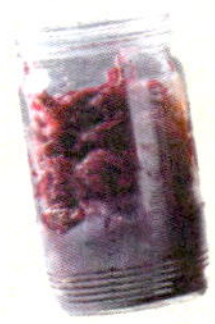
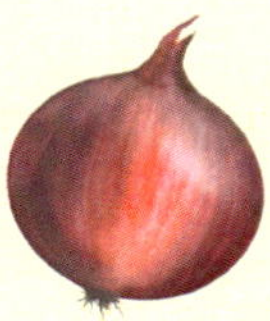
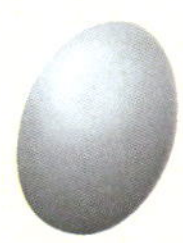
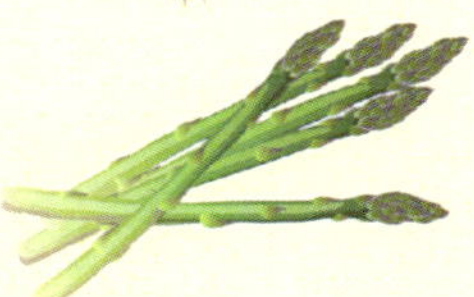
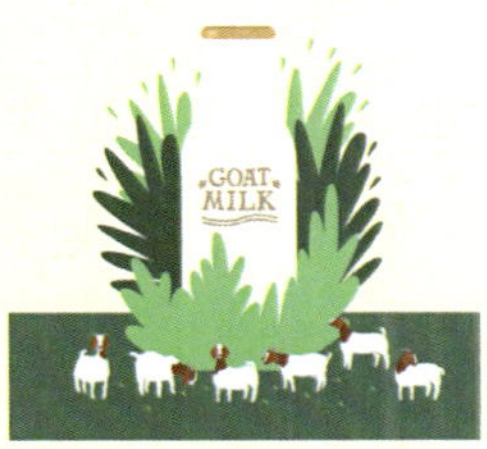

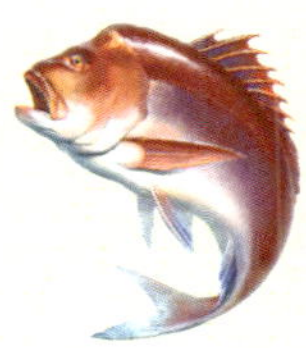

Maintain a shopping list

- Create a shopping list, perhaps based on the places where you get your foods, such as your garden, farmers market, or natural food co-op
(ref. **ACTIVITY BOOK** Shopping List)

The day before or the morning that you make and serve your meals

- Start bone broth to cook overnight
- Soak (potentially sprout or ferment) seeds, nuts, grains, legumes
- Take foods from the freezer and place them in the refrigerator to thaw
- Marinate fish, meat, vegetables
- Prepare ferments, such as sauerkraut
- Warm raw milk and place in the yogurt maker

Make extra batches, freezing, and storing

- Use large cookware or multiple pots
- Refrigerate or freeze meal-size portions for later, label and date
- Add fresh ingredients to leftover stocks, soups, stews
- In the refrigerator, store stalks of celery and herbs, such as parsley, standing up in clean, filtered water to stay fresh

Key Considerations for Food Preparation

- Raw foods to:
  - replenish the body's supply of enzymes and heat-sensitive vitamins, including water-soluble B and C vitamins

Discover which fermented foods are best for you?
Do you prefer them fermented for a short or long time?

- Fermented food–a small amount (one tablespoon or more) with meals or once per day
  - replenishes probiotics in the microbiome and enzymes for digestion and metabolism
  - provides in abundance of nutrients that are made more bioavailable through fermentation
- Cooking edible plants, mushrooms, and algae to:
  - reduce and neutralize their phyto, myco, and algal toxins
  - help break-down (predigest) the fiber
  - make certain nutrients more bioavailable
- Including different colors and tastes of foods
- Acid-forming (contracting) and alkaline-forming (expanding) foods
  - consider the unique properties of sea salt being alkaline-forming and astringent (contracting)
- Combining foods for optimal digestion based on their macro-nutrient composition of protein, lipids (fats and oils), and carbohydrates

If In Doubt, Throw It Out
If food ever does not smell, look, or taste right, discard it.

Is Food Combining Beneficial for Your Digestion?
To find out whether food combining makes a difference for you – Try and compare how you feel during and after eating these two meals (on two separate days):
On one day – eat a meal of seafood or meat with a starchy food (baked or cooked)
On another day – eat seafood or meat with non-starchy vegetables (raw or cooked)
(ref. the Food Combining Chart, pages 146-158 and NutritioninaNutshell.com/Shop Tapestry Books/Charts)

Traditionally-Prepared Natural Foods

The Weston A. Price Foundation developed the *Timeless Principles of Healthy Traditional Diets*, drawing from the research findings of Weston A. Price, D.D.S., below.[1]

"**Principle 1.** The diets of healthy, nonindustrialized peoples contain no refined or denatured foods or ingredients, such as refined sugar or high fructose corn syrup; white flour; canned foods; pasteurized, homogenized, skim or lowfat milk; refined or hydrogenated vegetable oils; protein powders; synthetic vitamins; or toxic additives and artificial colorings.

Principle 2. All traditional cultures consume some sort of animal food, such as fish and shellfish; land and water fowl; land and sea mammals; eggs; [raw] milk and milk products; reptiles; and insects. The whole animal is consumed—muscle meat, organs, bones and fat, with the organ meats and fats preferred.

Principle 3. The diets of healthy, nonindustrialized peoples contain at least four times the minerals and water-soluble vitamins, and TEN times the fat-soluble vitamins found in animal fats (vitamin A, vitamin D and Activator X, now thought to be vitamin K_2) as the average American diet.

Principle 4. All traditional cultures cooked some of their food but all consumed a portion of their animal foods raw.

Principle 5. Primitive and traditional diets have a high content of food enzymes and beneficial bacteria from lactofermented vegetables, fruits, beverages, [raw] dairy products, meats and condiments.

Principle 6. Seeds, grains and nuts are soaked, sprouted, fermented or naturally leavened to neutralize naturally occurring anti-nutrients such as enzyme inhibitors, tannins and phytic acid.

Principle 7. Total fat content of traditional diets varies from 30 percent to 80 percent of calories but only about 4 percent of calories come from polyunsaturated oils naturally occurring in grains, legumes, nuts, fish, animal fats and vegetables. The balance of fat calories is in the form of saturated and monounsaturated fatty acids.

Principle 8. Traditional diets contain nearly equal amounts of omega-6 and omega-3 essential fatty acids.

Principle 9. All traditional diets contain some [sea] salt.

Principle 10. All traditional cultures make use of animal bones, usually in the form of gelatin-rich bone broths.

Principle 11. Traditional cultures make provisions for the health of future generations by providing special nutrient-rich animal foods for parents-to-be, pregnant women and growing children; by proper spacing of children; and by teaching the principles of right diet to the young."

Reference

[1]WAPF. (1999). *Timeless principles of healthy traditional diets*. Washington, D.C.: The Weston A. Price Foundation. https://www.westonaprice.org/health-topics/abcs-of-nutrition/principles-of-healthy-diets-2.

Ideas for Meals – Applying the Principles Above (page 253)

Quality – organic, regenerative, humane, 100% pastured, free-range, wild harvested, traditionally-prepared

EXAMPLES

- Whole animal protein and fat – meat (especially organ meat), seafood (including fish & fish eggs), and land or waterfowl eggs – cooked in butter/ghee/tallow with herbs & sea salt
- Gelatin-rich bone broth added generously to cooked meals
- Raw salads of leafy greens, vegetables, and dressing with cold-pressed olive oil (maybe a little flax or sesame oil), lemon/lime juice or raw apple cider vinegar, herbs, and sea salt
- Raw-fermented side dish or a little added to a salad
- Vegetables and leafy greens cooked in butter/ghee/tallow, herbs, & sea salt – eaten on the side or added to a whole animal protein fat dish or cooled and added to a raw salad
- Raw milk yogurt, kefir, cheese, or cream eaten as a side dish; added to other dishes; or, if digested best alone, eaten as a separate meal; soaked or sprouted nuts or seeds
- Soaked (and rinsed), sprouted, fermented seeds and nuts (as a side or in a salad) with grains or legumes cooked with vegetables, butter/ghee/tallow/olive oil, herbs, and sea salt
- Raw fruits (simple carbohydrates) eaten alone for optimal digestion and health benefits. Small amounts of fruit, mostly berries, can be suitable for a low sugar/low glycemic diet

To fully enjoy traditionally-prepared homemade and artisan-made meals, it is helpful to sit comfortably and take time to be calm, benefiting the digestive and nervous systems. Eating slowly and chewing thoroughly facilitates nourishment and allows the aromas and flavors to reach the senses. Sourcing natural foods from the land (including freshwater ecosystems) and sea and preparing them at home connects us with nature and sharing meals together connects us with each other.

Benefits of Traditionally-Prepared Natural Foods

- Colorful phytonutrients – fruits, vegetables, leafy greens
- Enzyme-rich – raw, sprouted, & fermented foods (especially fermented raw)
- Probiotic – fermented foods
- Immune-building – garlic and onions, oranges (vitamin C and bioflavinoids), mushrooms
- Nutrient-dense – organ meats, fish roe, eggs
- Strengthening – animal protein fat, including seafoods, organ meats, eggs
- Easily-digested – gelatin-rich bone broth; foods combined for optimal digestion
- Locally adapted – heritage breeds and heirloom seeds
- With fiber – vegetables & fruits (especially raw); mushrooms; algae
- Healthy pH – example: animal protein fat (acid-forming) and non-starch vegetables (alkaline-forming)
- Hydrating – fruits, vegetables, gelatin-rich bone broth
- Cleansing – chlorella, leafy greens, herbs, fruits, vegetables
- Healing – gelatin-rich bone broth, raw & fermented foods, herbal remedies

Nourishment with whole natural foods enables the body to maintain and repair itself and build high immunity to disease. This includes tens of thousands of protective and restorative substances that can help the body prevent illness and heal. While there are specific nutritional and medicinal remedies, there are also many health benefits that are common among natural foods, including: anti-bacterial, anti-tumor, anti-oxidant, anti-inflammatory.

Animal Kingdom

Animal foods provide complete protein and fats that enhance the taste of food and contribute to satiety.

Seafoods and Meats

The sea and freshwater habitats

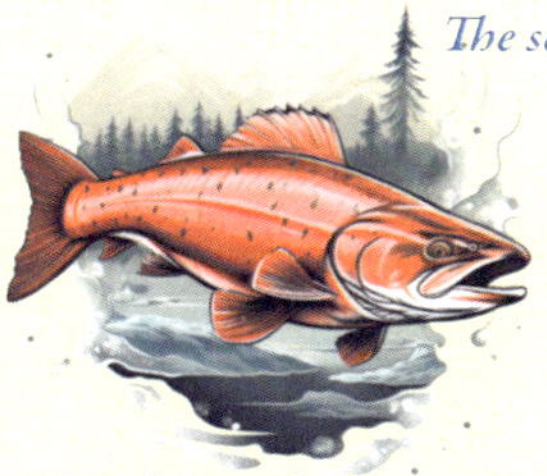

Sockeye Salmon

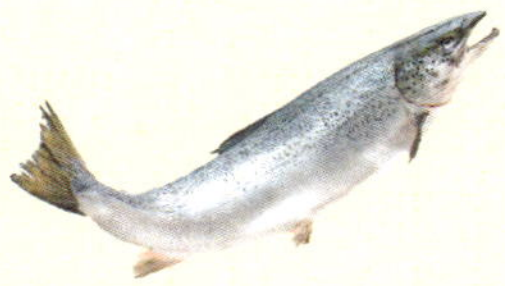

Freshwater Trout

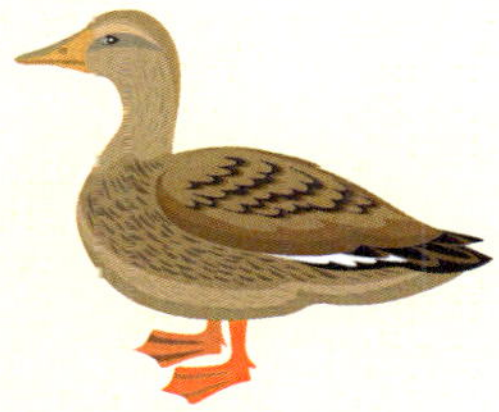

Duck

Browning (caramelizing) natural foods aids in digestion and enhances their color, aroma, and taste. As proteins, fats, and carbohydrates break down into amino acids, fatty acids, and simple sugars, they meld and create an array of flavors. Fine-tuning the temperature and moisture helps to discover delicious combinations of natural foods. Cooking vegetables on the stove-top, with some animal fat in the pan and the cover on, keeps the moisture in and allows vegetables to cook in their own juices at a low temperature. On the other hand, uncovered, open to the air, and at higher temperatures, vegetables will become crisp and brown more effectively.

Seafoods and Meats

For optimal digestion, seafoods and meat combine well with lemon and lime, non-starch vegetables, and animal fats.
It may be easier to digest one type of animal protein per day.

Organ Meats

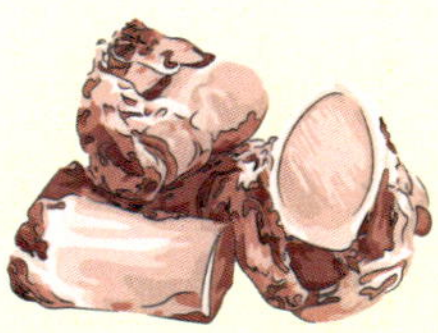

Bone Marrow

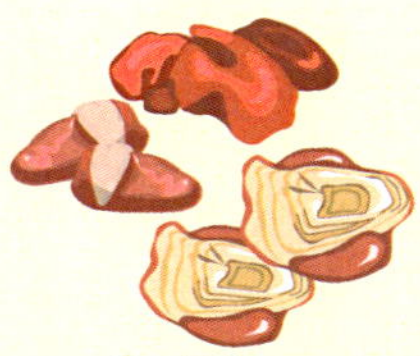

Gizzards, Liver, & Heart

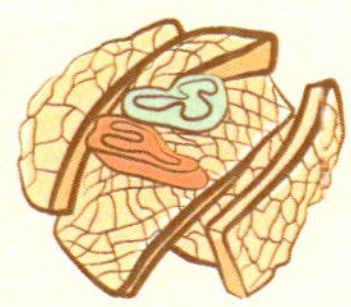

Offal

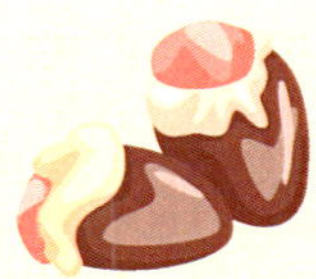

Organ Meats

<u>Example of how to prepare and cook organ meats</u>

- set in cold water, with sea salt (such as a brine) and lemon juice for two hours; discard the water when done. The brine draws out impurities, tenderizes, and moisturizes the meat.
- brown in animal fats on the stove-top until tender

Gelatin-Rich Bone Broths and Stocks

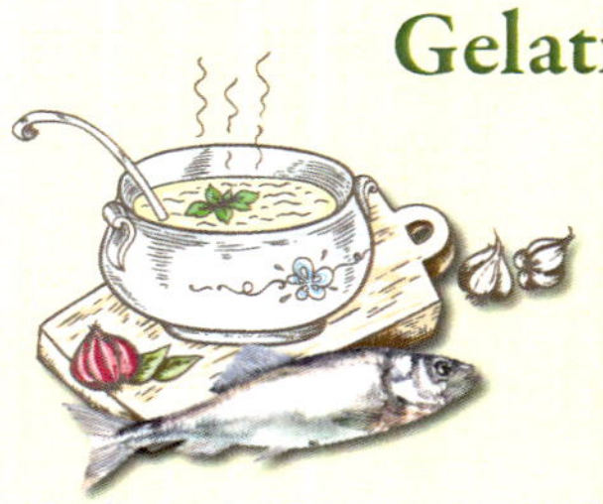

The gelatin in bone broth is a 'water-loving' (hydrophilic), colloidal substance that lubricates and soothes the intestinal lining and supports digestion.

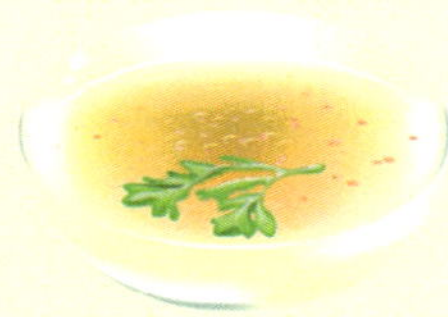

Seafood Bone Broth

(whole carcasses)
Cook for 4 to 24 hours

Bone Broth

(bones and cartilage from land animals and waterfowl)
Cook for 24 to 72 hours

Bone broth and stocks can be the base for soups or included in any savory dish for added nourishment.

When making broth or stock an 8-quart stockpot is often used with a heavy bottom (to prevent scorching), gripping handles, and high sides to limit evaporation.

The principle of 'like feeds like' applies to gelatin-rich bone broth. With its dissolved bone, cartilage, collagen, and marrow, bone broth contains the nutrients to repair and rejuvenate bone and connective tissue, including: the skeletal system and teeth, tendons, ligaments, cartilage, skin, hair, and nails. Broths provide the nutrients the body uses to develop strength and flexibility in the joints and arteries and nourish the corneas (which supports vision).[7] Major minerals in broth include: calcium, magnesium, phosphorus, potassium, sodium, and chloride in their ". . . ready-to-use ionized form as a true electrolyte solution."[8]

Resources
Nourishing Broth by Sally Fallon Morell and Kaayla T. Daniels
Nourishing Traditions by Sally Fallon Morell

Common Steps to Preparing Bone Broth

- wash and wipe bones dry, then brown in the oven
- set bones in pot and cover with cold, clean, filtered water
- add raw apple cider vinegar at the start, and let sit in cold water for 30 to 60 minutes (begins drawing out the minerals from the bones, bone marrow, and cartilage)
- slowly bring the water to a gentle simmer
- skim the foam that rises (with impurities) to the top
- add seasonings after skimming
- cook for 24 to 72 hours, depending on the type of bones

River Cottage Farm, Tennessee, Recommendation
"IMPORTANT: keep the simmer temperature at 200°F (93°C) or below. Higher temperatures will inhibit the release of the gelatin from the bones. Chicken Bones can be simmered 6-48 hours, Beef 12-72 hours."

"If your oven can be set to a low temperature that maintains the stock at 200°F (93°C) or lower just put your stock into the oven overnight. You can also use a crock pot."
(ref. www. rivercottagefarm.net/traditional-bone-broth)

Bone Broth Cooking and Cautions

In her books and workshops, Certified GAPS Practitioner, chef, and educator Monica Corrado describes that bone broth simmers long enough to allow the connective tissues to dissolve and the minerals to be drawn into the broth. For instance, chicken bone broth needs to cook 6–24 hours and beef and bison bone broth needs 24 to 72 hours for the cartilage and tendons to dissolve. A tremendous amount of glutamic acid is the result of such long cook times.

Corrado explains that glutamic acid and glutamate are highly regulated by the brain. As a result, she cautions that for people who have a leaky brain, as those with a leaky gut often do, high amounts of glutamic acid can trigger migraine headaches or seizures. Corrado further points out that children and adults with nervous system disorders (including: ADD, ADHD, Autism Spectrum Disorders, or autoimmune dysfunction) may have glutamic acid sensitivity, in which case, long-cooked bone broth may put them at risk for seizures or other health problems.[6]

Stocks

Seafood Stock

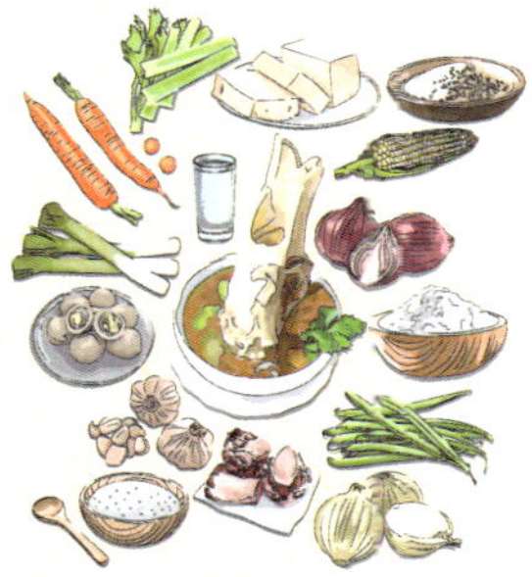

Meat Stock

Stocks are made in a similar fashion to broths, and are cooked from 4 to 24 hours. They include either seafood or meat, vegetables, and seasonings and, therefore, may be more flavorful than bone broth. Stock can be the basis for soups, stews, gravies, and sauces.

Raw Milk Products

Rennet Coagulates Milk for Cheese Making

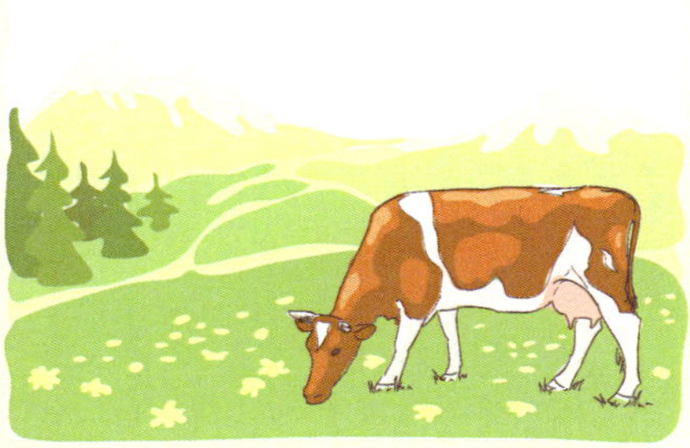

Raw, whole milk from heritage breeds, foraging in fresh pasture

Mammal Rennet

Rennet is composed of enzymes that are produced in the fourth stomach of young ruminant mammals suckling milk. These acidifying enzymes coagulate milk, facilitating digestion–especially the protease enzyme chymosin that breaks down the casein protein in milk, separating the curds (solids) from the whey (liquid).

Plant Rennet

In many countries, artisan cheese makers traditionally use the flower and/or leaf extract of milk thistle, nettle, or sorrel (that contain protease enzymes similar to chymosin) to coagulate milk, separating the curds from the whey.

Milk has been harvested from animals, including: antelope, water buffalo, yaks, camels, bison, cows, goats, and sheep for 30,000 or more years. Nomadic societies continue to travel with herds of herbivores, such as the indigenous Sámi people with reindeer (caribou) inhabiting the Sápmi region that extends across northern Norway, Sweden, Finland, and Russia.

Fresh cream and butter

- cream and butter are best added when served, to the bowl or plate, rather than in the pot on the stove where it would get too hot and lose enzymes, flavor, and quality
- the whey can be separated from the milk and used as a starter culture to provide lactic-acid producing bacteria in making lacto-ferments
- seasonings (such as cinnamon, cardamom, anise seeds) can be added when warming the milk to make yogurt and other fermented milk products for health-giving properties

Plantae Kingdom

Plant Foods

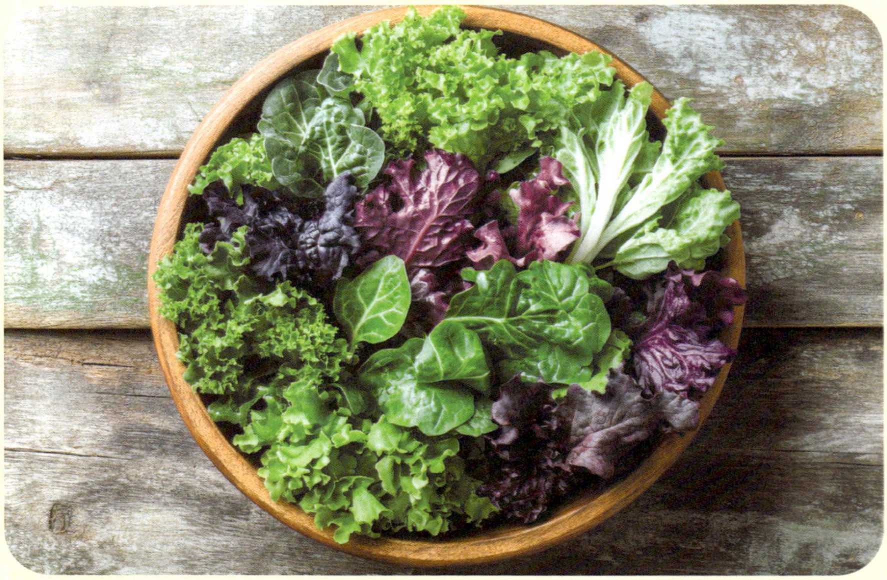

Photographer Yulia Gapeenko, Dreamstime

Springtime Salads

Starting with leafy greens

Select a variety of leafy greens, such as romaine, green leaf, and red leaf lettuces; endives, and perhaps a few leaves of bitter greens (for example, arugula, dandelion, escarole, and watercress) as a foundation for the salad.

Place lettuce; other leafy greens, including herbs; and flowers in a bin of cold water, gently wash, and soak for a few minutes to allow them to rehydrate. Lift from the water and either place in a salad spinner or spread out on towels and pat dry. These leafy greens can be used as the base for a salad or to wrap any kind of sandwich-type food items.

Tearing leafy greens

Tearing leafy greens by hand, into bite size pieces, naturally breaks the leaves along their outer cell walls, retaining their integrity and crispness. Using scissors or chopping them with a knife cuts through and damages the cell walls, exposing their inner tissue to the air which will cause them to wilt more easily; this is not a problem if you are going to eat your salad soon after making it.

Keeping Leafy Greens Crisp

To stay crisp for several days in the refrigerator, store leafy greens wrapped in towels and in airtight container (limited air causes leafy greens to slow their metabolism, reducing wilting).

Raw Foods – Enzymes, Vitamins, Minerals, Alkaline-Forming

The raw food in a fresh salad replenishes our enzymes, furnishing an array of vitamins and minerals and providing soluble and insoluble fiber. Leafy greens and vegetables are alkaline-forming. Animal fats, such as cream, yogurt, or cheese, and plant oils, such as olive oil, in the salad dressing facilitate the digestion, absorption, and assimilation of the fat-soluble vitamins, A, D_2, D_3, E, K_1, and K_2 in the vegetables and leafy greens.

Adding color and texture with raw vegetables

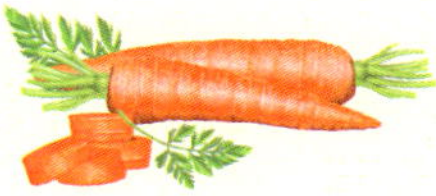
Carrot

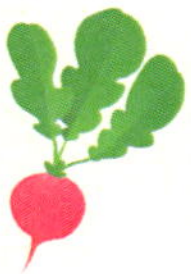
Radish

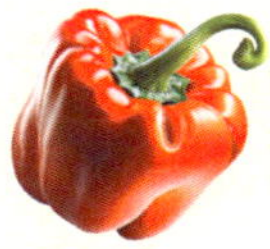
Bell Pepper (red)

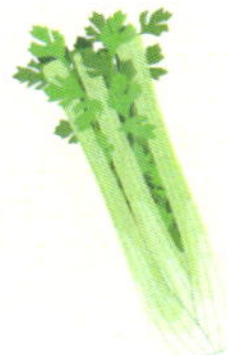
Celery

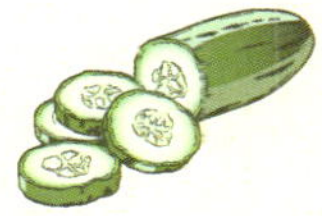
Cucumber

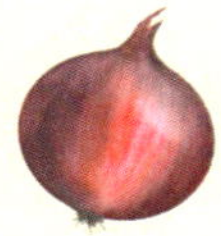
Onion (red)

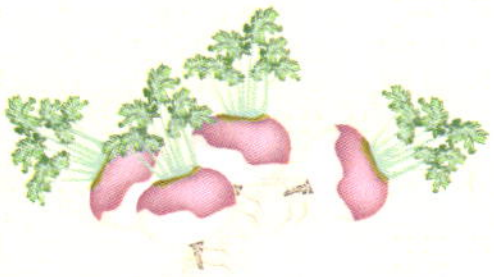
Turnips

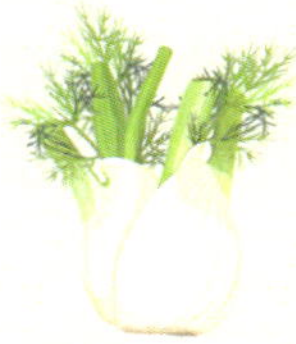
Fennel Bulb and Leaves

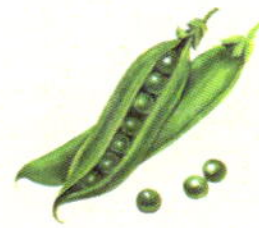
Peas (green)

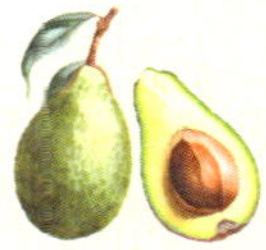
Avocado

Vegetables, sliced, diced (cubed), and chopped add color, such as: orange carrots, red radishes, tender purple turnips, red or orange bell peppers, green-white celery, green-white cucumbers, red-purple onions, the tender inside of white-green fennel bulb, fresh green peas, and yellow-green avocados.

Preparing vegetables

- wash with a vegetable wash (for example, gentle organic soap or baking soda dissolved in water) and natural bristle vegetable scrub brush
- cut off and compost any damaged, wilted, and moldy spots (the mold-free parts of vegetables are fine to eat). Place other tougher (fibrous), bruised, and wilted parts of the vegetables that are still appetizing in a 'save-for-soup' container or maybe a 'save-for-juicing/blending' container.
- shave off (with a vegetable peeler or small knife) the inedible outer covering of vegetables, like kohlrabi for compost
- chop for the salad the most appealing and tender parts of the vegetables–straight or diagonally sliced, diced (cubed), or julienned (the shape of match sticks)

Bitter Leafy Greens and Herbs

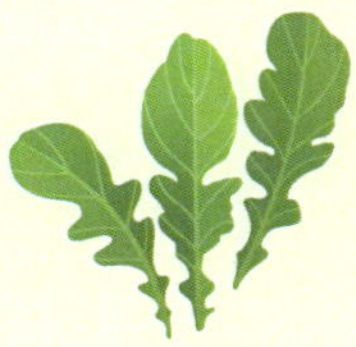
Arugula

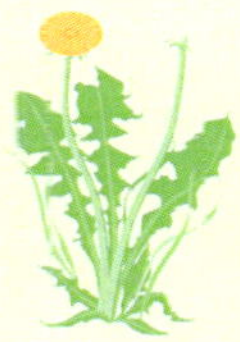
Dandelion

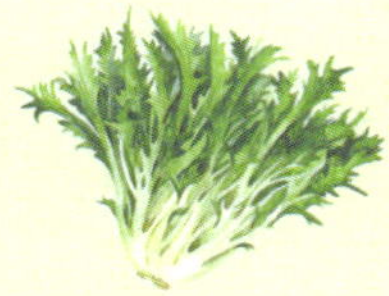
Escarole

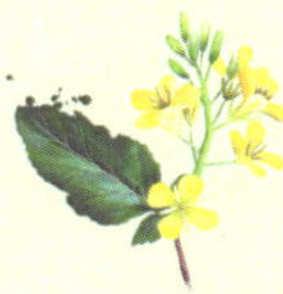
Mustard Greens

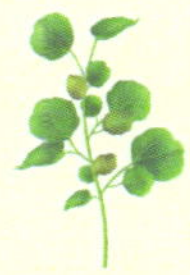
Watercress

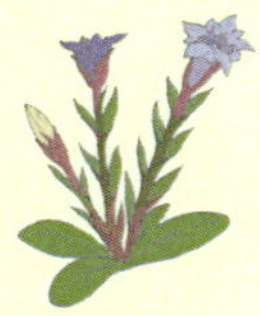
Gentian

Leafy greens and herbs with a distinct bitter taste, include: arugula, dandelion leaves, escarole, mustard greens, and watercress. Consuming a little bit of bitters, like well-known gentian root tea, and the leafy greens and herbs pictured above, supports digestion by promoting the production and secretion of digestive enzymes and bile; therein, they help digestion, reduce stagnation, and tone and strengthen the digestive tract. Bitters also support liver function, reduce sugar craving, and gently detoxify the body.

(ref. Tastes of Foods Chart on page 244)

Turning the salad into a whole meal

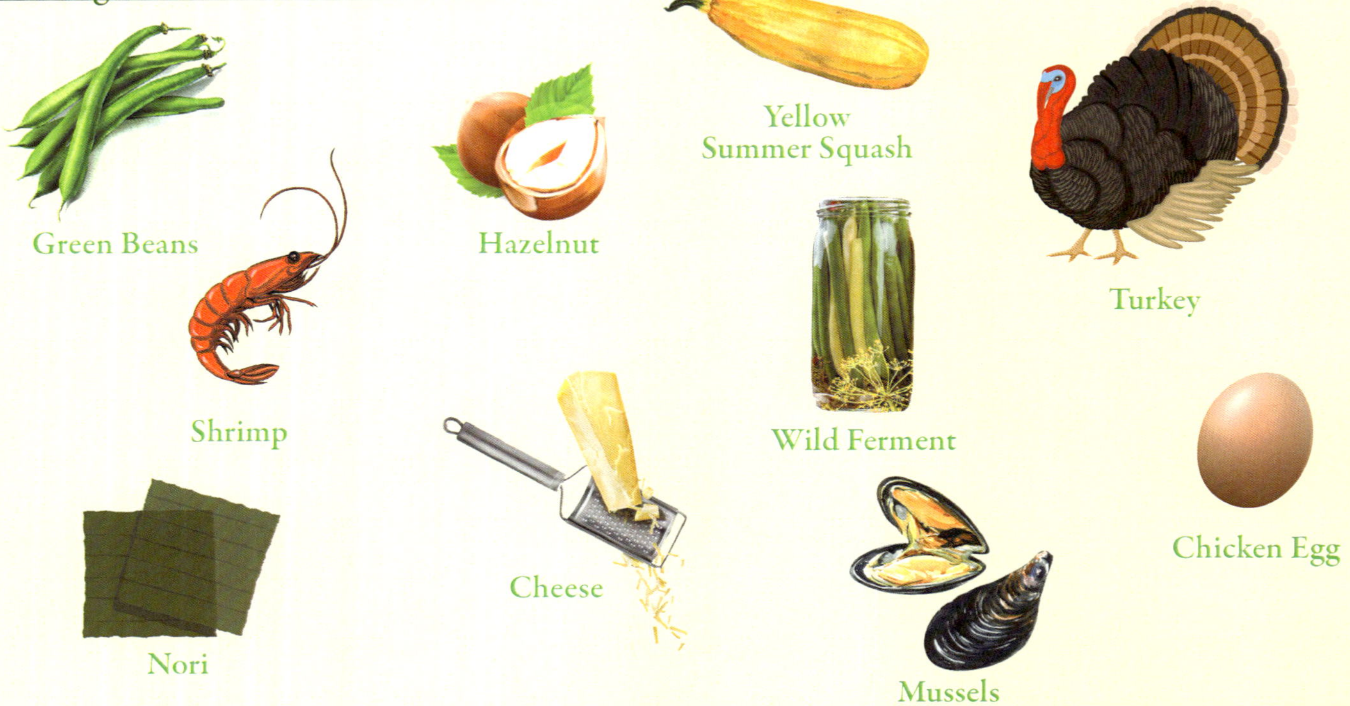

To make a 'whole meal salad,' add cold (previously cooked) seafoods, meats, or eggs. You could include parboiled vegetables, such as green beans and squash; they can be cooked, made cold in the refrigerator, and then chopped and added to the salad. Probiotic ferments could also be mixed into the salad or included in the meal as a side dish.

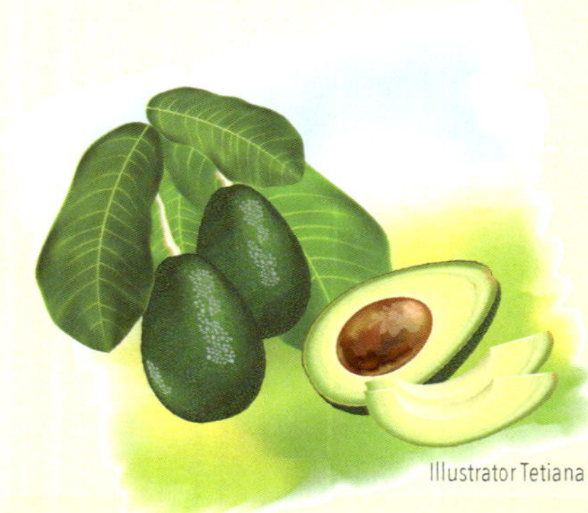

Illustrator Tetiana Kovalenko, Dreamstime

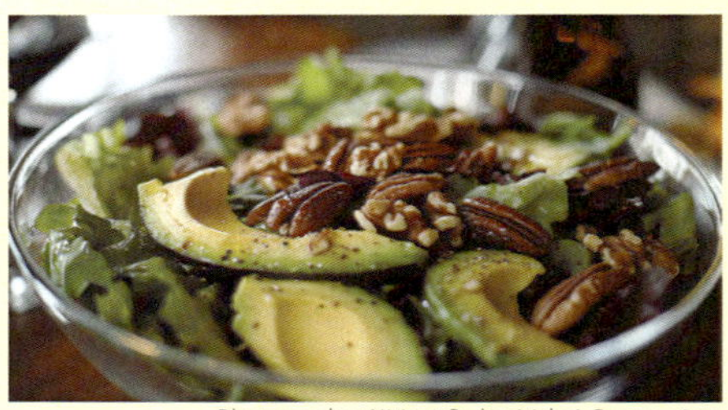

Photographer Nitipat Sadtasirichai, Dreamstime

Slicing Avocado

Holding an unpeeled avocado in the palm of one hand, slice the avocado in half the long way with a small knife. Keep the half with the pit in one hand and set the other half down.

Stick the tip of a small knife into the pit (seed) with the free hand, just enough to turn the knife slightly to loosen the pit, give it a little pull, and lift the pit out. Set this avocado half down and take the pit off the tip of the small knife and plant it in soil to grow an avocado tree or put it in the compost.

Holding one of the avocado halves (skin still on) in the palm of one hand, gently cut the inner avocado into slices or cubes. Do the same to the other avocado half. Lastly, use a large spoon to scoop out the avocado slices or cubes into a salad or onto a serving plate.

Making the Salad Dressing

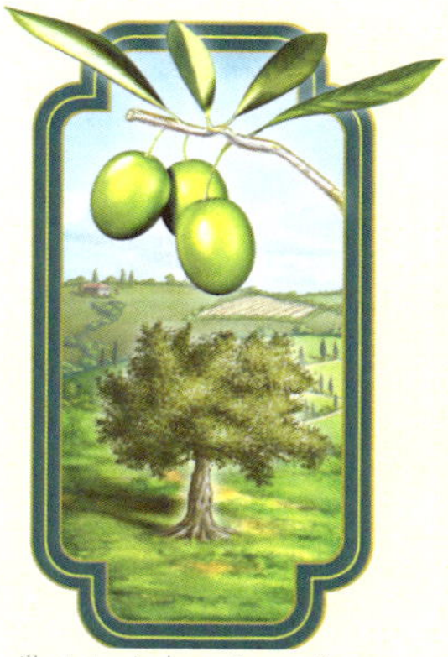

Illustrator Andreus, Dreamstime

Raw Olives and Olive Oil

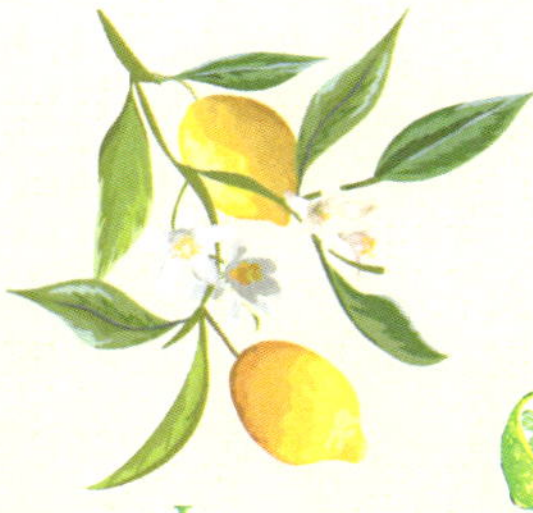

Lemon

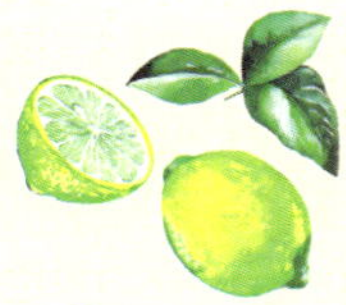

Lime

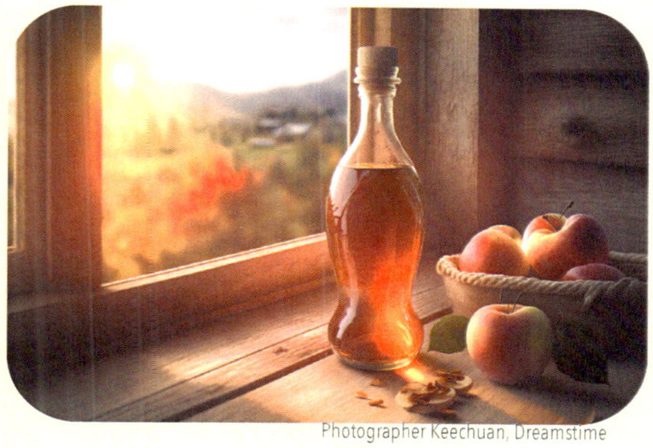

Photographer Keechuan, Dreamstime

Raw Apple Cider Vinegar

Cold-pressed virgin olive oil, with healthy monosaturated fats, and fresh-squeezed lemon/lime juice or raw, unfiltered apple cider vinegar (naturally probiotic) can be place in a glass salad dressing jar. Then, adding fresh herbs can make each salad dressing a unique creation. Add seasoning, such as, oregano, thyme, and rosemary.

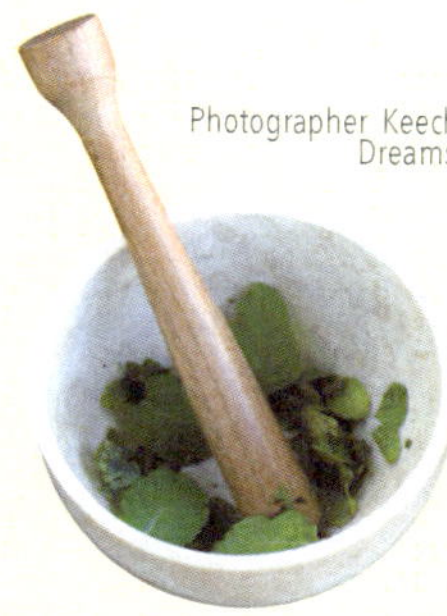

Photographer Keechuan, Dreamstime

Pestle and Mortar

Preparing the herbs:

- herb leaves can be removed by holding one end of the stem with one hand, and holding the other hand around the stem right below, and slide the hand (that is below) over the stem in the opposite direction of the way the leaves grow, gently pulling the leaves off with this hand
- herb leaves can be clipped small with the kitchen scissors, finely chopped with a chef's knife, or ground with a pastel and mortar. Note: unlike more delicate leafy greens, the benefit of crushing fresh herbs (breaking their cell walls) is that it releases their nutrients and distinct aromas and flavors into the salad dressing.
- adding a small amount of sea salt enhances the flavor of the dressing and provides electrolyte minerals

These ingredients can be stirred or shaken in the salad dressing jar and served. Or, for added fullness and creaminess, raw zucchini or other raw summer squashes, and any prior-cooked cold vegetable, can be blended smooth and included in the salad dressing.

The final step–adding toppings and sprinkles

Grated raw cheeses, raw soaked and sprouted seeds and nuts, and microgreens enrich a salad. Algae flakes, such as, dulse or nori, offer flavor and mineral nutrients. Ready to serve.

Protecting Plant Oils from Oxidative Damage

Salad dressing and plant oils, such as olive and coconut, should be stored in a tightly shut bottle in the dark because light, heat, and exposure to the air can damage them.

Juice from Lemons and Limes

When ripe, lemons and limes can be rolled and pressed with the palm of your hand before cutting and squeezing, to get more juice from them.

Olive Oil

High quality–extra virgin, cold-pressed, raw, freshly-harvested olive oil from regenerative orchards contains thiocanthal and thiocanthol. Being sulfur-derived, these compounds have a slightly acid-forming effect on the body and they are anti-inflammatory, anti-tumor, and neuro and cardiovascular protective.

Seeds – Soaking, Sprouting, and Growing Micro-Greens

Soaking and sprouting seeds and nuts increases their nutrient enzymes and digestibility

Stages of Broccoli – Seed Soaking to Maturity

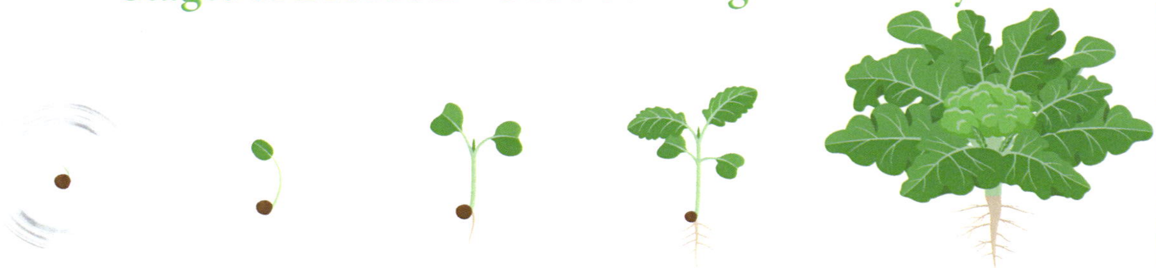

Bowl Photographer Anton Starikov, Dreamstime   IllustratorAndrii Bezervershenko, Dreamstime

A head of broccoli comprises thousands of flower buds.
Broccoli and cauliflower can be harvested before and after the flowers bloom.

Five Stages of Plant Growth

Grains and legumes are more digestible if they are soaked overnight and then rinsed (soak water discarded) before they are cooked. It is important to cook grain and legume sprouts for digestibility.

Nuts, grains, and legumes are all seeds. Here are five stages of plant growth:

1) Soaked seeds – seeds become active and grow
2) Sprouts – seeds germinate and grow into sprouts
3) Microgreens – plants grow their first leaves (cotyledons) and begin to photosynthesize and grow rudimentary roots (with the aid of bacteria and micro-fungi, they obtain mineral nutrients from the soil)
4) Baby greens – plant foods produce tender green leaves
5) Mature greens – tender baby greens grow into mature leafy greens

In a greenhouse or an outside garden, depending on the temperature, plant foods can be grown from seeds or seedlings to mature green leaves. The earlier stages of soaking seeds and growing sprouts, microgreens, and baby greens can easily be accomplished indoors, such as kitchen gardens.

Soaking Seeds, Nuts, Grains, and Legumes

Traditional practices entail soaking seeds, nuts, grains, and legumes to increase their digestibility. Mimicking their natural habitat, a small amount of 1) lemon/lime juice or raw apple cider vinegar, whey, yogurt, kefir, or buttermilk can be added to produce a slightly acidic medium or 2) sea salt or baking soda (dissolved in water) can be added to produce a slightly alkaline medium. Most nuts thrive in a slightly alkaline medium. Traditionally, corn/maize is soaked in a small amount of crushed/slaked limestone (calcium hydroxide) or wood ashes from cooking fires (alkaline); a process known as nixtamalization. After soaking overnight at room temperature, seeds should be rinsed; and if they are soaked longer, they should be rinsed at least once or twice per day. The water will be discolored because the seeds cast off their enzyme inhibitors and other phytotoxins, including tannins and phytic acid. Rinsing washes these wastes away.

Soaking Seeds and Nuts

In summary, soaking seeds and nuts involves these steps:

Step 1.
Submerge seeds or nuts in three times their volume in clean, filtered water; leave overnight

Optional steps
- add either a little acidifying or alkalinizing liquid to the soak water
- add a small amount of algae foods, such as dulse or nori flakes or a strip of kombu, to allow the seeds to absorb trace minerals and other nutrients

Step 2.
Rinse thoroughly once or twice per day–some seeds and nuts, such as walnuts, are ready to eat after one day and night of soaking; other kinds of seeds and nuts, such as almonds can be eaten after one day and night of soaking or they can continue to be rinsed; and they will sprout and be ready to eat.

Note: flax and chia seeds become mucilaginous. They cannot be rinsed; they are ready to eat or be cooked.

Having soaked overnight and absorbed water, some seeds, like walnuts, will grow to twice their original size and (after being rinsed) become crunchy and taste less bitter.

Soaking and Sprouting – Germination – the Transformation of Seeds

Once conditions are suitable for sprouting, such as the temperature, moisture, and pH, seeds cast off their enzyme-inhibitors and the sprouting action of enzymes begins: protease converts proteins into amino acids, lipase transforms lipids (plant oils) into fatty acids, and amylase breaks down carbohydrates into simple sugars. As a result, these macro-nutrients become more easily digested. When sprouting plants absorb minerals, they chelate them (bind them to amino acids), making the minerals more easily assimilated. Additionally, the phytotoxins in seed foods are neutralized or reduced through the sprouting process. As living (raw) foods, sprouts replenish our enzymes that we need for digestion and to metabolize food, cleanse, build, and regenerate the body.

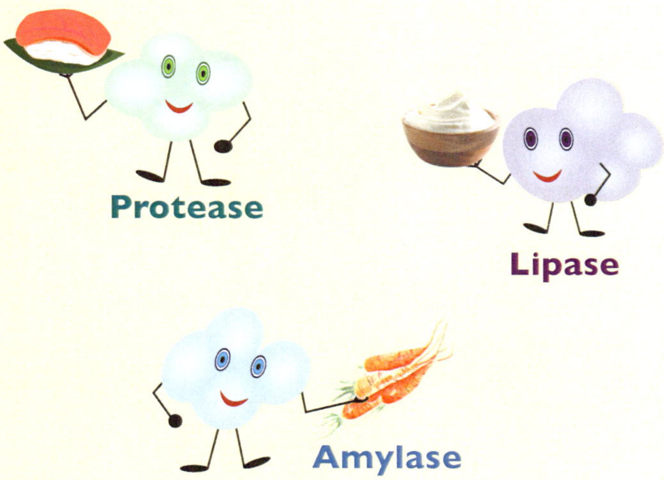

Seeds Remain Dormant Until Their Habitat is Suitable for Sprouting

Ancient seeds have been found that were safely kept dormant by their enzyme inhibitors for centuries and even thousands of years.
Once conditions were suitable (temperature and moisture), the seeds germinated.

Soaking, Sprouting, and Cooking Grains and Legumes

Sprouting Seeds

Just needs water

Step 1.
Place seeds in wide-mouth glass jar and fill with clean, filtered water

Step 2.
Soak overnight, then pour off the water

Step 3.
Rinse well and let drain with the jar upside down at an angle and allow air to circulate

Step 4.
Cover and place in the refrigerator or continue to rinse and drain twice daily for another day or two and then cover and store in refrigerator

Step 5.
At this stage, most sprouts are not easily digested, and should be cooked. They can be baked, for instance, at ~250° F (121° C).[2] Sprouts can be ground into sprout dough for making sprouted breads and crackers. Sprouts can also be added to soups and casseroles. Very small sprouts, such as broccoli sprouts can be eaten raw on a salad.

Caution: Susceptibility to Mold

Grains, legumes, and alfalfa seeds are susceptible to mold especially when stored in damp conditions.

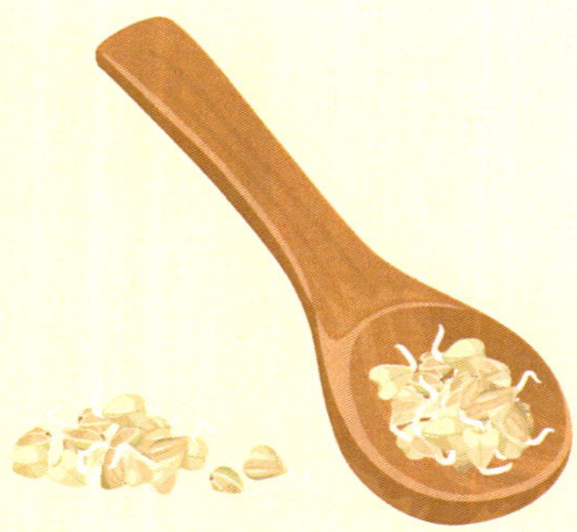

Illustrator Tetiana Gutnyk, Dreamstime

Buckwheat Sprouts

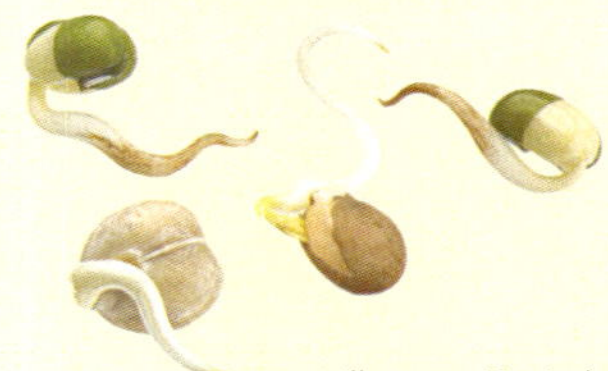

Illustrator Max Lashcheuski, Dreamstime

Mung Bean and Chick Pea Sprouts

Edible Seeds – Including Nuts, Grains, and Legumes

Edible seeds are embryos that develop into plants. The endosperm that surrounds them provides the nutrition the embryo needs during germination, until leaves and roots develop to obtain nutrients from the environment. The seed embryo and endosperm are covered by their protective seed coat. Tree nut seeds are protected in shells, grains (grass seeds) by hulls, and legumes (beans and peas) by pods.

In flowering plants, edible seeds are embedded in fruit. Some fruits are single-seeded, such as apricots, peaches, and plums, while others have many seeds, such as grapes, kiwis, and watermelons. Lacking a sweet taste, cucumbers, summer and winter squashes, and bell peppers, are multi-seeded fruits too. The seeds of herbaceous plants are tiny and generally have tough seed coats, for example, anise, caraway, and chia seeds.

Growing Micro-Greens and Baby Greens

Small tender plants that can be eaten raw

These plant foods, with little leaves and roots, grow best in soil

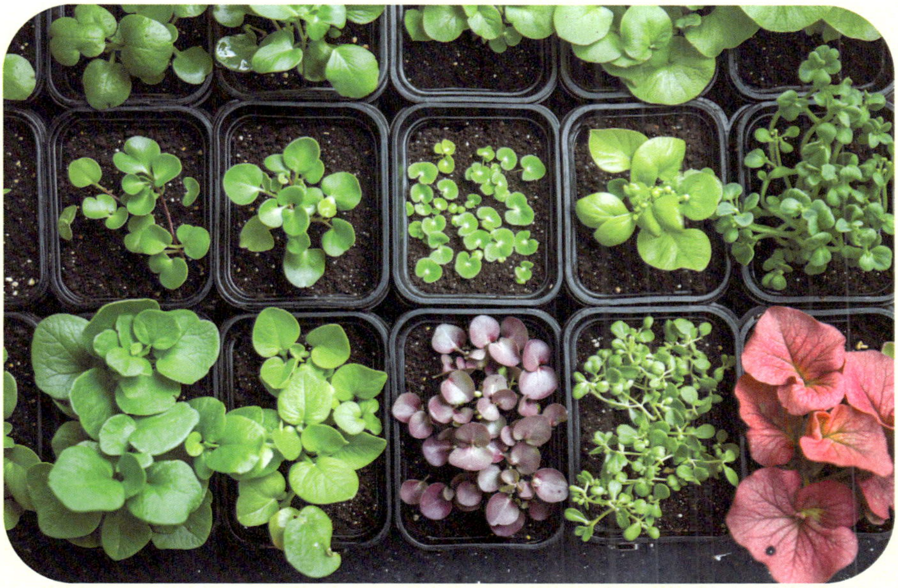

Photographer Valentyn640, Dreamstime

Microgreens and baby greens are young seedlings and herbs with tender stems and leaves that are edible raw. To harvest microgreens, cut them at the base, above their roots. They can be mild, bitter, spicy, or sour and their texture may be juicy or crunchy. Their colors vary greatly depending on the species of plant.

Families of microgreens and baby greens, for example, may include:

- *Amaranthaceae* – amaranth, beet, and chard
- *Amaryllidaceae* – garlic, onion, and leek
- *Apiaceae* – celery, fennel, and parsley
- *Asteraceae* – dandelion, lettuce, and sunflower
- *Brassicaceae* – broccoli, cabbage, cauliflower
- *Cucurbitaceae* – cucumber, squashes, and watermelon
- *Lamiaceae* – basil, mint, and rosemary
- *Fabaceae* – fenugreek, green bean, and pea

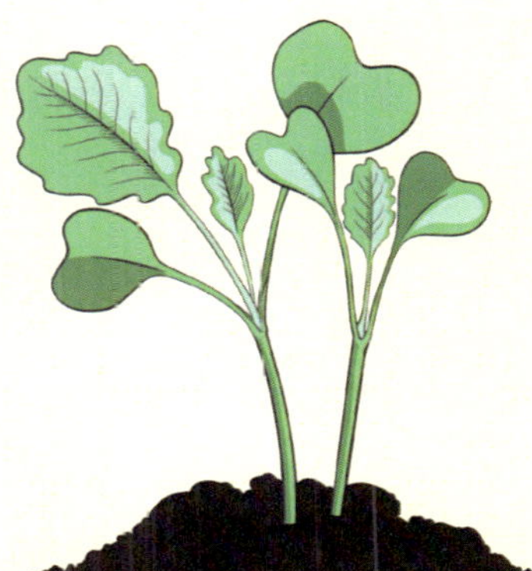

Illustrator Daria Likhodedova, Dreamstime

Broccoli Microgreens

Mature leafy greens such as lettuces and spinach can be grown in a kitchen or outdoor garden.

Juicing Fresh Vegetables, Leafy Greens, Fruits

Nutrients and natural fibers are plentiful in vegetables, leafy greens, and fruits

The anti-oxidant effect of phytonutrients, such as quercetin and anthocyanin found in many vegetables and fruits, is enhanced when they are consumed together.

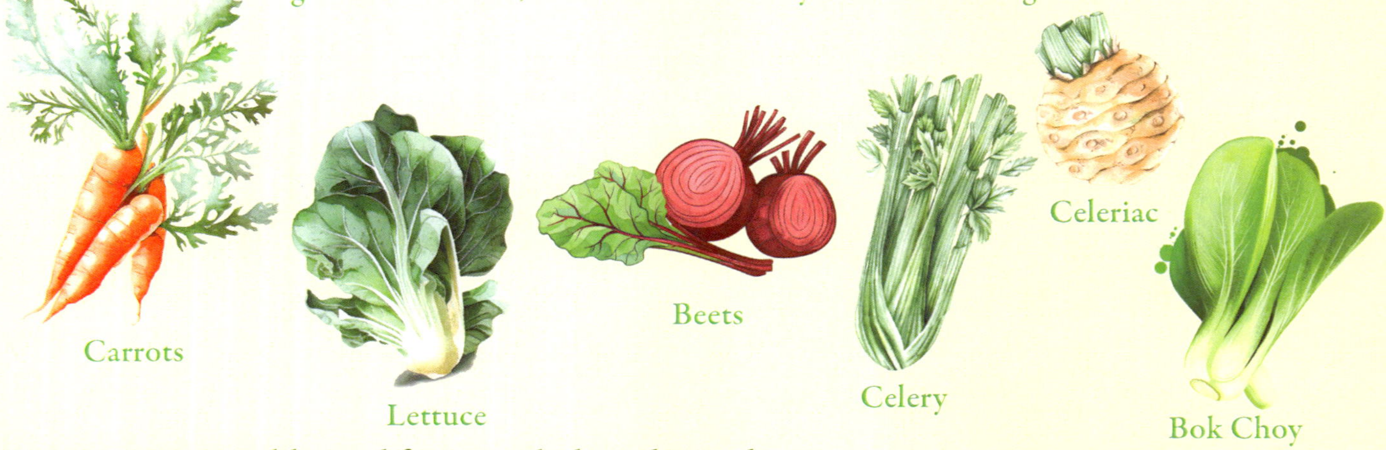

Consuming vegetables and fruits – whole and juiced

Juicing vegetables or fruits separates the pulp, including soluble and insoluble fiber, from the juice. Without the fiber, juices are especially abundant in vitamins, minerals, colorful phytonutrients, and enzymes. Juices are much more beneficial when consumed fresh because they begin to oxidize as soon as they are exposed to the air. Some fruits have skins that may be tough to chew, such as plums or grapes; in this case, juicing may help make the skins, which are loaded with phytonutrients, more digestible and absorbable.

It's important to remove any labels, and pits on the inside. Also, remove apple and pear seeds because they contain arsenic. Watermelon, grapefruit, lemon, and lime seeds are beneficial–cleansing and anti-microbial. Whole watermelon juice can include the dark green rind as well as the seeds.

Limonene is a phytonutrient present in the white pithy part next to the rind on the inside of citrus fruits, such as lemons, limes, grapefruit, and oranges. It has been found to help dissolve gallstones and contains substantial anti-oxidant, anti-microbial, and anti-tumor properties.

Vegetables and fruits can be washed in clean water and scrubbed gently with a vegetable brush and non-toxic vegetable wash, such as baking soda dissolved in water.

Juicing Releases Enzymes, Vitamins, and Trace Minerals

Notably, juices are a plentiful source of inorganic trace minerals which we need in quantities less than 100 milligrams per day. Important trace minerals include; boron, cobalt, copper, chromium, iodine, iron, manganese, molybdenum, selenium, silicon, vanadium, and zinc. Michael T. Murray, N.D. and Joseph E. Pizzorno, N.D. explain in their book, *The Encyclopedia of Healing Foods*, that plants incorporate these trace minerals from the soil into their tissues and complex them with organic molecules, making the trace minerals more absorbable; and juicing liberates the trace minerals, providing them in a highly bioavailable form.[3]

CAUTION
Juicing and Blood Sugar

Juicing, which removes the fiber and concentrates the natural sugars in sweet fruits and some vegetables, such as beets and carrots, can significantly raise blood sugar and feed pathogenic micro-organisms such as *Candida* (yeast infections) and parasites associated with degenerative diseases. On the other hand, juicing non-sweet, non-starch vegetables support stable blood sugar levels.

Juice Ideas – non-sweet, non-starch

Celery; cucumber; romaine and other lettuces; green beans, asparagus, and bok choy; leafy greens, such as dandelion, parsley, and watercress; fresh herbs (a small amount), such as oregano, rosemary, thyme, and sage; burdock, ginger, and turmeric (stains an orange color) roots; and soaked overnight and rinsed seeds, such as chia and flax seeds.

Note: Given that juicing concentrates nutrients and other compounds, juices can be diluted with water as much as 50% or more to reduce the quantity of natural sugars or strong tastes (ref., Tastes Chart on page 244).

Fresh Fruits – Eaten Whole

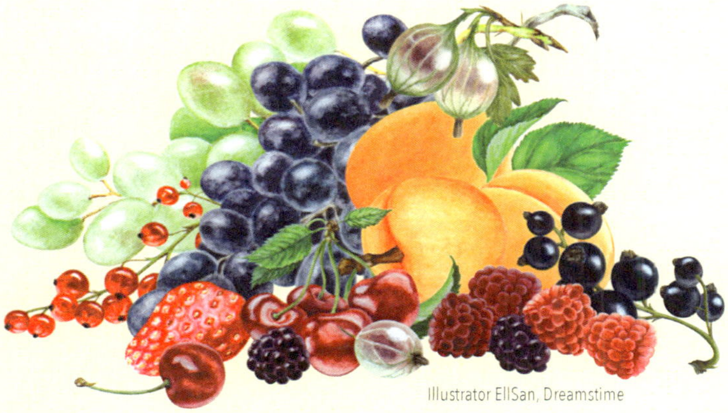

Illustrator EllSan, Dreamstime

When ripe, fruits are especially delicious, hydrating, easy to digest, alkaline-forming, expanding (loosening), and cleansing

Infusing sliced fruit, such as berries and/or herbs in filtered, clean water can enhance the flavor of drinking water

Fruit freezes well as an easy snack, particularly grapes, blueberries, and peaches

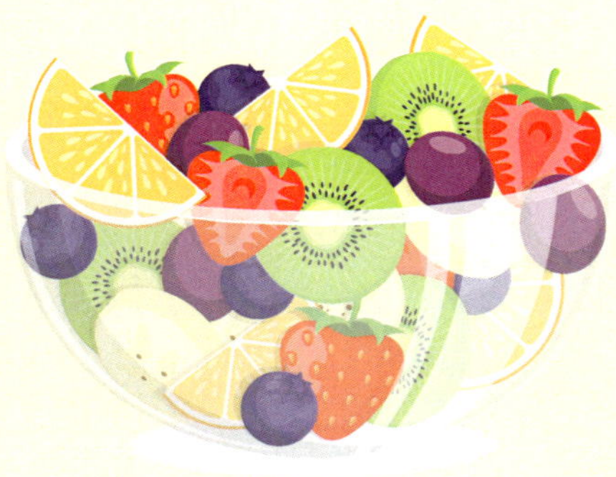

Illustrator Chuhail, Dreamstime

Acid Fruits and Tooth Enamel

Acidic foods, such as lemons, limes, and apple cider vinegar, while they are cleansing and aid in digestion, they can also dissolve tooth enamel. Swishing the mouth with baking soda in water or salt water can wash away the acids.

Spiralizing Raw Vegetable Noodles

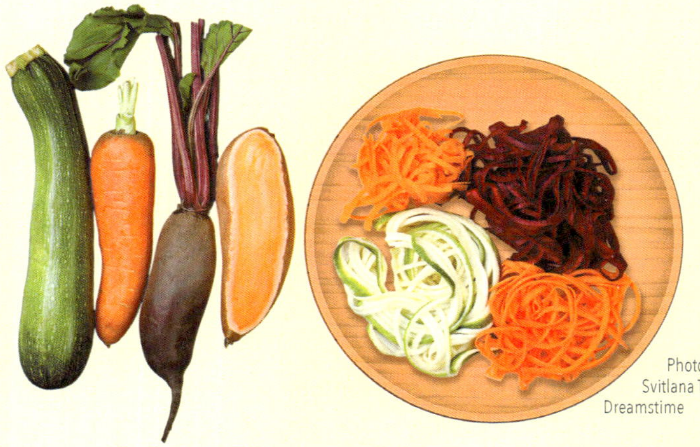

Photographer Svitlana Tereshchenko, Dreamstime

In addition to salads, spiralized vegetable noodles incorporate raw food enzymes and the water-soluble B and C vitamins into a meal. The spiralizer tool makes raw 'vegetable noodles,' such as zucchini (often called 'zoodles'), carrots, cucumbers, jicama, and tender inside of fennel bulbs. Peeled and deseeded as needed, raw vegetables that are hard or semi-hard are easier to spiralize, for example: beets, celeriac (celery root), kohlrabi, parsnips, mature turnips, and yams. Once spiralized into noodles, these vegetables digest better when cooked.

Cooked seafoods, meats, and eggs can be placed onto raw or cooked spiralized noodles. Then, various sauces and toppings can be added for a complete meal. Home chef Ali Maffucci, in her book, *Spiralized*, provides inspiring recipes and instructive tips on using a spiralizer, including ideas on how to make spiral noodle sauces.[5] Spiralized vegetables hold up well when they are cooked and can be the foundation for delicious dishes for a wide array of meals.

Vegetable Cooking Tips

Phytonutrients

The carotenoids in carrots, beets, and asparagus; lycopene in tomatoes; and quercetin and organo-sulfur compounds in garlic and onions become more bioavailable when they are lightly cooked.

Removing thin skins

Place thin, tough-skinned vegetables, such as tomatoes in boiling water for a few seconds, then place in cold water where the skin will peel off easily.

Preparing Vegetables for Cooking

Vegetables cook more evenly when they are sliced, diced (cubed), or chopped equal in size and shape.

Sautéing vegetables in their own juices

With the cover on, at a low temperature (slowly) on the stove-top, in a small amount of fat or oil (such as ghee or olive oil) spread across the bottom of the pan, vegetables cook very well in their own juices–optionally with sea salt and herbs. A great variety of vegetables, for example, onions, celery, carrots, zucchini, broccoli, cauliflower, green beans, okra, asparagus, Brussels sprouts, Bok choy, and many others can be chopped and sautéed this way. Once they are cooked, the vegetables can be eaten by themselves or added to soups or any other savory dish.

Baking winter squash

Spread ghee on baking dish and add filtered water to keep moist. Then, cut winter squashes in half and place, with the inside facing down on the baking dish; wherein, the dome-shaped outer skin serves as an 'oven' to keep in the moisture.

Fiddlehead ferns and prickly pear cactus

Wild foods, fiddlehead ferns (natural brown papery coverings removed) and prickly pear cactus pads (thorns removed) and fruits, can be sautéed in animal fats or olive/coconut oil until tender or simmered in water, stock, or broth until soft.

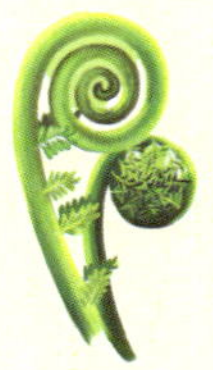

Fiddlehead Fern

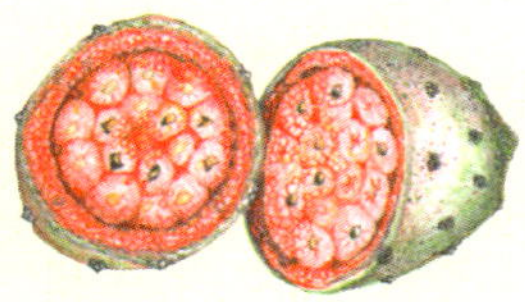

Prickly Pear Cactus

Fiddlehead Ferns

The coiled tender tips of young ostrich fiddlehead ferns (*Matteuccia struthiopteris*) are edible; whereas, most other fiddlehead ferns are inedible due to the toxic compound ptaquiloside. Ostrich fiddlehead ferns have been consumed by Indigenous people for centuries throughout the northeastern United States and Canada. Fiddlehead ferns grow in the woods, forests, and along the banks of brooks and streams.

Prickly Pear Cactus

Prickly pear cactus (*Opuntia*, many species) pads (nopales) and ripe fruit (tunas) are edible once the thorns and small 'glochids' under the thorns have been removed. Leather gloves and tongs are sometimes used to collect the pads and fruits from the cactus. Prickly pear are among the many traditional foods indigenous people harvest in the desert during summer and autumn.

Fungi Kingdom

Mushrooms (macro-fungi)

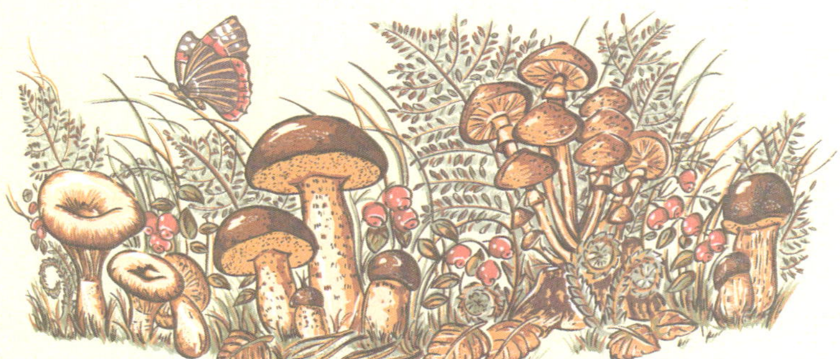

Illustrator Nearbirds, Dreamstime

Mushrooms should be cooked to breakdown fiber, facilitate digestion, and neutralize naturally-occurring myco-toxins

CAUTION **Edible and Poisonous Mushroom Look-Alikes**

There are many edible mushrooms that look like poisonous mushrooms; therefore, it is very important to accurately identify them before consuming them. Poisonous mushrooms are still poisonous when cooked.

Edible mushrooms are particularly nutritious when wild-harvested from pristine temperate and boreal forests. They can also be grown on the logs from their native trees or in organic, regenerative soil. Mushrooms obtain phytonutrients from the standing or fallen trees they live on or the regenerative soils they live in. This gives them distinct flavors and earthy aromas, such as chaga from birch or other deciduous hardwood trees and chanterelles from the forest floor. Like adaptogenic plant foods, such as ginseng and astragalus root, edible mushrooms have a normalizing effect on physiological functions, supporting the body in maintaining homeostasis. From a culinary standpoint, mushrooms are versatile, blending nicely with a wide range of flavors and enhancing virtually any savory dish, such as casseroles, sauces, roasts, omelets, tarts, and pies.

Preparing to cook with mushrooms

- brush lightly with a cloth to remove soil on the mushrooms and wash them clean
- trim the tough stem off the bottom part of the mushroom; it can be used for stocks and soups
- chop, dice (cube), or slice the mushrooms (they can be cut easily with an egg slicer)
- to facilitate browning (caramelizing) mushrooms and to prevent them from absorbing too much fat or oil from the cooking pan, first steam or simmer them in water and sea salt (just enough water to cover them) with the lid off; once the water has evaporated, the mushrooms are ready for cooking

Cooking mushrooms

- braise or grill (larger mushrooms); if cooking whole mushrooms, season the underside
- sauté with onions, herbs, and sea salt; eat as is or add to soups and stews
- bake and broil: stuffed mushrooms with chopped vegetables, leafy greens, cheese, and seasonings
- barbeque mushrooms skewered with vegetables, seafood, and/or meat

Storage

- store mushrooms for later use, unwashed, in a paper bag (if damp, wrap in paper towel)
- use mushrooms as soon as possible for best nutrition and flavor
- freeze mushrooms (raw or cooked)

Plantae and Chromista Kingdoms

Green, Red, and Brown Algae Foods

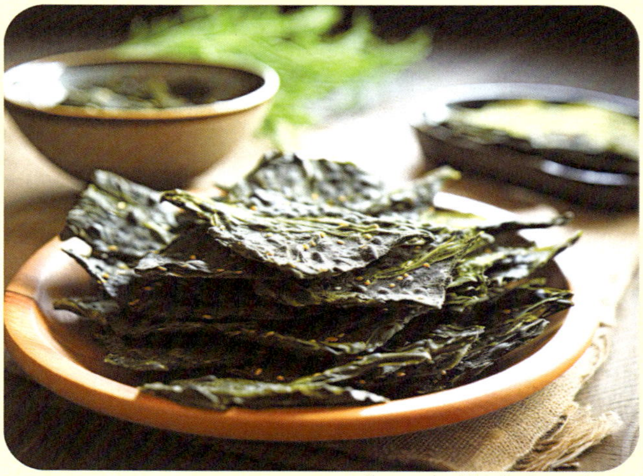

Photographer Airinsalev, Dreamstime

Algae (Seaweed) Chips

Seaweeds of the Oceans

Among the hundreds of different kinds of edible, salt water algae that grow on ocean shores (seaweeds), only a few species are widely known, such as: arame, dulse, hijiki, kelp, kombu, nori, and wakame. Chlorella is a unique algae food in that it is single-celled and mostly found in freshwater. Although algae foods are wet when harvested, they are typically purchased dried. They can easily be rehydrated by soaking them in filtered or spring water.

Absorbing water, algae may double or triple in size. It can be used soon after it has been rehydrated. Fresh wakame and dulse can be included in salads. They can also be roasted, crumbled, and then sprinkled on top of a variety of savory dishes, for example, furikake, a common Japanese dish made with dried fish, sesame seeds, chopped seaweed, and sea salt. Algae foods are often added to soups; stocks; broths; sautéed with onions, carrots, garlic, ginger; and eaten as salads with wasabi and soy sauce, avocado, and cucumber. Kombu can be soaked overnight and then cooked as a mineral rich broth.

Nori comes in dried sheets and is often used as a wrap for seafood and vegetables; it can also be used as a wrap for rice and vegetable combinations. To make nori crispier, it can be briefly heated in the oven. Once toasted, nori can be crushed into flakes and added to salads, dressings, casseroles, omelets, sauces, soups, stocks, and broths. Thin seaweeds can rehydrate during cooking. When sea/Irish moss simmers, it becomes gelatinous and can be used in jellies and soups. Dried or flaked sea lettuce can be sprinkled on savory dishes. Arame comes in fine strips. It has a mild taste. After soaking for 10 to 15 minutes, arame can be chopped raw into small pieces and put in a salad. It is delicious, too, when sautéed with onions and carrots. Hijiki is a thicker type of algae. It can be soaked overnight and then simmered for 45 minutes to an hour to soften. Then, it can be chopped and added to soups. Algae sea salt can be an artful combination of algae, such as chlorella or spirulina; flakes of dulse or nori, ground herbs, and sea salt.

Caution: Excess Iodine

In consuming marine algae, make sure iodine levels do not get too high in the body.

Tips to Reduce Excess Sea Salt

To reduce the salt that sometimes accumulates on algae, soak the algae for a few minutes in filtered water and then discard the soak water. If too much sea salt was added to a soup or stew, there is a solution–place a cut, peeled potato into the pot and cook for a few minutes, allowing the potato to absorb the excess salt. Then, discard the potato in the compost.

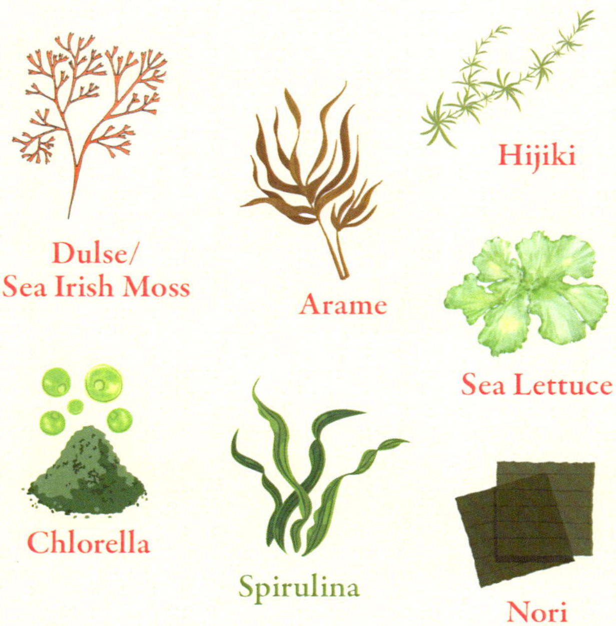

Algae Probiotics

People who have been consuming seaweeds for generations or for many years may naturally possess algae probiotics (that feed on algae) in their microbiome, which are different from other probiotics. For instance, a common probiotic marine bacteria, *Zobellia galactanivorans*, is found feeding on edible red algae and aids in digesting algae. Those who are unaccustomed to eating edible algae may initially have some difficulty digesting the algae-specific carbohydrates, such as, alginate and laminarin, until the algae probiotics become a natural part of their microbiome.

Cooking Methods for Natural Foods

Tallow

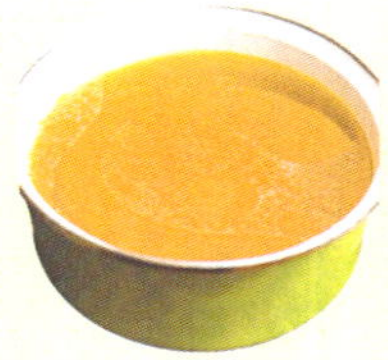

Chicken, Duck, Goose Fat

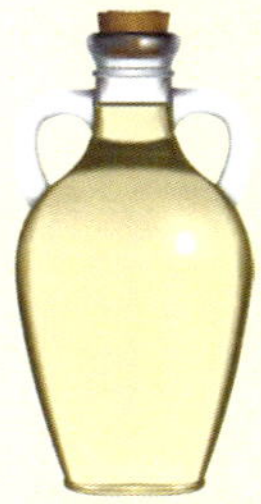

Emu Oil

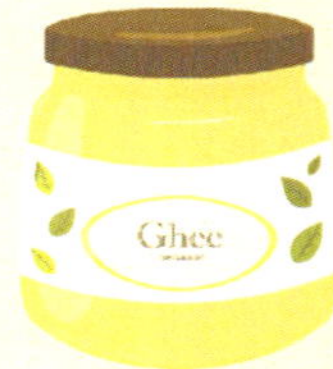

Ghee

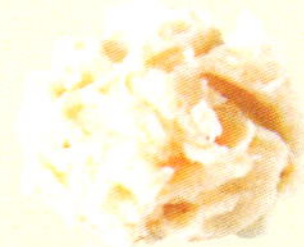

Pork Lard

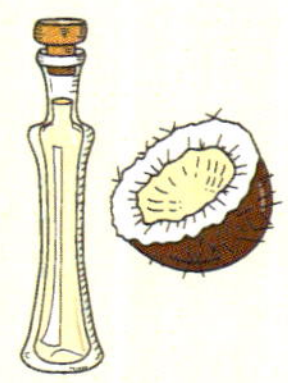

Coconut Oil

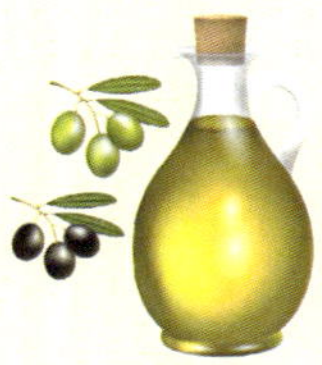

Emu Oil

Animal Fat and Plant Oil Smoke Points

Every fat and oil has a smoke point at which the heat begins to alter its molecular structure and potentially produce harmful compounds. Example smoke points are:

- ghee ~485° F (~252° C),
- beef tallow ~480° F (~250° C)
- avocado oil ~482° F (~251° C)
- coconut oil ~350° F (~177° C)
- olive oil ~405° F (~207° C)

Cook on stove-top or in the oven with high smoke point animal fats, plant oils, or with stocks or broths. Raw and cooked fats are satiating and enhance the flavors in natural foods.

Cooking with Animal Fats or Plant Oils

Preparing Animal Foods for Cooking

- Marinating may entail placing food in a seasoned liquid, such as lemon/lime, tamari, and/or herbs to tenderize and impart flavor before cooking. The acids in the lemons and limes and probiotic foods, like tamari, help break down the food, facilitating digestion.
- Pat dry seafoods and meats before sautéing or searing (cooking at high temperature) on the stove-top or roasting in the oven to facilitate browning. Fats and oils are sensitive to heat; thus, heating the pan before adding fats or oils is preferable, exposing them to the heat for less time.

Cooking with Water or Liquid and Heat

- Braising or roasting involves browning foods at relatively high temperatures
- Stewing is like braising, though, with less liquid
- Boiling occurs when water reaches 212°F (100 °C)
- Simmering maintains the temperature of the water, stock, broth, or sauces that food is being cooked in, just below the boiling point of water/until the liquid reaches ~180–200°F (82–93°C); this may entail having the burner on the stove between low to medium-low heat–this allows the flavors to develop gradually; lower temperatures also help keep proteins from becoming tough or rubbery
- Poaching involves cooking food in water, stock, or broth at a lower temperature than simmering: ~160–175 °F (70–80 °C) for gentler cooking
- Steaming vegetables briefly, such as broccoli, maintains the bright green color without losing many nutrients; the steam-water in the pot can be added to soups
- 'Reducing' is to thicken a liquid mixture by heating in an uncovered pot or pan, reducing the excess liquid

Caution: Concerns with Cooking at Too High of a Temperature

When seafood and meat burn, char, or blacken, they can generate harmful chemicals, including acrylamide and heterocyclic amines (HCA). If the fat or juices drip into an open flame, they may produce polycyclic aromatic hydrocarbons (PAHs) which can be carried up with the smoke into the air and onto the food.

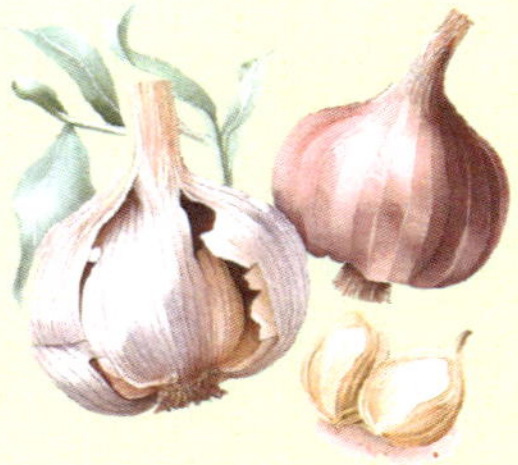

Garlic – Producing Allicin

The nutrient allicin is found in all members of the onion (*Allium*) family. It is anti-microbial, anti-oxidant, and anti-tumor, supporting the immune system. Crushing garlic and allowing it to sit for several minutes or more gives the enzyme alliinase a chance to catalyze the formation of allicin. Add raw garlic last when cooking to maintain enzymes and benefits of allicin.

Garlic and Onion Peel Seasoning

This nutritious *Allium* (Onion Family) seasoning enhances the flavor of savory dishes, such as salads, omelettes, sauces, casseroles, stews, soups, broths, and stocks.

Basic Recipe:

Step 1) Save the garlic and onion skins you peel off when you cook; place them in a dry glass jar

Step 2) Once you have plenty of them, wash in a bowl of water with a splash of white vinegar; let sit for a few minutes, stir with your hands, and rinse in a colander under clean running water

Step 3) Spread the garlic and onion skins out to dry on paper towels

Step 4)To make crunchy, place the dry garlic and onion skins on parchment paper; and cook lightly at a low heat in the oven for a few minutes

Step 5) Blend until powdery in a blender, food processor, or herb grinder (sea salt and dried herbs can be added before blending)

Step 6) Place in a dry glass jar, cover with a top, and store for use as a seasoning

Cooking with Dry Heat

- Glazing (brushing the surface of the food before, during, or after baking) with a beaten egg, ghee/butter, or honey–moistens and gives a glossy look
- Baking involves dry heat, cooking food in an oven, over hot ashes, or on hot stones, with the temperature generally ~300°F (150 °C); the heat works its way from the outside to the inside of the food
- Broiling is a dry heat, at a high temperature of ~550° F (288° C)
- Roasting with dry heat from an open flame or oven evenly cooks all sides with temperatures of at least 300° F (150° C); caramelization/browning occurs on the surface of the food
    - basting/spooning involves pouring its own juices over the food while roasting, keeping the food moist and imparting flavor
    - gravies can be made with the fat from roasting, thickened with arrow root and seasoned with herbs, cream, or butter
    - seafood or meat juices can be used in stews, soups, or sauces
- Dehydrating is a traditional way of preserving food; wherein, the water in the food evaporates, concentrating flavor and creating a chewy or crunchy texture. The temperature used to dehydrate, depends on the type of food. Generally, as long as the temperature remains at or below 117° F (47° C)–enzymes in the food remain viable, replenishing the enzymes needed to nourish us, repair cells and tissues, and produce energy (ref. Enzyme Chart, pages 161-163).

Bacteria, Fungi, and Plantae Kingdoms

Probiotic Bacteria, Micro-fungi, and Plant Foods

Ferments

Virtually any natural food can be fermented to increase enzymes, probiotics, nutrients, and preserve the food for a long time

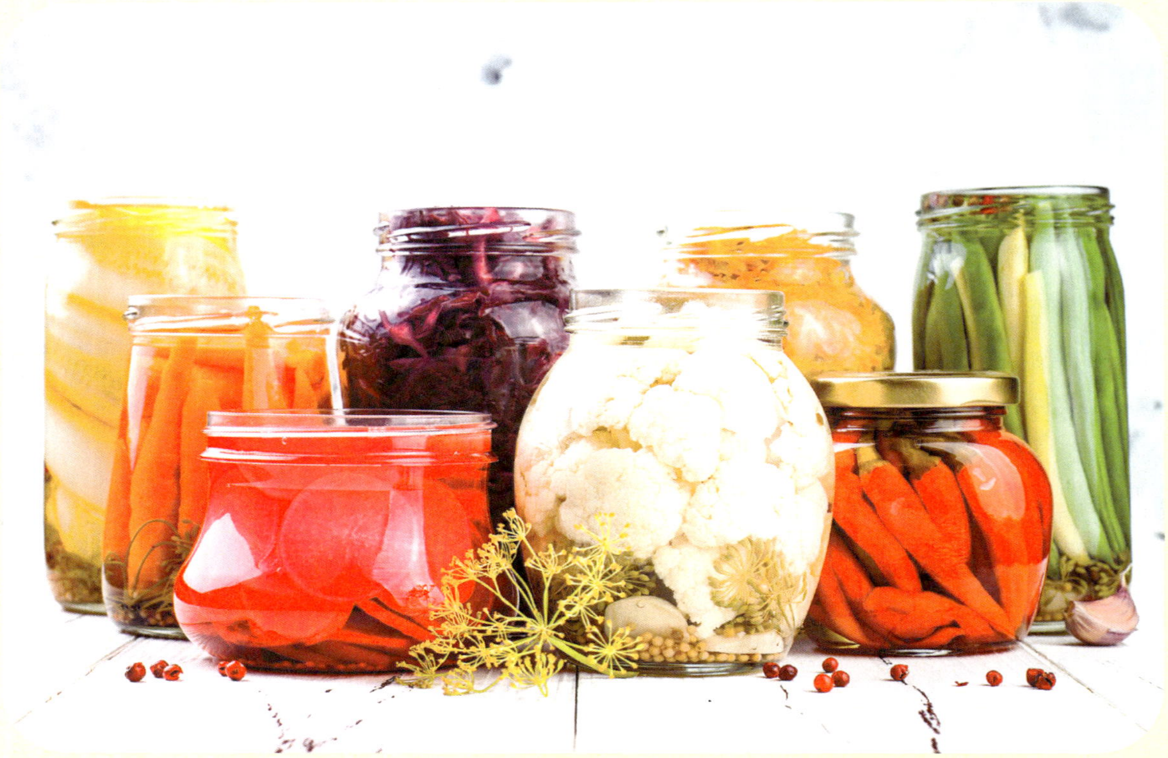

Illustrator Svitlana Tereshchenko, Dreamstime

Variety of Fermented Vegetables

Consuming a small quantity of fermented foods each day can help the body develop and maintain a healthy microbiome. Fermentation takes place when the food is entirely submerged in liquid (anaerobic conditions) at room temperature when micro-organisms actively consume (break down) natural foods. The probiotic micro-organisms naturally present on foods are the starter cultures for wild ferments. Sea salt draws out the moisture in the foods and creates more liquid helping to keep the fermented food submerged. Additionally, sea salt's antiseptic properties help guard against pathogens. Probiotic bacteria and micro-fungi species in wild ferments and starter cultures help us digest the foods. These probiotic micro-organisms produce lactic acid, increase the enzyme and nutrient content, and make the food more digestible and bioavailable. Ferments can develop over a few days, months, or years; and their taste changes over time. Fermentation specialist Sandor Katz explains how the probiotics produce lactic acid and acetic acid which act as 'bio-preservatives' that prevent spoilage.[4]

Resource

Cultures for Health - Learn

https://culturesforhealth.com/blogs/learn

Making ferments – vegetable example

Supplies – vegetables, sea salt, cutting board, knife, peeler, wooden pounder, wide-mouth jar, tray, and ceramic weight (optional)

Basic steps and concepts:

- wash, chop, and ideally grate vegetables–to increase the surface area for fermentation
- add and mix in sea salt, to help draw out the juice from the vegetables and prevent pathogenic bacteria (brines are ferments with a higher concentration of sea salt)
- add fresh or dried herbs, such as caraway or cumin seeds, or algae foods (optional), for more nutrition and health benefits
- pound the chopped and/or grated vegetables to further release the juices in the vegetables
- place in wide-mouth jar and add water as needed to fully cover the vegetables, leaving one inch of air space at the top for the fermenting juice to expand; making sure liquid covers all the vegetables ensures anaerobic conditions necessary for fermentation–a ceramic weight can be used to weigh the vegetables down, keeping them under the liquid; set jar in tray to catch any overflow of liquid
- gently cover jar with loose jar lid or special ferment airlock lid or cabbage leaf, allowing the carbon dioxide released from the ferments to escape
- taste each day to determine (based on taste) when the ferment is ready to eat
- keep at room temperature during fermentation
- when done fermenting, place in the refrigerator

Ferments that are started with cultures or wild-ferments include: sauerkraut, sour beets, borscht, kvass, kimchi, brined garlic, miso, buttermilk, yogurt, kefir, cheeses, seed milks and cheese, chutneys, sourdough bread and crackers, rejuvelac, kombucha, and raw apple cider vinegar. Raw foods from all the kingdoms of life can be fermented, including: algae, mushrooms, and animal foods (seafoods, meats, and eggs). Even more than soaking and sprouting seeds, fermenting neutralizes or reduces phytotoxins, including: oxalic acid, phytic acid, nitrosamines, and glucosides in leafy greens, grains, legumes, and other plant foods. Ferments are high in enzymes, supporting our microbiome, improving digestion and the absorption of nutrients into the blood and lymph, promoting overall health, and strengthening the immune system. With respect to our health, making and consuming fermented foods connects us with natural processes in nature.

Raw Foods and Low-Temperature Cooking Preserves Heat-Sensitive Enzymes and Vitamins

Enzymes, B vitamins, and vitamin C are heat sensitive. They do not generally survive above 117° F (47° C). This is the temperature at which food begins to feel hot to the touch.

If In Doubt, Throw It Out

When making ferments, keep in mind that food can spoil at room temperature. If a ferment ever does not smell, look, or taste right, discard it.

Meal Presentation

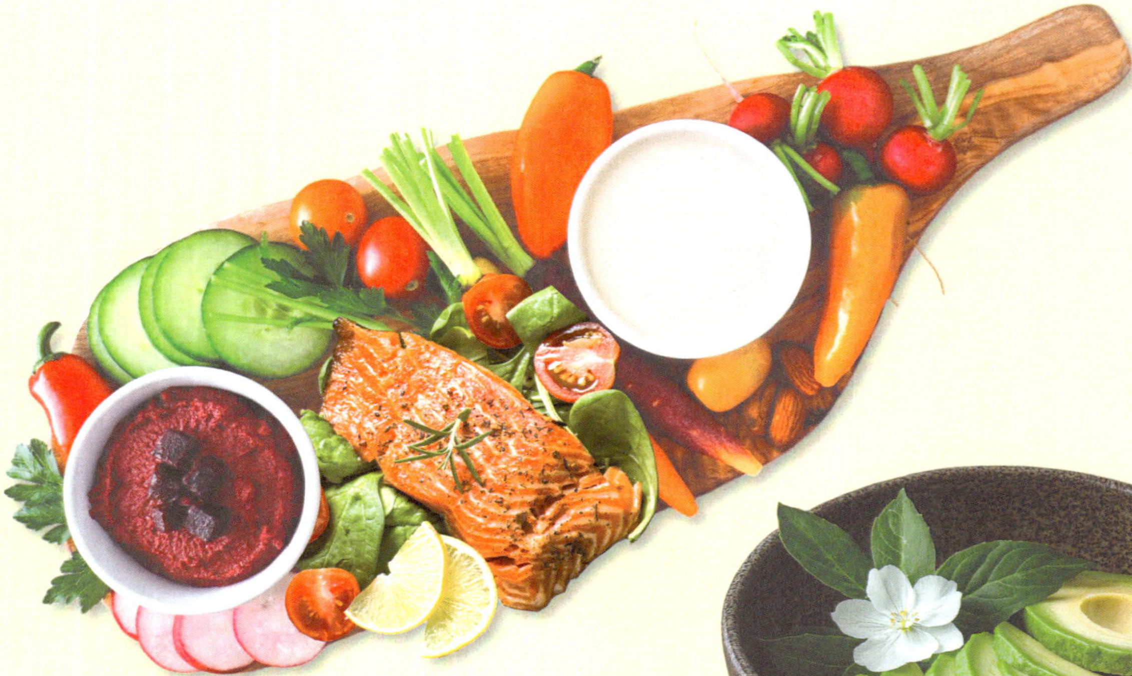

Photographers Jenifoto406 & Nadianb, Dreamstime

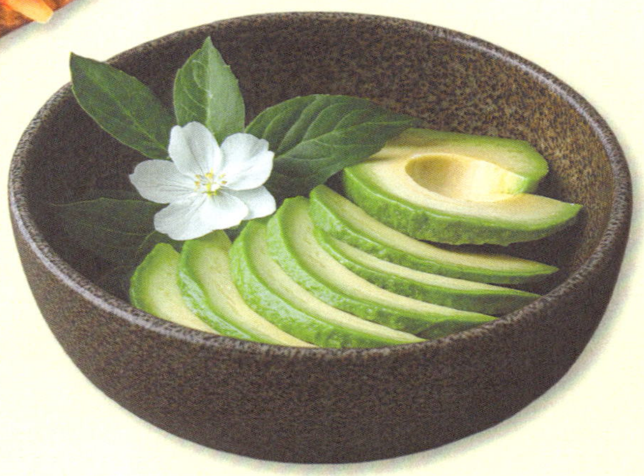

Photographer Adamnizol, Dreamstime

Providing a meal to family and friends is a opportunity to offer a presentation with a variety of colors, textures, and designs. For instance, create an array of delicious natural foods on beautiful wooden serving boards made of walnut, maple, and/or cherry. A buffet style could include full meals or simply appetizers. Some foods could be placed directly on charcuterie boards or platters, such as carrots, celery, onion rings, radishes, and snow peas. Sauces, dips, and toppings can be set in small plates and bowls on the charcuterie boards, while other dishes could be handhelds–stuffed mushrooms, cut vegetables, and sandwich wraps. Attractive ways to display natural foods include cutting vegetables against their natural grain, along the equator, such as red onions, tomatoes, and purple cabbage. A decorative arrangement might include cucumber ribbons, radishes cut into the shape of flowers, and garnishes, such as parsley, microgreens, and slices of lemon.

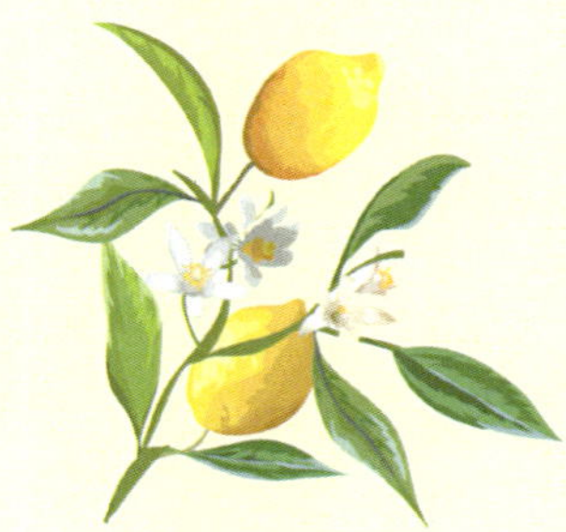

Natural Foods – Delicious and Deeply Nourishing

References

[1]WAPF. (1999). *Timeless principles of healthy traditional diets*. Washington, D.C.: The Weston A. Price Foundation. https://www.westonaprice.org/health-topics/abcs-of-nutrition/principles-of-healthy-diets-2.

[2]Meyerowitz, S. (1999). *Sproutman's Kitchen Garden Cookbook* (p. 223–235). Great Barrington, MA: Sproutman Publications.

[3]Murray, M. T. & Pizzorno, J. E. (2005). *The Encyclopedia of Healing Foods* (p. 116). New York, NY: Atria Books.

[4]Katz, S. E. (2003). *Wild Fermentation* (p. 5). White River Junction, VT: Chelsea Green Publishing.

[5]Maffucci, A. (2015). *Inspiralized* (p. 22). New York, NY: Clarkson Potter/Publishers.

[6]Corrado, M. (2015, August 27). *The Dark Side of Bone Broth*. Fort Collins, CO: Selene River Press. https://www.seleneriverpress.com/the-dark-side-of-bone-broth.

[7]Fallon Morell, S. & Daniels, K. T. (2014). *Nourishing Broth* (p. 9). New York, NY: Grand Central LifeStyle.

[8]Fallon Morell, S. (2001). *Nourishing Traditions* (p. 41). Washington, D.C.: NewTrends Publishing, Inc.

Additional Resources

Boynton, H. & Brackett, M. (2014). *The Heal Your Gut Cookbook*. White River Junction, VT: Chelsea Green Publishing.

Campbell-McBride, N. (2023) *Natural digestive healing* (website). https://www.gapsdiet.com.

Coleman, E. (2018). *The New Organic Grower* (30th Anniversary Edition). White River Junction, VT: Chelsea Green Publishing.

Cooksley, V. G. (2018). *Seaweed: Nature's Secret to Balancing Your Metabolism, Preventing Disease, and Revitalizing Body and Mind*. The Woodlands, TX: Floramed Publishing.

Corrado, M. (2019). *The Complete Techniques for the GAPS Diet*. Fort Collins, CO: Selene River Press.

D'Adamo, P. J. (2001). *Live Right for Your Type*. New York, NY: G. P. Putnam's Sons.

Debuigne, G. & Couplan, F. (2024). *100 Plants That Heal*. Exeter, England: Pynes Hill. Davidandcharles.com.

Eng, S. N. (2023). *Building A Nourishing Asian Kitche*n. White River Junction, VT: Chelsea Green Publishing.

Fung, J., Mayer, E., Ramos, M. (2020). *Life in the Fasting Lane*. New York, NY: HarperCollins Publishers.

Gates, D. (2011). *The Body Ecology Diet*. Carlsbad, CA: Hay House, Inc.

Gedgaudas, N. (2017). *Primal Fat Burner*. New York, NY: Atria.

Isokauppila, T. (2017). *Healing Mushrooms*. New York, NY: Penguin Random House LLC.

Katz, S. E. (2012). *The Art of Fermentation*. White River Junction, VT: Chelsea Green Publishing.

Livers, E. (2018). *Revitalize Digestion*. Little Elm, TX: Brainy Babe Micro Pub.

Marciano, M. & Vizniak, N. (2012). *Botanical Medicine*. (2nd Edition). Prohealthsys.com

McIntyre, A. (2000). *Drink to Your Health*. New York, NY: Simon and Schuster, Inc.

McNamee, T. (2007). *Alice Waters and Chez Panisse*. New York, NY: The Penguin Press.

Mars, B. (2004). *Rawsome!* Laguna Beach, CA: Basic Health Publications, Inc.

Murray, M. T. (1998). *The Complete Book of Juicing*. New York, NY: Three Rivers Press.

Nienhiser, J. (2000). *Characteristics of traditional diets*. The Weston A. Price Foundation. https://www.westonaprice.org/health-topics/abcs-of-nutrition/characteristics-of-traditional-diets/#gsc.tab=0.

Price, W.A. (2019). *Nutrition and Physical Degeneration*. (8th ed.). Lemon Grove, CA: Price-Pottenger.

Quillin, P. (2020). *Beating Cancer with Nutrition*. Carlsbad, CA: Nutrition Times Press, Inc.

RMI. (2024). *About raw milk*. Raw Milk Institute. https://www.rawmilkinstitute.org/about-raw-milk ACRM. Milk as medicine. A Campaign for Raw Milk. https://www.realmilk.com/milk-as-medicine/; audio and video (2015, December 10) https://www.realmilk.com/audio-and-video/ (11:42 minutes).

Sakai, S. (2019). *Japanese home cooking*. Boulder, CO: Roost Books.

Schindler, B. (2021). *Eat Like a Human*. New York, NY: Little, Brown Spark.

Warwick-Evans, C. & Van Berkel, T. V. (2022). *The Seaweed Cookbook*. Wwwannesspublishing.com: Anness Publishing Ltd.

Wigmore, A. (1986). *The Sprouting Book*. Wayne, NJ: Avery Publishing Group, Inc.

PART X
Inspiration

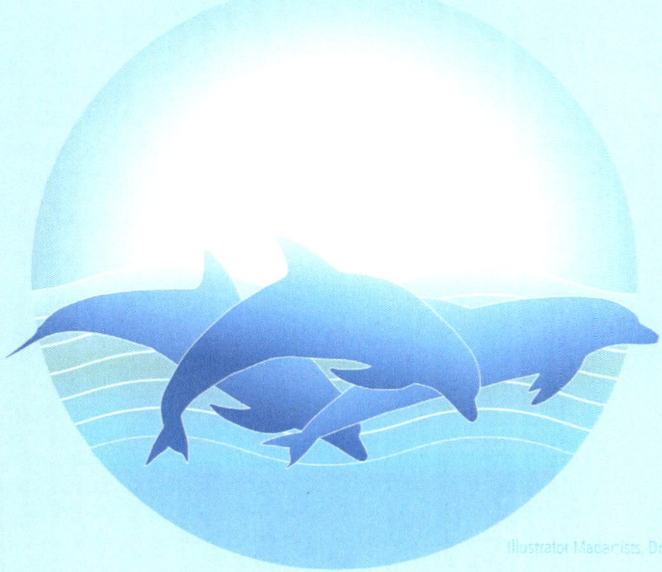

Illustrator Macarists, Dreamstime

Conserving nature and looking out for one another across the world

Appendix: Federal Natural Resources Conservation Statutes

Includes excerpts from Federal Statutes enacted by the Senate and House of Representatives of the United States of America in Congress assembled

SPECIES AND ECOSYSTEM CONSERVATION

1) Endangered Species Act

"SEC. 2 (b) PURPOSES.—

The purposes of this Act are to provide a means whereby the ecosystems upon which endangered species and threatened species depend may be conserved, to provide a program for the conservation of such endangered species and threatened species, and to take such steps as may be appropriate to achieve the purposes of the treaties and conventions set forth in subsection (a) of this section."

Notices of federal agency actions under the statutes are published in the Federal Register, including public hearings and comment periods.

(ref. https://www.federalregister.gov.)

"(c) POLICY.—(1) It is further declared to be the policy of Congress that all Federal departments and agencies shall seek to conserve endangered species and threatened species and shall utilize their authorities in furtherance of the purposes of this Act. (2) It is further declared to be the policy of Congress that Federal agencies shall cooperate with State and local agencies to resolve water resource issues in concert with conservation of endangered species."

2) Migratory Bird Conservation Act

"SEC. 10.
(a) Areas of lands, waters, or interests therein acquired or reserved pursuant to this Act shall, unless otherwise provided by law, be administered by the Secretary of the Interior under rules and regulations prescribed by him to conserve and protect migratory birds in accordance with treaty obligations with Mexico, Canada, Japan, and the Union of Soviet Socialist Republics, and other species of wildlife found thereon, including species that are listed pursuant to section 4 of the Endangered Species Act of 1973 as endangered species or threatened species, and to restore or develop adequate wildlife habitat."

3) Marine Mammal Protection Act

"Title I—Conservation and Protection of Marine Mammals Moratorium on taking and importing marine mammals and marine mammal products 16 U.S.C. 1371 Sec. 101. (a) [Imposition; exceptions.] — There shall be a moratorium on the taking and importation of marine mammals and marine mammal products, commencing on the effective date of this Act, during which time no permit may be issued for the taking of any marine mammal and no marine mammal or marine mammal product may be imported into the United States except in the following cases:
(b) Conservation Plans; preparation and implementation —
(C) as soon as possible, for any species or stock designated as depleted under this title, except that a conservation plan need not be prepared if the Secretary determines that it will not promote the conservation of the species or stock."

Marine Mammal Protection Act is administered by:

National Marine Fisheries Service, National Oceanographic and Atmospheric Administration, Department of Commerce for cetaceans, sea lions, and seals

U.S. Fish and Wildlife Service, Department of the Interior for walruses, manatees, dugongs, sea cows, sea otters, and polar bears

"(2) Each plan shall have the purpose of conserving and restoring the species or stock to its optimum sustainable population. The Secretary shall model such plans on recovery plans required under section 4(f) of the Endangered Species Act of 1973 (16 U.S.C. 1533(f))."

4) Anadromous Fish Conservation Act

"16 U.S.C. 757a That (a) for the purpose of conserving, developing, and enhancing within the several States the anadromous fishery resources of the Nation that are subject to depletion from water resources developments and other causes, or with respect to which the United States has made conservation commitments by international agreements, and for the purpose of conserving, developing, and enhancing the fish in the Great Lakes and Lake Champlain that ascend streams to spawn, the Secretary of the Interior is authorized to enter into cooperative agreements with one or more States, acting jointly or severally, that are concerned with the development, conservation, and enhancement of such fish, . . ."

The Wildlife and Sport Fish Restoration Program is administered by the U.S. Fish and Wildlife Service under the three statutes:

5) Fish and Wildlife Conservation Act

Grants monies to states and tribes under the *Nongame* Act may be used for developing fish and wildlife conservation plans and actions, and for other purposes.

6) Federal Aid in Sport Fish Restoration Act, and

7) Federal Aid in Wildlife Restoration Act

Grant monies to states and tribes under these two Federal Aid statutes may be used to address research needs, fish and wildlife surveys, species recovery, habitat management, and monitoring activities identified in State Wildlife Action Plans.

8) Fish and Wildlife Act

"(B) PROJECTS AND PROGRAMS.—Subject to the requirements of the National Wildlife Refuge System Administration Act of 1966 (16 U.S.C. 668dd et seq.) and other applicable law, and such terms and conditions as the Secretary determines to be appropriate, the Secretary may approve projects and programs for a refuge or complex of geographically related refuges that— (i) promote the stewardship of resources of the refuge through habitat maintenance, restoration, and improvement, biological monitoring, or research;"

9) Fish and Wildlife Coordination Act

"SEC. 2. ø16 U.S.C. 662¿ (a) Except as hereafter stated in subsection (h) of this section, whenever the waters of any stream or other body of water are proposed or authorized to be impounded, diverted, the channel deepened, or the stream or other body of water otherwise controlled or modified for any purpose whatever, including navigation and drainage, by any department or agency of the United States, or by any public or private agency under Federal permit or license, such department or agency first shall consult with the United States Fish and Wildlife Service, Department of the Interior, and with the head of the agency exercising administration over the wildlife resources of the particular State wherein the impoundment, diversion, or other control facility is to be constructed, with a view to the conservation of wildlife resources by preventing loss of and damage to such resources as well as providing for the development and improvement thereof in connection with such water-resource development."

10) National Fish and Wildlife Foundation Establishment Act

"(b) PURPOSES.—The purposes of the Foundation are— (1) to encourage, accept, and administer private gifts of property for the benefit of, or in connection with, the activities and services of the United States Fish and Wildlife Service; and (2) to undertake and conduct such other activities as will further the conservation and management of the fish, wildlife, and plant resources of the United States, and its territories and possessions, for present and future generations of Americans."

11) Convention on International Trade in Endangered Species of Wild Fauna and Flora

CITES: https://cites.org/eng/disc/text.php

AIR, WATER, & SOIL

12) Clean Air Act

"SEC. 101 b) The purposes of this title are—
(1) to protect and enhance the quality of the Nation's air resources so as to promote the public health and welfare and the productive capacity of its population;"

13) Clean Water Act

"DECLARATION OF GOALS AND POLICY
SEC. 101. (a) The objective of this Act is to restore and maintain the chemical, physical, and biological integrity of the Nation's waters."

"SEC. 131.12(a)(l), or "Tier 1," protecting "existing uses," provides the absolute floor of water quality in all waters of the United States. This paragraph applies a minimum level of protection to all waters.

SEC. 131.12(a)(2), or "Tier 2," applies to waters whose quality exceeds that necessary to protect the section 101(a)(2) goals of the Act. In this case, water quality may not be lowered to less than the level necessary to fully protect the "fishable/swimmable" uses and other existing uses and may be lowered even to those levels only after following all the provisions described in section 131.12(a)(2).

SEC. 131.12(a)(3), or "Tier 3," applies to Outstanding National Resource Waters (ONRW) where the ordinary use classifications and supporting criteria may not be sufficient or appropriate. As described in the preamble to the Water Quality Standards Regulation, "States may allow some limited activities which result in temporary and short-term changes in water quality," but such changes in water quality should not impact existing uses or alter the essential character or special use that makes the water an ONRW."

"SEC. 303(c), states, territories, and tribes may:

- adopt, review, and revise water quality standards and implementation procedures in a public process. U.S. Environmental Protection Agency (EPA) must approve the standards which can be more stringent than EPA recommends.
-may certify that federally licensed activities that may result in any discharge to their waters meet these approved water quality standards"
https://www.epa.gov/sites/default/files/2014-10/documents/handbook-chapter4.pdf.

14) Watershed Protection and Flood Prevention Act

"Sec. 1011. Watershed restoration and enhancement agreements (a) In general For fiscal year 1997 and each fiscal year thereafter, appropriations made for the Bureau of Land Management may be used by the Secretary of the Interior for the purpose of entering into cooperative agreements with the heads of other Federal agencies, tribal, State, and local governments, private and nonprofit entities, and landowners for the protection, restoration, and enhancement of fish and wildlife habitat and other resources on public or private land and the reduction of risk from natural disaster where public safety is threatened that benefit these resources on public lands within the watershed."

15) Soil and Water Resources Conservation Act

"SEC. 2. The Congress finds that: (1) There is a growing demand on the soil, water, and related resources of the Nation to meet present and future needs. (2) The Congress, in its concern for sustained use of the resource base, created the Soil Conservation Service of the United States Department of Agriculture which possesses information, technical expertise, and a delivery system for providing assistance to land users with respect to conservation and use of soils; plants; woodlands; watershed protection and flood prevention; the conservation, development, utilization, and disposal of water; animal husbandry; fish and wildlife management;"

16) Land and Water Conservation Fund Act

"(b) PURPOSES.—. . . ";(1) providing funds for and authorizing Federal assistance to the States in planning, acquisition, and development of needed land and water areas and facilities and (2) providing funds for the Federal acquisition and development of certain lands and other areas."

NATIONAL ENVIRONMENTAL POLICY

17) National Environmental Policy Act

"An Act to establish a national policy for the environment, to provide for the establishment of a Council on Environmental Quality, and for other purposes."

"Purpose Sec. 2

The purposes of this Act are: To declare a national policy which will encourage productive and enjoyable harmony between man and his environment; to promote efforts which will prevent or eliminate damage to the environment and biosphere and stimulate the health and welfare of man; to enrich the understanding of the ecological systems and natural resources important to the Nation; and to establish a Council on Environmental Quality."

"Sec. 101 [42 USC § 4331]. (a) The Congress, recognizing the profound impact of man's activity on the interrelations of all components of the natural environment, particularly the profound influences of population growth, high-density urbanization, industrial expansion, resource exploitation, and new and expanding technological advances and recognizing further the critical importance of restoring and maintaining environmental quality to the overall welfare and development of man, declares that it is the continuing policy of the Federal Government, in cooperation with State and local governments, and other concerned public and private organizations, to use all practicable means and measures, including financial and technical assistance, in a manner calculated to foster and promote the general welfare, to create and maintain conditions under which man and nature can exist in productive harmony, and fulfill the social, economic, and other requirements of present and future generations of Americans.

(b) In order to carry out the policy set forth in this Act, it is the continuing responsibility of the Federal Government to use all practicable means, consist with other essential considerations of national policy, to improve and coordinate Federal plans, functions, programs, and resources to the end that the Nation may –
1. fulfill the responsibilities of each generation as trustee of the environment for succeeding generations;
2. assure for all Americans safe, healthful, productive, and aesthetically and culturally pleasing surroundings;
3. attain the widest range of beneficial uses of the environment without degradation, risk to health or safety, or other undesirable and unintended consequences;
4. preserve important historic, cultural, and natural aspects of our national heritage, and maintain, wherever possible, an environment which supports diversity, and variety of individual choice;
5. achieve a balance between population and resource use which will permit high standards of living and a wide sharing of life's amenities; and
6. enhance the quality of renewable resources and approach the maximum attainable recycling of depletable resources. (c) The Congress recognizes that each person should enjoy a healthful environment and that each person has a responsibility to contribute to the preservation and enhancement of the environment."

Cumulative Effects
https://ceq.doe.gov/docs/ceq-publications/ccenepa/sec1.pdf.
Incorporating Biodiversity
https://ceq.doe.gov/docs/ceq-publications/Incorporating_Biodiversity_1993.pdf.
Council on Environmental Quality, Executive Office of the President

REGULATIONS For Implementing The Procedural Provisions Of The NATIONAL ENVIRONMENTAL POLICY ACT Reprint 40 CFR Parts 1500-1508 (2010)

"40 CFR § 1500.1 Purpose.

> (a) The National Environmental Policy Act (NEPA) is our basic national charter for protection of the environment. . . .
> (b) NEPA procedures must insure that environmental information is available to public officials and citizens before decisions are made and before actions are taken. The information must be of high quality. Accurate scientific analysis, expert agency comments, and public scrutiny are essential to implementing NEPA. Most important, NEPA documents must concentrate on the issues that are truly significant to the action in question, rather than amassing needless detail."

"40 CFR § 1508.18 Major Federal action.
"Major Federal action" includes actions with effects that may be major and which are potentially subject to Federal control and responsibility."

18) National Historic Preservation Act

"54 U.S.C. § 300101. Policy

It is the policy of the Federal Government, in cooperation with other nations and in partnership with States, local governments, Indian tribes, Native Hawaiian organizations, and private organizations and individuals, to— (1) use measures, including financial and technical assistance, to foster conditions under which our modern society and our historic property can exist in productive harmony and fulfill the social, economic, and other requirements of present and future generations; (2) provide leadership in the preservation of the historic property of the United States and of the international community of nations and in the administration of the national preservation program; (3) administer federally owned, administered, or controlled historic property in a spirit of stewardship for the inspiration and benefit of present and future generations; (4) contribute to the preservation of non-federally owned historic property and give maximum encouragement to organizations and individuals undertaking preservation by private means; (5) encourage the public and private preservation and utilization of all usable elements of the Nation's historic built environment; and (6) assist State and local governments, Indian tribes and Native Hawaiian organizations, and the National Trust to expand and accelerate their historic preservation programs and activities."

RESTORATION OF INJURED NATURAL RESOURCES

The Natural Resource Damage Assessment and Restoration (NRDAR) process is used by federal, state, and tribal agencies to determine whether public natural resources have been injured, destroyed, or lost as a result of a release of hazardous substances or oil and to identify the actions and funds needed to restore these resources.
The NRDAR process is authorized by the Clean Water Act and the two statutes below:

19) Comprehensive Environmental Response, Compensation, and Liability Act (CERCLA or Superfund)

20) Oil Pollution Act

These statutes designate federal, state and tribal government officials to act as 'trustees" on behalf of the public to recover damages from responsible parties to restore injured, destroyed, or lost natural resources. Damages can include money for trustee implementation of restoration actions and/or work undertaken by responsible parties with trustee oversight.

The goal of the NRDAR Program is restoration of injured natural resources. This drives the damage assessment process and provides the basis for the damage claim. Over ninety percent of all funds received from natural resource damage case settlements and judicial agreements are designated as restoration funds. After the development of a publicly-reviewed restoration plan, the NRDAR Program and co-trustees implement restoration projects, often in partnership with non-governmental groups, local governments, and sometimes the responsible party. Through these actions, injured natural resources and the services they provide are restored at the expense of the responsible party, not the taxpaying public.

21) Partners for Fish and Wildlife Act

"SEC. 2. FINDINGS AND PURPOSE.

(a) FINDINGS.—Congress finds that—
(7) since 1987, the Partners for Fish and Wildlife Program has exemplified cooperative conservation as an innovative, voluntary partnership program that helps private landowners restore wetland and other important fish and wildlife habitat; and
(8) through 33,103 agreements with private landowners, the Partners for Fish and Wildlife Program has accomplished the restoration of 677,000 acres of wetland, 1,253,700 acres of prairie and native grasslands, and 5,560 miles of riparian and in-stream habitat since 1987, demonstrating much of that success since only 2001.

(b) PURPOSE.—The purpose of this Act is to provide for the restoration, enhancement, and management of fish and wildlife habitats on private land through the Partners for Fish and Wildlife Program, a program that works with private landowners to conduct cost-effective habitat projects for the benefit of fish and wildlife resources in the United States."

LAND MANAGEMENT

22) Wild and Scenic Rivers Act

"(b) It is hereby declared to be the policy of the United States that certain selected rivers of the Nation which, with their immediate environments, possess outstandingly remarkable scenic, recreational, geologic, fish and wildlife, historic, cultural, or other similar values, shall be preserved in free-flowing condition, and that they and their immediate environments shall be protected for the benefit and enjoyment of present and future generations. The Congress declares that the established national policy of dam and other construction at appropriate sections of the rivers of the United States needs to be complemented by a policy that would preserve other selected rivers or sections thereof in their free-flowing condition to protect the water quality of such rivers and to fulfill other vital national conservation purposes."

"SECTION 6. (a) (1) The Secretary of the Interior and the Secretary of Agriculture are each authorized to acquire lands and interests in land within the authorized boundaries of any component of the national wild and scenic rivers system designated in section 3 of this Act, or hereafter designated for inclusion in the system by Act of Congress, which is administered by him, but he shall not acquire fee title to an average of more than 100 acres per mile on both sides of the river."

23) The Wilderness Act

"AN ACT To establish a National Wilderness Preservation System for the permanent good of the whole people, and for other purposes."

WILDERNESS SYSTEM ESTABLISHED STATEMENT OF POLICY

"SECTION 2. (a) In order to assure that an increasing population, accompanied by expanding settlement and growing mechanization, does not occupy and modify all areas within the United States and its possessions, leaving no lands designated for preservation and protection in their natural condition, it is hereby declared to be the policy of the Congress to secure for the American people of present and future generations the benefits of an enduring resource of wilderness. For this purpose there is hereby established a National Wilderness Preservation System to be composed of federally owned areas designated by Congress as "wilderness areas", and these shall be administered for the use and enjoyment of the American people in such manner as will leave them unimpaired for future use and enjoyment as wilderness, and so as to provide for the protection of these areas, the preservation of their wilderness character, and for the gathering and dissemination of information regarding their use and enjoyment as wilderness; and no Federal lands shall be designated as "wilderness areas" except as provided for in this Act or by a subsequent Act."

24) North American Wetlands Conservation Act

"AN ACT To conserve North American wetland ecosystems and waterfowl and the other migratory birds and fish and wildlife that depend upon such habitats."

"SEC. 9. RESTORATION, MANAGEMENT, AND PROTECTION OF WETLANDS AND HABITAT FOR MIGRATORY BIRDS ON FEDERAL LANDS. The head of each Federal agency responsible for acquiring, managing, or disposing of Federal lands and waters shall, to the extent consistent with the mission of such agency and existing statutory authorities, cooperate with the Director of the United States Fish and Wildlife Service to restore, protect, and enhance the wetland ecosystems and other habitats for migratory birds, fish, and wildlife within the lands and waters of each such agency."

25) Bureau of Land Management – Federal Land Management Policy and Management Act

"DECLARATION OF POLICY

Sec. 102. The Congress declares that it is the policy of the United States that–
(8) the public lands be managed in a manner that will protect the quality of scientific, scenic, historical, ecological, environmental, air and atmospheric, water resource, and archaeological values; that, where appropriate, will preserve and protect certain public lands in their natural condition; that will provide food and habitat for fish and wildlife and domestic animals; and that will provide for outdoor recreation and human occupancy and use;"

26) National Park Service – National Park System Organic Act

"Subtitle I—National Park System

DIVISION A—ESTABLISHMENT AND GENERAL ADMINISTRATION
CHAPTER 1001—GENERAL PROVISIONS
§100101. Promotion and regulation

(a) In General.—The Secretary, acting through the Director of the National Park Service, shall promote and regulate the use of the National Park System by means and measures that conform to the fundamental purpose of the System units, which purpose is to conserve the scenery, natural and historic objects, and wild life in the System units and to provide for the enjoyment of the scenery, natural and historic objects, and wild life in such manner and by such means as will leave them unimpaired for the enjoyment of future generations."

27) U.S. Fish and Wildlife Service – National Wildlife Refuge System Administration Act

"(2) The mission of the System is to administer a national network of lands and waters for the conservation, management, and where appropriate, restoration of the fish, wildlife, and plant resources and their habitats within the United States."

28) U.S. Forest Service – National Forest Management Act

"Renewable Resource Program"
"(C) recognize the fundamental need to protect and where appropriate, improve the quality of soil, water, and air resources;
(D) state national goals that recognize the interrelationships between and interdependence within the renewable resources;"

Special Thank You

Author's Acknowledgements

A special thank you to each of you for your ideas, inspiration, love, and support, to my colleagues: Vivian Vergara, Holistic Wellness Specialist, Sarasota, Florida, and Eleanor Tison, Co-Director, Green Mountain Center for Sustainability, Prescott College, Arizona; Kristin Little, close friend; and to my family: Shelley Ehrlich, Leah Wing, Deepika Marya, Jesse Wing, Monica Harris, Olivia Wing, and Elle Wing.

With Great Appreciation to These Talented Illustrators and Photographers at ©Dreamstime.com

1evgeniya1
7active Studio
7vect0r
Abel Tumik
Adamnizol
Adisak Rungjaruchai
Adogslifephoto
Agami Photo Agency
Ahmad Safarudin
Ajafoto
Akinshin
Aleksandr Andrushkiv
Alessandra Rc
Alexander Babich
Alexander Konoplyov
Alexander Pokusay
Alexander Raths
Alexey Stiop
Alexoakenman
Alexokov
Allegro7
Allexxandar
Altitudevs
Altitudevs
Amnat Buakeaw
Anastasia Darii
Anastasiia Zabolotna
Anatoly Repin
Andegraund548
Andjelka Simic
Andreistanescu
Andreuma3
Andreus
Andrey
Andrey Golubtsov
Andrii Bezvershenko
Anemad
Anggraeni Sri Rahayu
Anico G. Enderle
Anikasalsera
Ann Moore
Anna
Anna Bergbauer
Anna Komisarenko
Anna Kucherova
Anna Lopatina
Anna Puhan
Anna Rusan
Anna Sedneva
AnnaMartinskaya
Annzabella
Araya Pacharabandit
Ariadna De Raadt
Arkela
Arloofs
Artem Efimov
Artex67
Artness
ArtoPhotoDesignoStudio
Artur Balitskii
Artur Kutskyi
Asetrovaann
Athapet Piruksa
Aviag7
Ayutaka
Azot Susila
Beata Jana Filarova
Beautifulblossom
Beinluck
Belusuab
Bert Folsom
Bianca Wisseloo
Biancaoddi
Blackphoenix1980
Bobyramone
Bohdan Skrypnyk
Boonmee
Bruce Macqueen
Canan Baris
Candace Schoner
Captivatinglightphotos
Casejustin
Castecodesign
Catarii
Charmaine Paulson
Chase Dekker
Chernetskaya
Chinook203
Chon Kit Leong
Chumporn Chophwan
Cleverson Felix
Cobia
Colin Buckland
Colorcocktail
Compsachen
Conceptcafe
Cookamoto
Corey A Ford
Corina Tintila
Cornelius20
Daisuke Kurashima
Daria Likhodedova
Dave Massey
David Cornelius
davidhoffmannphotography
Dayzeren
Debrahughes
Denis Kostroma
Dennis Jacobsen
Designua
Diana Eller
Diidik
Dipak Talati
Dj0038
Djvstock
Dmitry Krikun
Dmstudio
dorsetgirl2001
Dpimborough
Dracozlat
Duc Hong
dvoriankin
Eak Kem
Ekaterina Efanova
Ekaterina Glazkova
Ekaterina Mikheeva
Ekaterina Romenskaia
Elena
Elena Borisova
Elena Elisseeva
Elena Medvedeva
Eleonora Ivanova
Elina Yakhontova
Elizaveta Poroshina
Elokuu
Ennjee
Erik Zunec
Erika Norris
Erinphoto10
Ernest Akayeu
Ethan Daniels
Evamask
Evgeniia Parkhomenko
Evgeniya Grishkina
Ezumeimages
Famveldman
Farinoza
Fascinadora
Flashvector
Foster
Fotografiecor
Foxyliam
Francesco Pussumato
Frank Fichtmueller
Fredweiss
Freeprintbq
Friesart
Galina Malareva
Gary Gray
Georgii Dolgykh
Gijsvdabeele
Gl0ck33
Gloria Rosazza
Godruma
Golden Sikorka
Gorgulias
Grant Phillips
Grazia Natalotto
Green earth with leaves
Gribnick
Hanna Hryharenka
Harijanto Suwarno
Hartnett2007
Heather Jones
Henk Wallays
Honourableandbold
Hsiu Chuan Yu
Iamnee
Idey
Ievgen Melamud
Igor Tokalenko
Igor Zakharevich
Ihor Svetiukha
Ilja Enger Tsizikov
Ilya Golubev
Ilyakalinin
Imaginiac
Info11778
Inkdropcreative1
Inna Feshchyn
Inspirationupload
Ipolstock
Iquacu
Ira529
Iricat
Irina Belokrylova
Irinafotina
Irinav
Iryna Lukashuk
Iryna Zaichenko
Ivandzyuba
Ivansabo
Izanbar
Izonda
J2
Jairo Souza
James Mahan
Jan Havlicek
Jason Hindman
Jason Ondreicka
Jean Landry
Jedimaster
jeff waibel
Jehsomwang
Jenifoto406
Jianghongyan
Jixin Yu
Jminka
Joachim Berschauer
Joannatkaczuk
John Anderson
John Sirlin
Jon Bilous
Jose Mathew
Juan Moyano
Julian Popov
Juliengrondin
Justlight
Jyothi
Kamenuka
Kannan Sundaram
Karen Foley
Karl Ander Adami
Karl Umbriaco
Katarinochka
Kateryna Kon
Katrinshine
Keechuan
Kinek00
Kingan
Kitti Kahotong
Konstantin
Konstantin Gerasimov
Konstantin Kostan
Kostiantyn Kravchenko
Kotina
Kristof Lauwers
Ksena Shu
Ksenyasavva
Kurylo54
Kutukupretkw2
Leekkk
Lehmanphotos
Lesia Pavlenko
Lesichkadesign
Lhall49
Lianainasaridze
Lightkeeper
Liliya Shlapak
Lim Seng Kui

With Great Appreciation to These Talented Illustrators and Photographers at ©Dreamstime.com

Liskonogaleksey
Llopartic
Lnsdes
Loflo69
Loreena
Lorna Jane
Luayana
Luis Echeverri Urrea
Lukaves
Lyubov Tolstova
Maart
Macrovector Art
Madartists
Maksim Bazarov
Maksim Pauliukevich
Mappingz01
Marazem
Margarita Vais
Margaritashi
Margo555
Maria Bobrova
Maria Kalashnik
Mariia Bogdanova
Mariia Domnikova
Mariia Sultanova
Marilyn Gould
Marina Vorontsova
Marinodenisenko
Mariusz Prusaczyk
Mark Hryciw
Martin ProchÃ¡zka
Mary Salen
Maryna Hlushko
Maryna Lahereva
Massimo Parisi
Mast3r
Max Lashcheuski
Md Khurshid Alam
Michael Gray
Michael Woodruff
Mike Monahan
mikrobiuz
Mila130189
Miloart
Mirecca
Miriam Doerr
Mogilevchik
Mohammad Shirani
Molekuul
Monika Adamczyk
Moonkin
Mr E J Wilde
Mr.siwabud Veerapaisarn
Mrjpeg
Mudwalker
Muradin
Nadezhda Shoshina
Nadiaforkosh
Nadiia Havryliuk Kharzhevska
Nahhan
Natalia Kazakova
Natalie Shmeleva
Nataliia Darmoroz
Nataliia Demydenko
Nataliia Vladymyrova
Natasha55
NatashaBreen
Natis76
Ncl
Nedim Bajramovic
Nehru
Nenilkime
Nerss
Nevinates
Nextmars
Nina Firsova
Nitipat Sadtasirichai
Nitr
Norbert Buchholz
Nurma Agung
Oksana Ermak
Oksana Smyshliaeva
Oksanabratanova
Oleksandra Martiukova
Oleksiy Kovalenko
Olena Danileiko
Olena Troshchak
Olesh
Olesya Turchuk
Olga Hmelevskaya
Olga Kriger
Ondrej
onnada srilawong
Orxpikdesign
Pairoj Sroyngern
Pascal Halder
Passiveaggressive
Patarajan
Pattarawit Chompipat
Pavel Naumov
Pavlo Syvak
Penchan Pumila
Peter Leahy
Phanuchat Prasertpol
Pheby
Philipp Schlüter
Photogallet
Picture Partners
Pimonpim Tangosol
Pisicasfioasa
Pisotckii
Piyapong Thongdumhyu
Pkzphotos
Pleshko74
Pnwnature
Polelya
Portraitquo
Potatushkina
Potysiev
Ppy2010ha
Pram Samnak
Premyuda Yospim
Pressmaster
Ptasha
Rainer
Raman Maisei
Ramilf
Rawpixelimages
Richard Carey
Rima Al Turk
Rinus Baak
Riverlim
Rob Jorg
Roberto Scandola
Robin Nelson
Rolandtopor
Roman Ivaschenko
Romana Anji
Ruslan Batiuk
Russieseo
Rvlsoft
Sabelskaya
Sarawut Samansup
Sarsmis
Sasha Kircanski
Sasha Kondr
Satheesh Rajh Rajagopalan
Sayda Nargish Parvin
Sburel
Scott Karcich
Seadam
Seamartini
Sean Steininger
Selentaoriart
Selvam Raghupathy
Sergey Kolesnikov
Serjio74
Setory
Siarhei Nosyreu
Siberica27
Sikth
Silvionka
Slowmotiongli
Snitovets
Soleilc
Somesun
Sonulkaster
Spelagranda
Stefano Ember
Stephan Pietzko
Stephen Moehle
Steve Byland
Steven Melanson
Stockeeco
Stu Porter
Styranets Oksana
Sumikophoto
Suriya Siritam
Sutichak
Svetlana Gardus
Svitlana Tereshchenko
Svitlana Vilhauk
Swee Ming Young
Takan Kaewswangsap
Tamara Didenko
Tanaphong Sattayamit
Tanyapeliustka
Tartilastock
Taseret
Tatiana Belova
Tatiana Pankova
Teekaygee
Teirin
Terrence Allison
Tetiana Gutnyk
Tetiana Kovalenko
Thanarat Boonmee
Themorningglory
Theresa
Thitinai Permsawat
Thongchai Anothai
THPStock
Tuja
Tural Mammadzada
Tyler Olson
Ueapun
Usersam2007
Vaivirga
Valentin Balan
Valentyn640
Valiva
Varvara Sharovatova
Vasyl Duda
Vasyl Kosolovskyy
VectorMine
Veronika Kornienko
Vgrebelskiy
Viacheslav Besputin
Viacheslav Dubrovin
Viennetta
Viktoria Kabanova
Viniciussouza06
Vismax
Vita30
Vitor Hugo Artigiani Filho
VittoriaChe
Vivilweb
Vladimir Ceresnak
Voislav Kolevski
Volha Paulava
Volodymyr Byrdyak
Volodymyr Markin
Volodymyr Ovcharov
Volodymyr Shevchuk
Wanlop Phuengyoi
Webpainterstd
Welcomia
Woodhouse84
Xsviatx
Yamasanphoto0708
Yamix
Yaroslav Borysovych
Yasonya
Yehor
Yelena Panyukova
Yin21205
Ylivdesign
Yodke67
Yodsawaj Suriyasirisin
Yolfran
Ys7485
Yuliia Inshyna
Yuliya Shevchenko
Yunaco
Yuri Arcurs
Yuriy Brykaylo
Zeechinchun
Zeninaasya
Zkruger

REFERENCE *for* COMPANION ACTIVITY BOOK

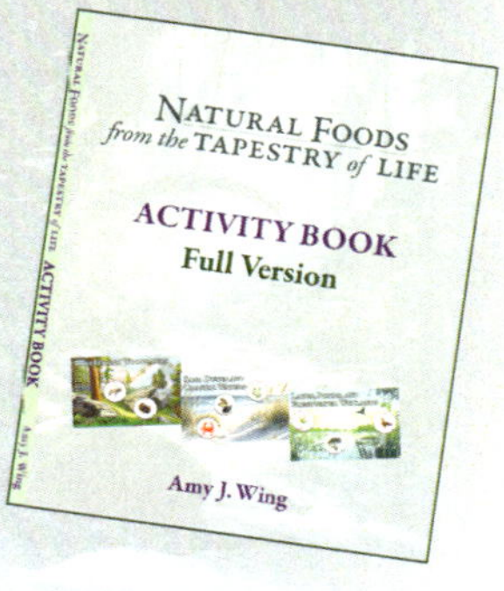

Common Food Groups
(Stickers for Activities)

Seafoods	Seeds
Meats	Seasonings
Milk Products	Vegetables
Land & Water Fowl Eggs	Leafy Greens
Animal Fats	Plant Oils
Fruits	Mushrooms
Grains	Seaweeds & Chlorella (Algae)
Legumes	Cyanobacteria
Nuts, Bark, Saps	Probiotic Ferments (Bacteria & Micro-Fungi)

Seafoods

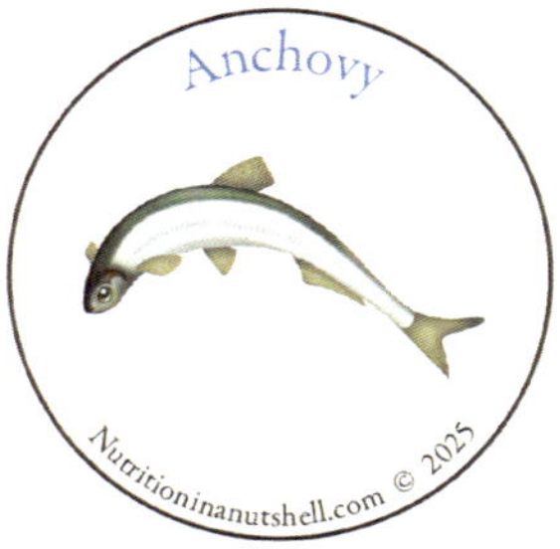
Anchovy
Nutritioninanutshell.com © 2025

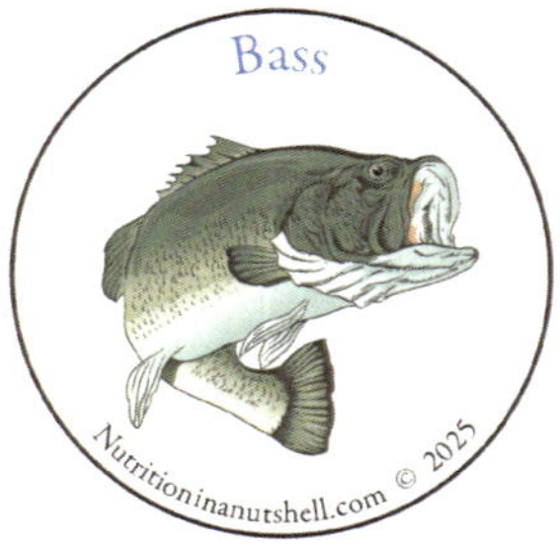
Bass
Nutritioninanutshell.com © 2025

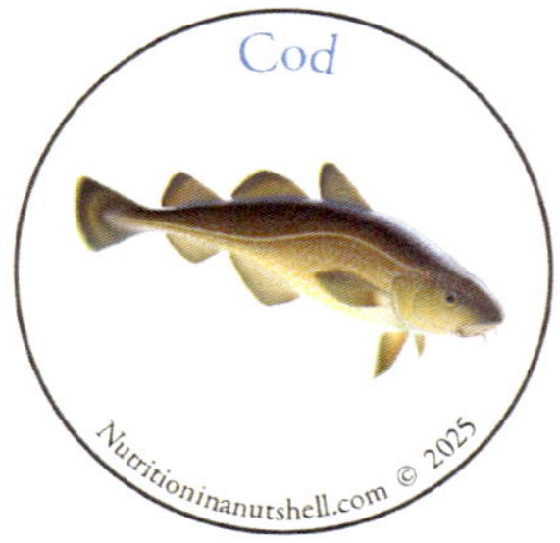
Cod
Nutritioninanutshell.com © 2025

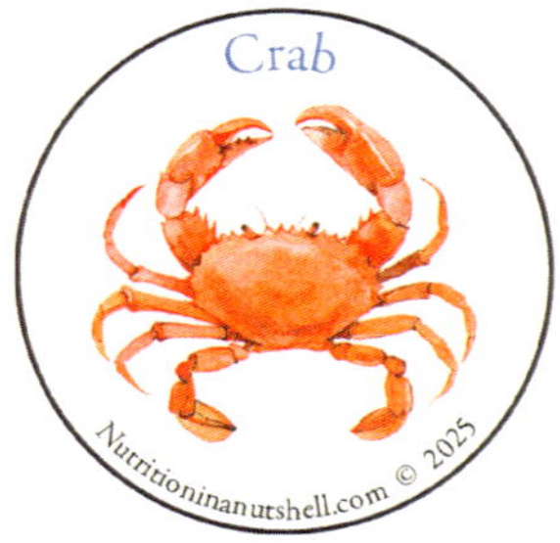
Crab
Nutritioninanutshell.com © 2025

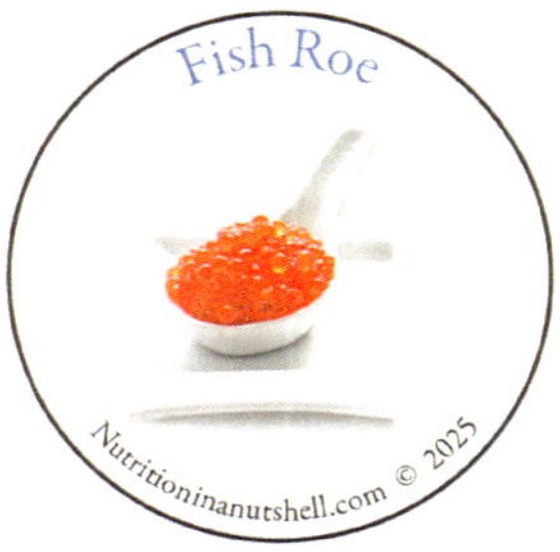
Fish Roe
Nutritioninanutshell.com © 2025

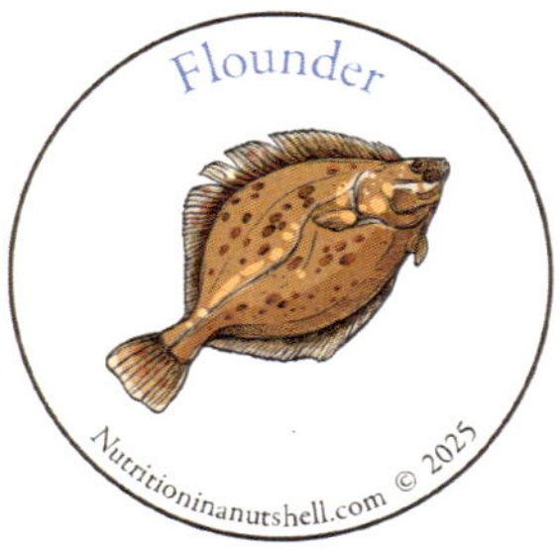
Flounder
Nutritioninanutshell.com © 2025

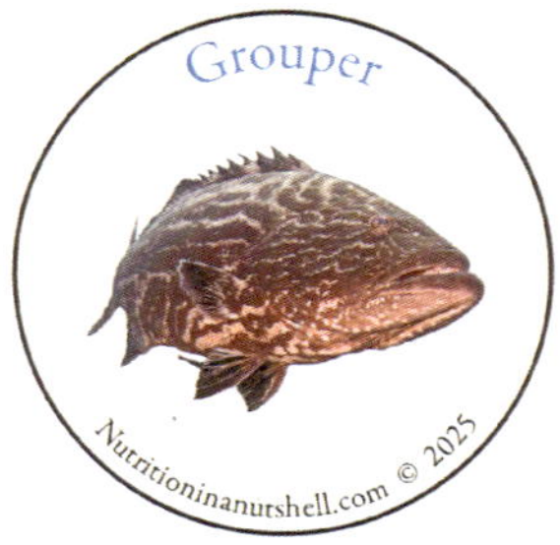
Grouper
Nutritioninanutshell.com © 2025

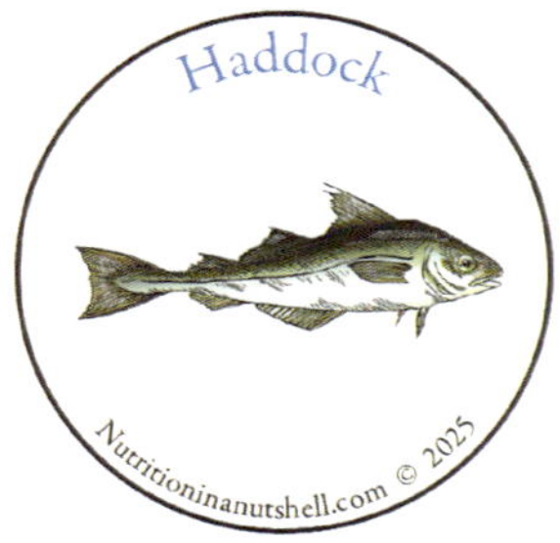
Haddock
Nutritioninanutshell.com © 2025

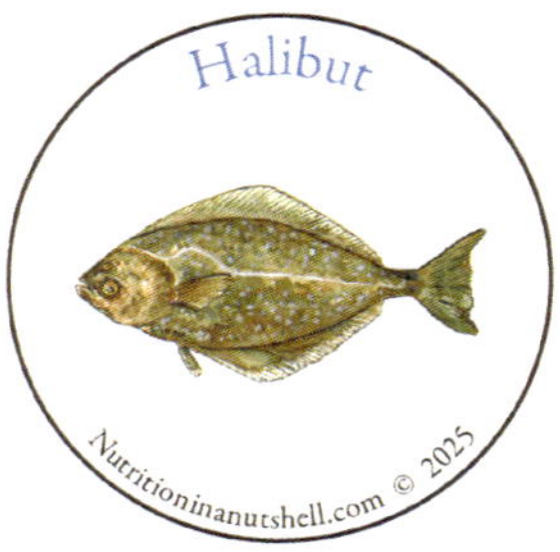
Halibut
Nutritioninanutshell.com © 2025

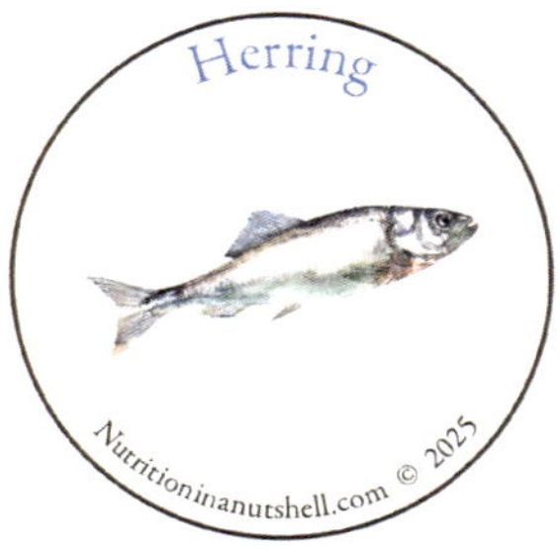
Herring
Nutritioninanutshell.com © 2025

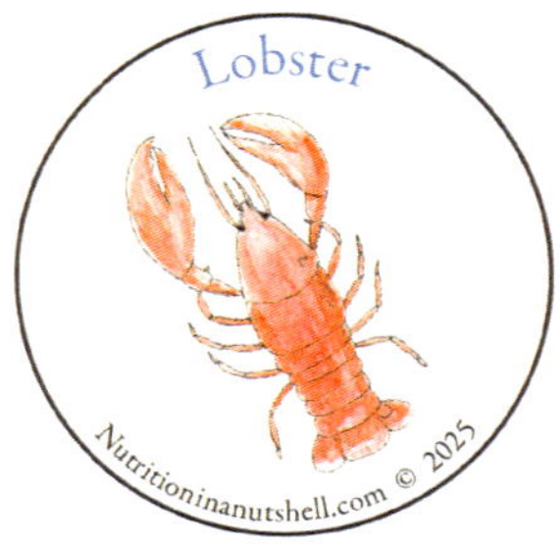
Lobster
Nutritioninanutshell.com © 2025

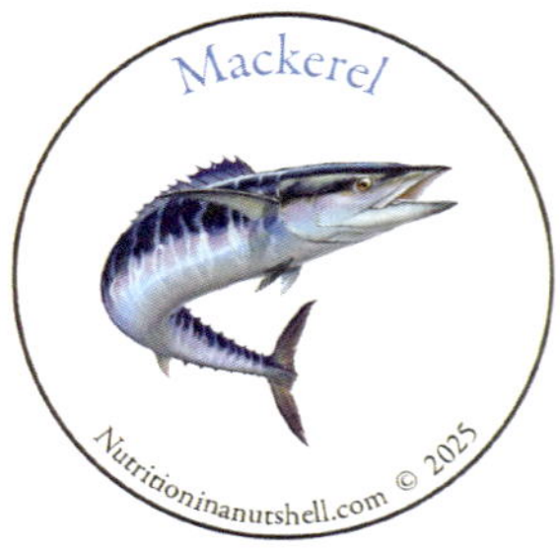
Mackerel
Nutritioninanutshell.com © 2025

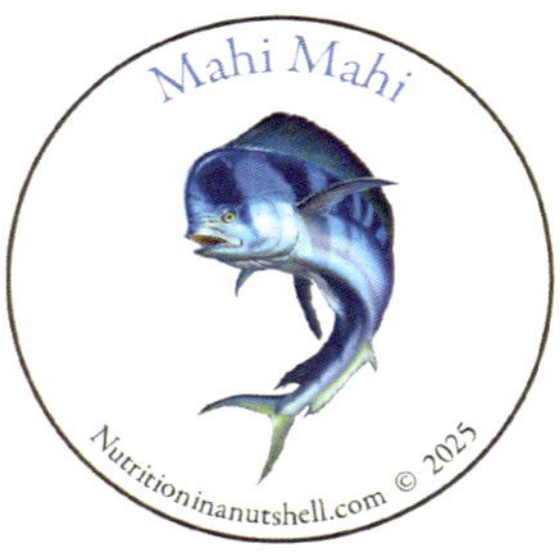
Mahi Mahi
Nutritioninanutshell.com © 2025

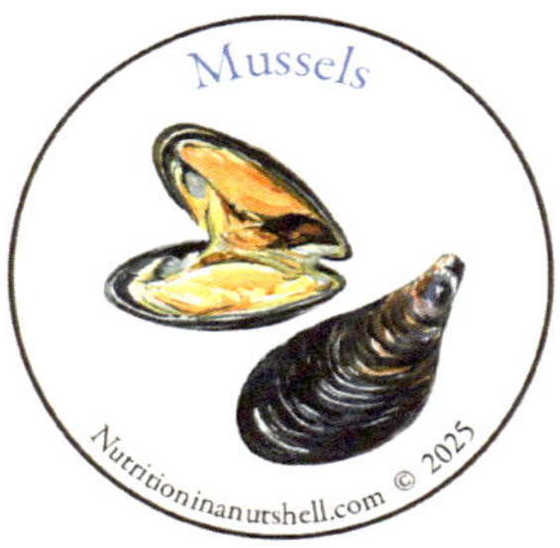
Mussels
Nutritioninanutshell.com © 2025

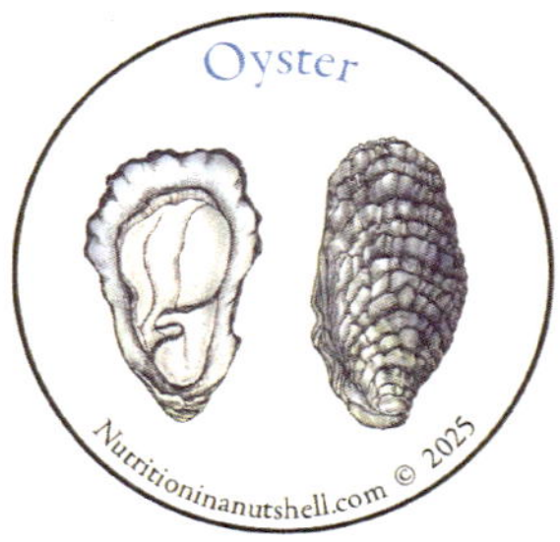
Oyster
Nutritioninanutshell.com © 2025

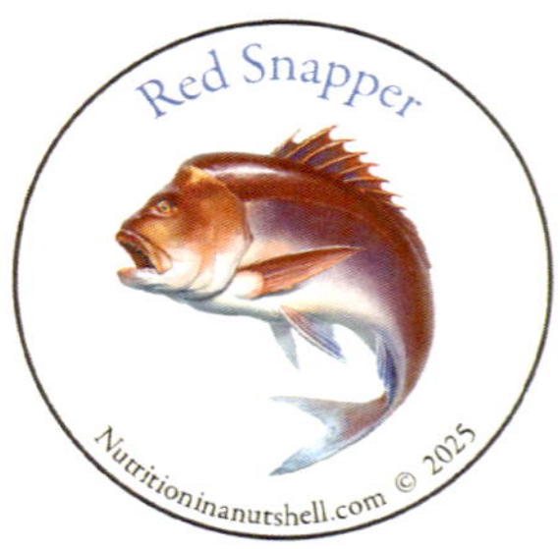
Red Snapper
Nutritioninanutshell.com © 2025

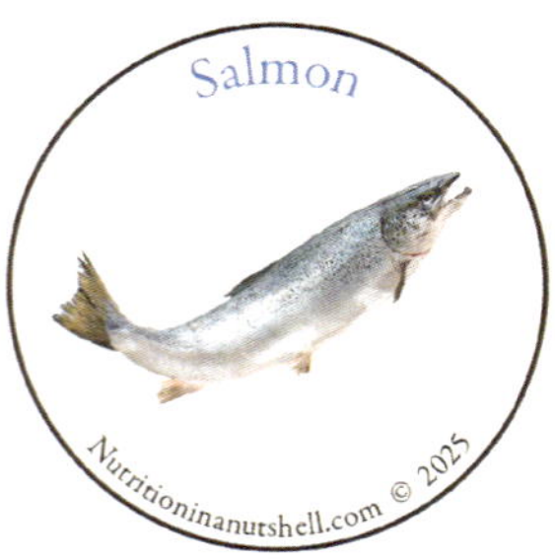
Salmon
Nutritioninanutshell.com © 2025

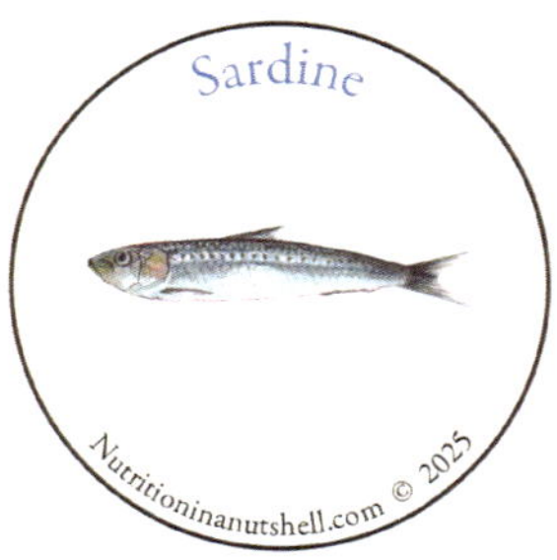
Sardine
Nutritioninanutshell.com © 2025

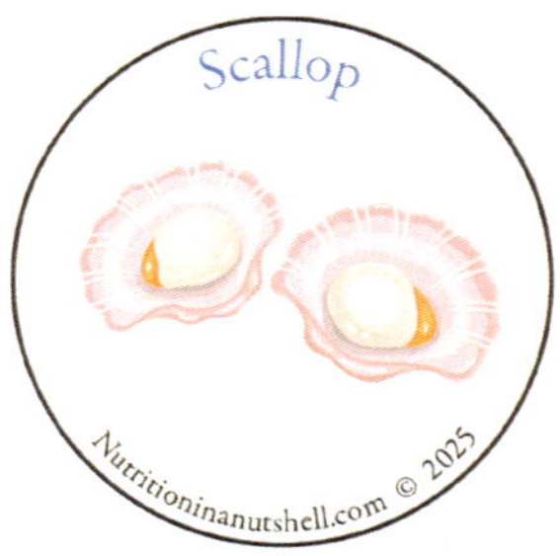
Scallop
Nutritioninanutshell.com © 2025

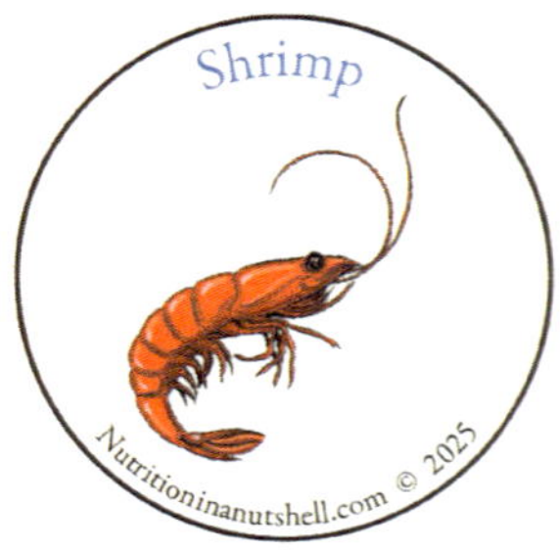
Shrimp
Nutritioninanutshell.com © 2025

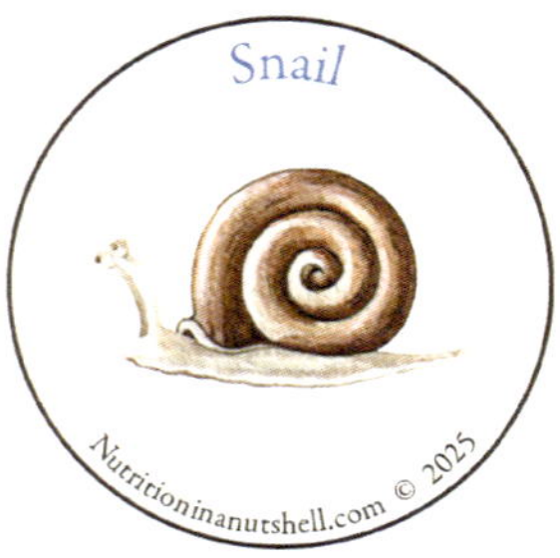
Snail
Nutritioninanutshell.com © 2025

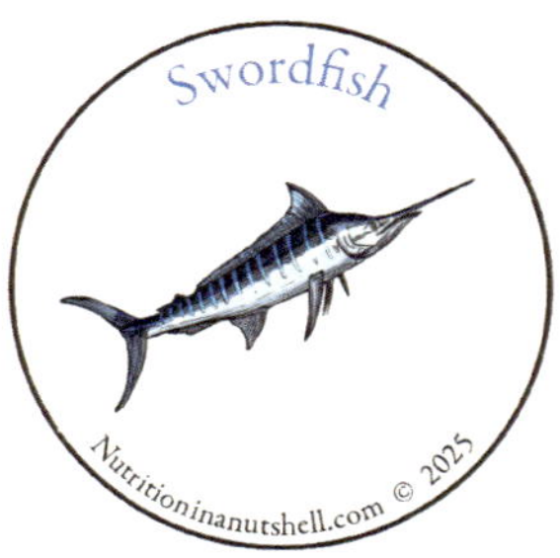
Swordfish
Nutritioninanutshell.com © 2025

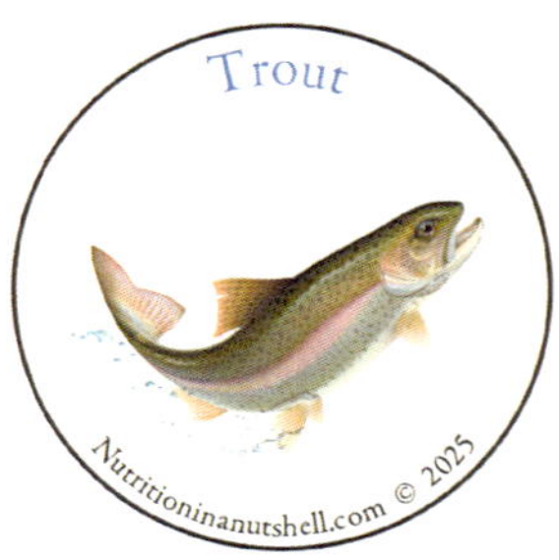
Trout
Nutritioninanutshell.com © 2025

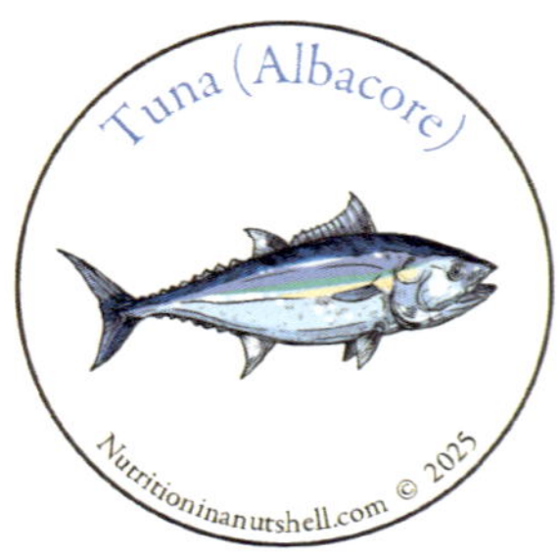
Tuna (Albacore)
Nutritioninanutshell.com © 2025

Seafoods

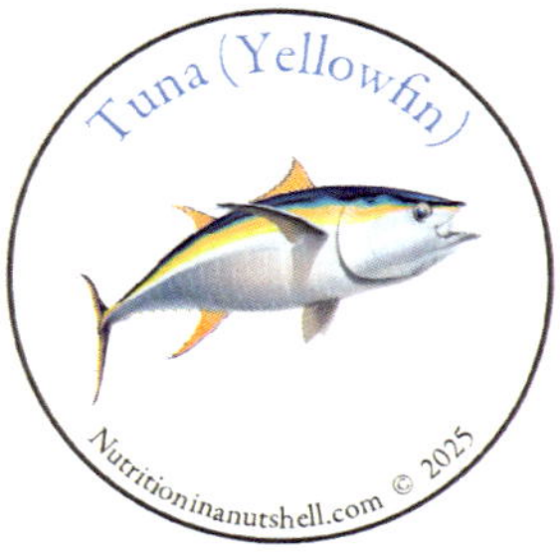
Tuna (Yellowfin)
Nutritioninanutshell.com © 2025

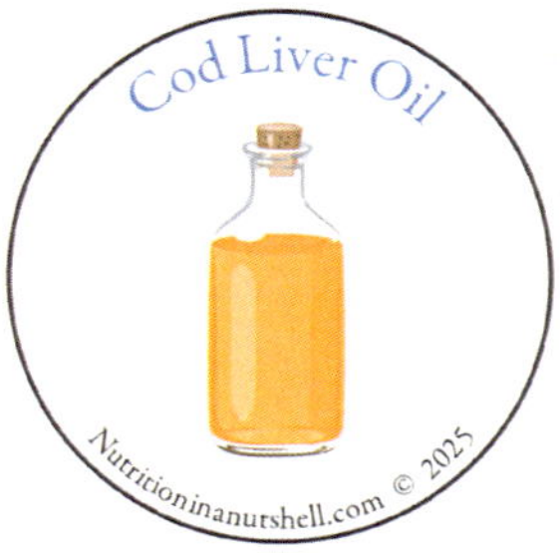
Cod Liver Oil
Nutritioninanutshell.com © 2025

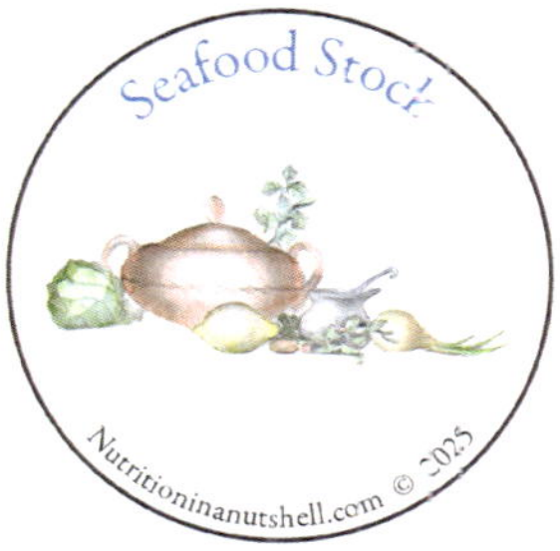
Seafood Stock
Nutritioninanutshell.com © 2025

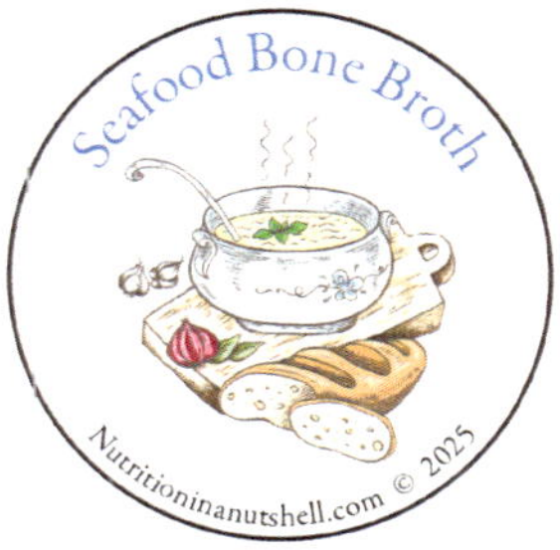
Seafood Bone Broth
Nutritioninanutshell.com © 2025

Meats

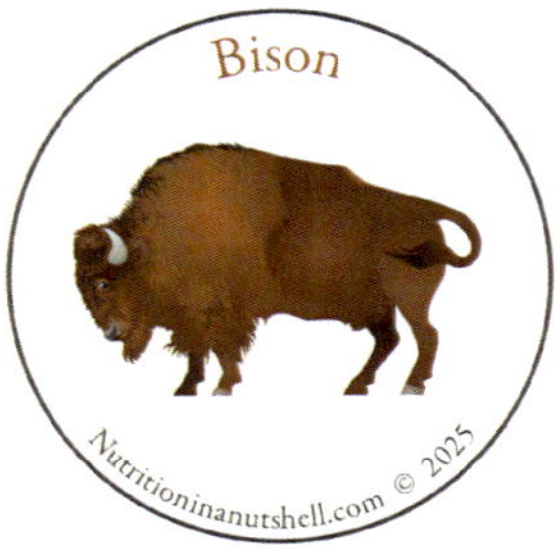
Bison
Nutritioninanutshell.com © 2025

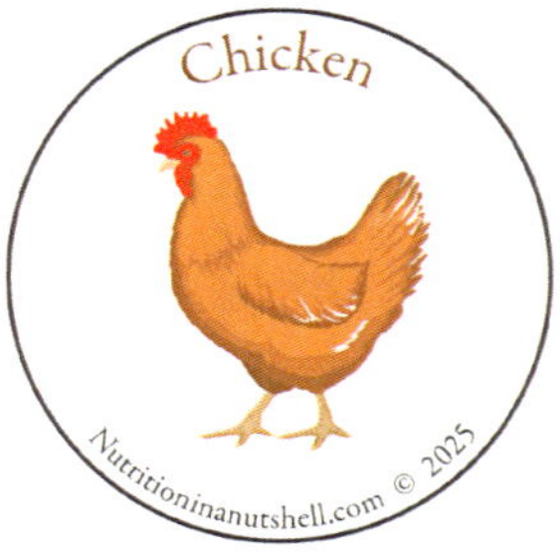
Chicken
Nutritioninanutshell.com © 2025

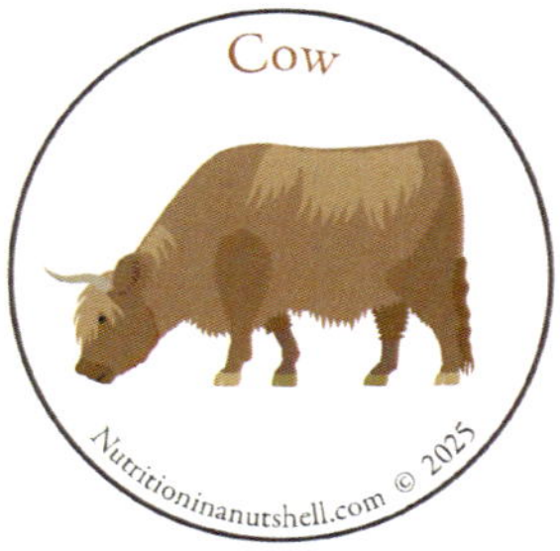
Cow
Nutritioninanutshell.com © 2025

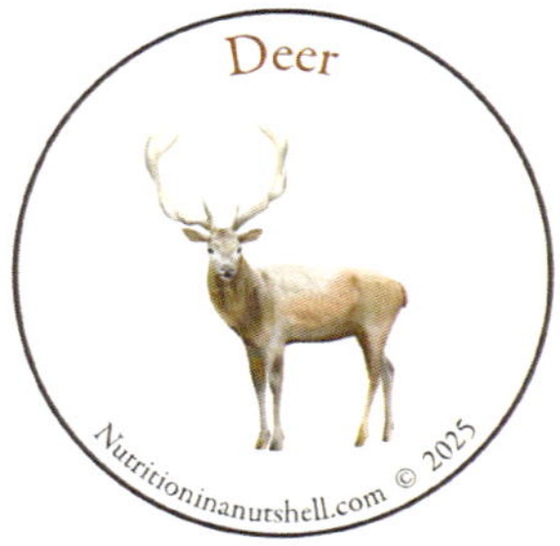
Deer
Nutritioninanutshell.com © 2025

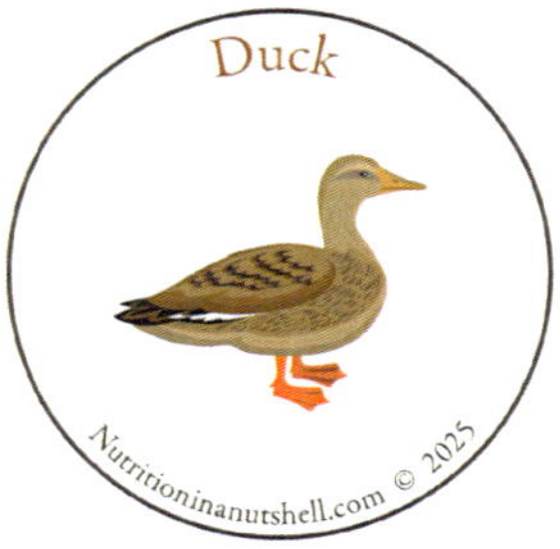
Duck
Nutritioninanutshell.com © 2025

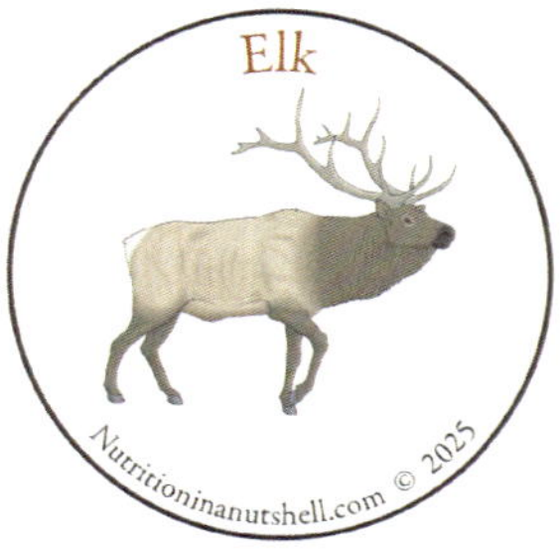
Elk
Nutritioninanutshell.com © 2025

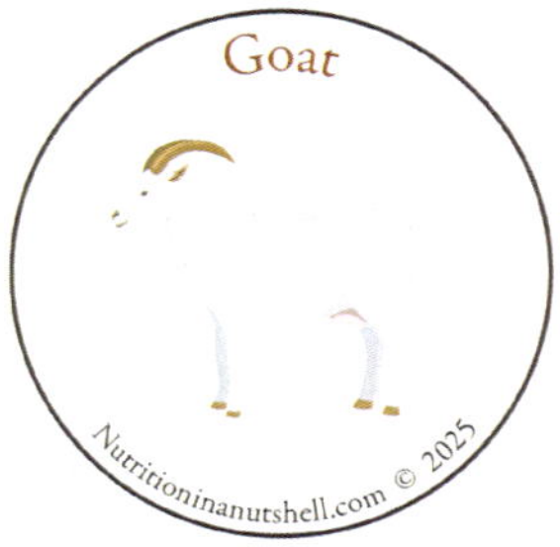
Goat
Nutritioninanutshell.com © 2025

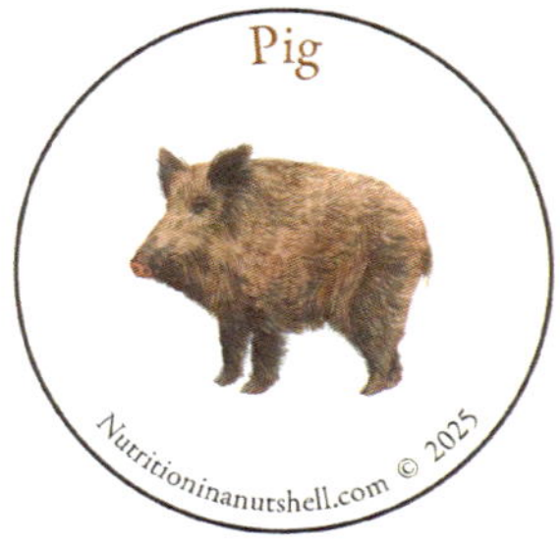
Pig
Nutritioninanutshell.com © 2025

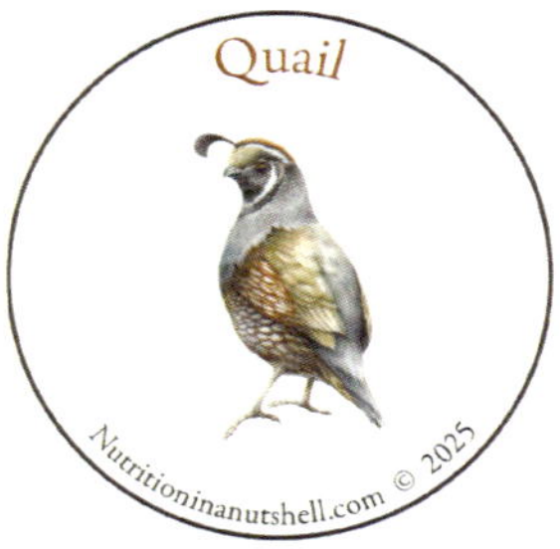
Quail
Nutritioninanutshell.com © 2025

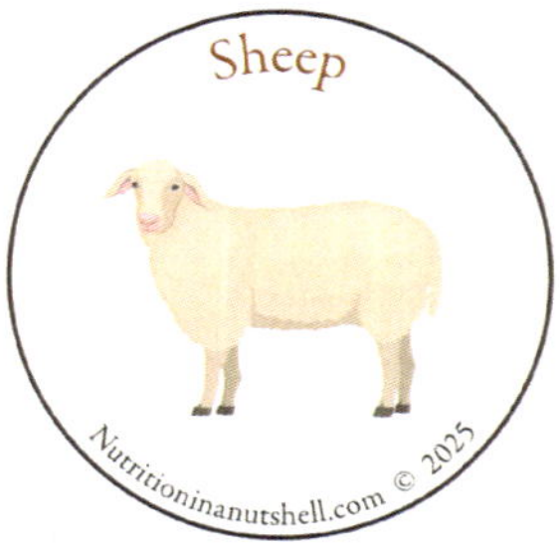
Sheep
Nutritioninanutshell.com © 2025

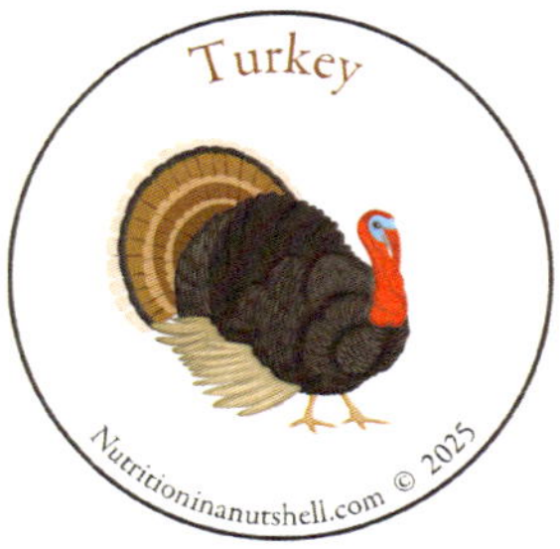
Turkey
Nutritioninanutshell.com © 2025

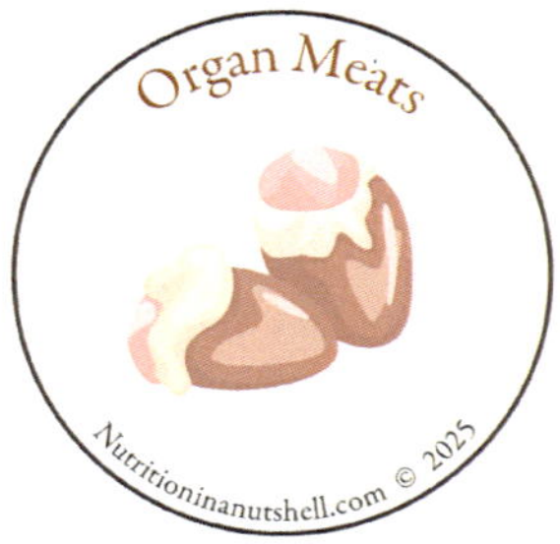
Organ Meats
Nutritioninanutshell.com © 2025

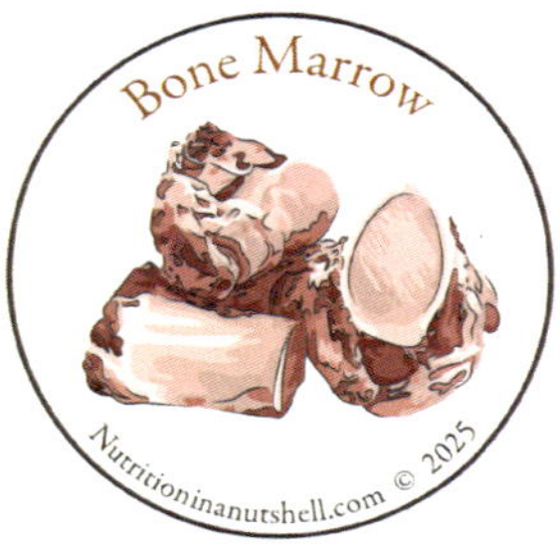
Bone Marrow
Nutritioninanutshell.com © 2025

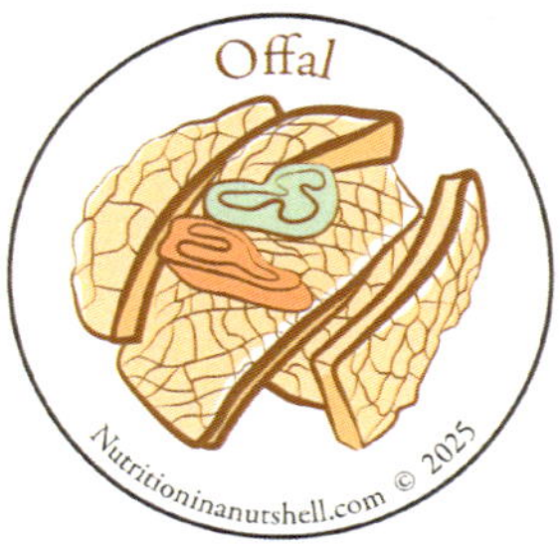
Offal
Nutritioninanutshell.com © 2025

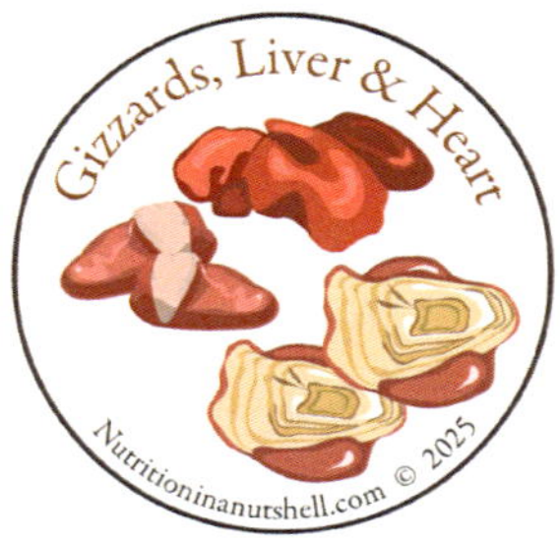
Gizzards, Liver & Heart
Nutritioninanutshell.com © 2025

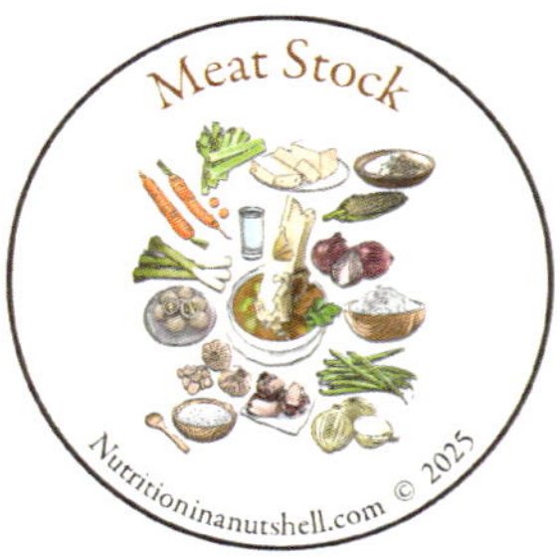
Meat Stock
Nutritioninanutshell.com © 2025

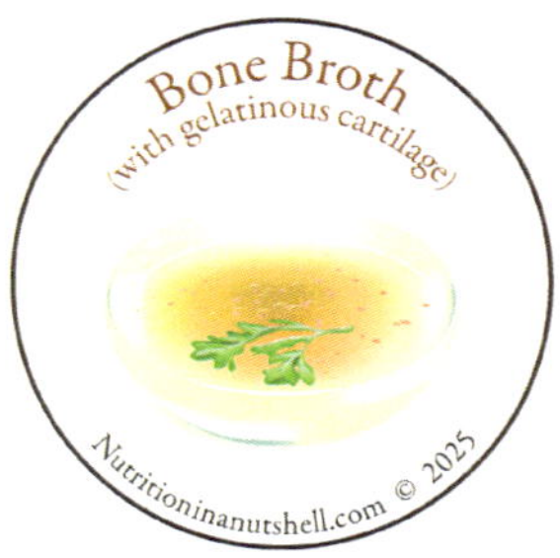
Bone Broth
(with gelatinous cartilage)
Nutritioninanutshell.com © 2025

Milk Products

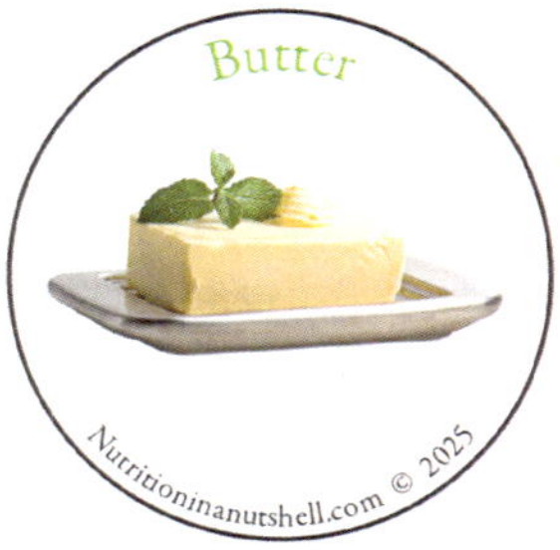

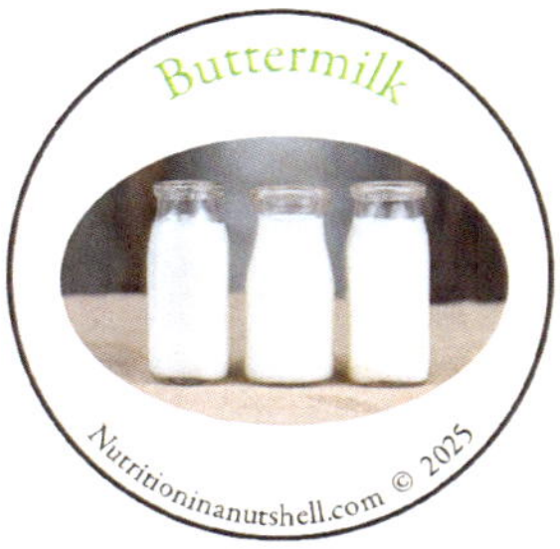

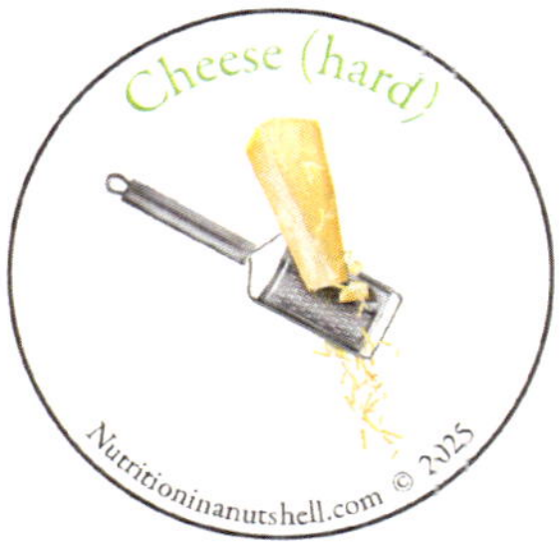

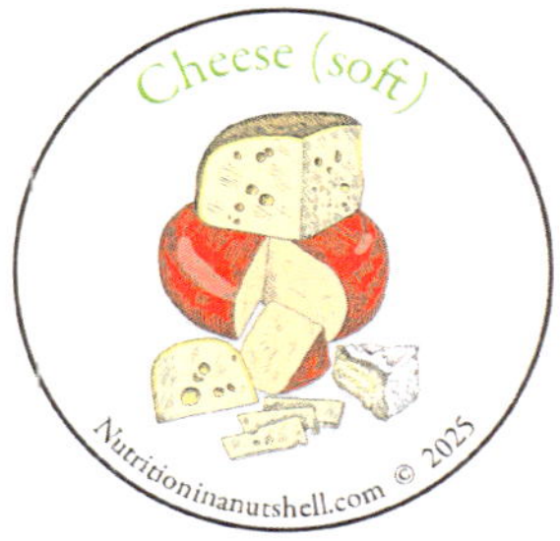

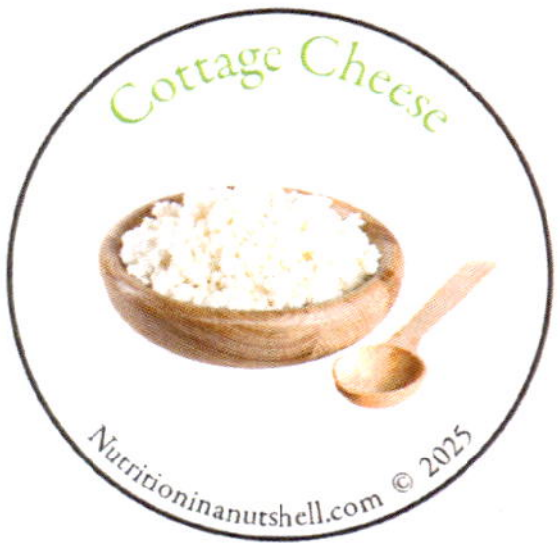

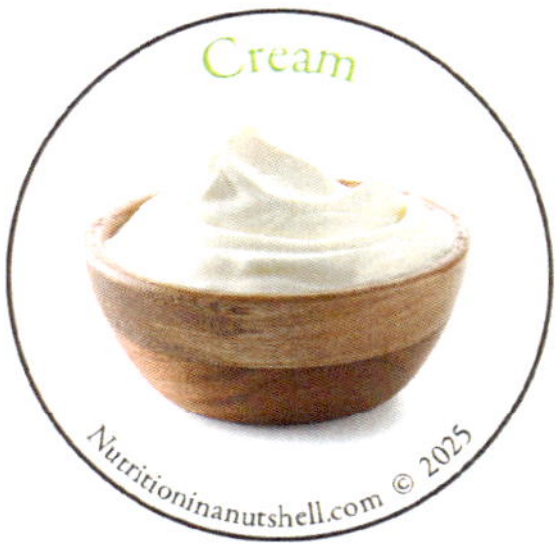

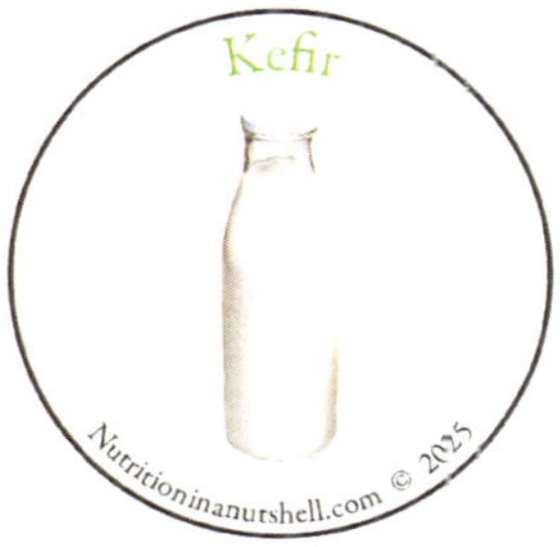

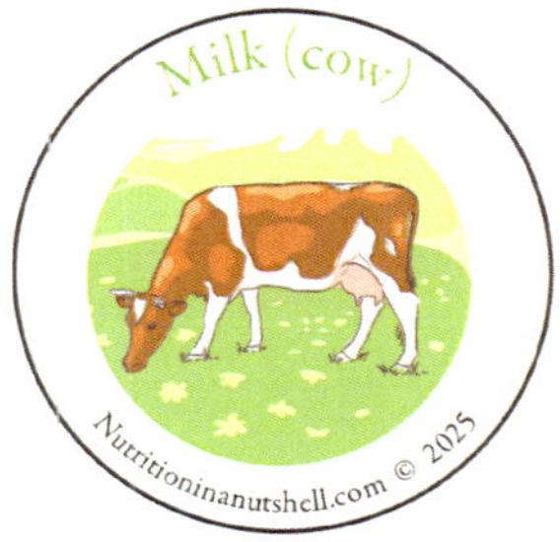

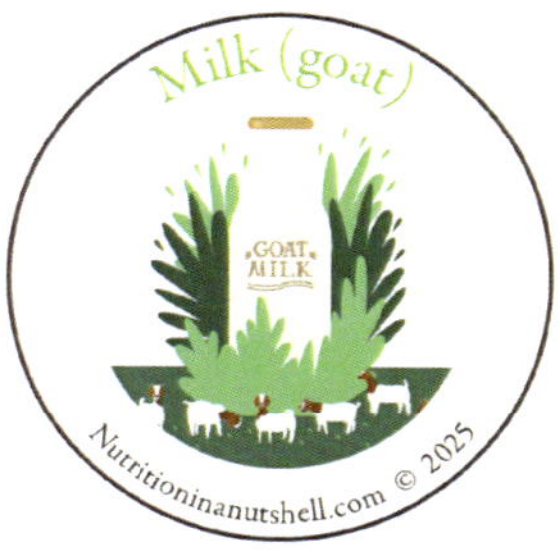

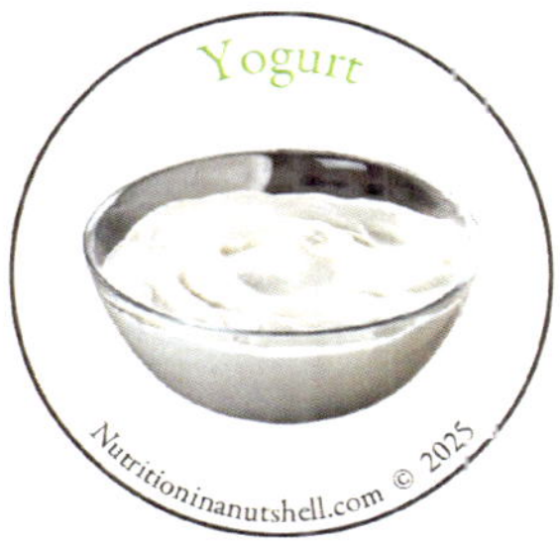

Land & Waterfowl Eggs

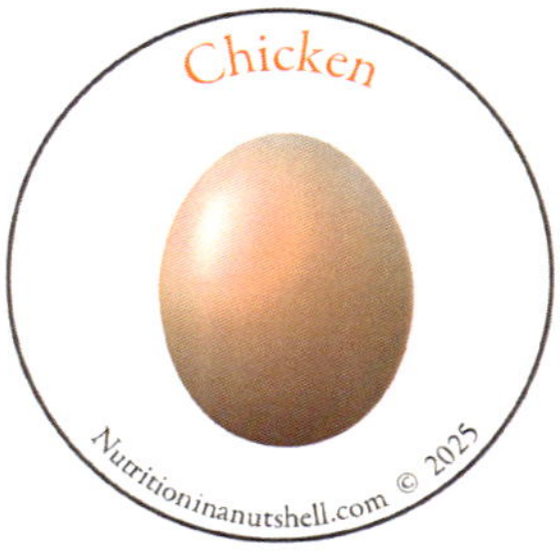

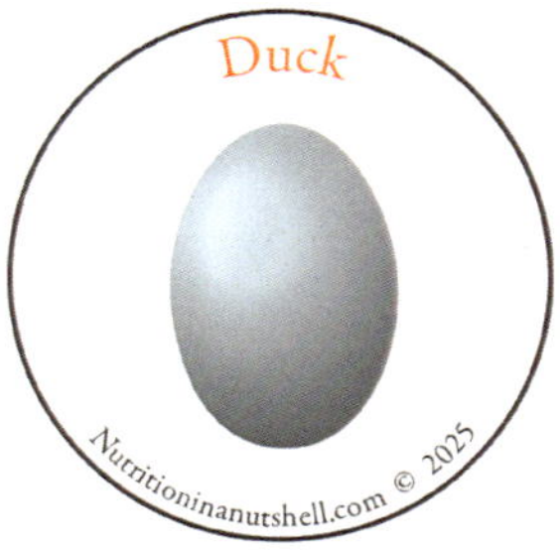

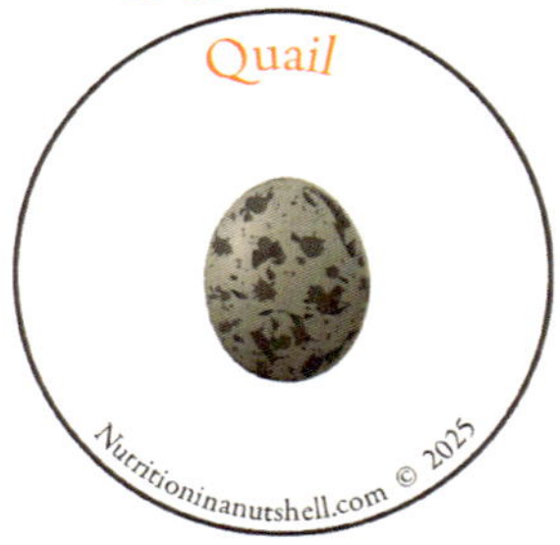

Animal Fats

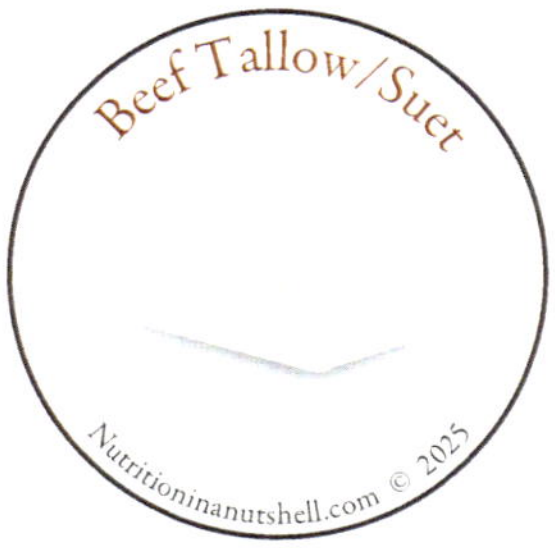
Beef Tallow/Suet
Nutritioninanutshell.com © 2025

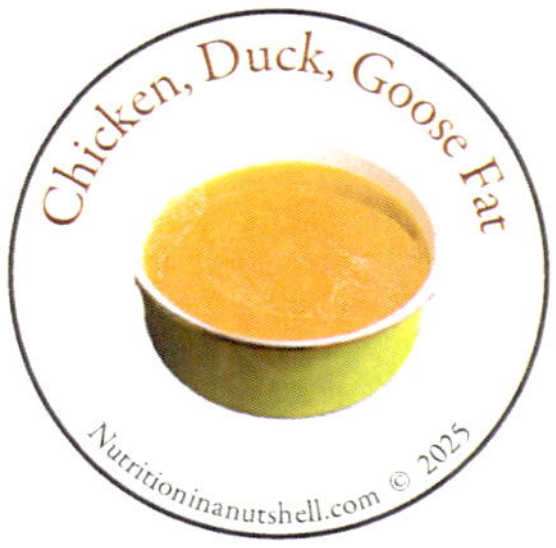
Chicken, Duck, Goose Fat
Nutritioninanutshell.com © 2025

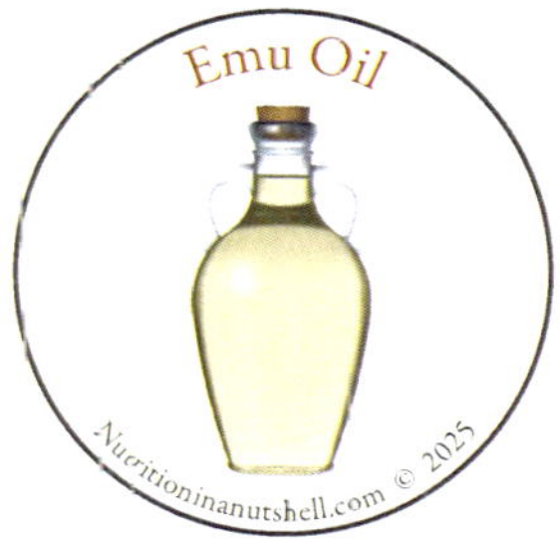
Emu Oil
Nutritioninanutshell.com © 2025

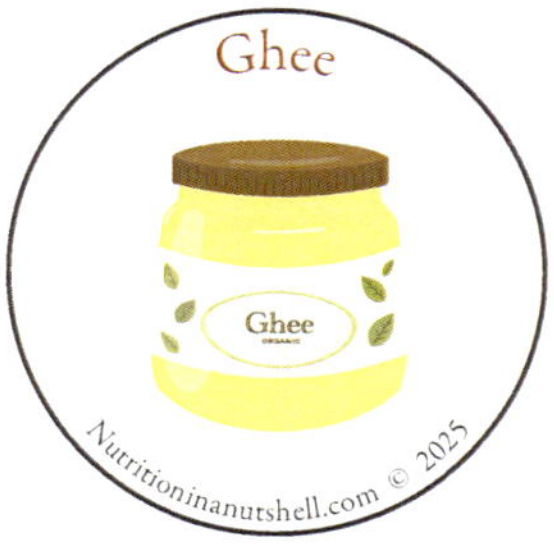
Ghee
Ghee
Nutritioninanutshell.com © 2025

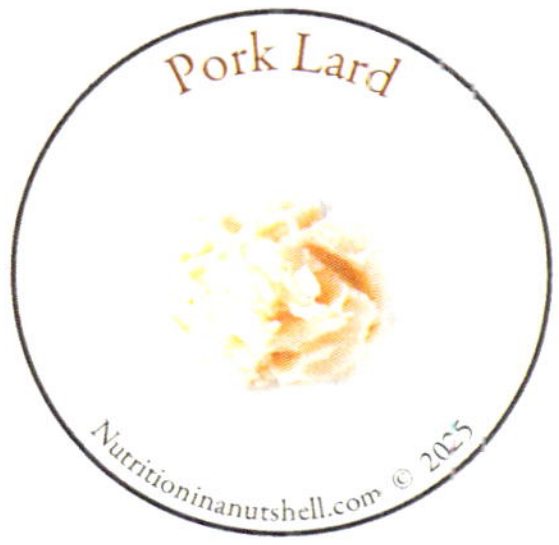
Pork Lard
Nutritioninanutshell.com © 2025

Fruits

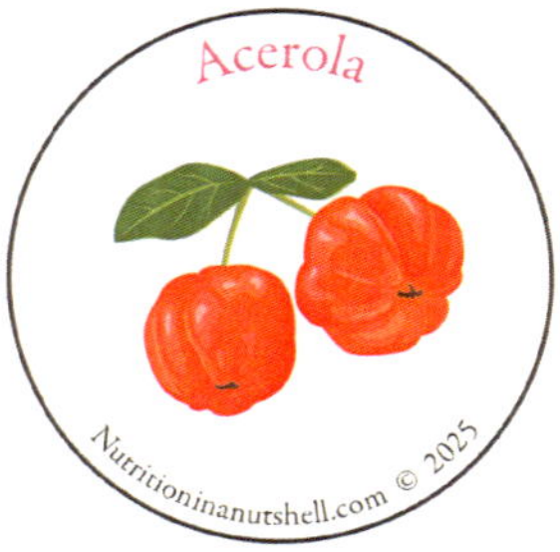
Acerola
Nutritioninanutshell.com © 2025

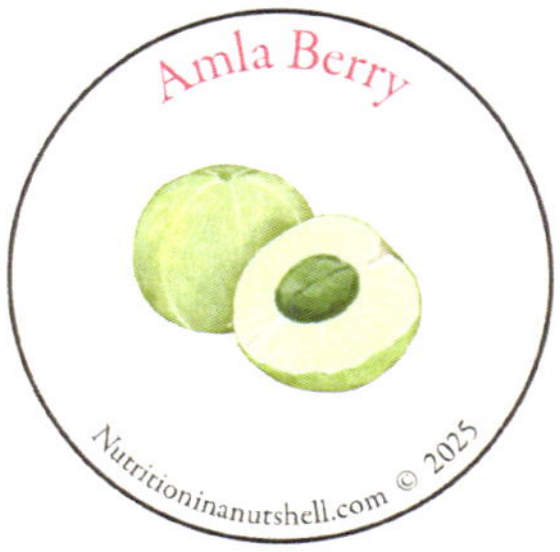
Amla Berry
Nutritioninanutshell.com © 2025

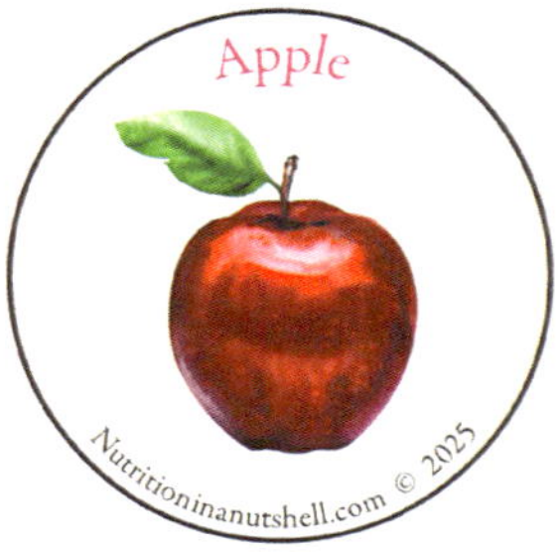
Apple
Nutritioninanutshell.com © 2025

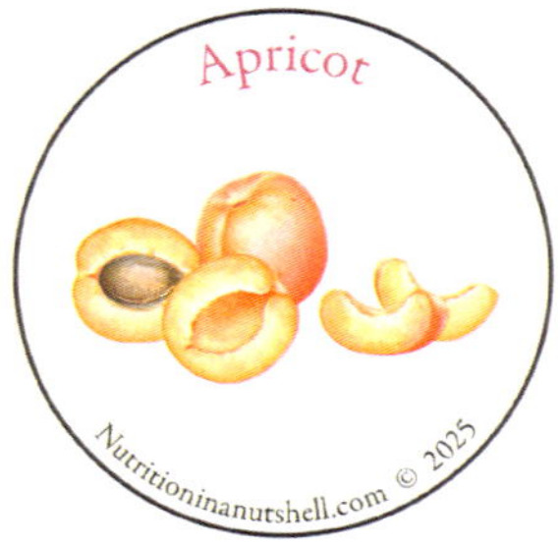
Apricot
Nutritioninanutshell.com © 2025

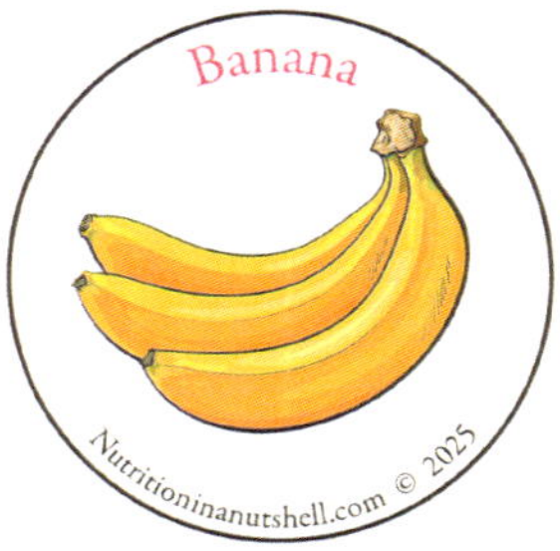
Banana
Nutritioninanutshell.com © 2025

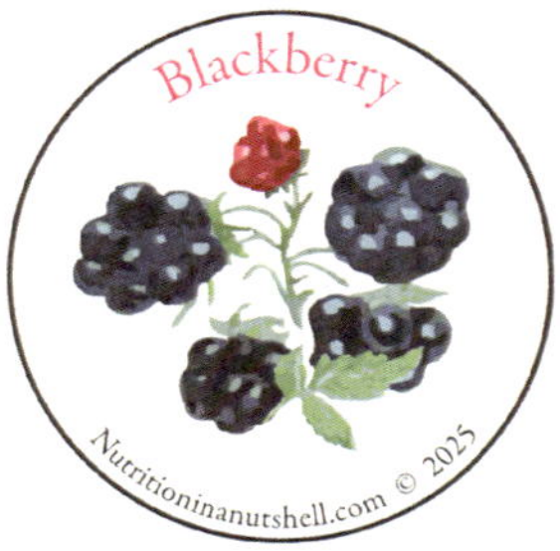
Blackberry
Nutritioninanutshell.com © 2025

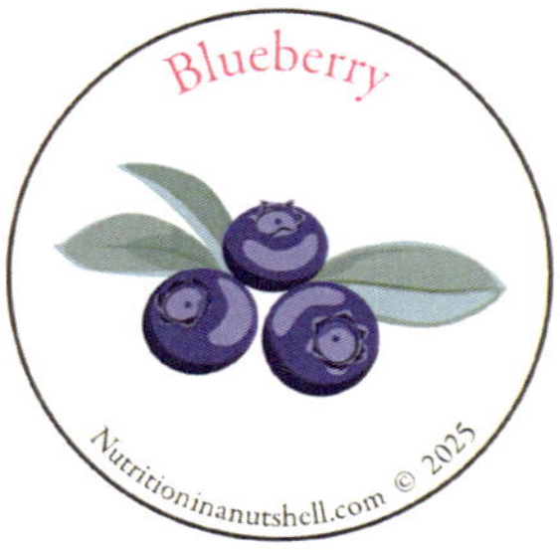
Blueberry
Nutritioninanutshell.com © 2025

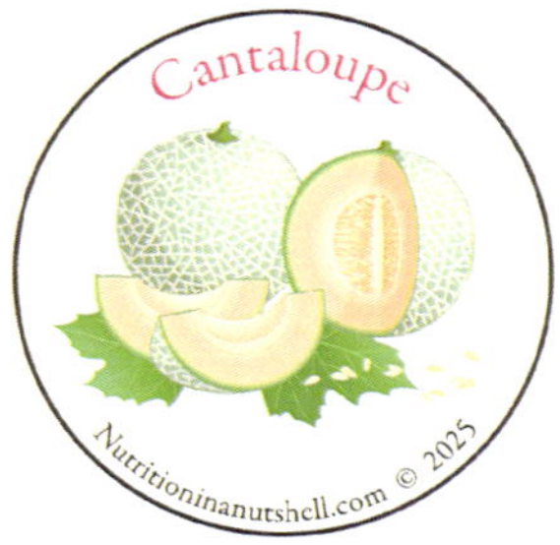
Cantaloupe
Nutritioninanutshell.com © 2025

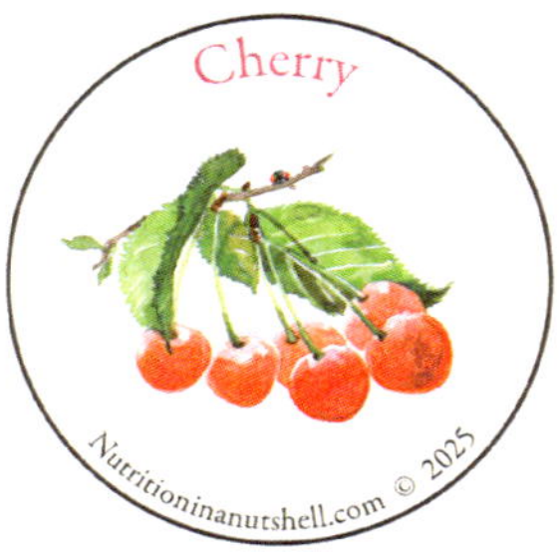
Cherry
Nutritioninanutshell.com © 2025

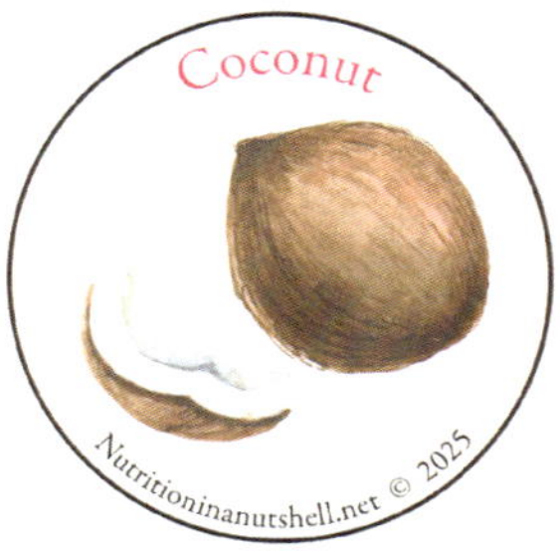
Coconut
Nutritioninanutshell.net © 2025

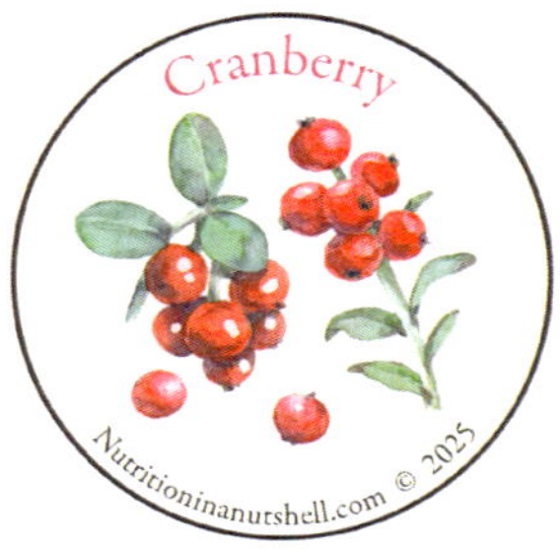
Cranberry
Nutritioninanutshell.com © 2025

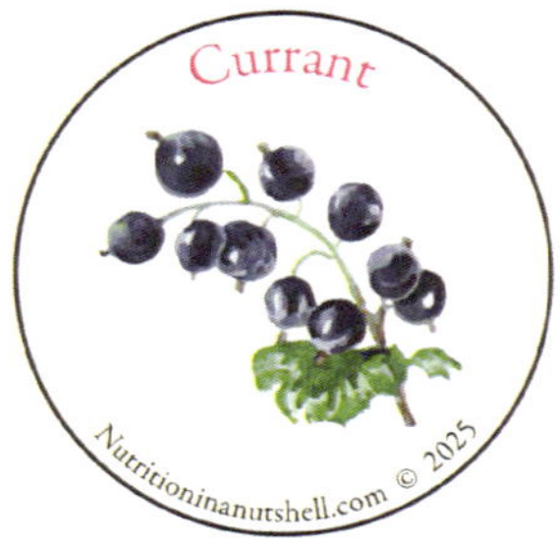
Currant
Nutritioninanutshell.com © 2025

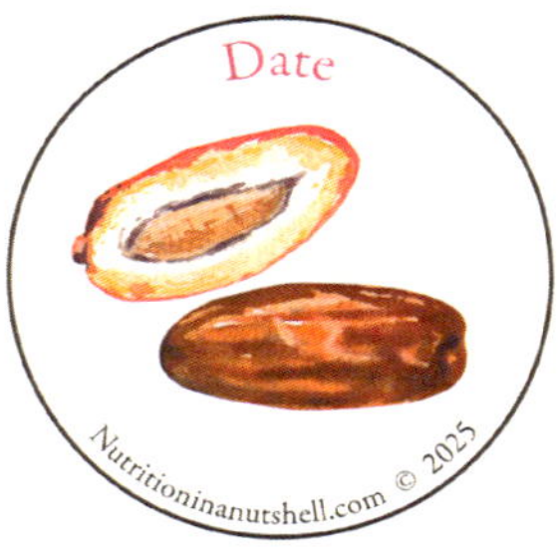
Date
Nutritioninanutshell.com © 2025

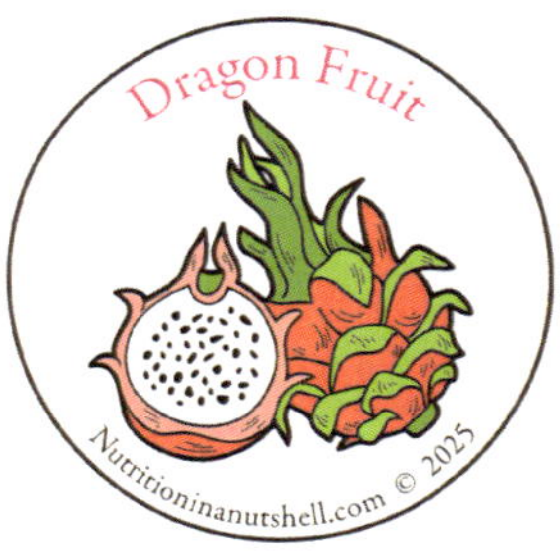
Dragon Fruit
Nutritioninanutshell.com © 2025

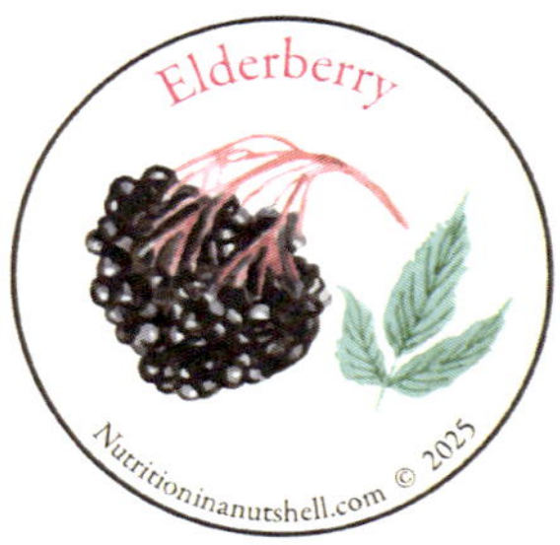
Elderberry
Nutritioninanutshell.com © 2025

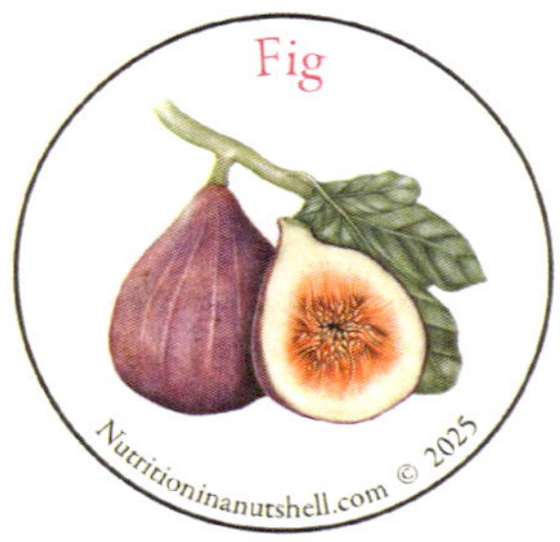
Fig
Nutritioninanutshell.com © 2025

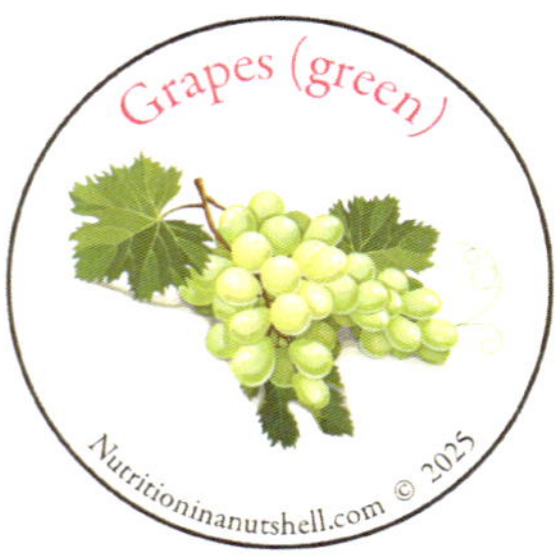
Grapes (green)
Nutritioninanutshell.com © 2025

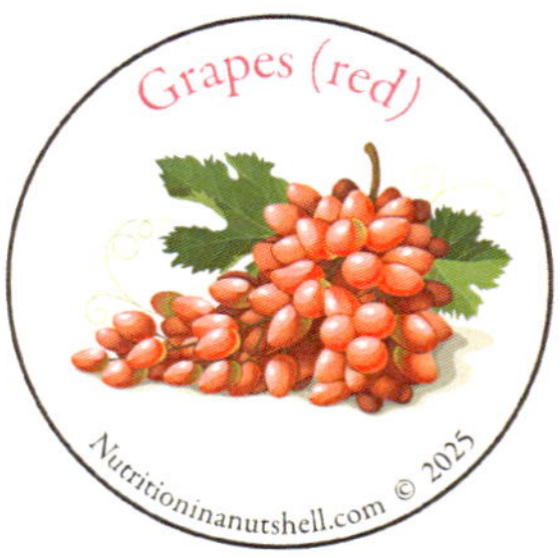
Grapes (red)
Nutritioninanutshell.com © 2025

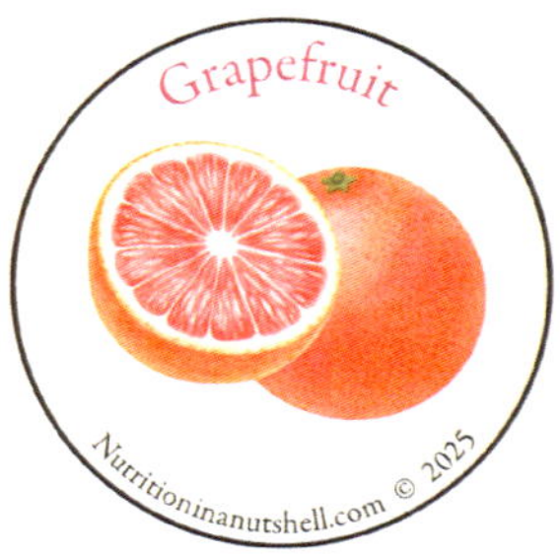
Grapefruit
Nutritioninanutshell.com © 2025

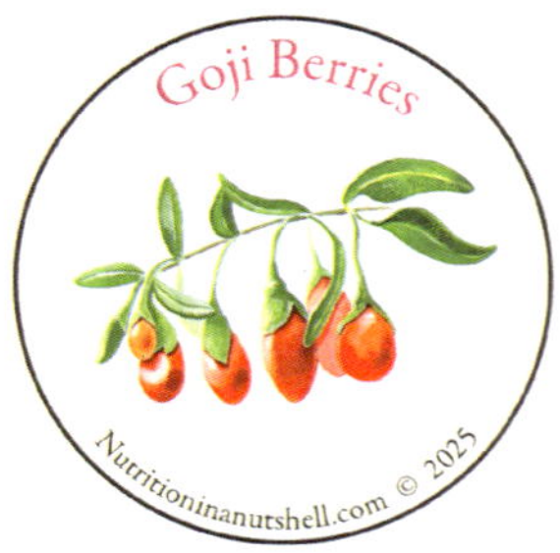
Goji Berries
Nutritioninanutshell.com © 2025

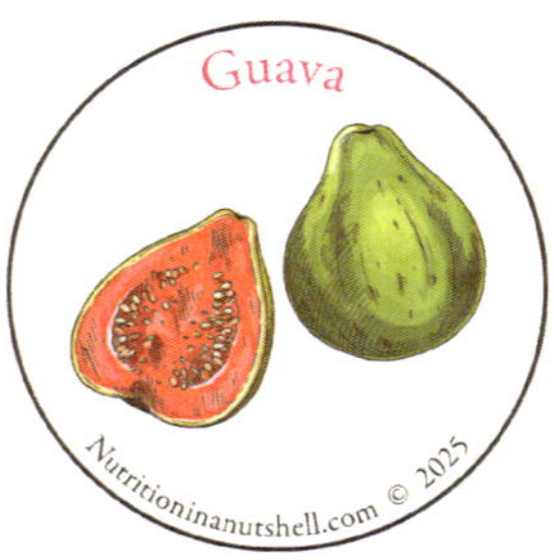
Guava
Nutritioninanutshell.com © 2025

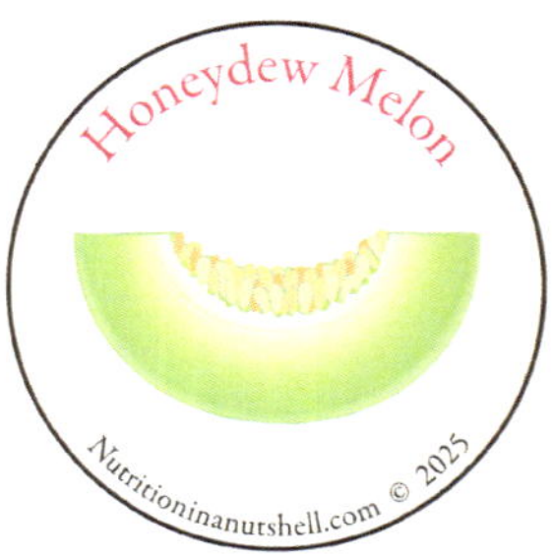
Honeydew Melon
Nutritioninanutshell.com © 2025

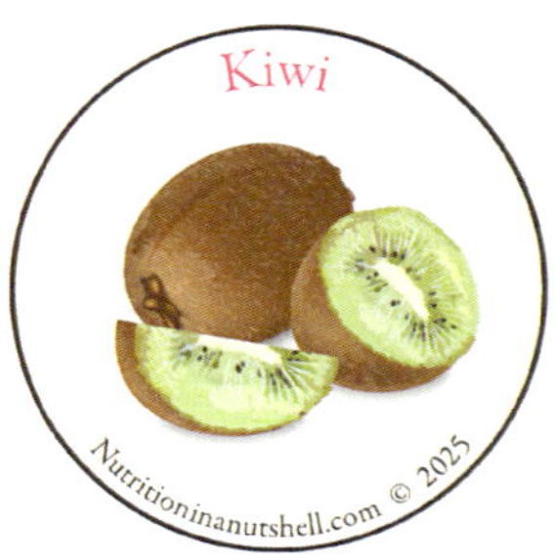
Kiwi
Nutritioninanutshell.com © 2025

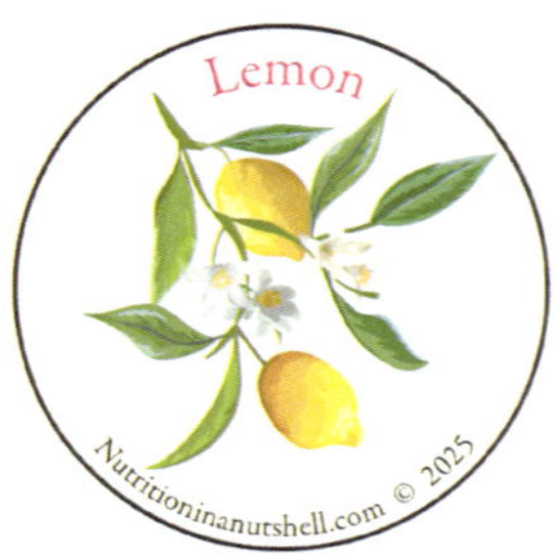
Lemon
Nutritioninanutshell.com © 2025

Fruits

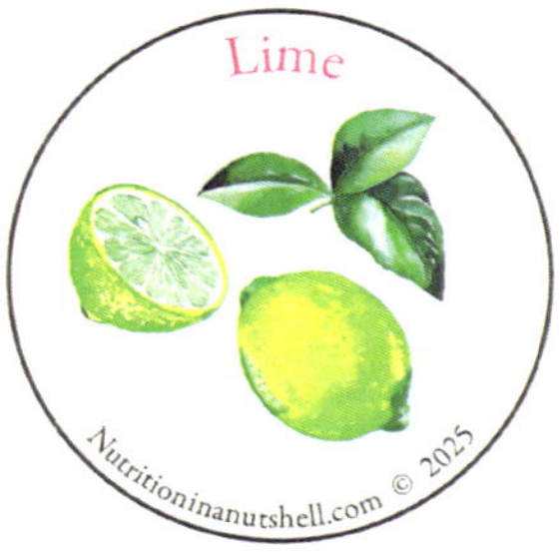
Lime
Nutritioninanutshell.com © 2025

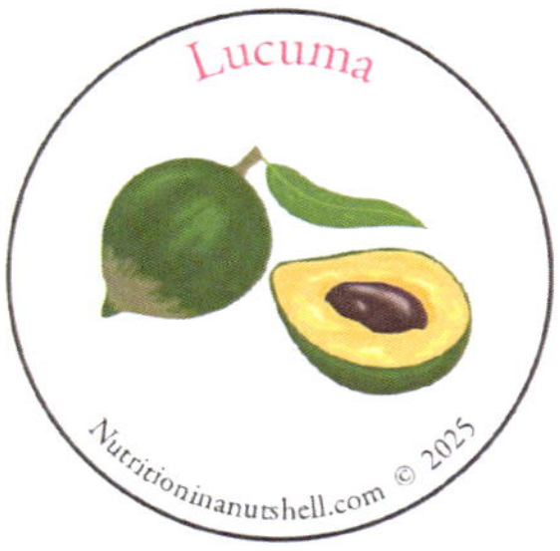
Lucuma
Nutritioninanutshell.com © 2025

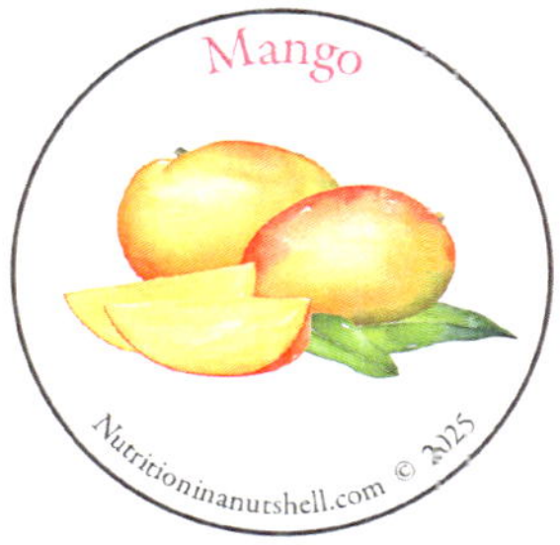
Mango
Nutritioninanutshell.com © 2025

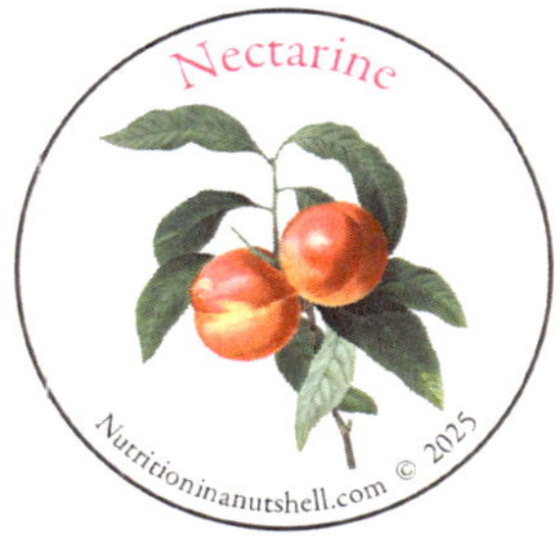
Nectarine
Nutritioninanutshell.com © 2025

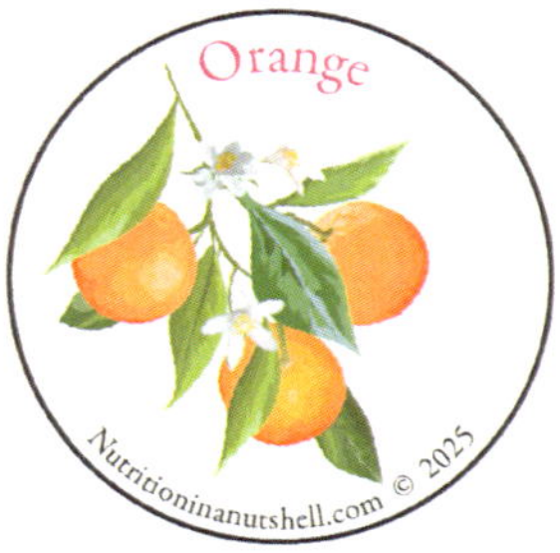
Orange
Nutritioninanutshell.com © 2025

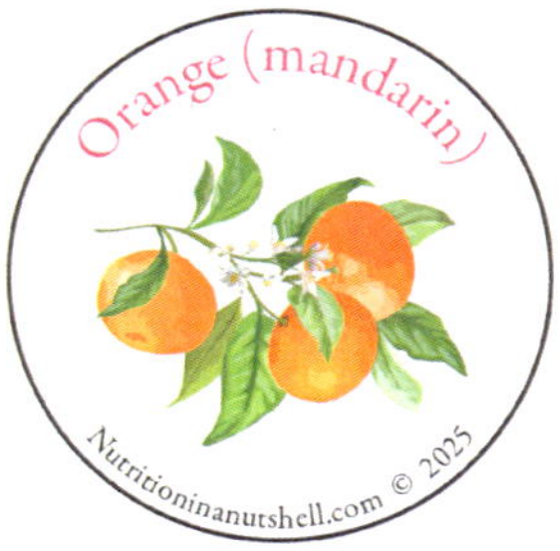
Orange (mandarin)
Nutritioninanutshell.com © 2025

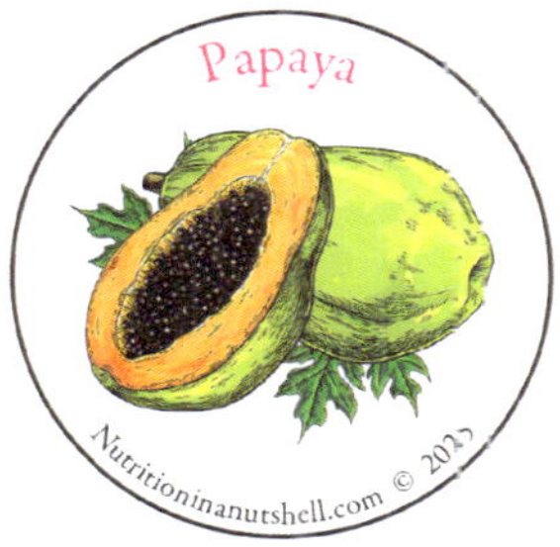
Papaya

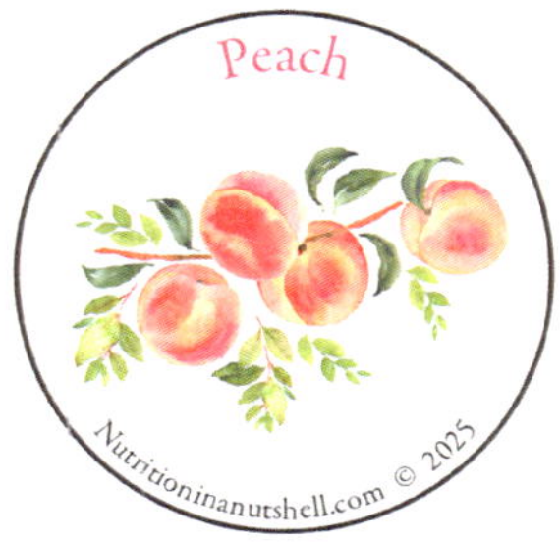
Peach
Nutritioninanutshell.com © 2025

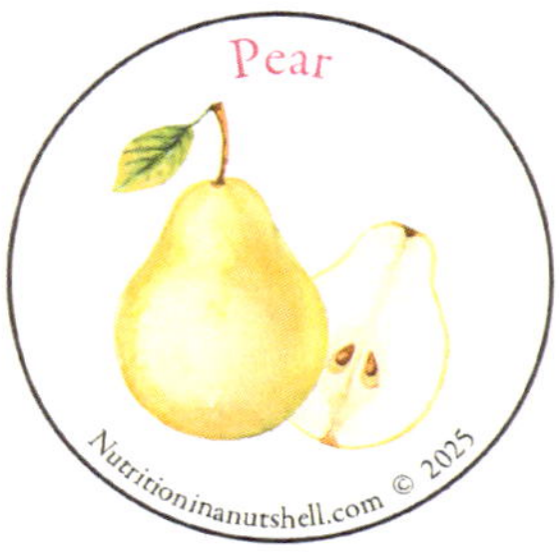
Pear
Nutritioninanutshell.com © 2025

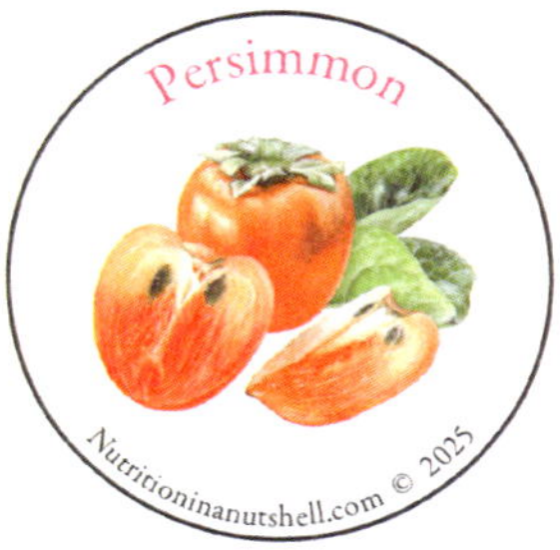
Persimmon
Nutritioninanutshell.com © 2025

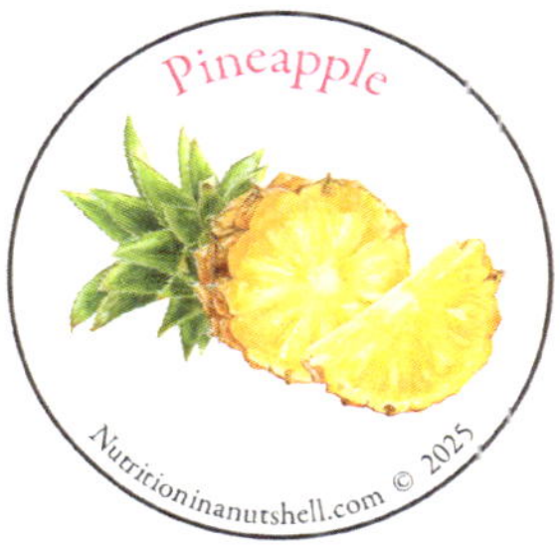
Pineapple
Nutritioninanutshell.com © 2025

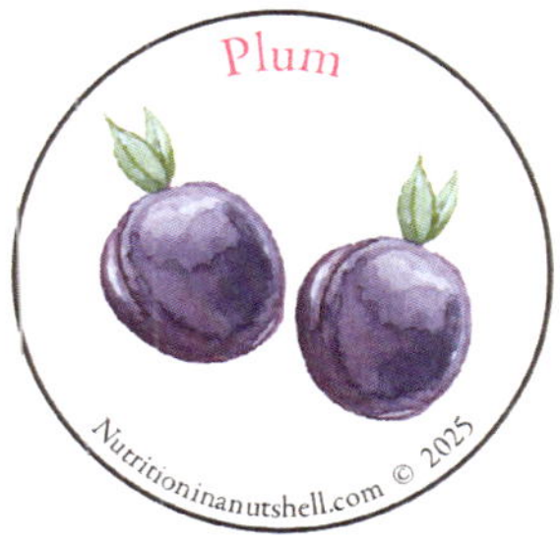
Plum
Nutritioninanutshell.com © 2025

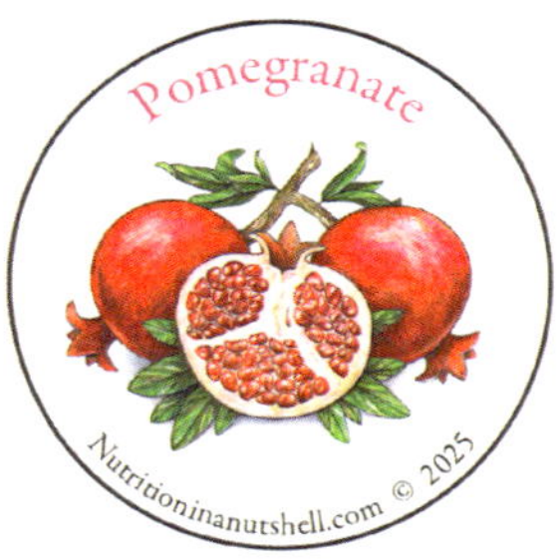
Pomegranate
Nutritioninanutshell.com © 2025

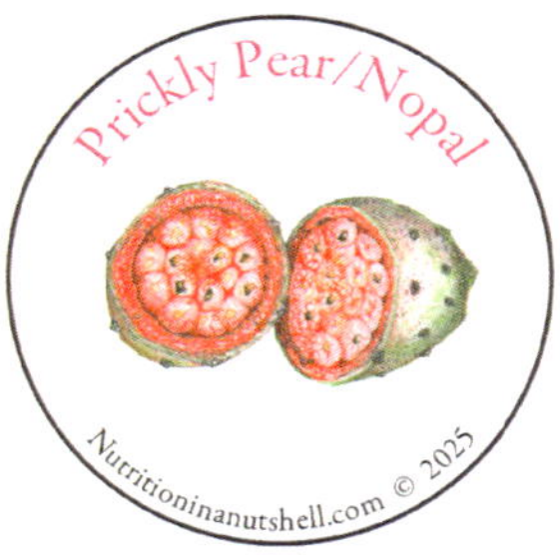
Prickly Pear/Nopal
Nutritioninanutshell.com © 2025

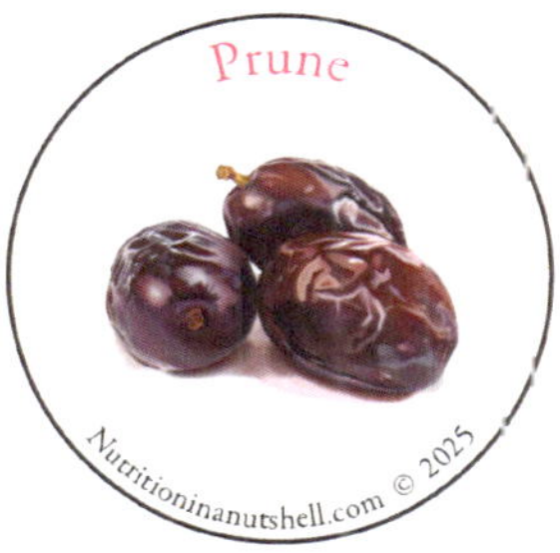
Prune
Nutritioninanutshell.com © 2025

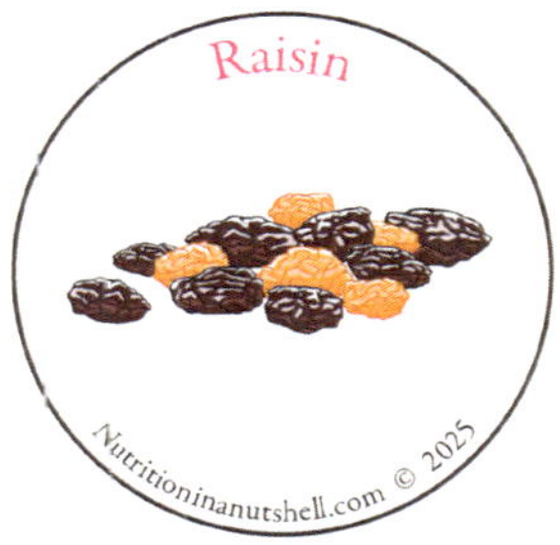
Raisin
Nutritioninanutshell.com © 2025

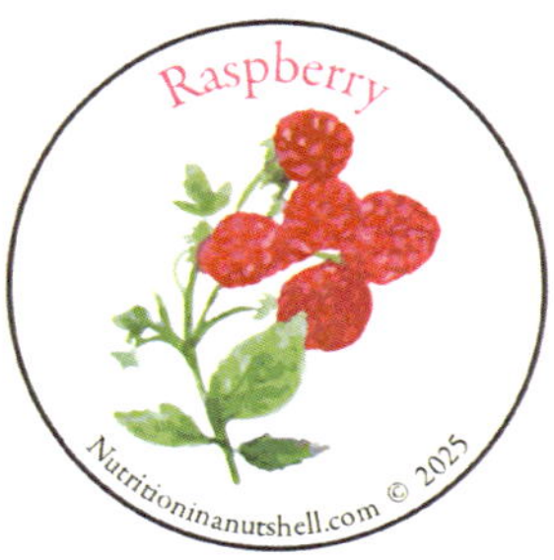
Raspberry
Nutritioninanutshell.com © 2025

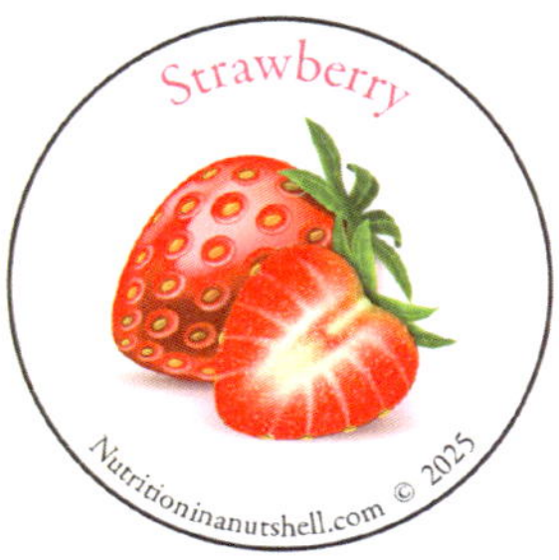
Strawberry
Nutritioninanutshell.com © 2025

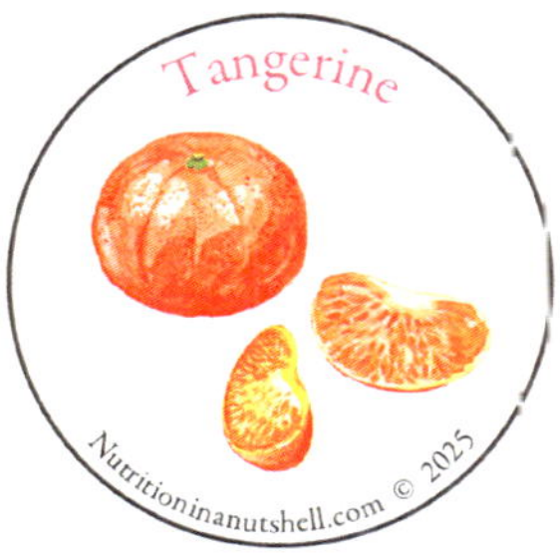
Tangerine
Nutritioninanutshell.com © 2025

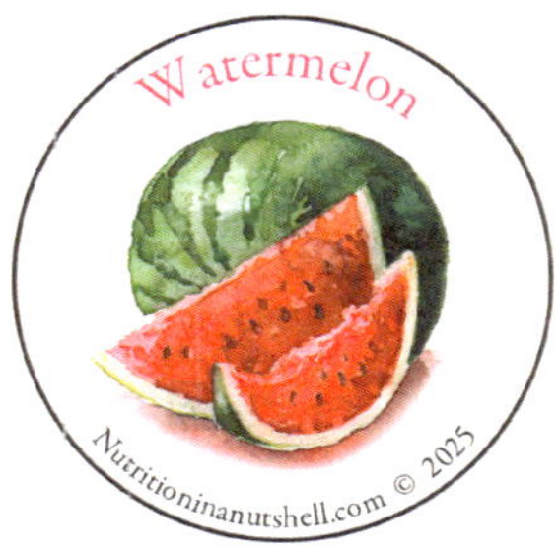
Watermelon
Nutritioninanutshell.com © 2025

Grains

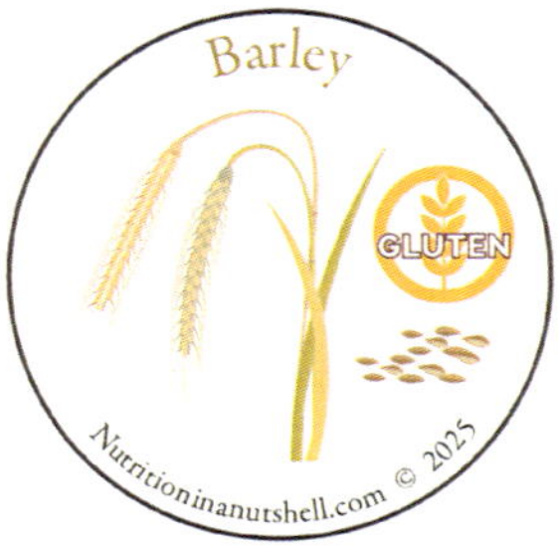
Barley
GLUTEN
Nutritioninanutshell.com © 2025

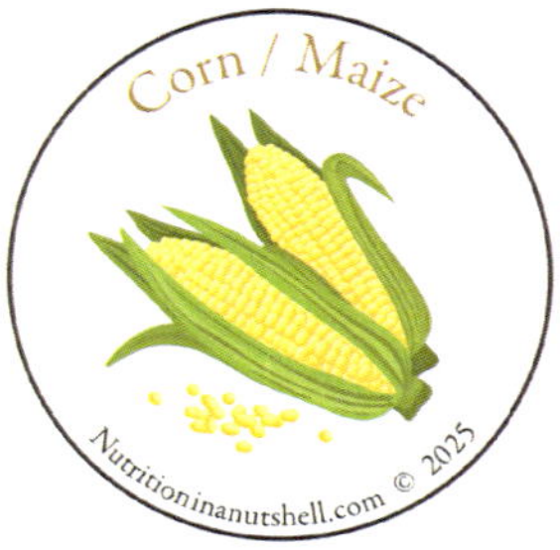
Corn / Maize
Nutritioninanutshell.com © 2025

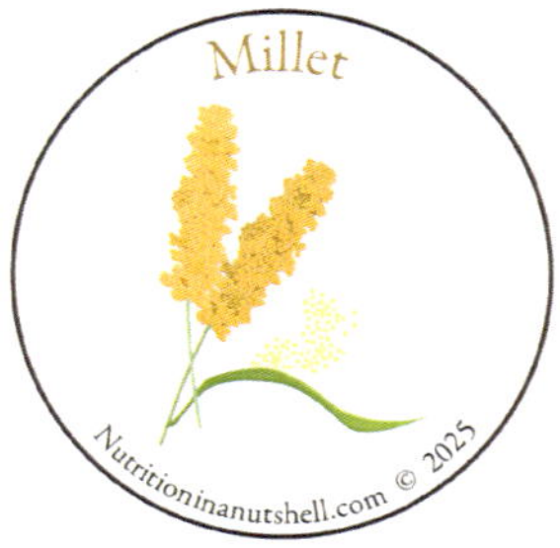
Millet
Nutritioninanutshell.com © 2025

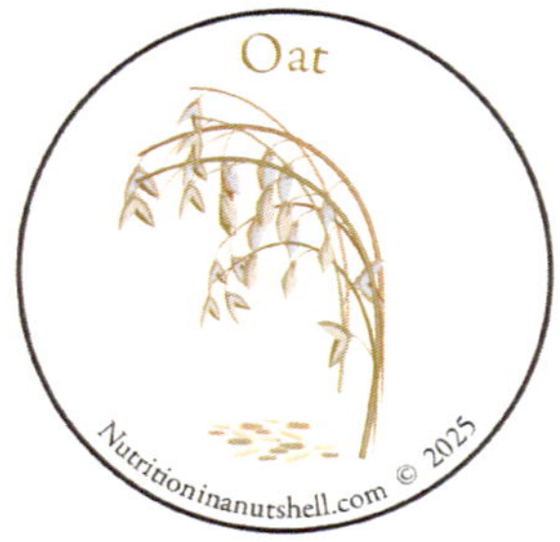
Oat
Nutritioninanutshell.com © 2025

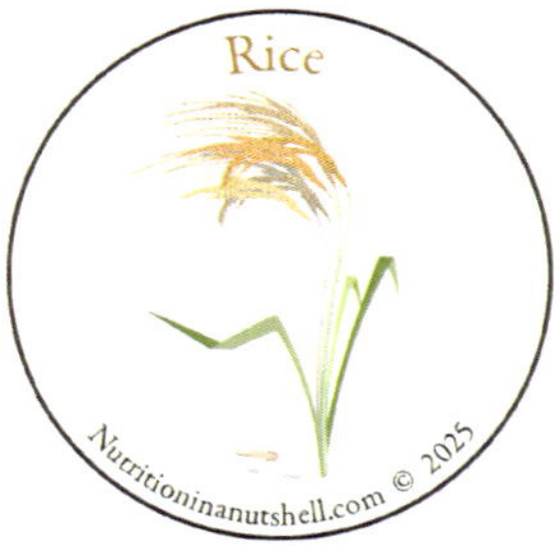
Rice
Nutritioninanutshell.com © 2025

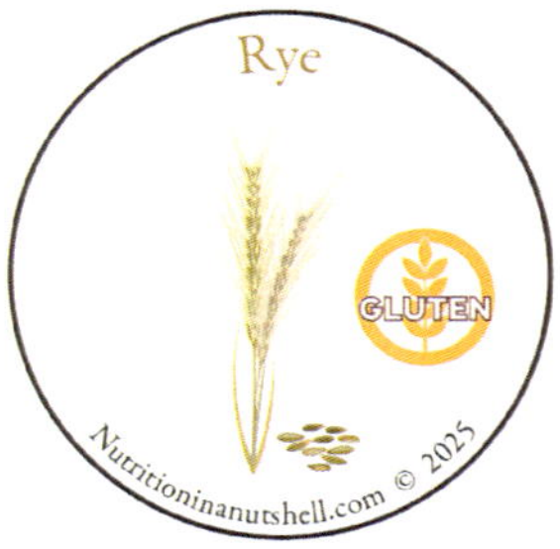
Rye
GLUTEN
Nutritioninanutshell.com © 2025

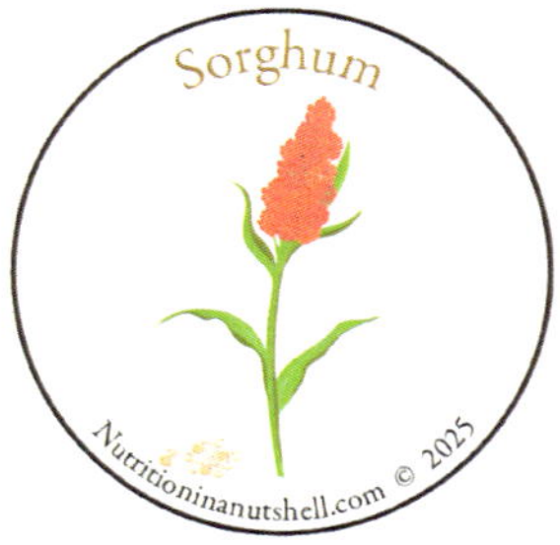
Sorghum
Nutritioninanutshell.com © 2025

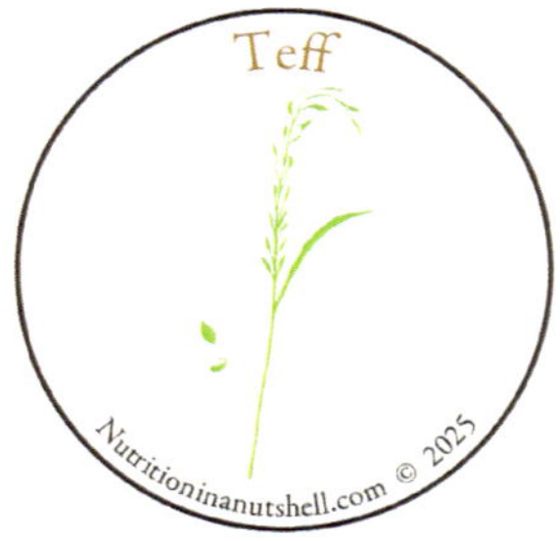
Teff
Nutritioninanutshell.com © 2025

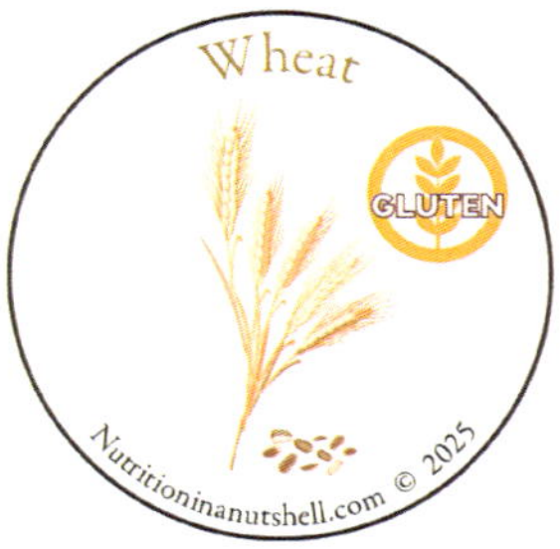
Wheat
GLUTEN
Nutritioninanutshell.com © 2025

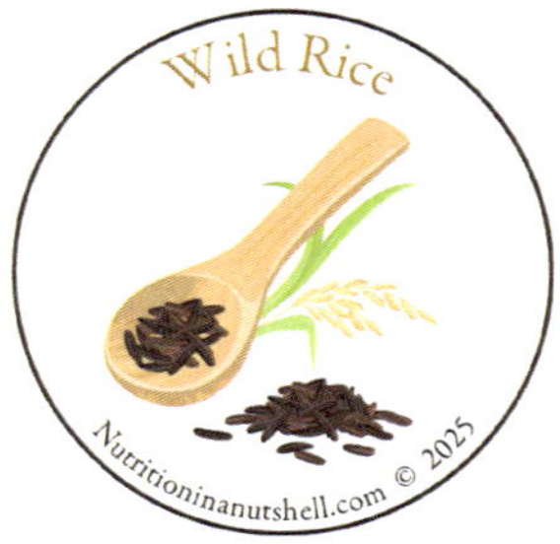
Wild Rice
Nutritioninanutshell.com © 2025

Legumes

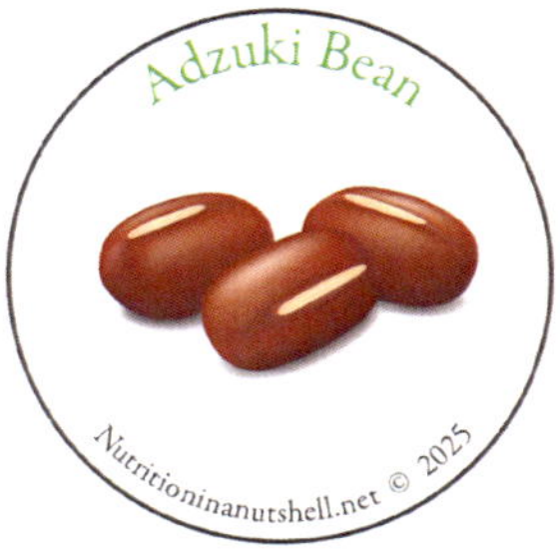
Adzuki Bean
Nutritioninanutshell.net © 2025

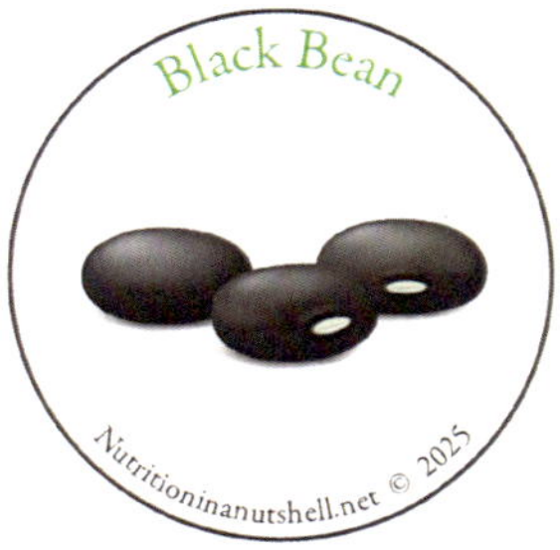
Black Bean
Nutritioninanutshell.net © 2025

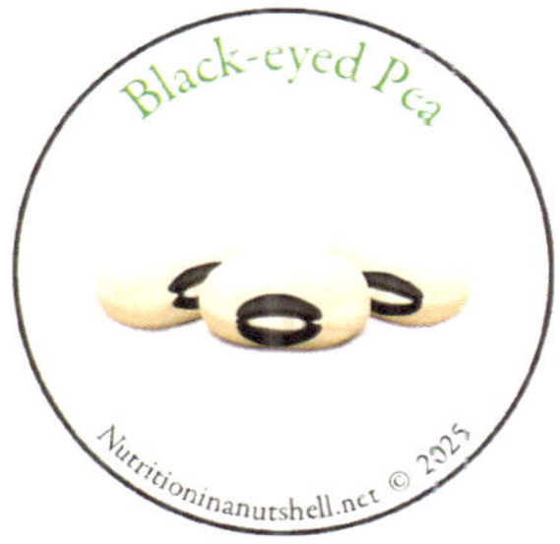
Black-eyed Pea
Nutritioninanutshell.net © 2025

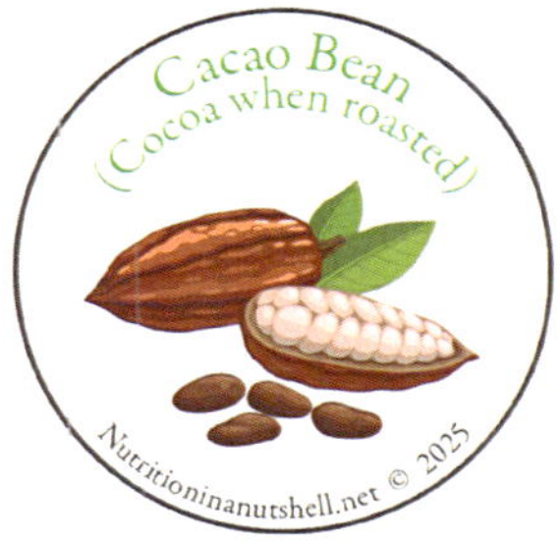
Cacao Bean
(Cocoa when roasted)
Nutritioninanutshell.net © 2025

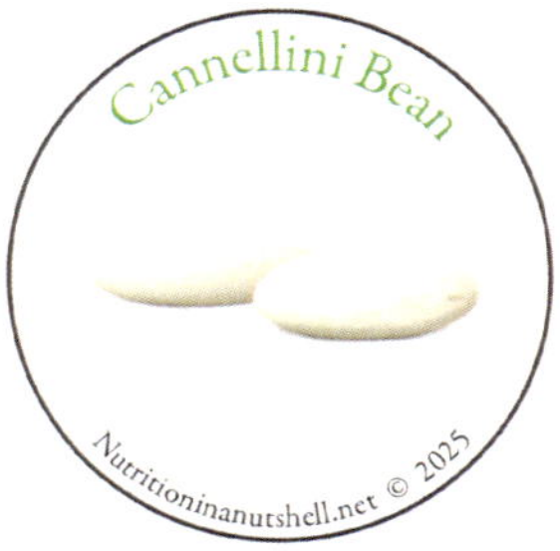
Cannellini Bean
Nutritioninanutshell.net © 2025

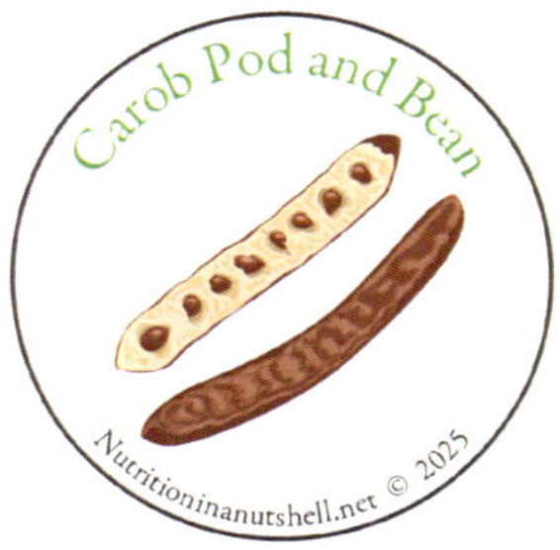
Carob Pod and Bean
Nutritioninanutshell.net © 2025

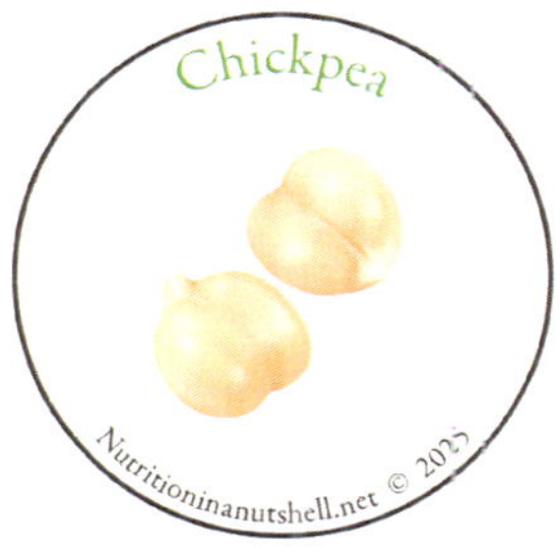
Chickpea
Nutritioninanutshell.net © 2025

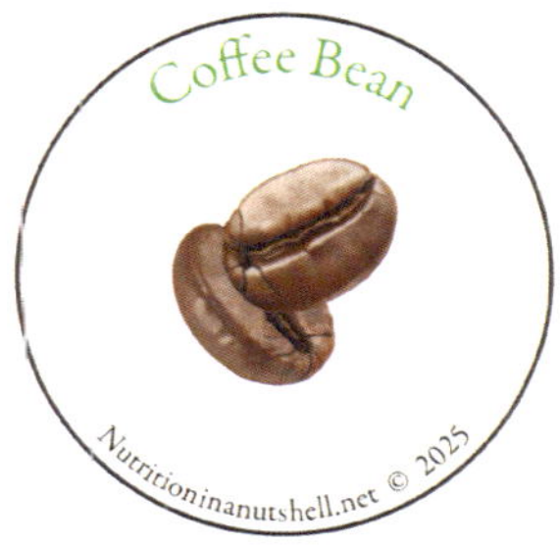
Coffee Bean
Nutritioninanutshell.net © 2025

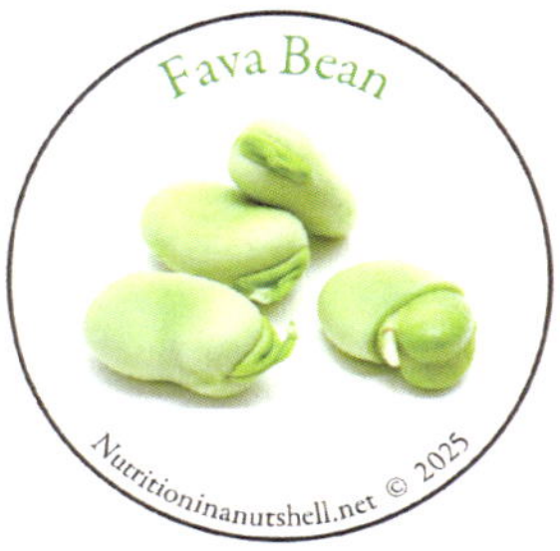
Fava Bean
Nutritioninanutshell.net © 2025

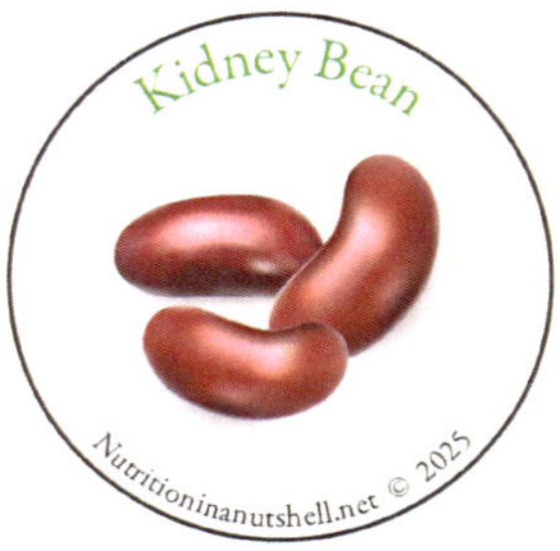
Kidney Bean
Nutritioninanutshell.net © 2025

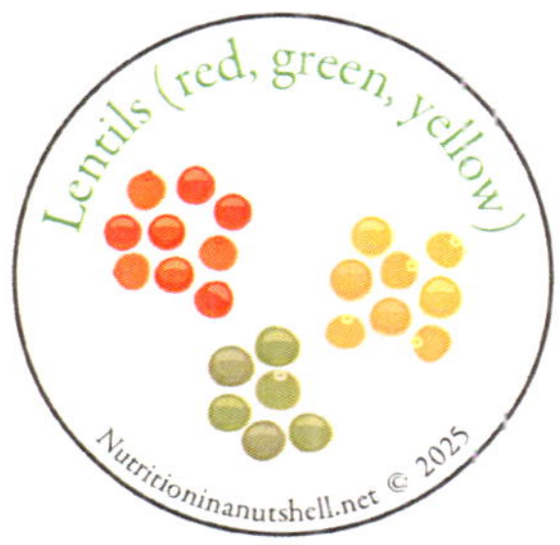
Lentils (red, green, yellow)
Nutritioninanutshell.net © 2025

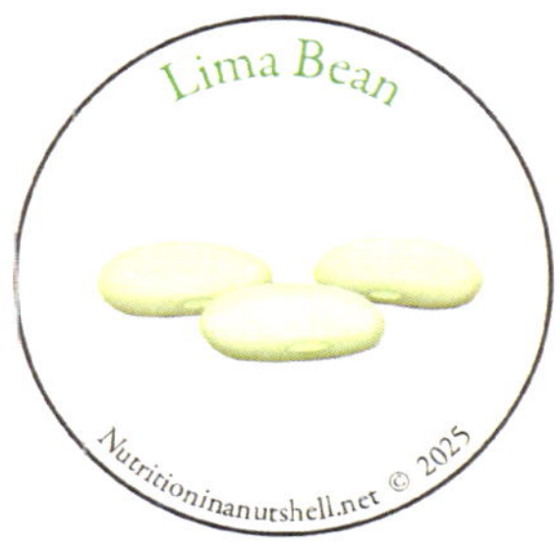
Lima Bean
Nutritioninanutshell.net © 2025

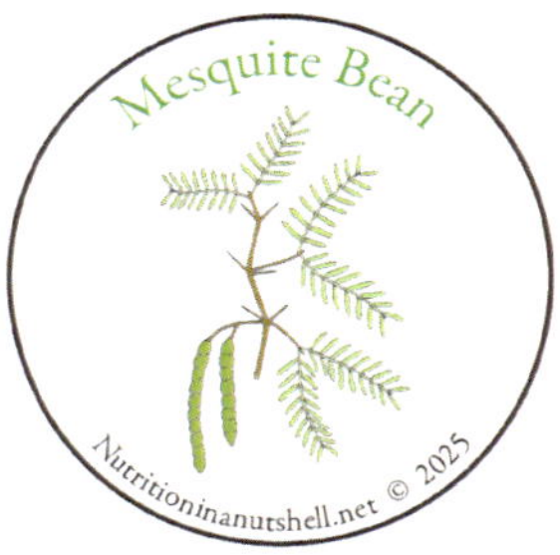
Mesquite Bean
Nutritioninanutshell.net © 2025

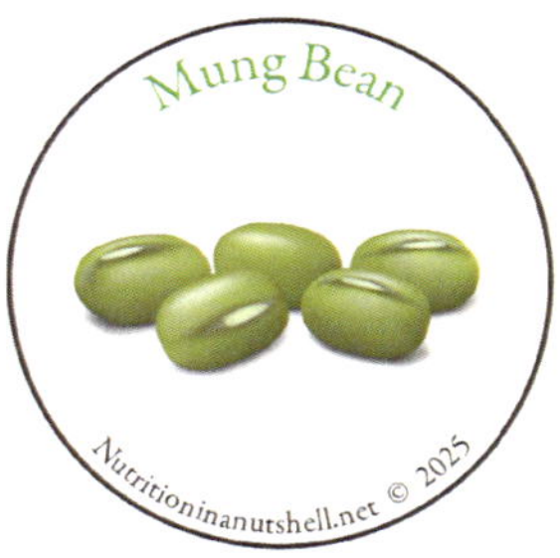
Mung Bean
Nutritioninanutshell.net © 2025

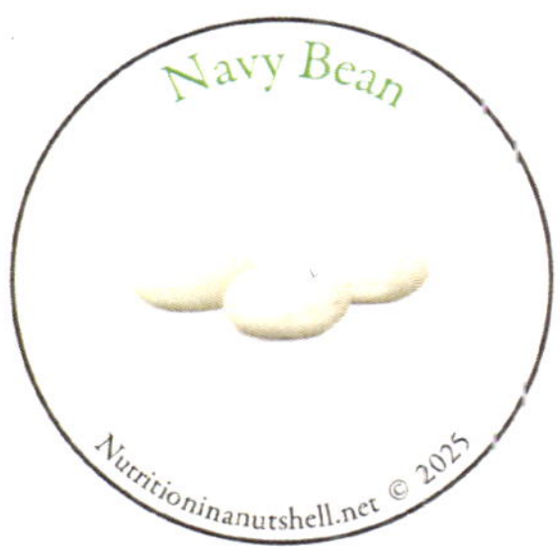
Navy Bean
Nutritioninanutshell.net © 2025

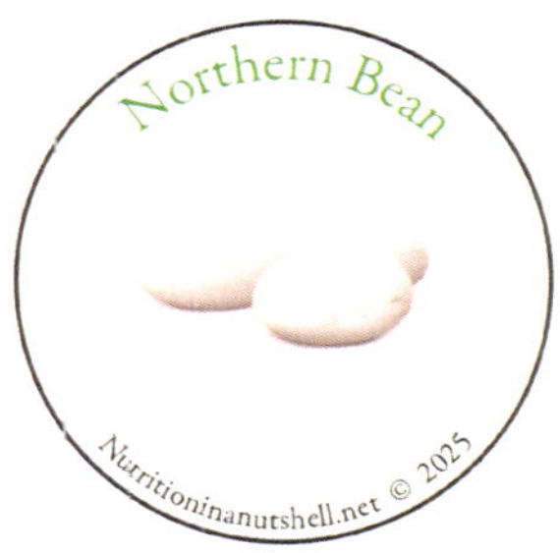
Northern Bean
Nutritioninanutshell.net © 2025

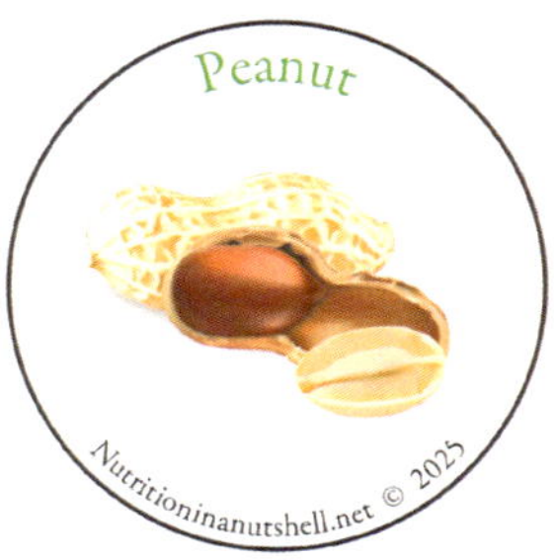
Peanut
Nutritioninanutshell.net © 2025

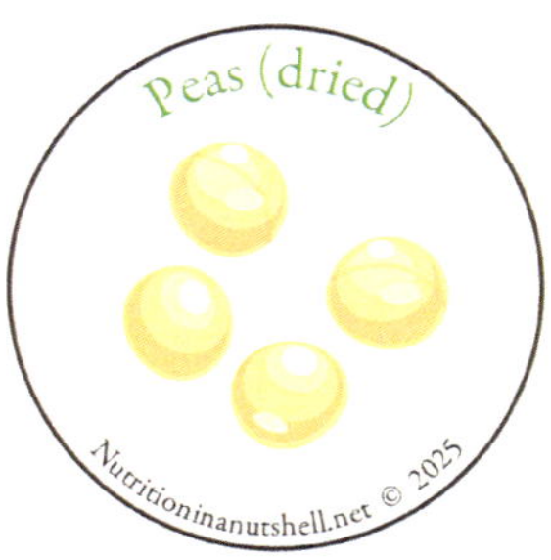
Peas (dried)
Nutritioninanutshell.net © 2025

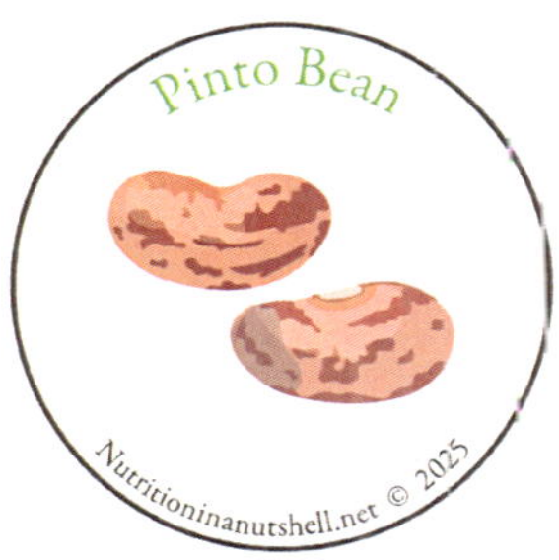
Pinto Bean
Nutritioninanutshell.net © 2025

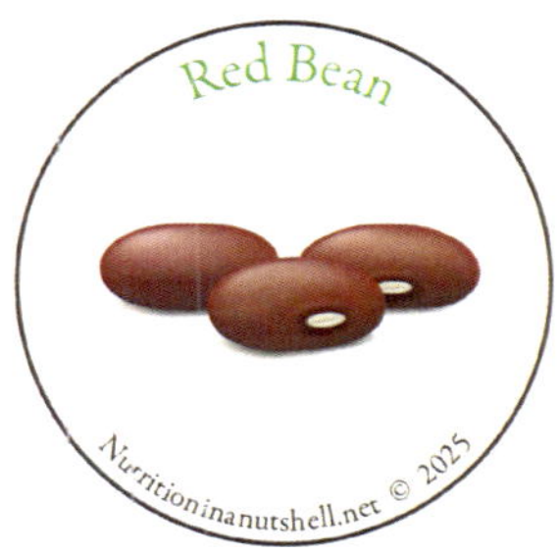
Red Bean
Nutritioninanutshell.net © 2025

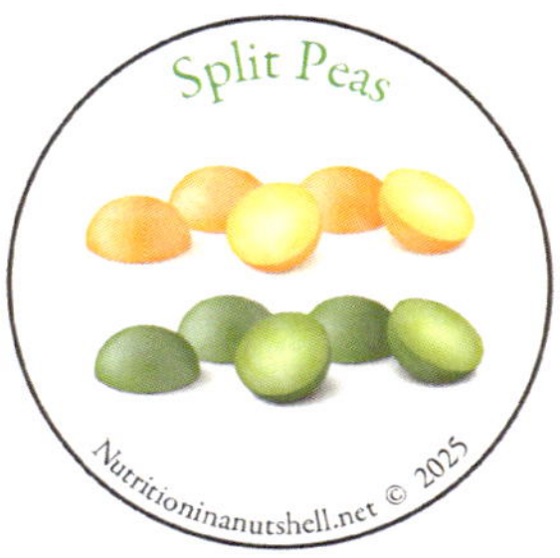
Split Peas
Nutritioninanutshell.net © 2025

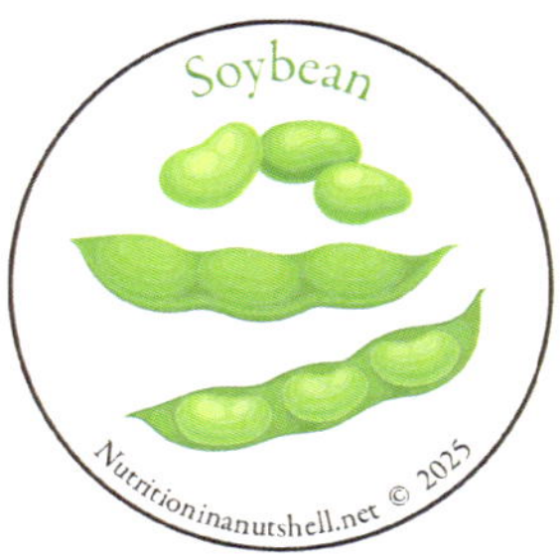
Soybean
Nutritioninanutshell.net © 2025

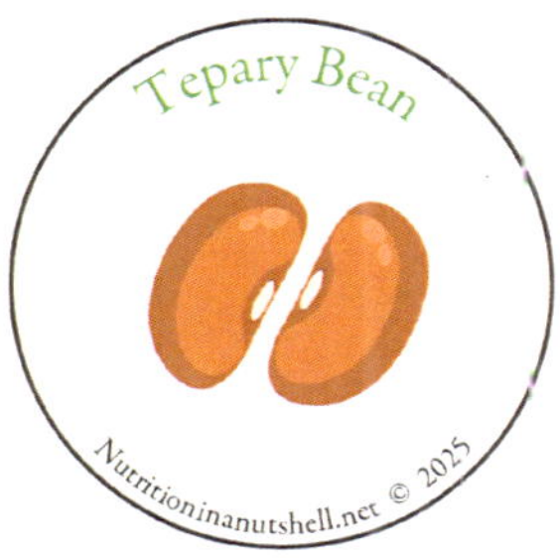
Tepary Bean
Nutritioninanutshell.net © 2025

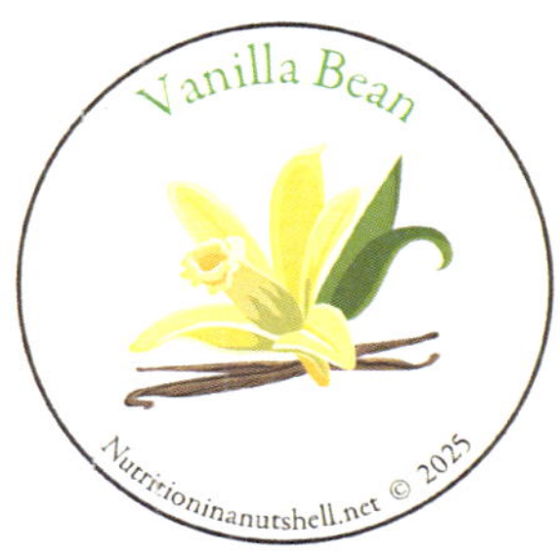
Vanilla Bean
Nutritioninanutshell.net © 2025

Tree Nuts

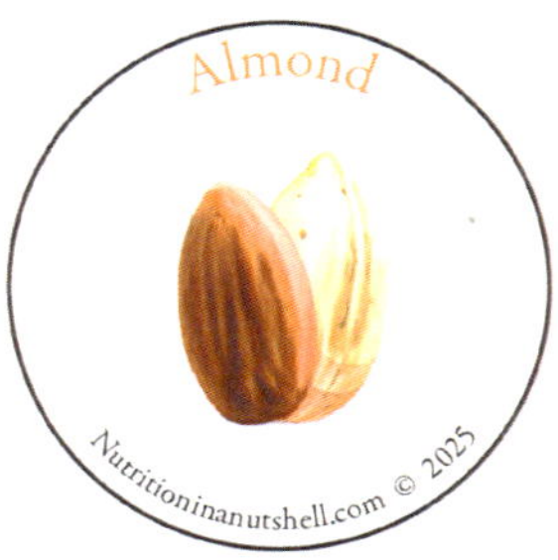

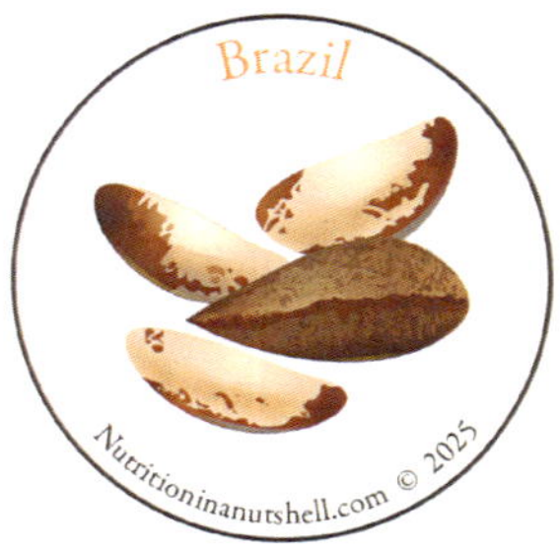

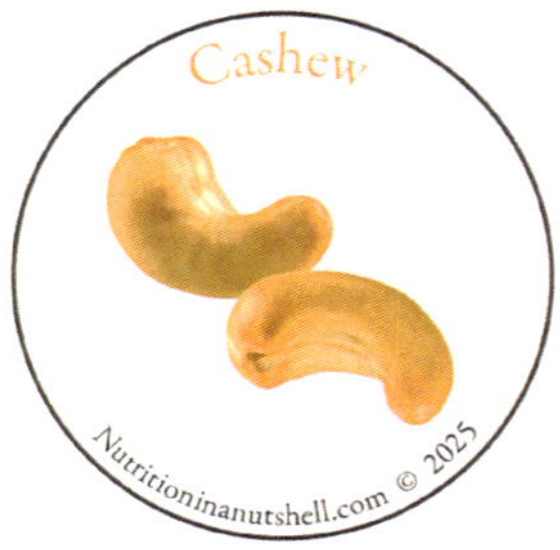

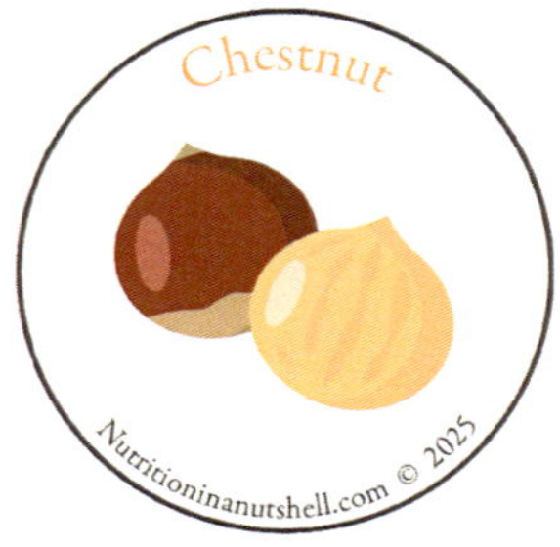

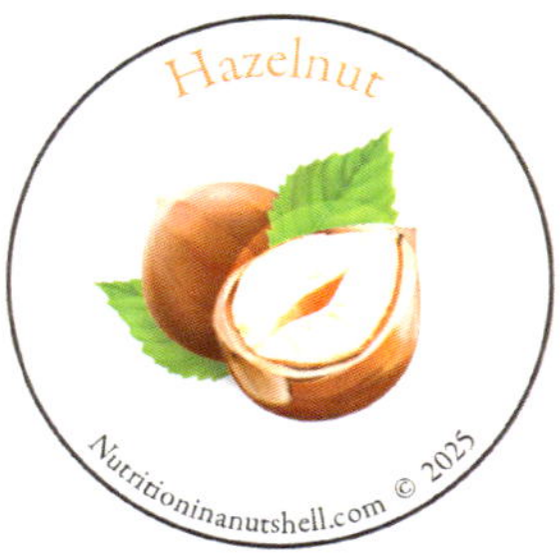

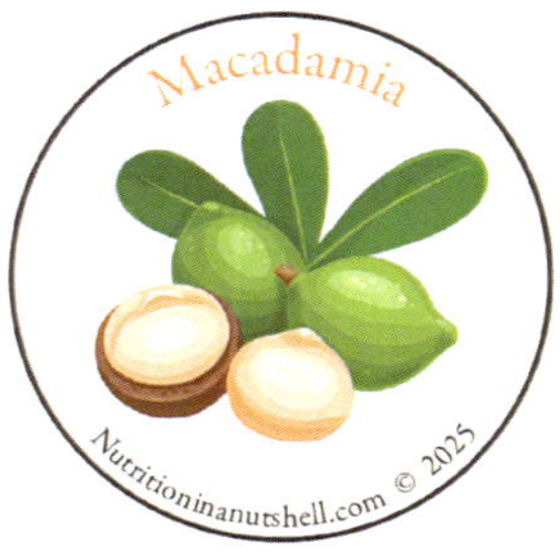

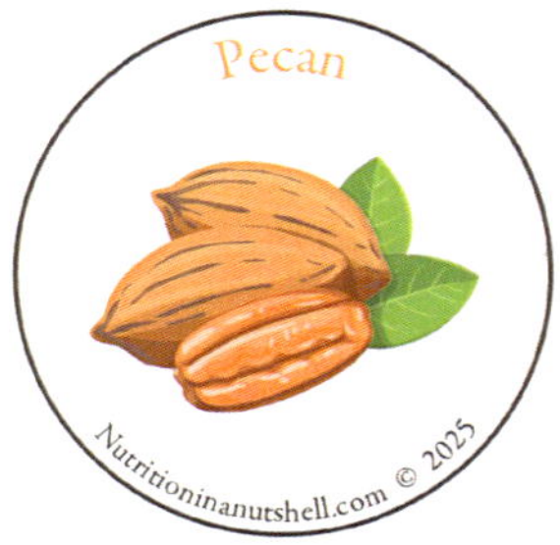

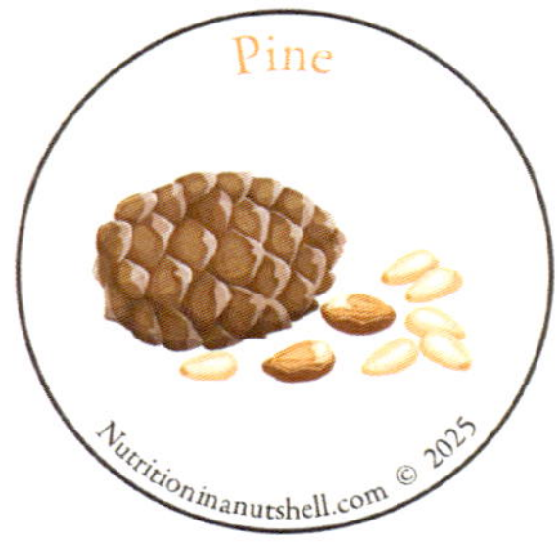

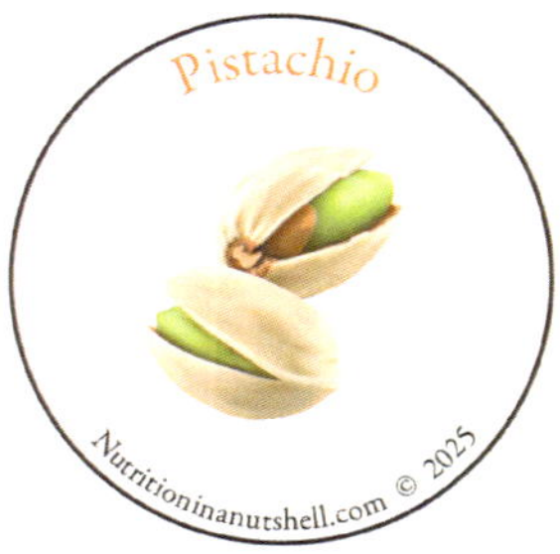

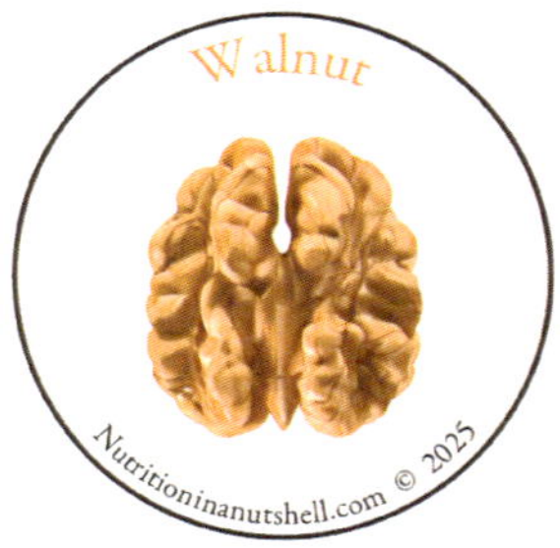

Bark & Saps

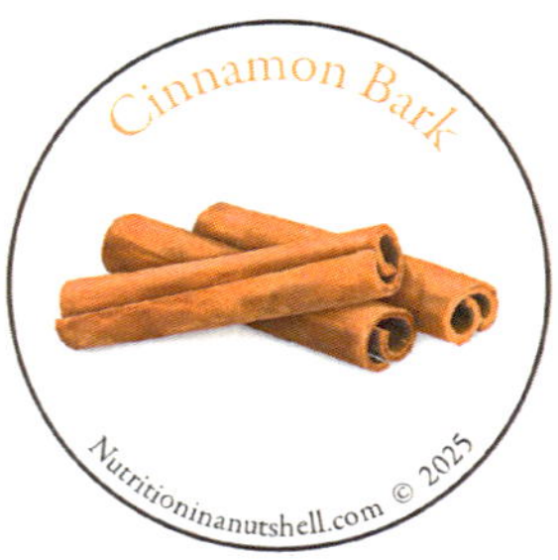

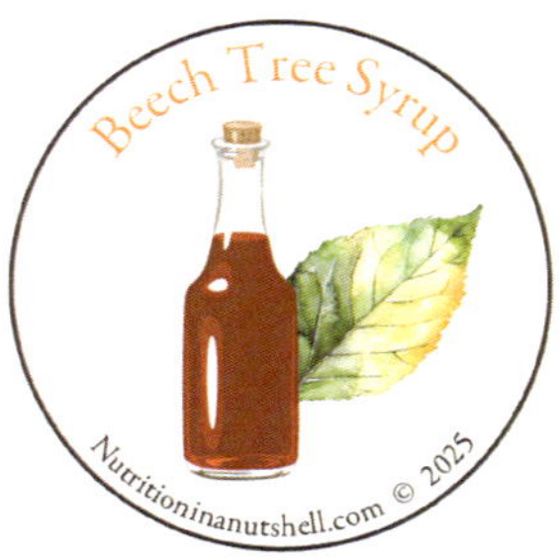

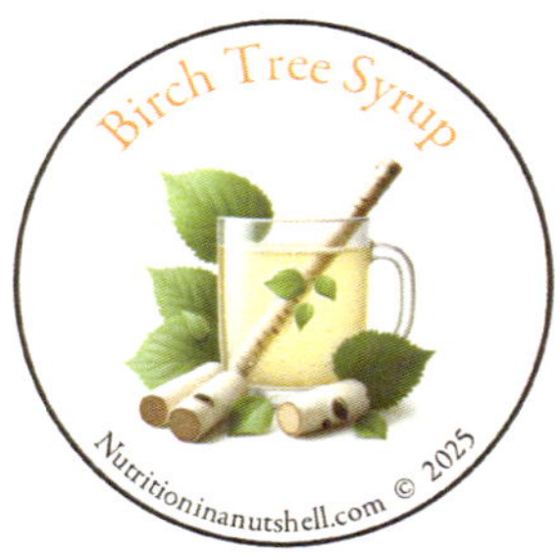

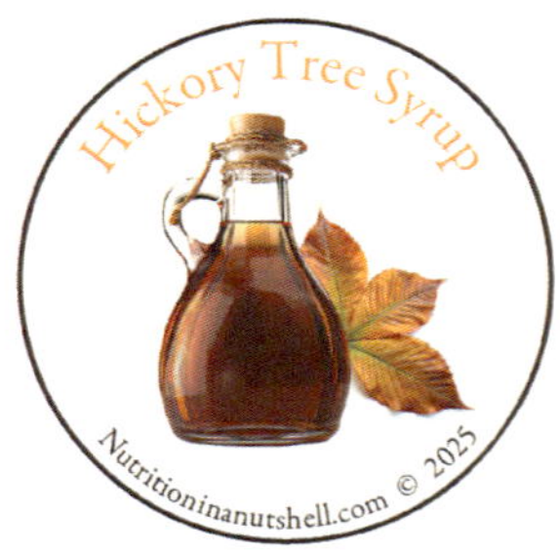

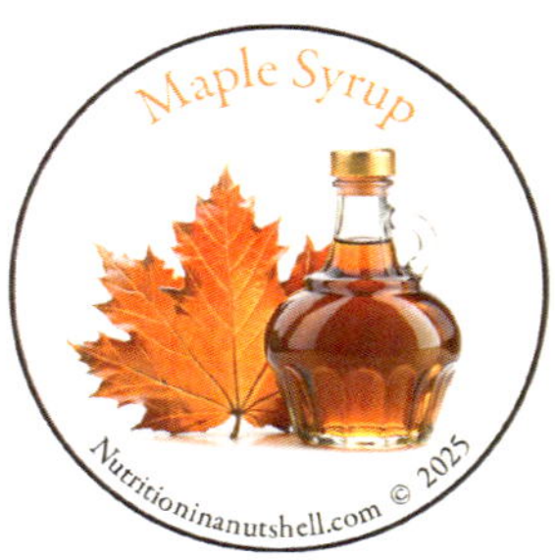

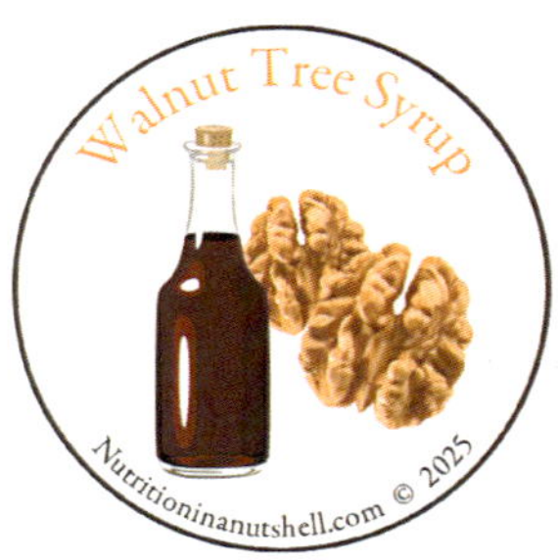

Seeds

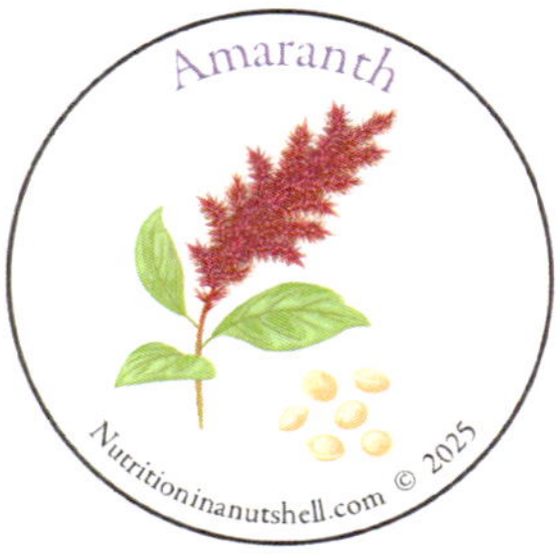
Amaranth
Nutritioninanutshell.com © 2025

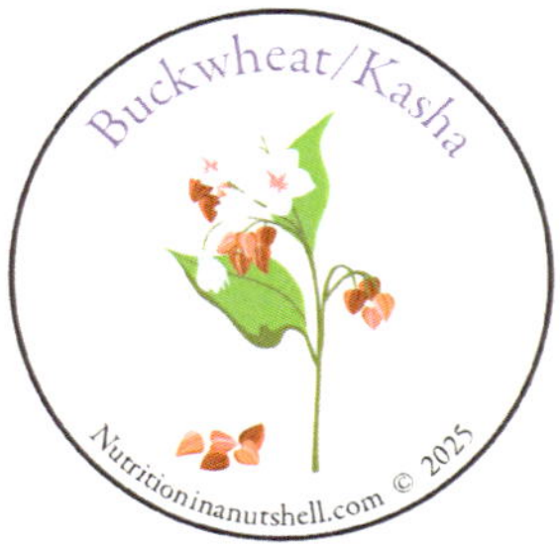
Buckwheat/Kasha
Nutritioninanutshell.com © 2025

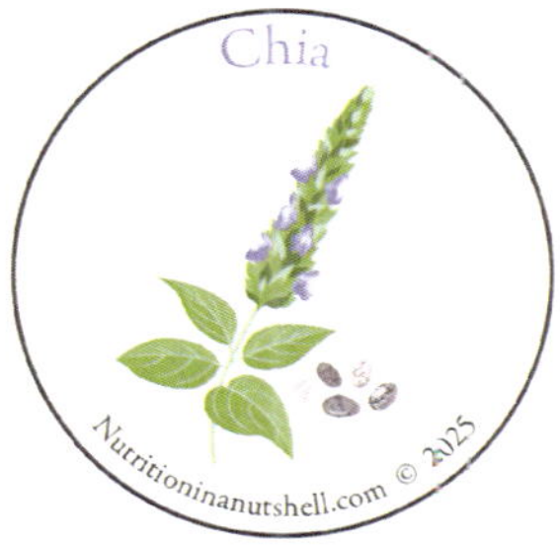
Chia
Nutritioninanutshell.com © 2025

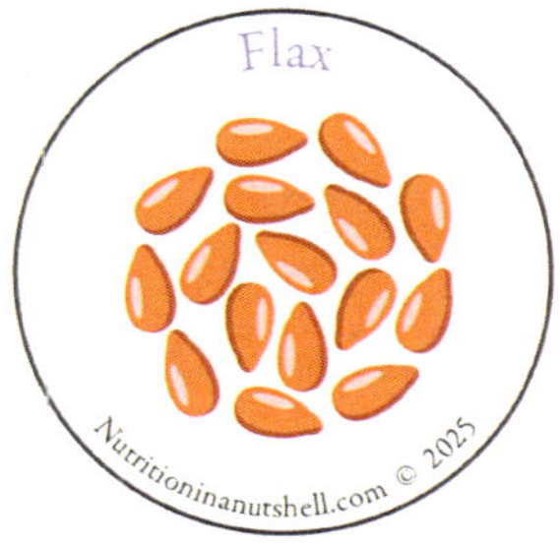
Flax
Nutritioninanutshell.com © 2025

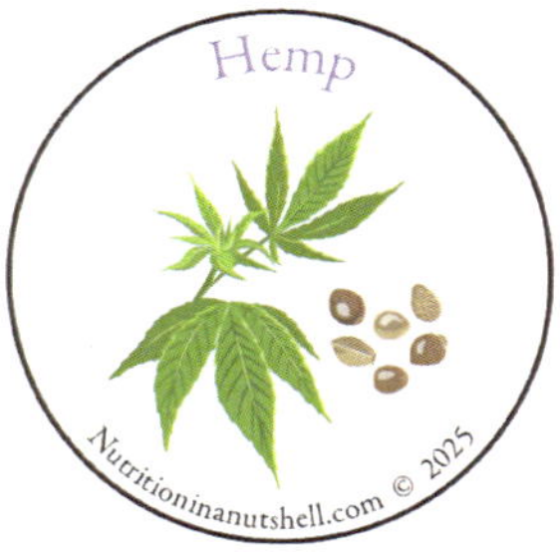
Hemp
Nutritioninanutshell.com © 2025

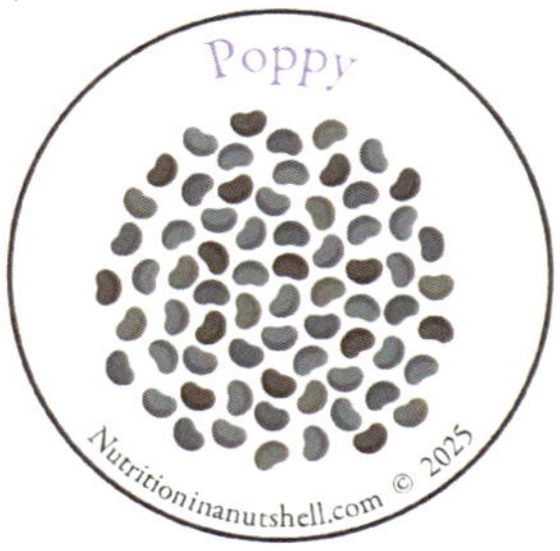
Poppy
Nutritioninanutshell.com © 2025

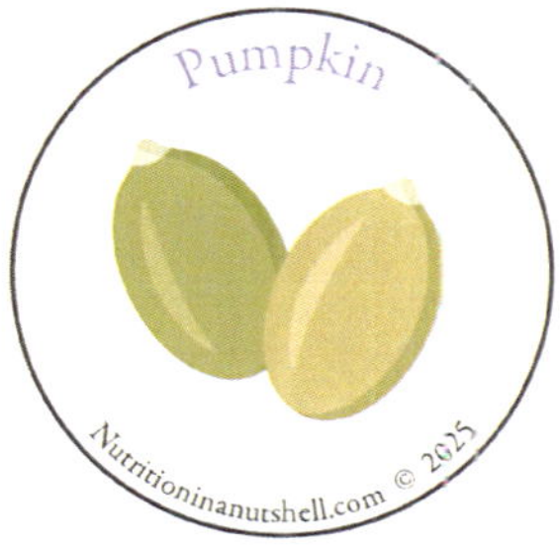
Pumpkin
Nutritioninanutshell.com © 2025

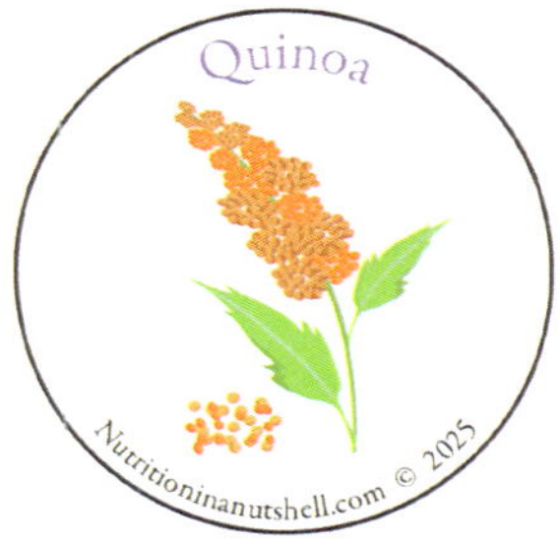
Quinoa
Nutritioninanutshell.com © 2025

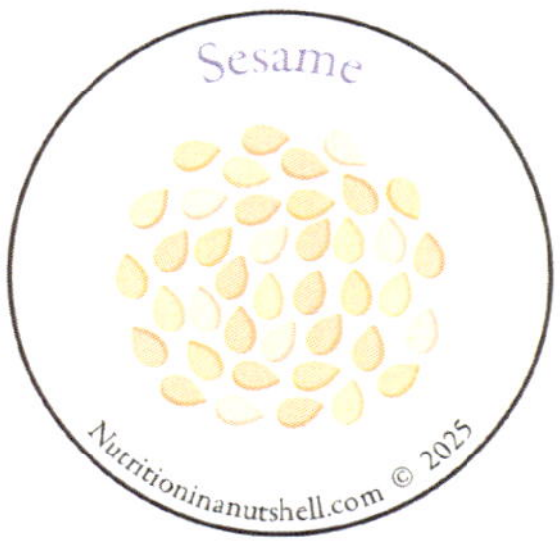
Sesame
Nutritioninanutshell.com © 2025

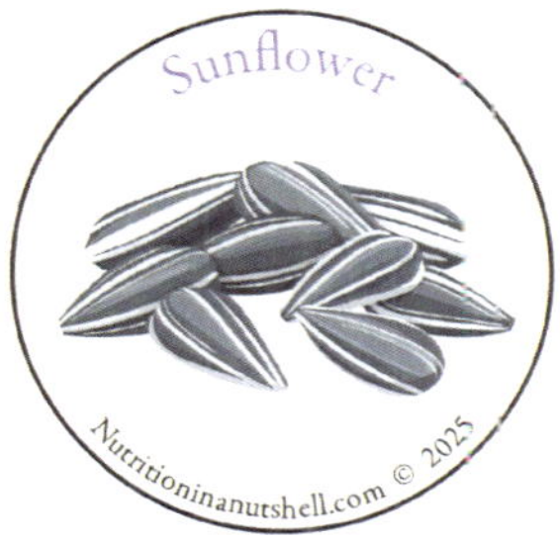
Sunflower
Nutritioninanutshell.com © 2025

Seasonings

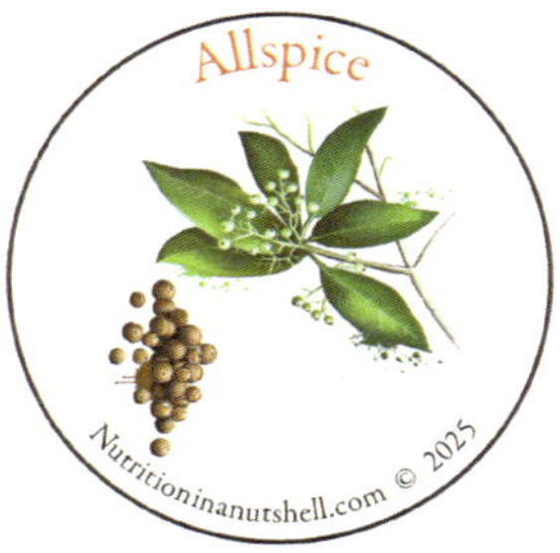
Allspice
Nutritioninanutshell.com © 2025

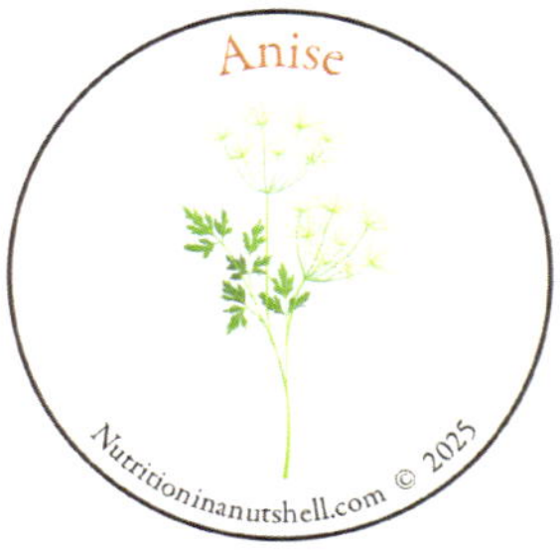
Anise
Nutritioninanutshell.com © 2025

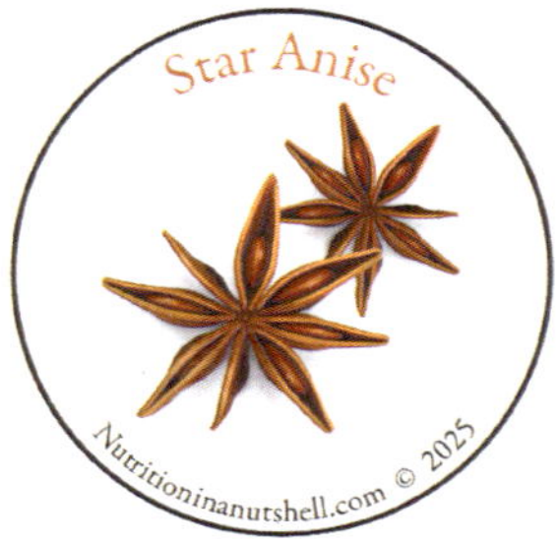
Star Anise
Nutritioninanutshell.com © 2025

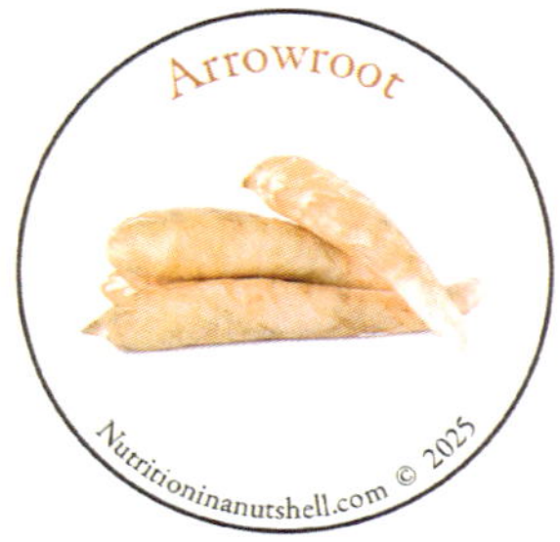
Arrowroot
Nutritioninanutshell.com © 2025

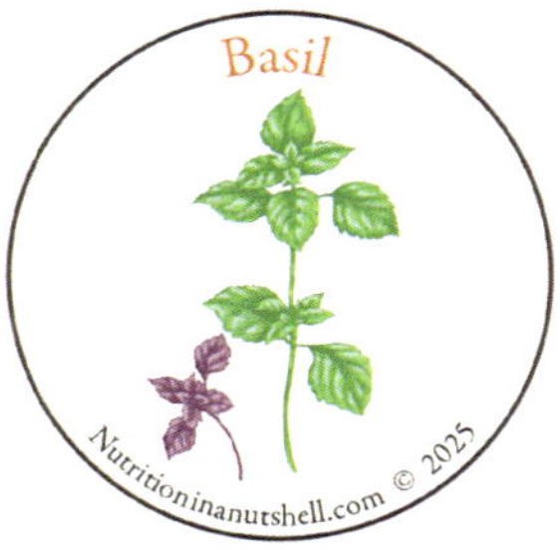
Basil
Nutritioninanutshell.com © 2025

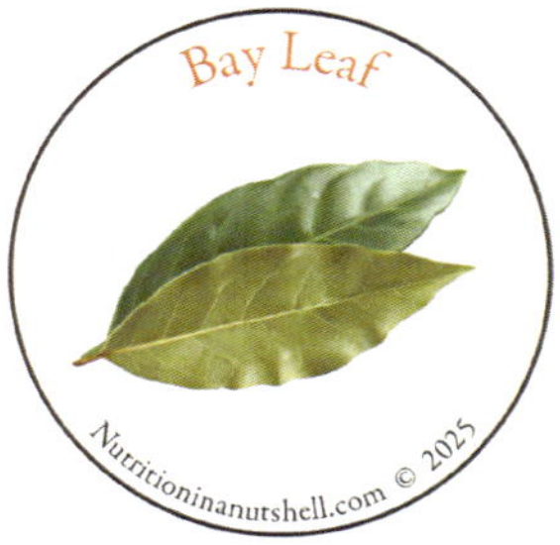
Bay Leaf
Nutritioninanutshell.com © 2025

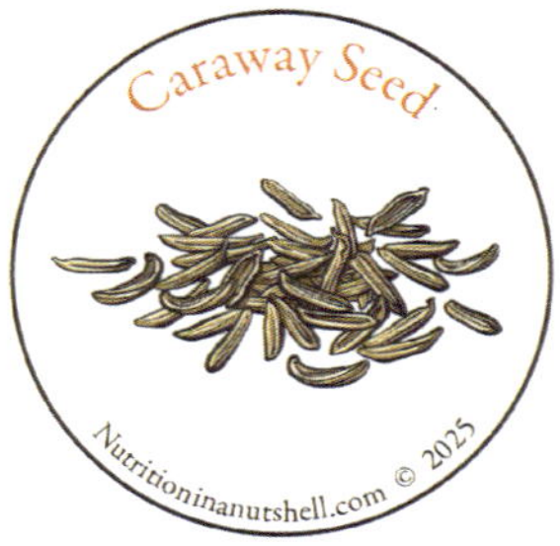
Caraway Seed
Nutritioninanutshell.com © 2025

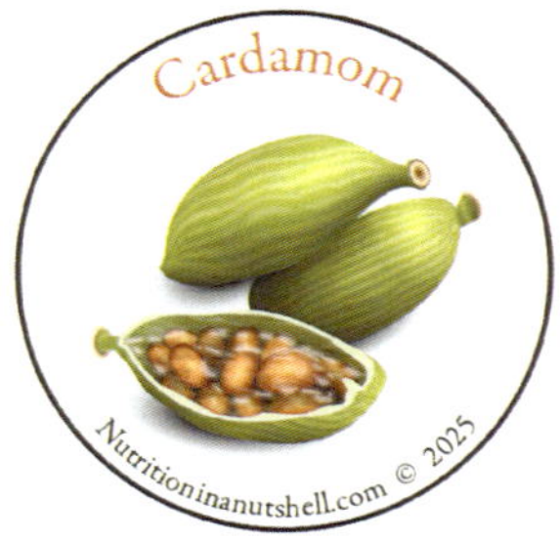
Cardamom
Nutritioninanutshell.com © 2025

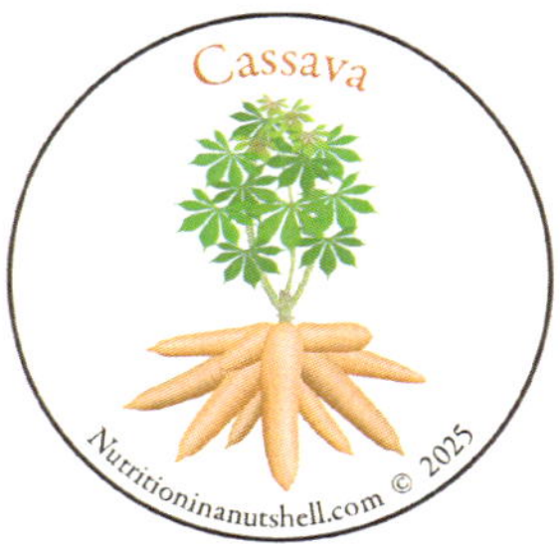
Cassava
Nutritioninanutshell.com © 2025

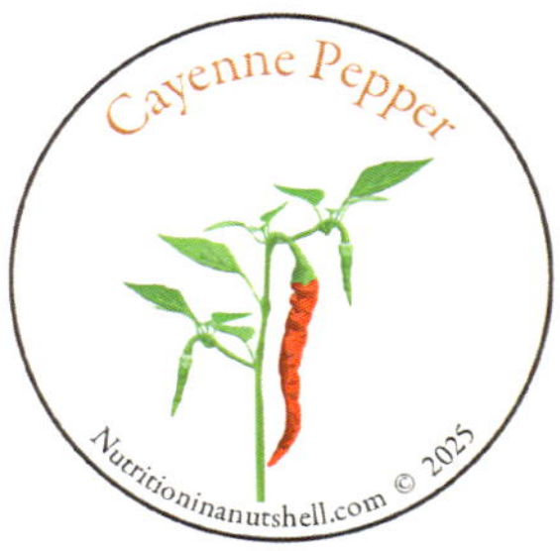
Cayenne Pepper
Nutritioninanutshell.com © 2025

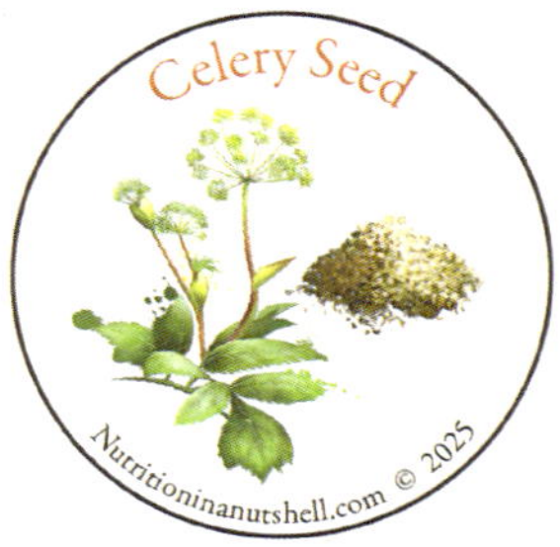
Celery Seed
Nutritioninanutshell.com © 2025

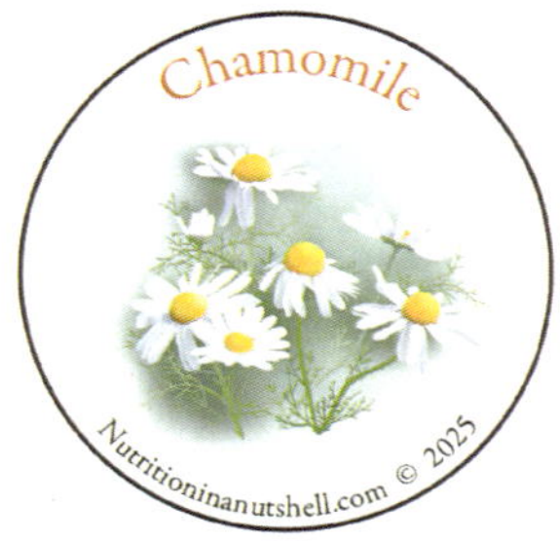
Chamomile
Nutritioninanutshell.com © 2025

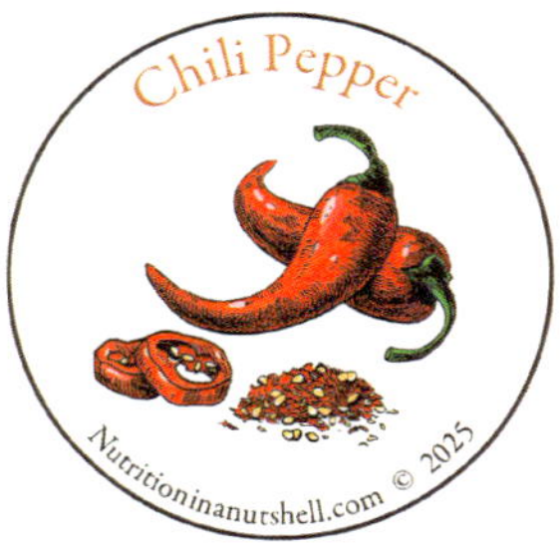
Chili Pepper
Nutritioninanutshell.com © 2025

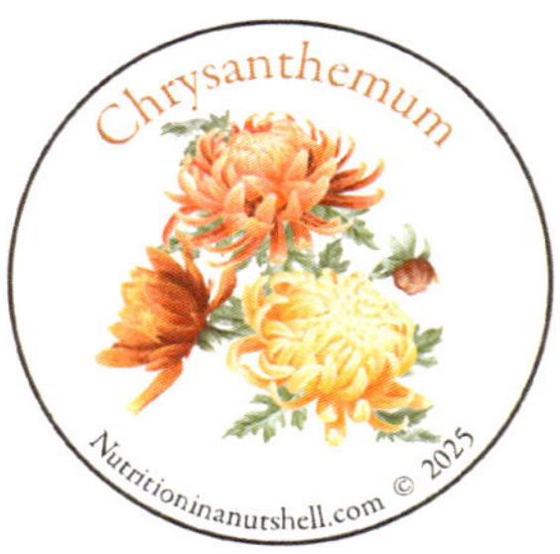
Chrysanthemum
Nutritioninanutshell.com © 2025

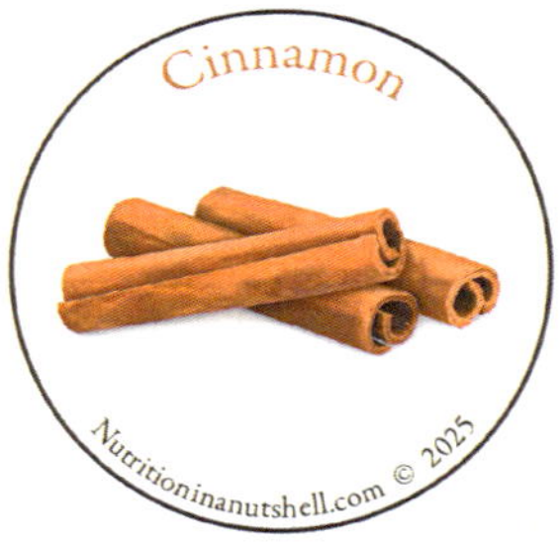
Cinnamon
Nutritioninanutshell.com © 2025

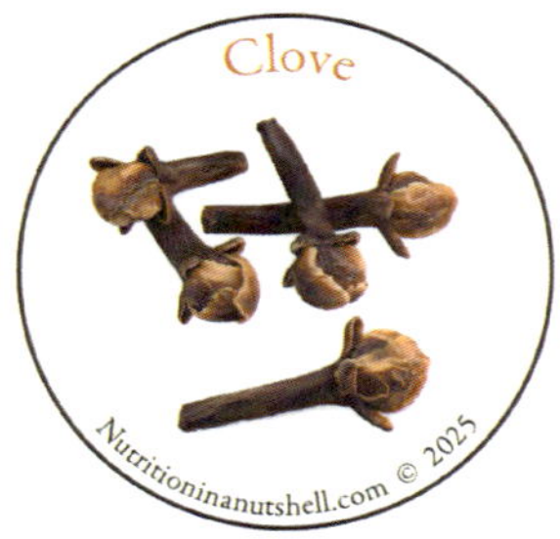
Clove
Nutritioninanutshell.com © 2025

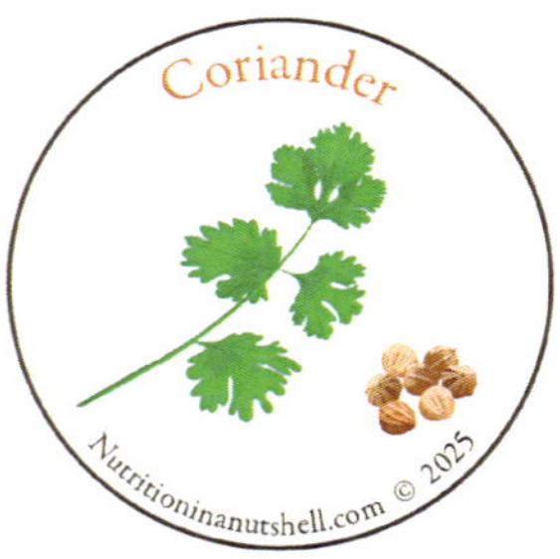
Coriander
Nutritioninanutshell.com © 2025

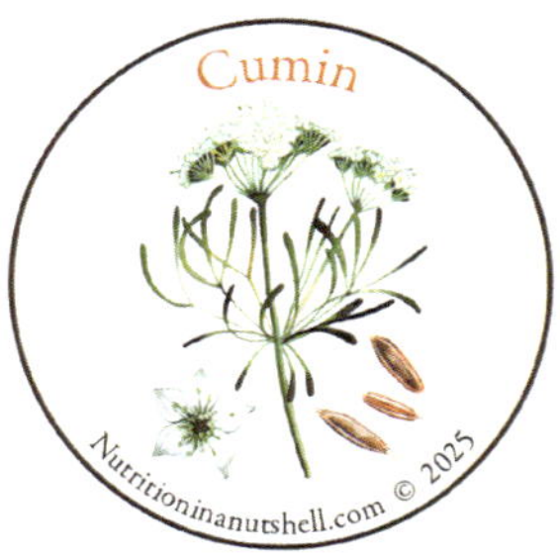
Cumin
Nutritioninanutshell.com © 2025

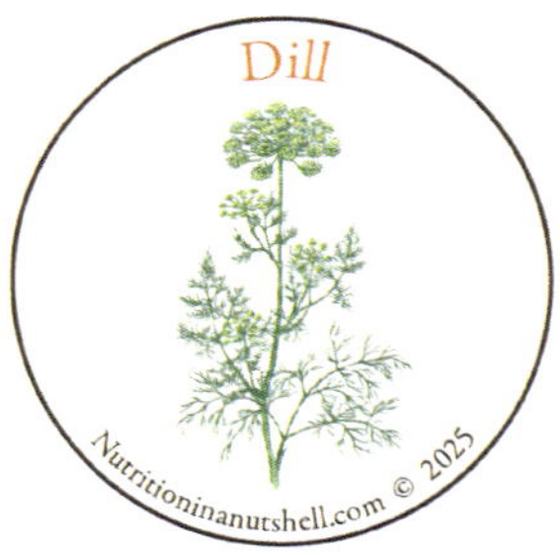
Dill
Nutritioninanutshell.com © 2025

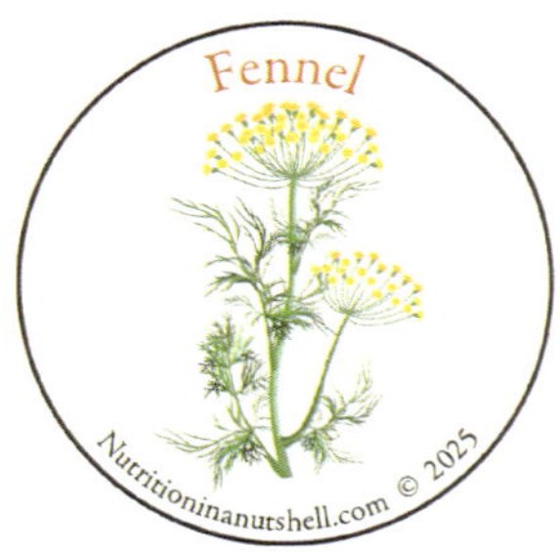
Fennel
Nutritioninanutshell.com © 2025

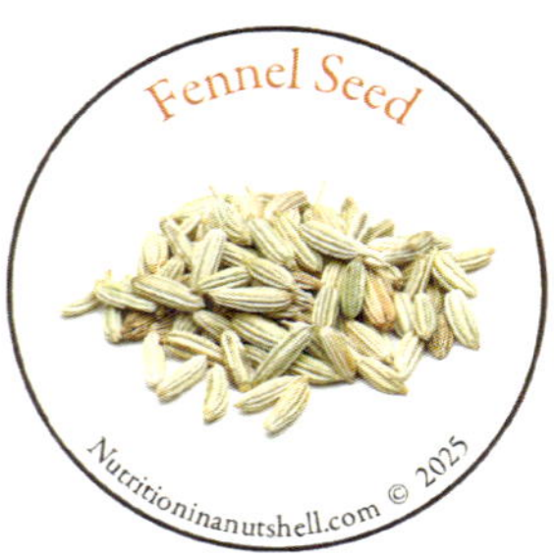
Fennel Seed
Nutritioninanutshell.com © 2025

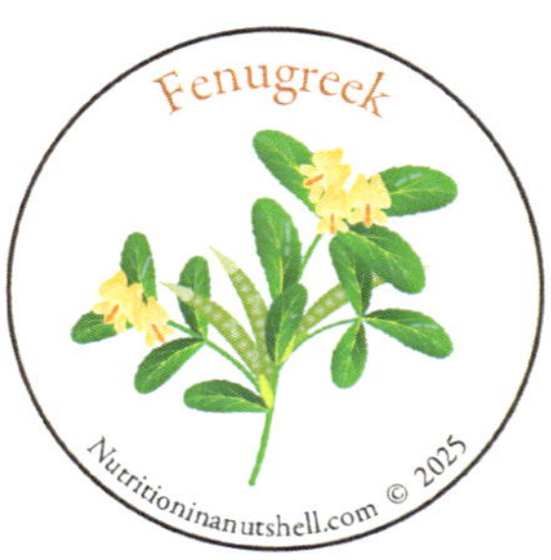
Fenugreek
Nutritioninanutshell.com © 2025

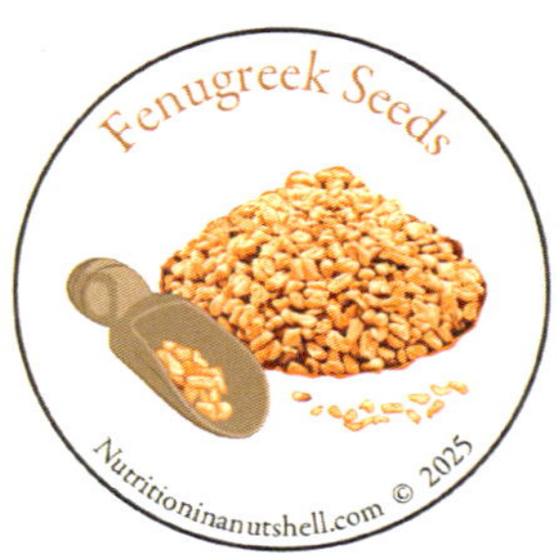
Fenugreek Seeds
Nutritioninanutshell.com © 2025

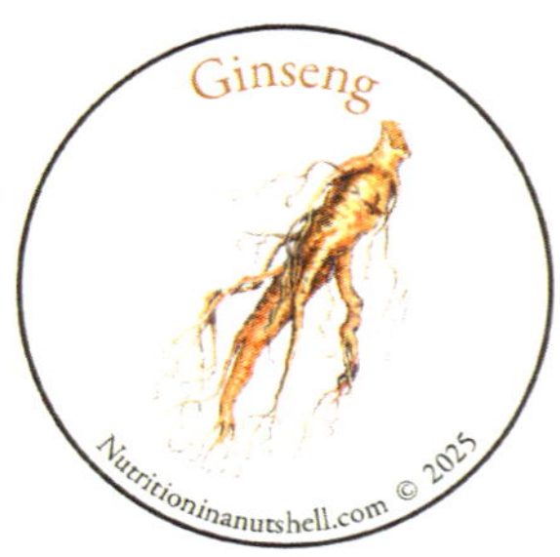
Ginseng
Nutritioninanutshell.com © 2025

Seasonings

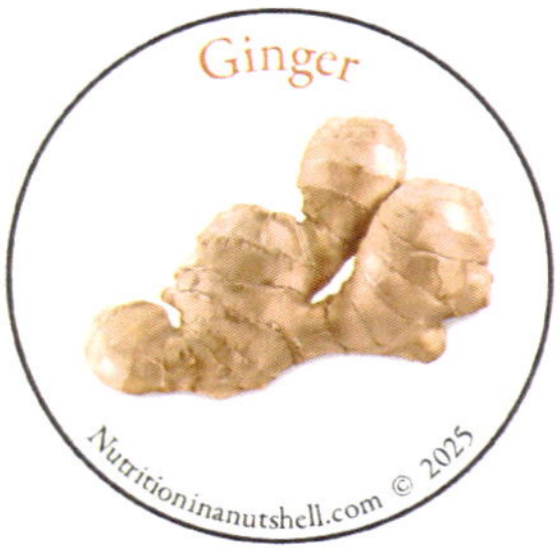
Ginger
Nutritioninanutshell.com © 2025

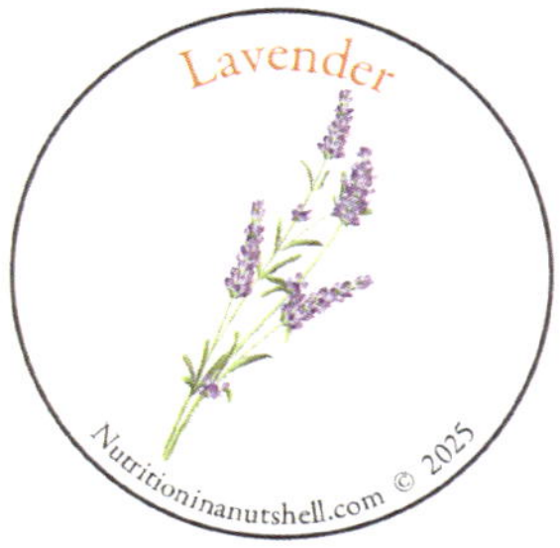
Lavender
Nutritioninanutshell.com © 2025

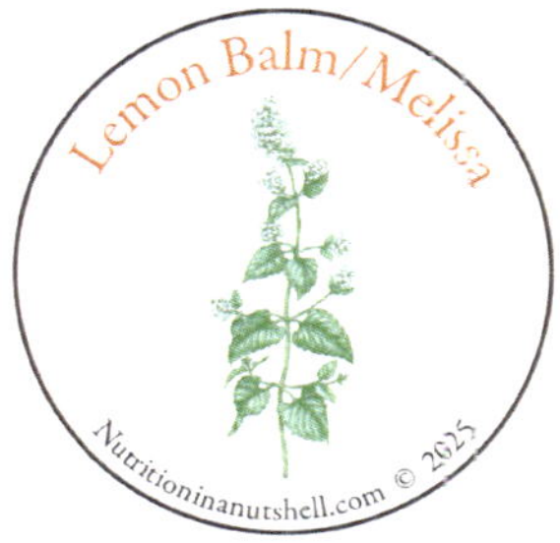
Lemon Balm/Melissa
Nutritioninanutshell.com © 2025

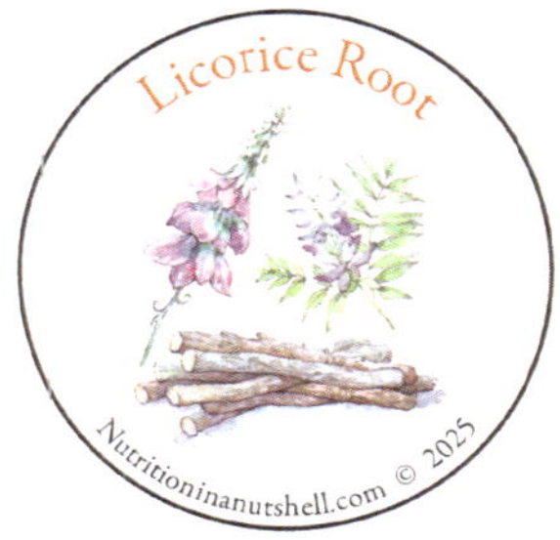
Licorice Root
Nutritioninanutshell.com © 2025

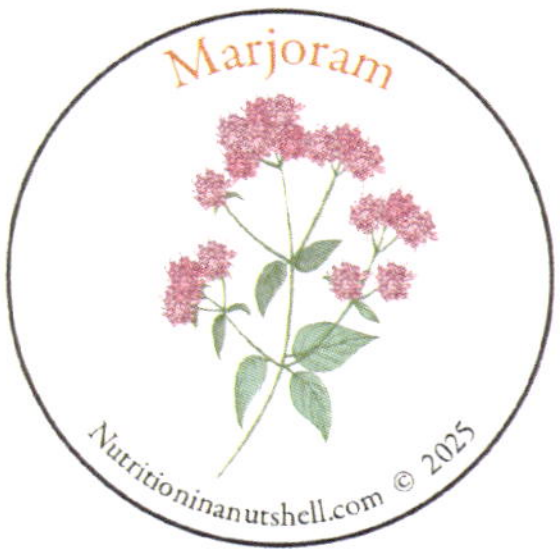
Marjoram
Nutritioninanutshell.com © 2025

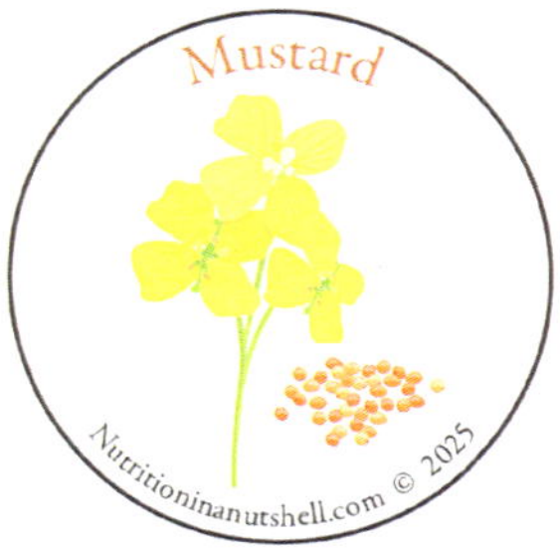
Mustard
Nutritioninanutshell.com © 2025

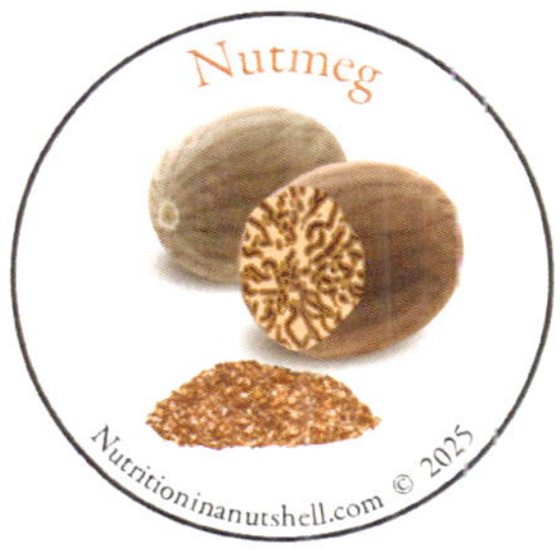
Nutmeg
Nutritioninanutshell.com © 2025

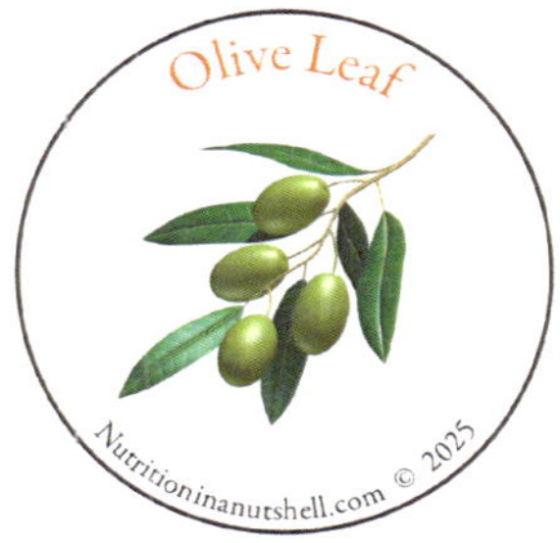
Olive Leaf
Nutritioninanutshell.com © 2025

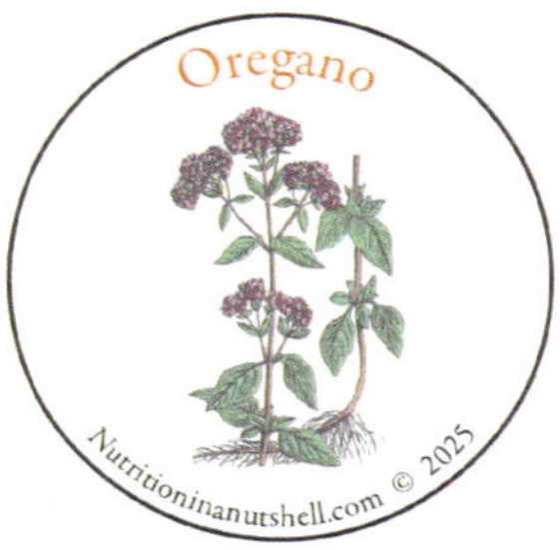
Oregano
Nutritioninanutshell.com © 2025

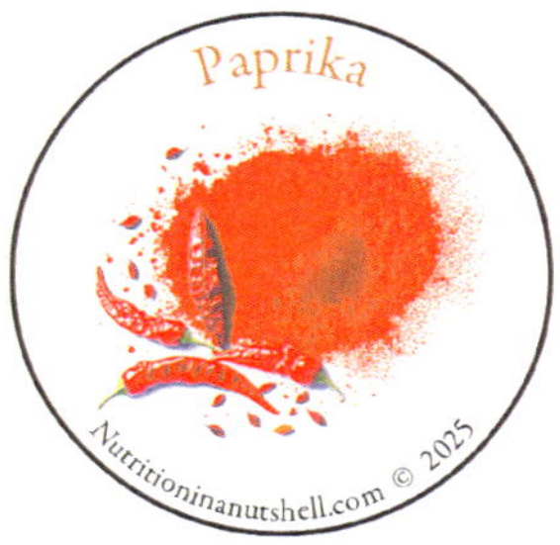
Paprika
Nutritioninanutshell.com © 2025

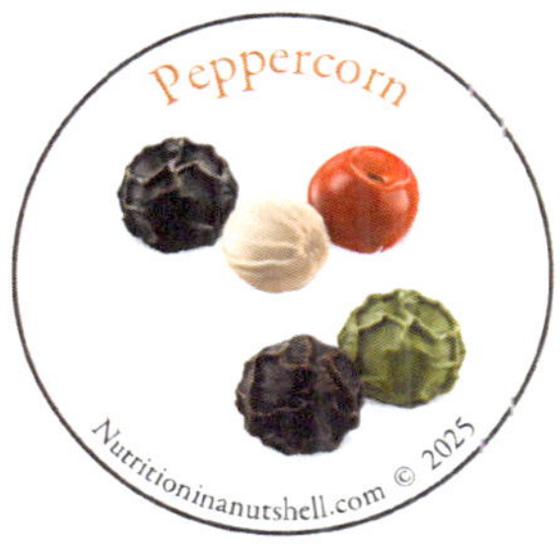
Peppercorn
Nutritioninanutshell.com © 2025

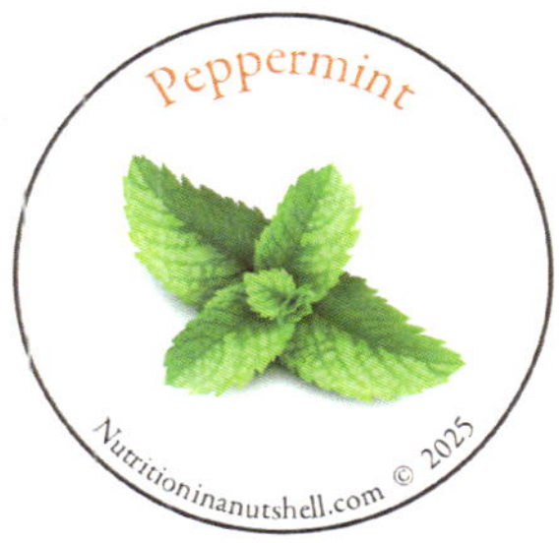
Peppermint
Nutritioninanutshell.com © 2025

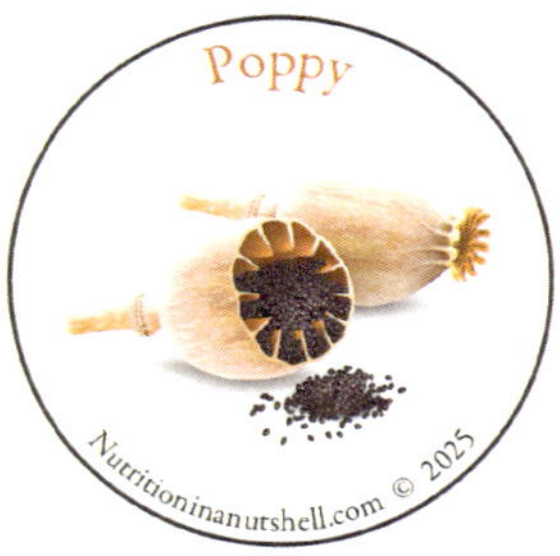
Poppy
Nutritioninanutshell.com © 2025

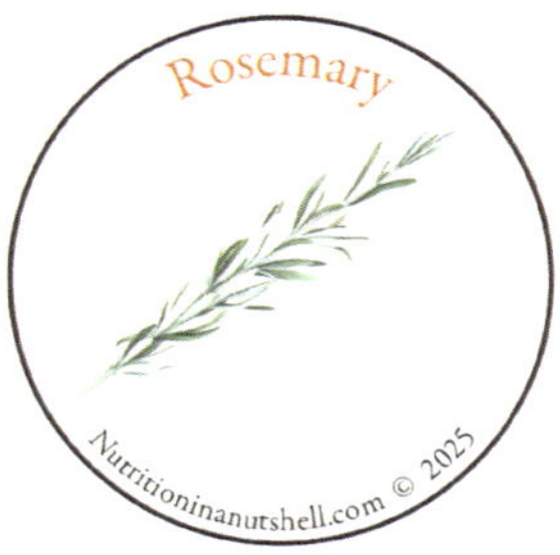
Rosemary
Nutritioninanutshell.com © 2025

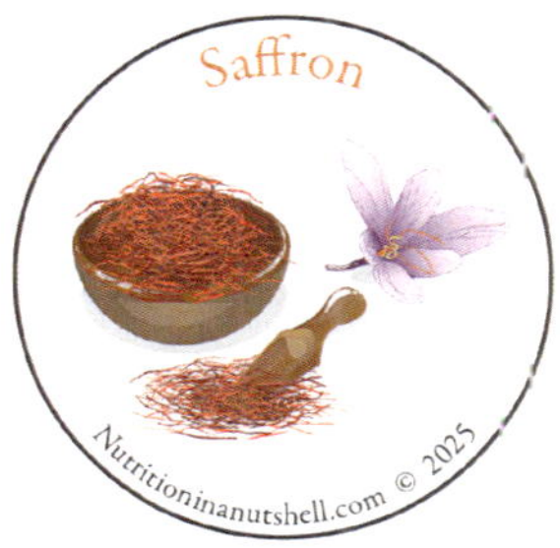
Saffron
Nutritioninanutshell.com © 2025

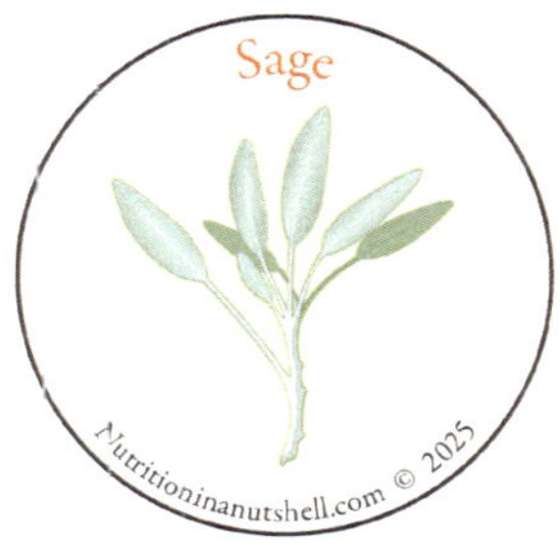
Sage
Nutritioninanutshell.com © 2025

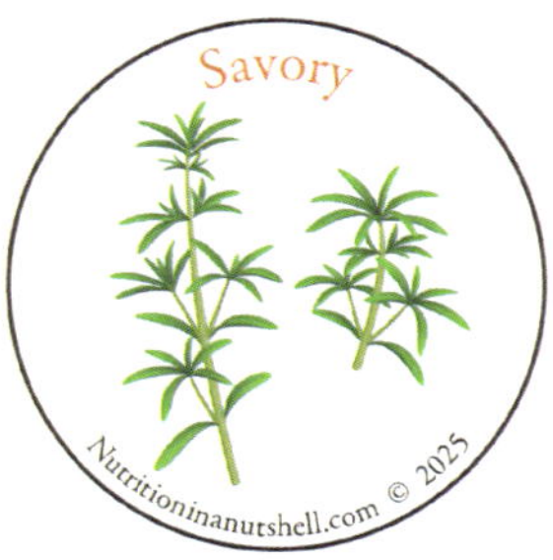
Savory
Nutritioninanutshell.com © 2025

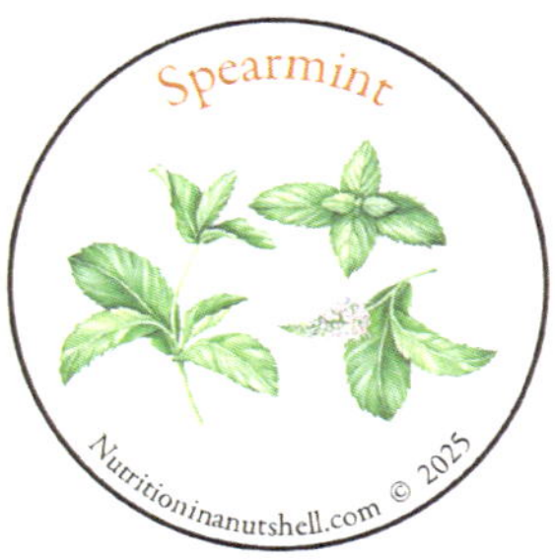
Spearmint
Nutritioninanutshell.com © 2025

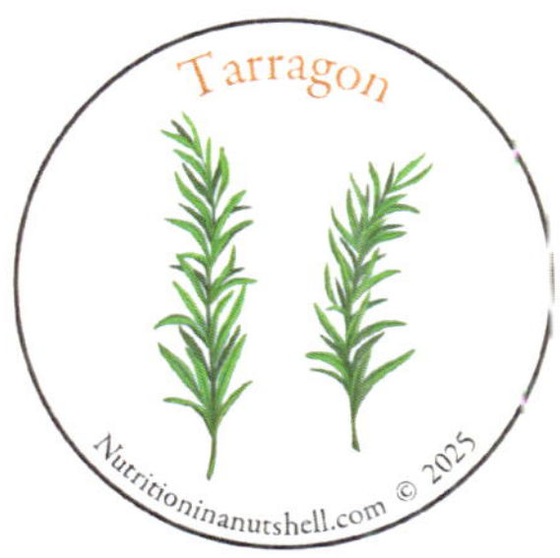
Tarragon
Nutritioninanutshell.com © 2025

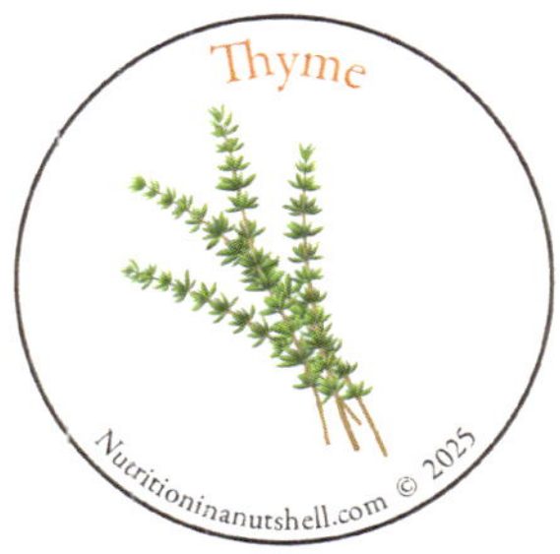
Thyme
Nutritioninanutshell.com © 2025

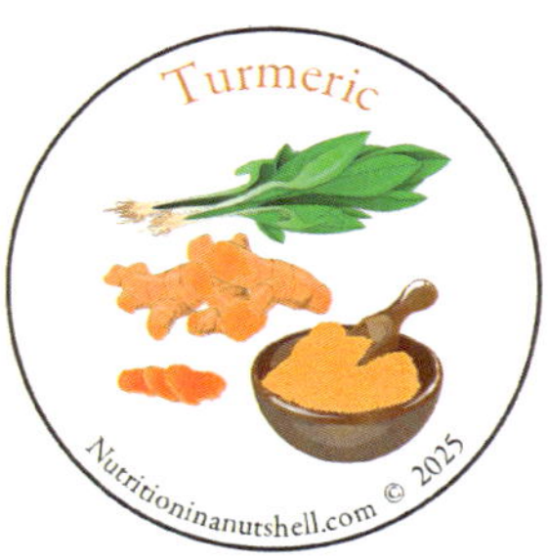
Turmeric
Nutritioninanutshell.com © 2025

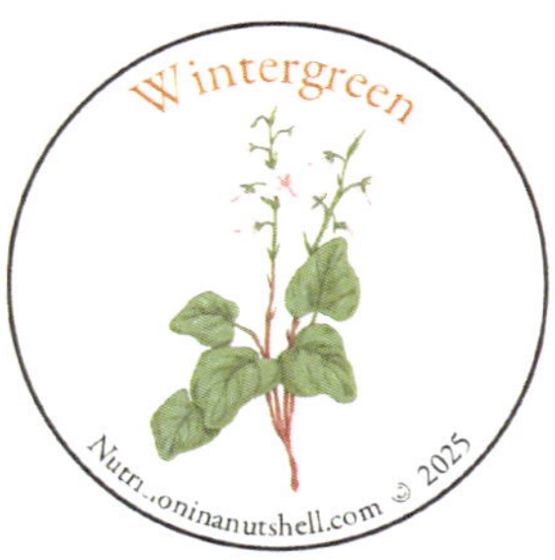
Wintergreen

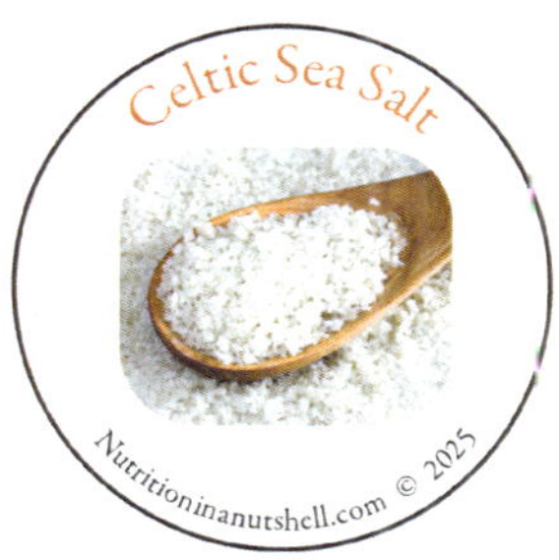
Celtic Sea Salt
Nutritioninanutshell.com © 2025

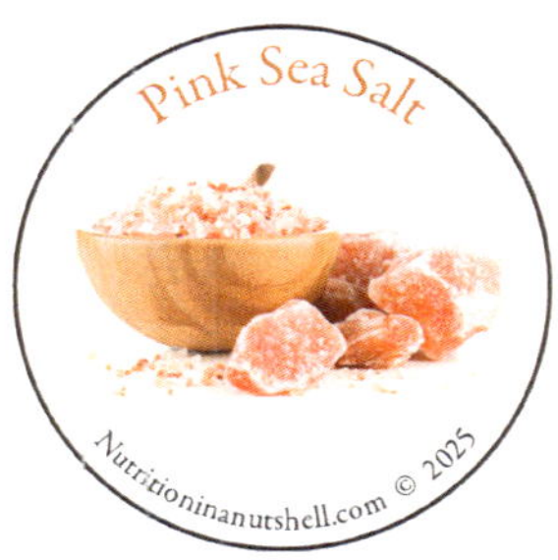
Pink Sea Salt
Nutritioninanutshell.com © 2025

Vegetables

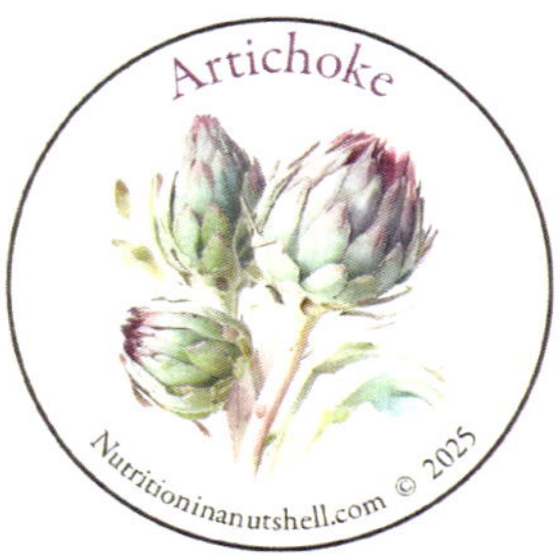
Artichoke
Nutritioninanutshell.com © 2025

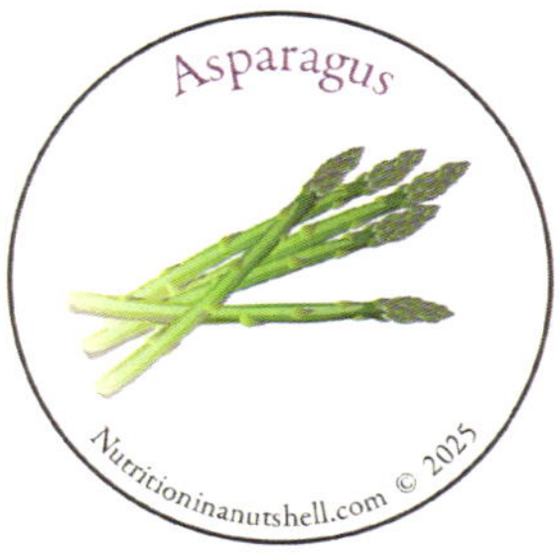
Asparagus
Nutritioninanutshell.com © 2025

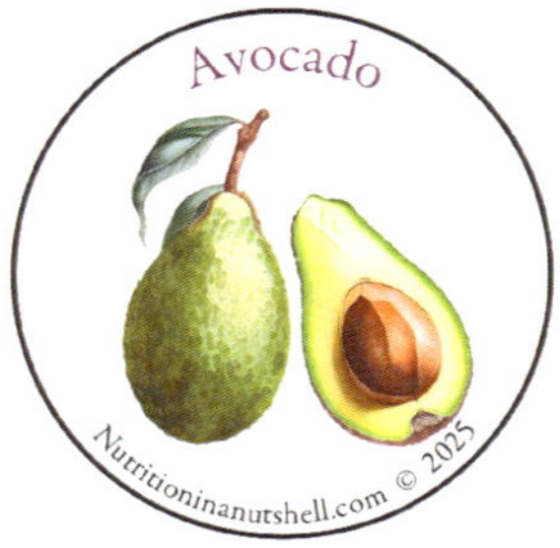
Avocado
Nutritioninanutshell.com © 2025

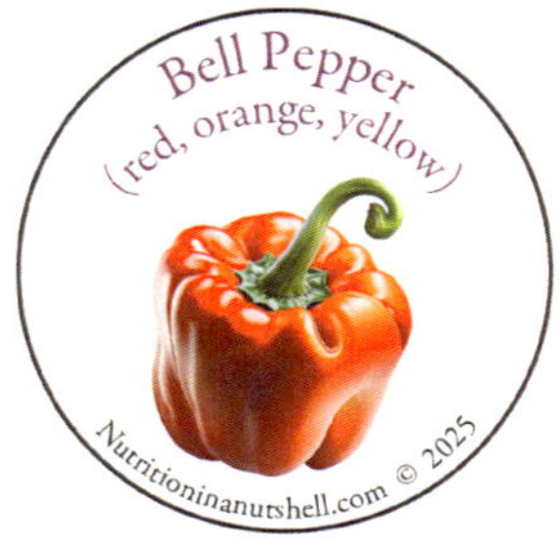
Bell Pepper
(red, orange, yellow)
Nutritioninanutshell.com © 2025

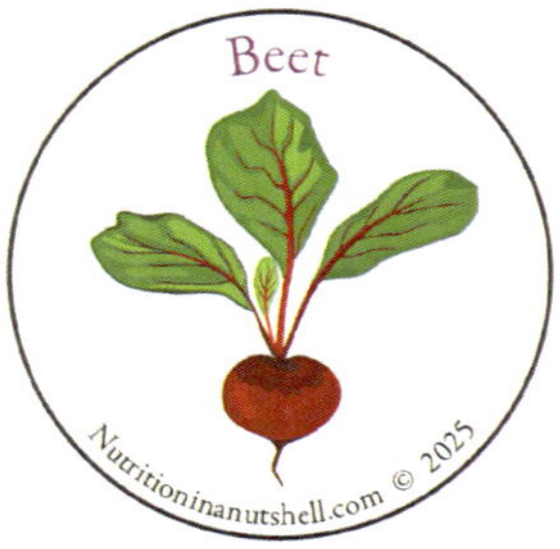
Beet
Nutritioninanutshell.com © 2025

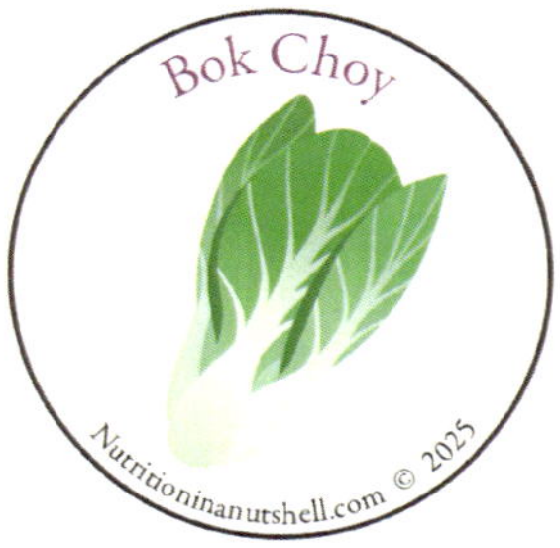
Bok Choy
Nutritioninanutshell.com © 2025

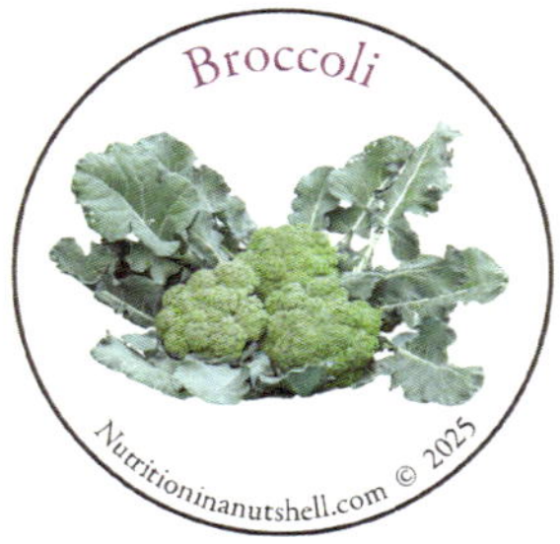
Broccoli
Nutritioninanutshell.com © 2025

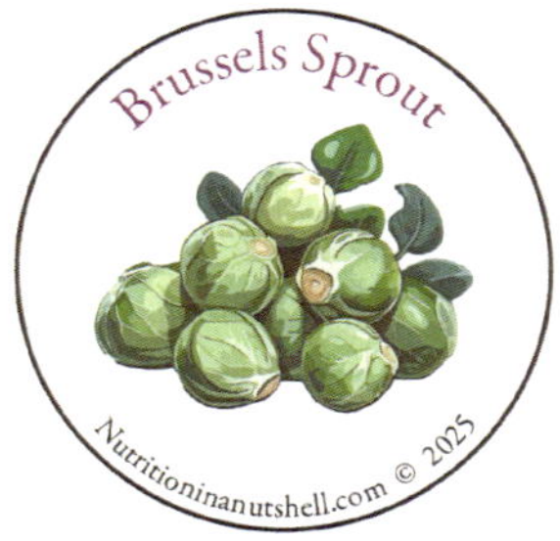
Brussels Sprout
Nutritioninanutshell.com © 2025

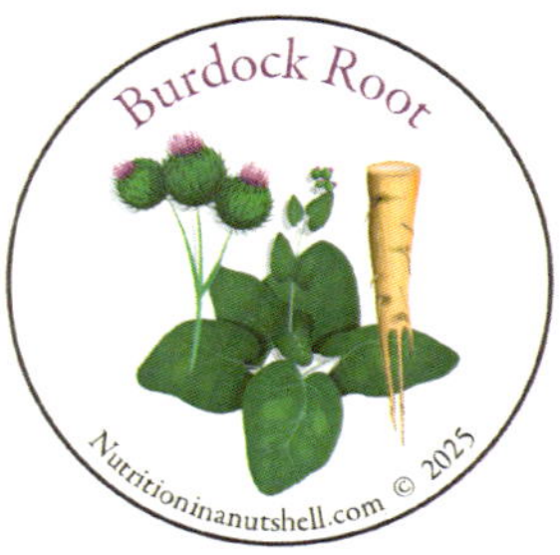
Burdock Root
Nutritioninanutshell.com © 2025

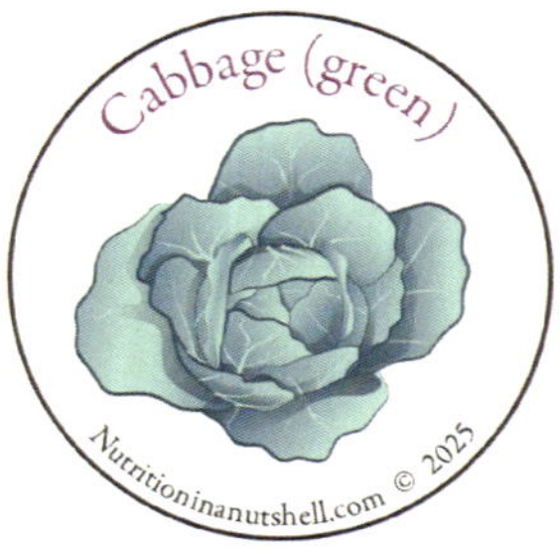
Cabbage (green)
Nutritioninanutshell.com © 2025

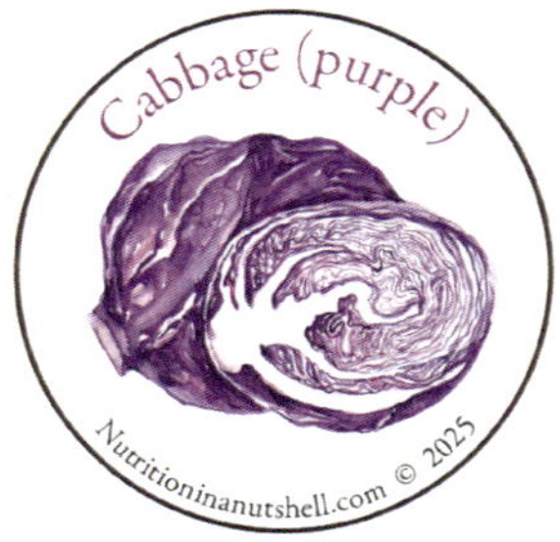
Cabbage (purple)
Nutritioninanutshell.com © 2025

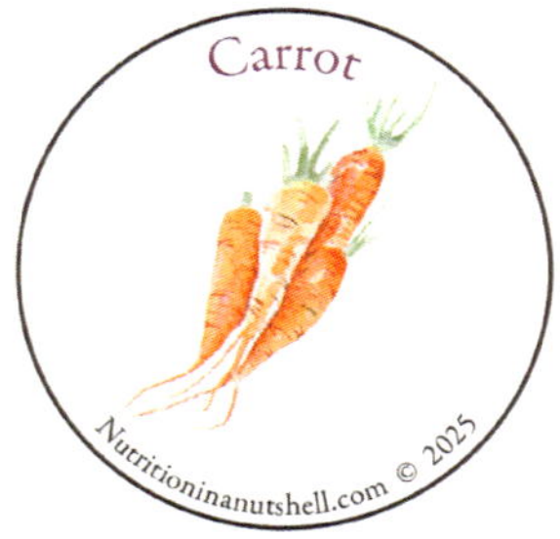
Carrot
Nutritioninanutshell.com © 2025

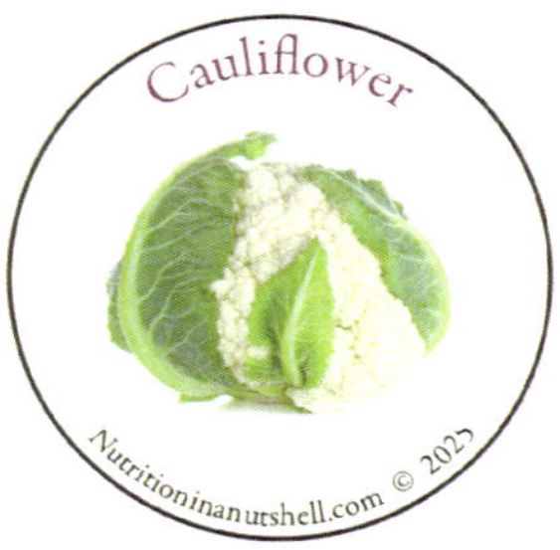
Cauliflower
Nutritioninanutshell.com © 2025

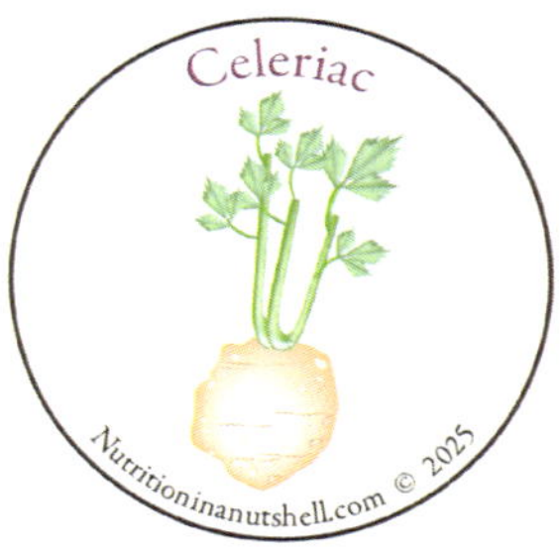
Celeriac
Nutritioninanutshell.com © 2025

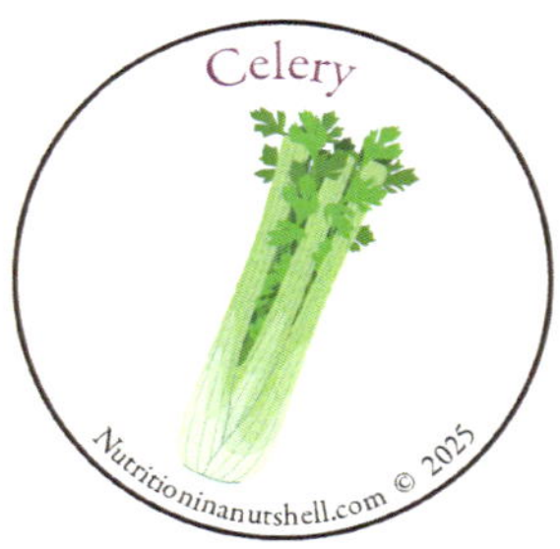
Celery
Nutritioninanutshell.com © 2025

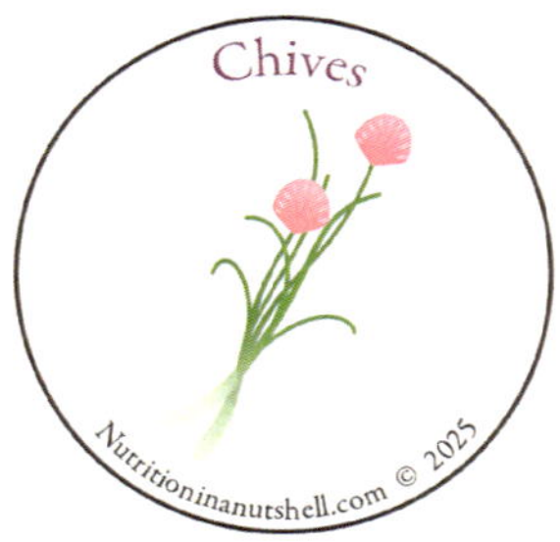
Chives
Nutritioninanutshell.com © 2025

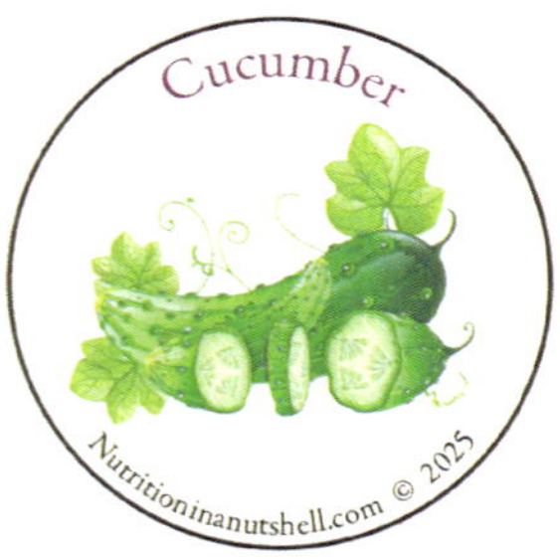
Cucumber
Nutritioninanutshell.com © 2025

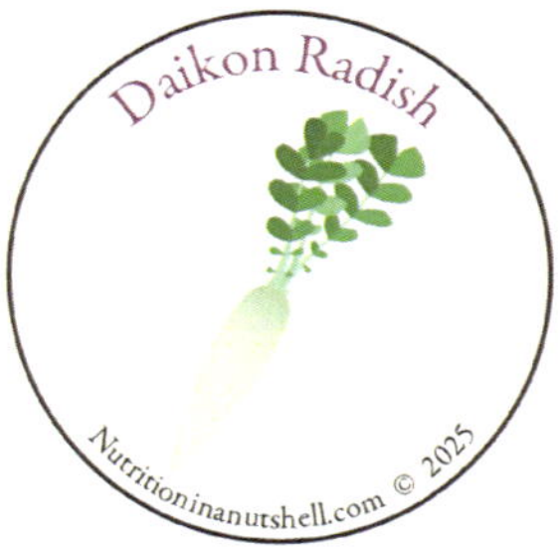
Daikon Radish
Nutritioninanutshell.com © 2025

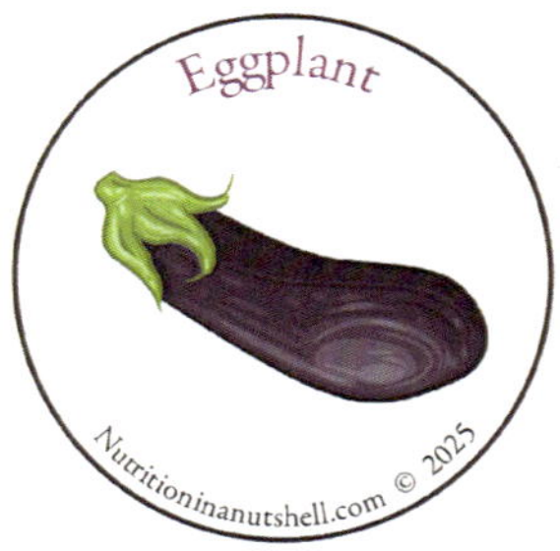
Eggplant
Nutritioninanutshell.com © 2025

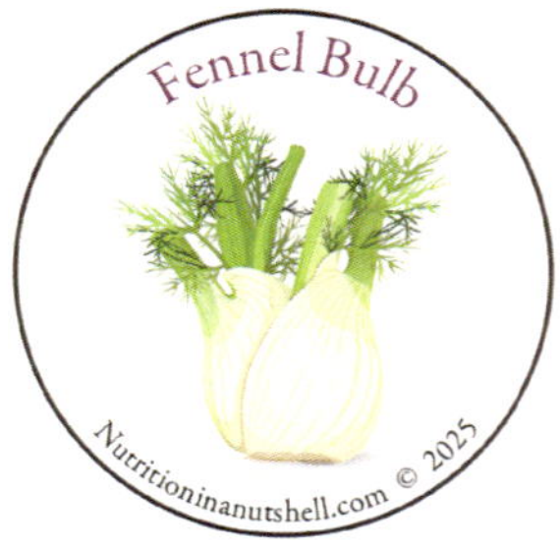
Fennel Bulb
Nutritioninanutshell.com © 2025

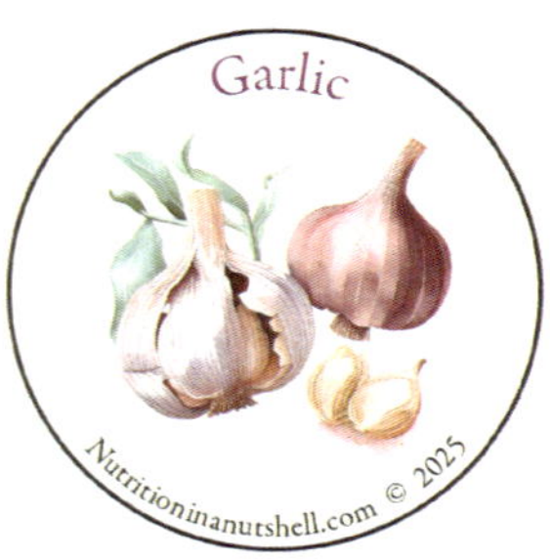
Garlic
Nutritioninanutshell.com © 2025

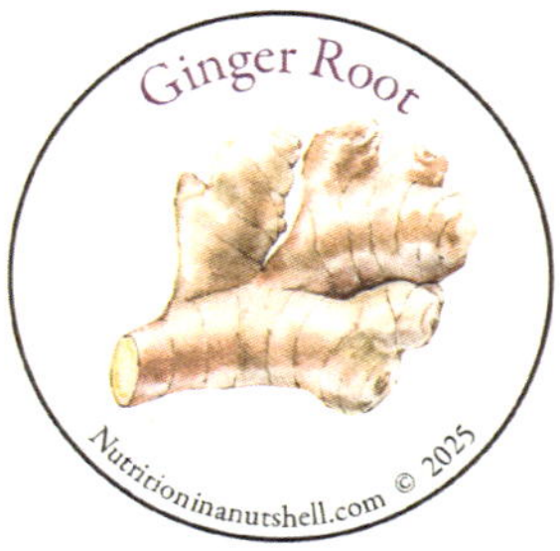
Ginger Root
Nutritioninanutshell.com © 2025

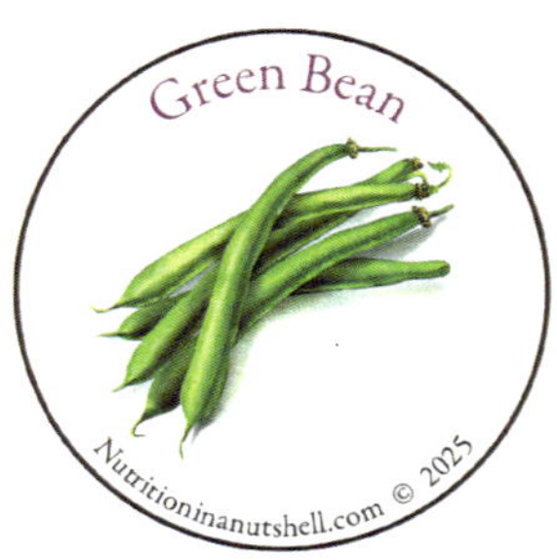
Green Bean
Nutritioninanutshell.com © 2025

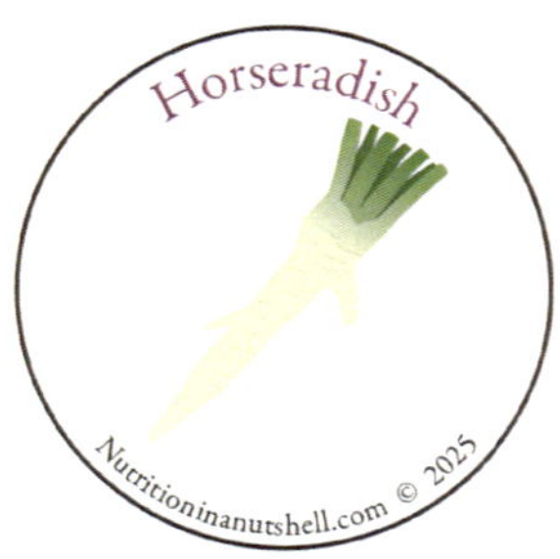
Horseradish
Nutritioninanutshell.com © 2025

Vegetables

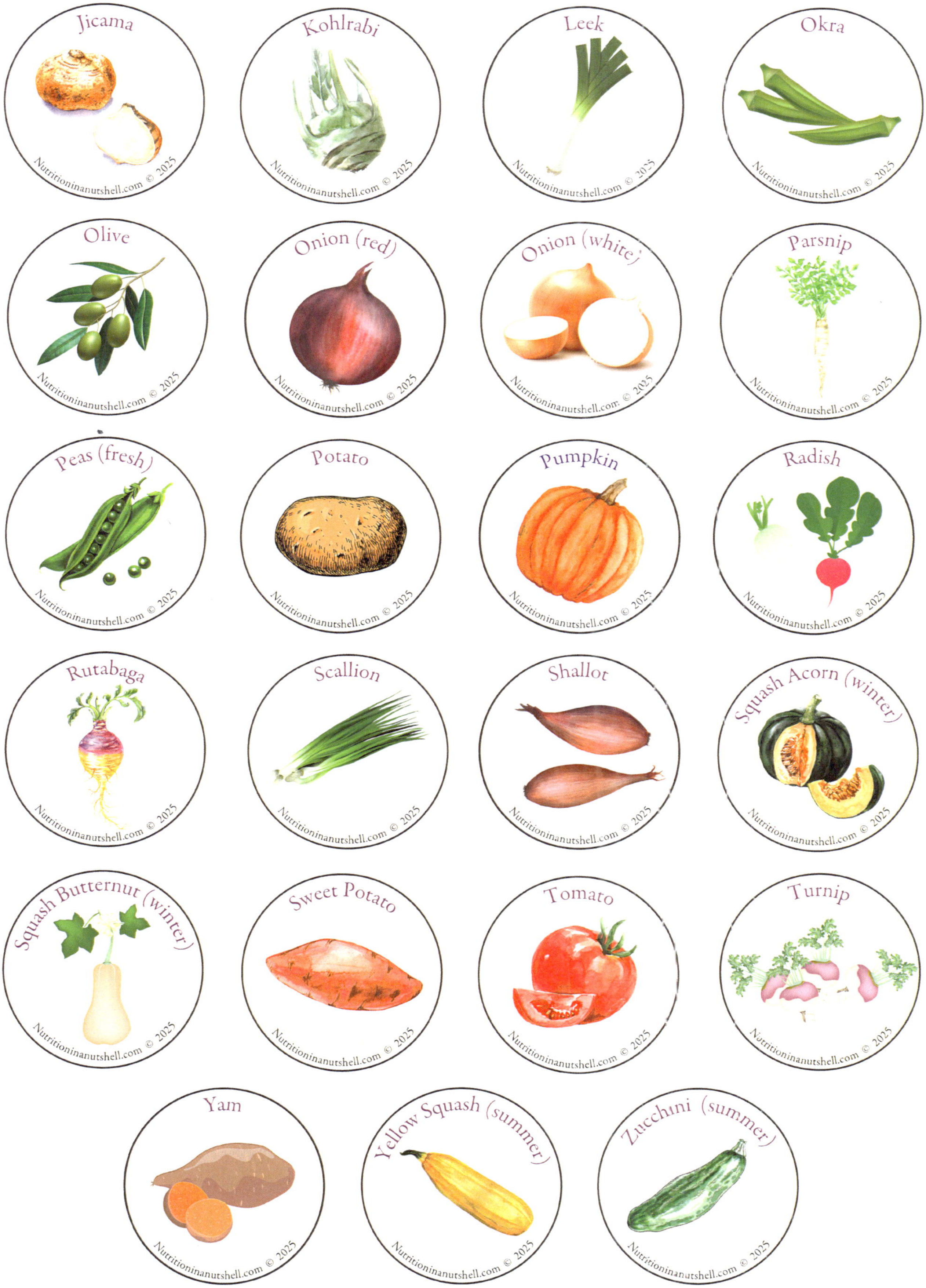
Jicama
Kohlrabi
Leek
Okra
Olive
Onion (red)
Onion (white)
Parsnip
Peas (fresh)
Potato
Pumpkin
Radish
Rutabaga
Scallion
Shallot
Squash Acorn (winter)
Squash Butternut (winter)
Sweet Potato
Tomato
Turnip
Yam
Yellow Squash (summer)
Zucchini (summer)
Nutritioninanutshell.com © 2025

Leafy Greens

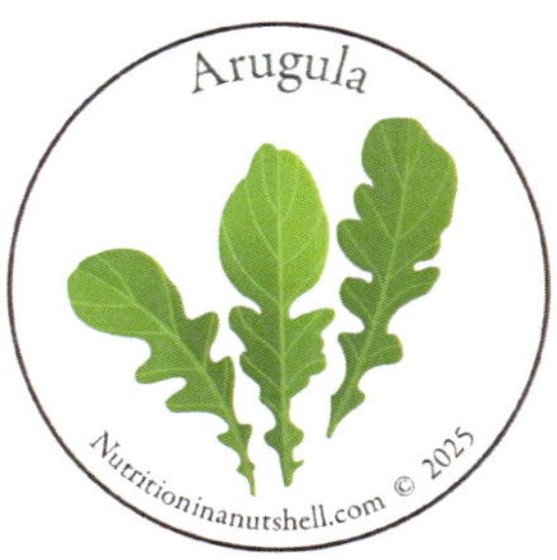

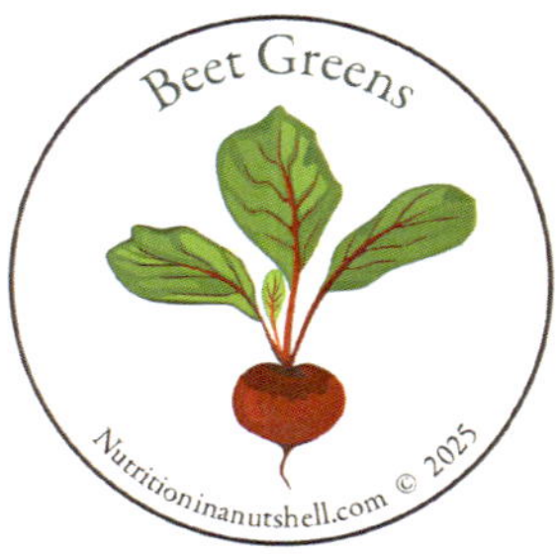

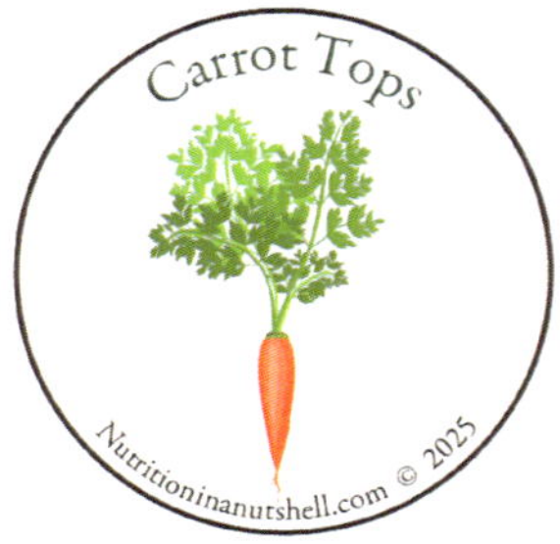

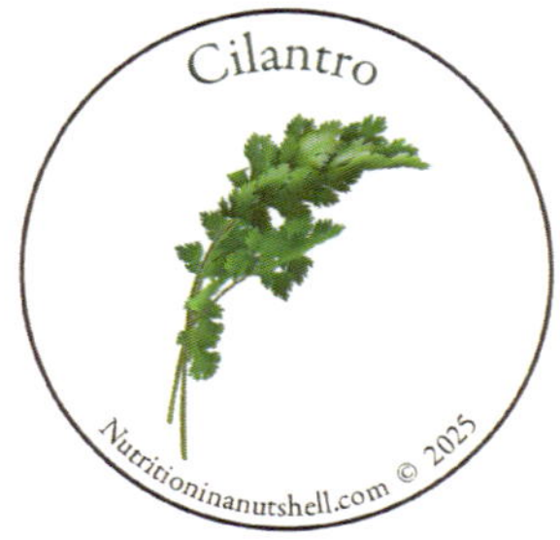

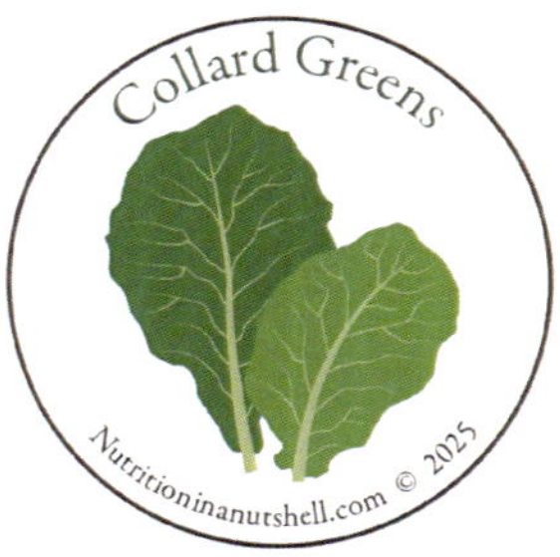

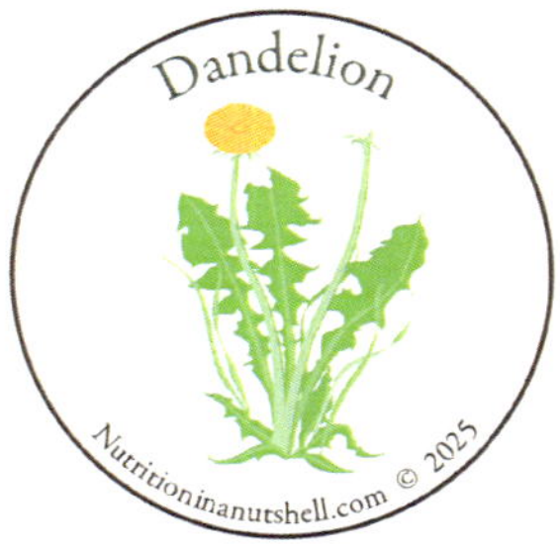

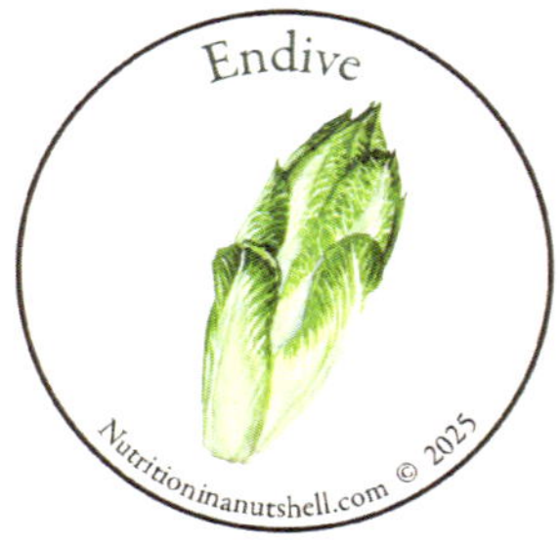

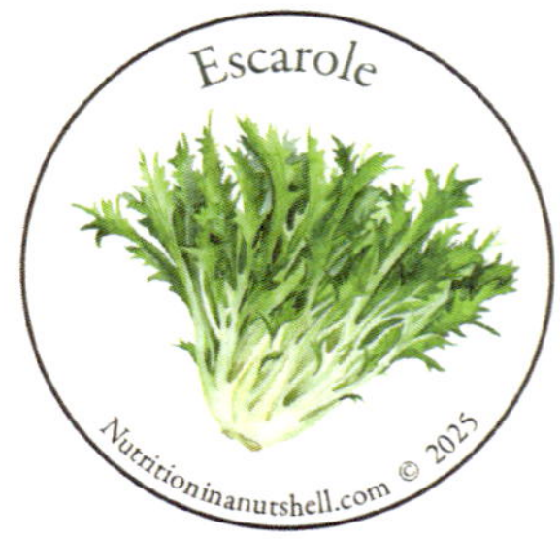

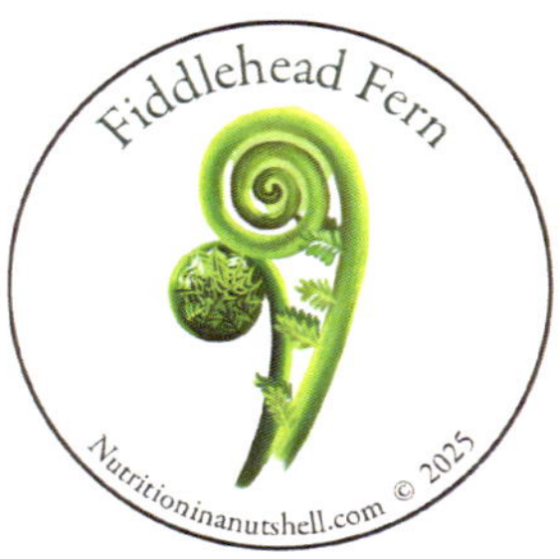

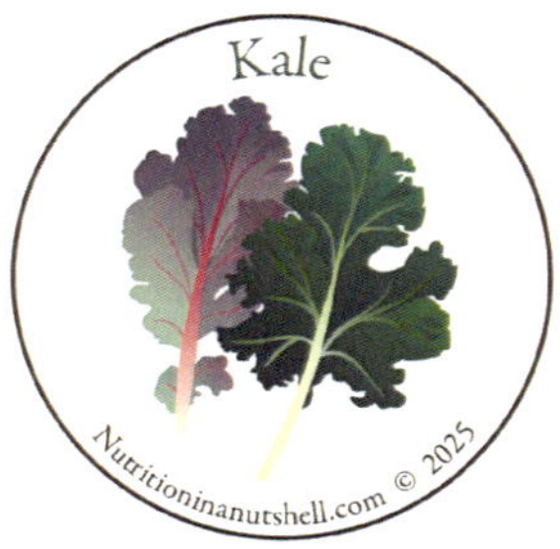

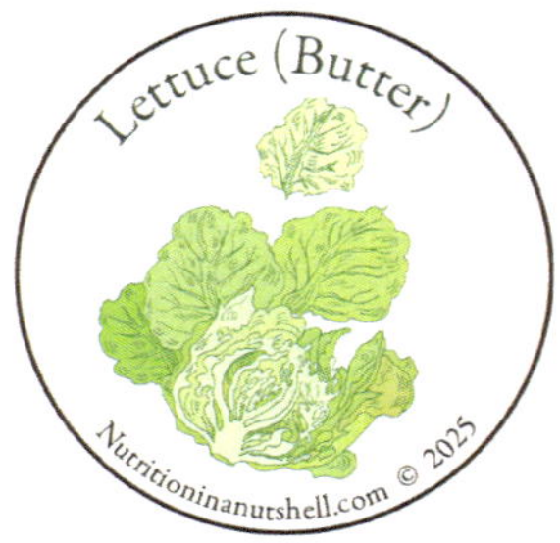

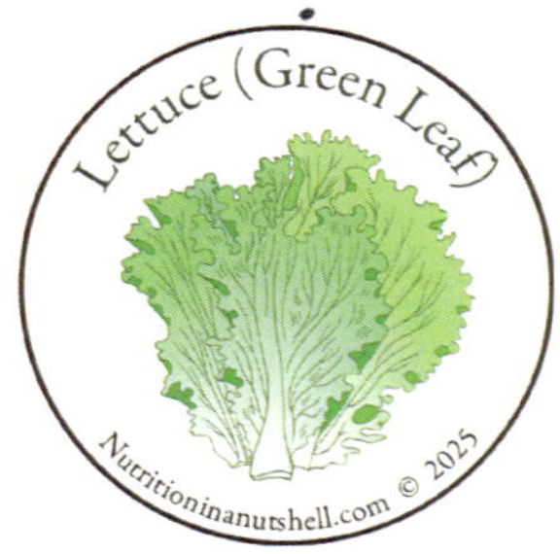

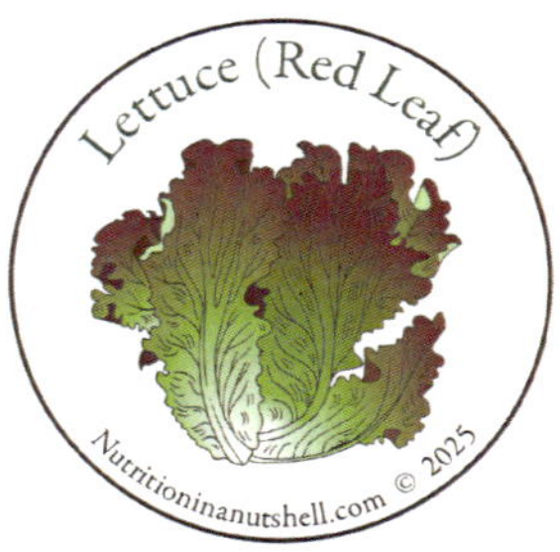

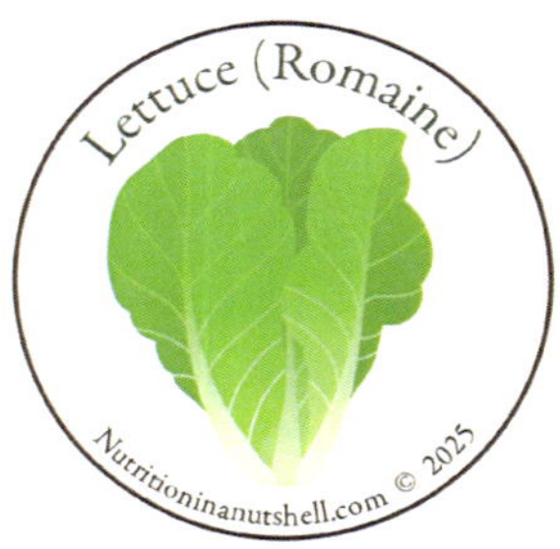

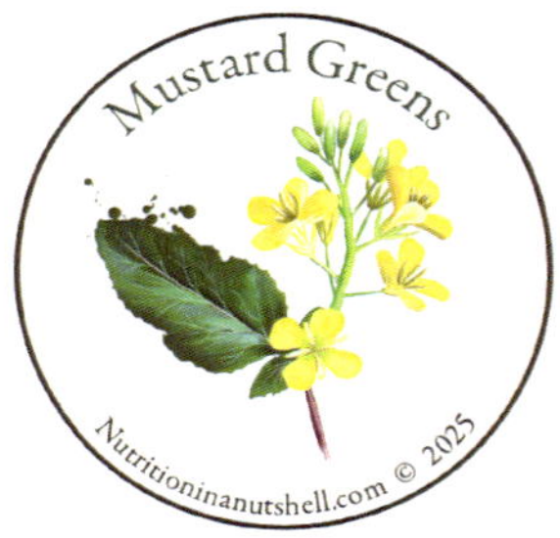

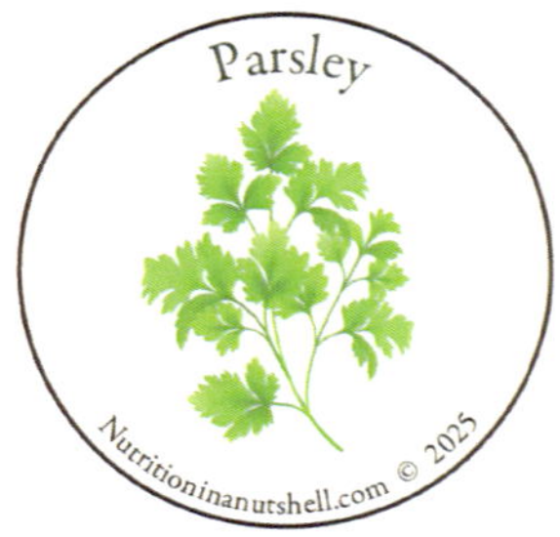

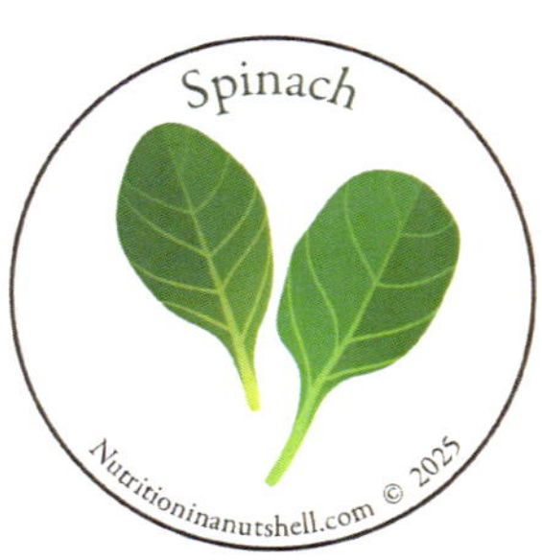

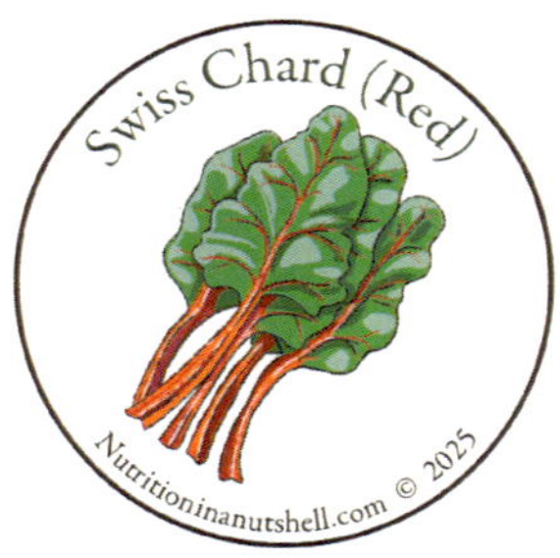

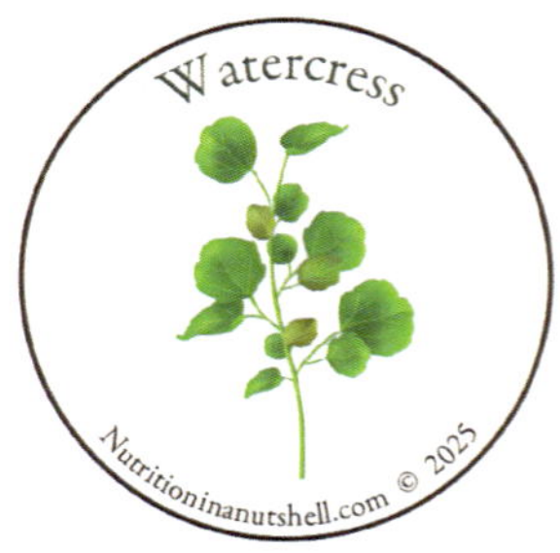

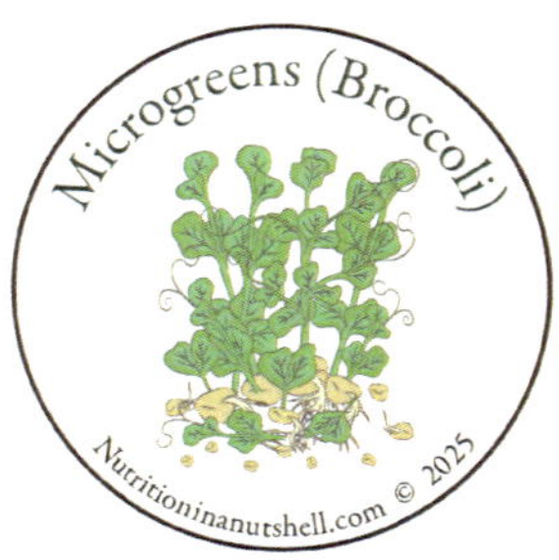

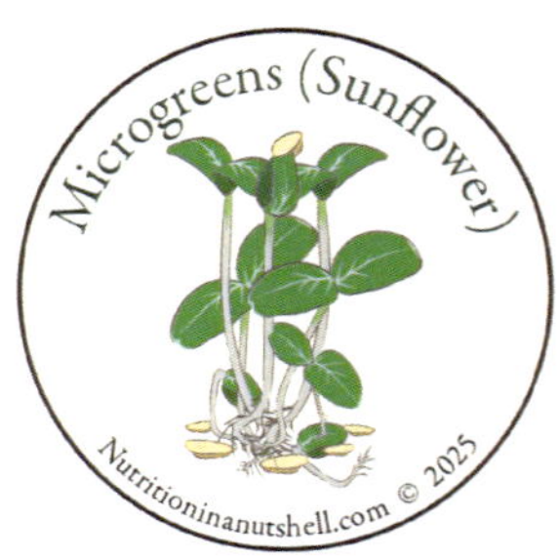

Plant Oils

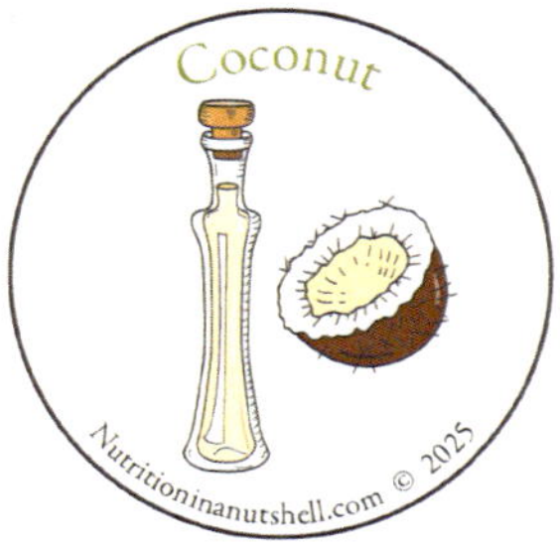
Coconut
Nutritioninanutshell.com © 2025

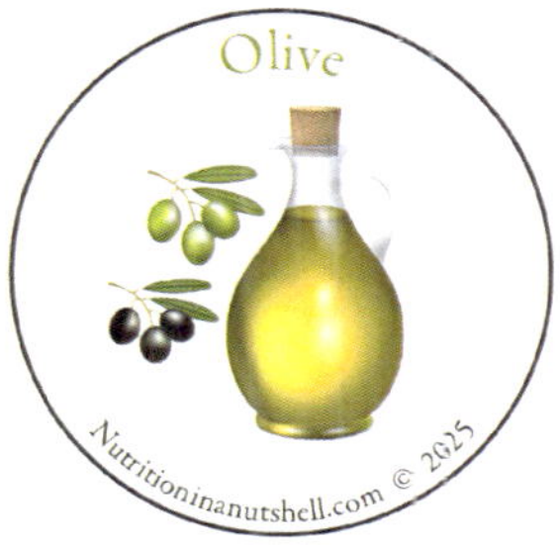
Olive
Nutritioninanutshell.com © 2025

Mushrooms

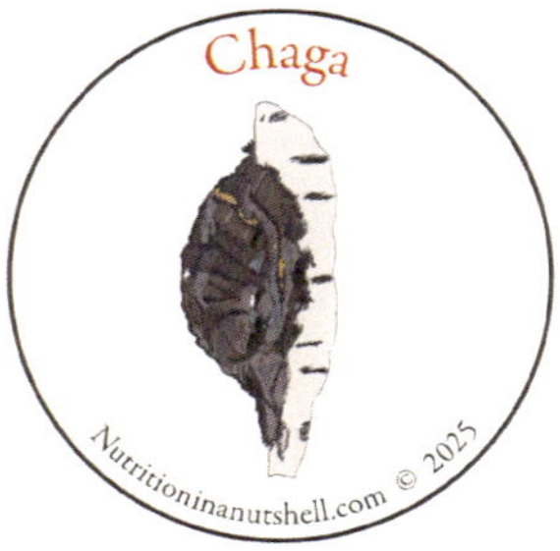
Chaga
Nutritioninanutshell.com © 2025

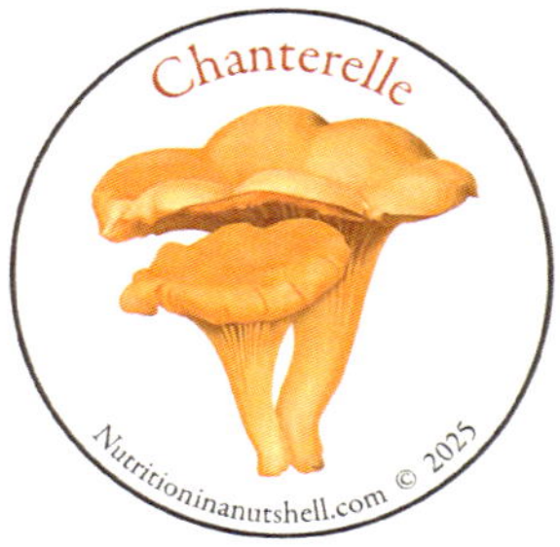
Chanterelle
Nutritioninanutshell.com © 2025

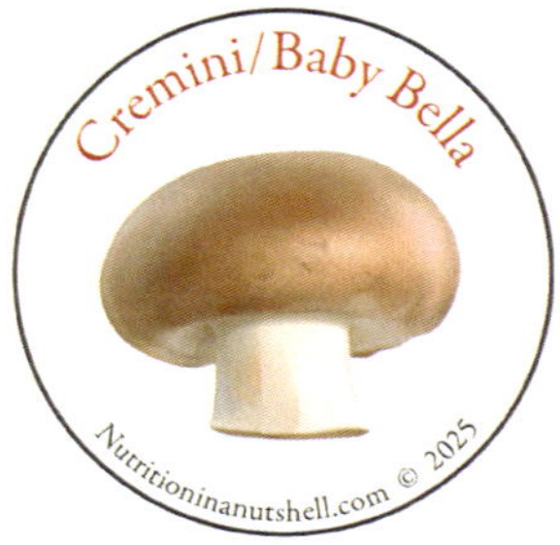
Cremini/Baby Bella
Nutritioninanutshell.com © 2025

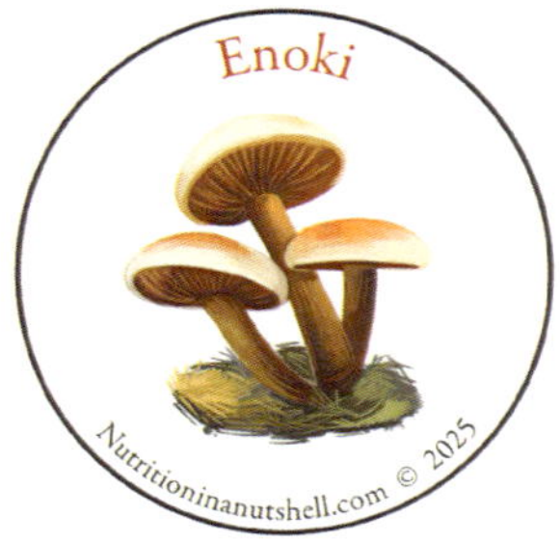
Enoki
Nutritioninanutshell.com © 2025

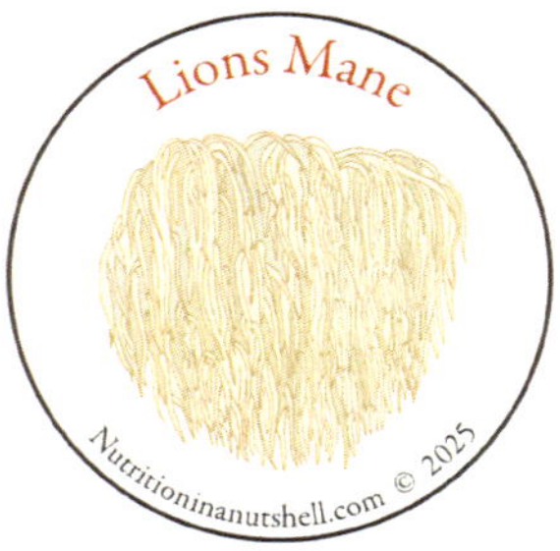
Lions Mane
Nutritioninanutshell.com © 2025

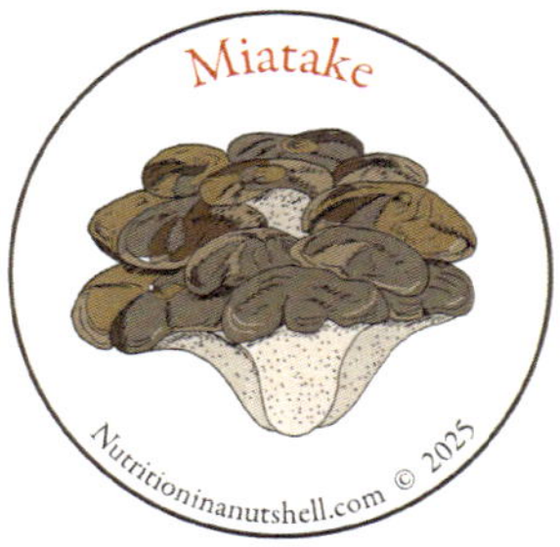
Miatake
Nutritioninanutshell.com © 2025

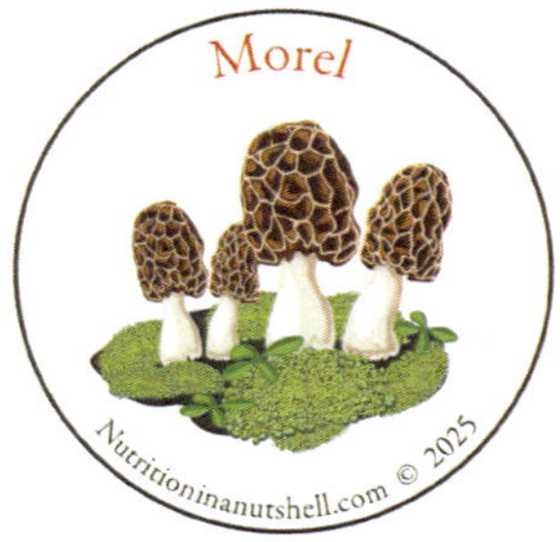
Morel
Nutritioninanutshell.com © 2025

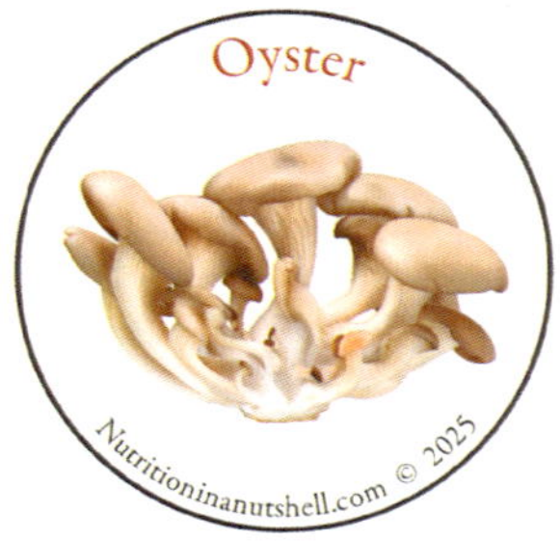
Oyster
Nutritioninanutshell.com © 2025

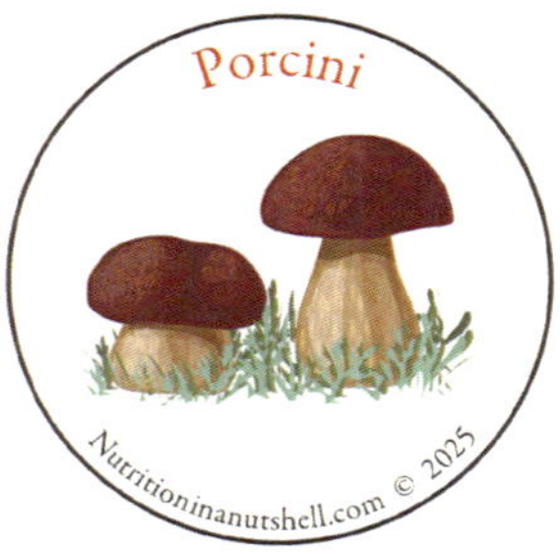
Porcini
Nutritioninanutshell.com © 2025

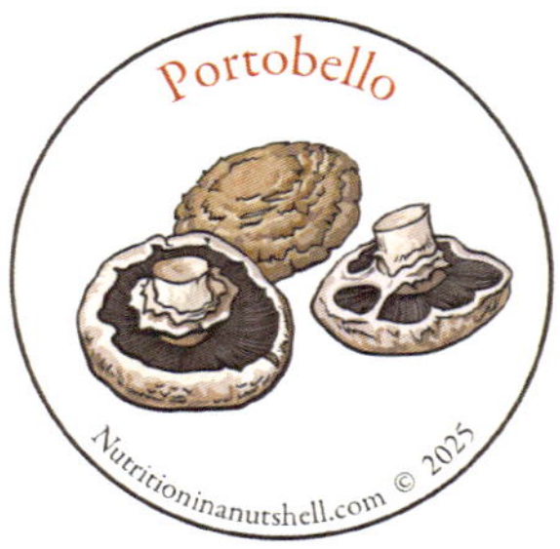
Portobello
Nutritioninanutshell.com © 2025

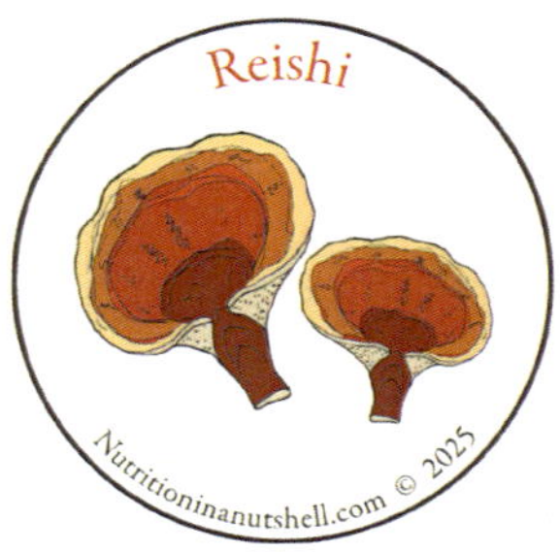
Reishi
Nutritioninanutshell.com © 2025

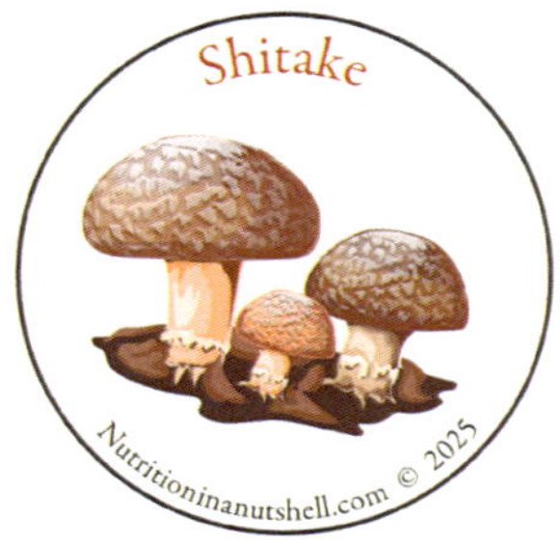
Shitake
Nutritioninanutshell.com © 2025

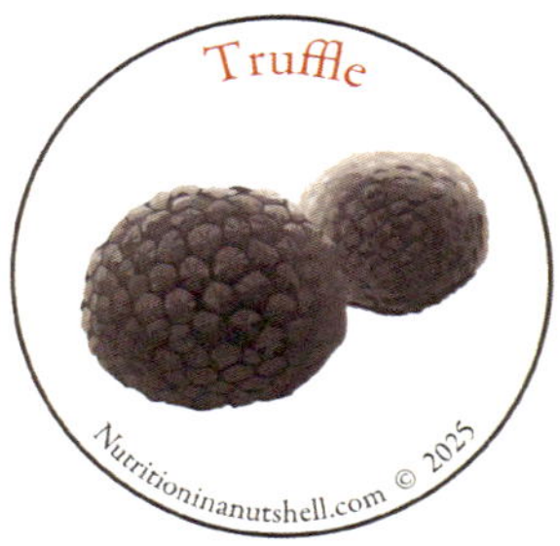
Truffle
Nutritioninanutshell.com © 2025

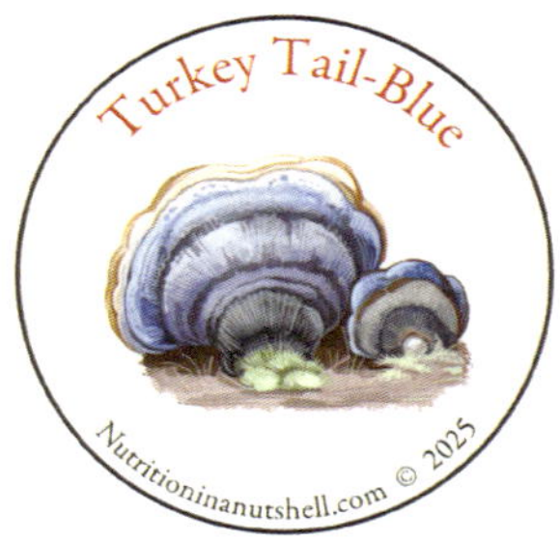
Turkey Tail-Blue
Nutritioninanutshell.com © 2025

Seaweeds & Chlorella (Algae)

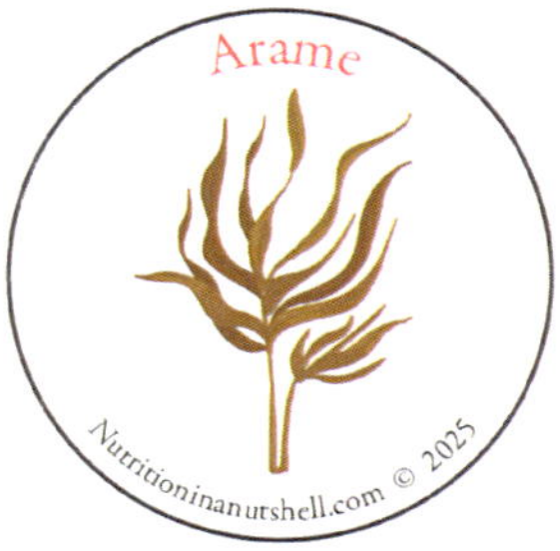

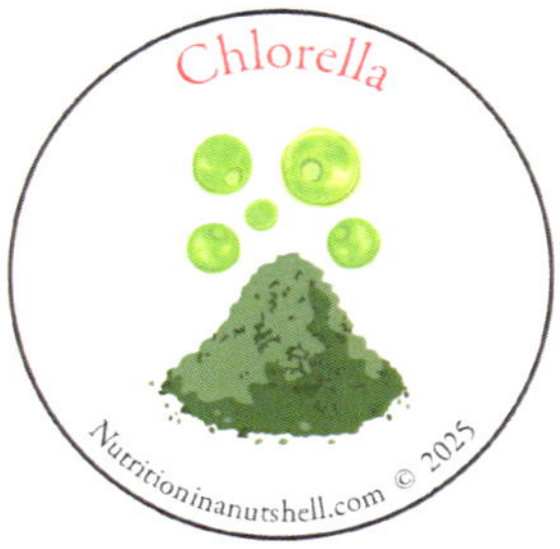

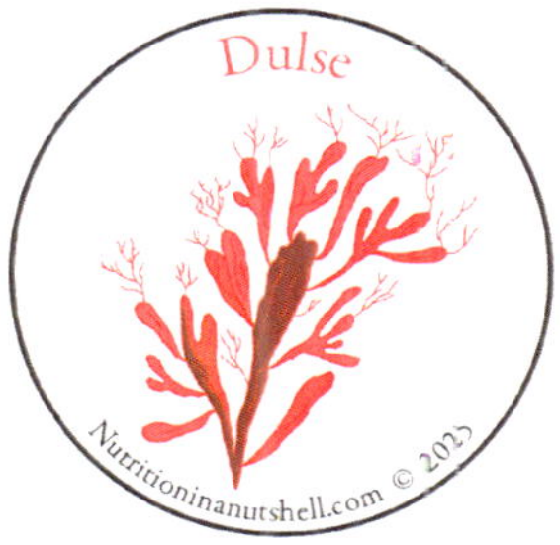

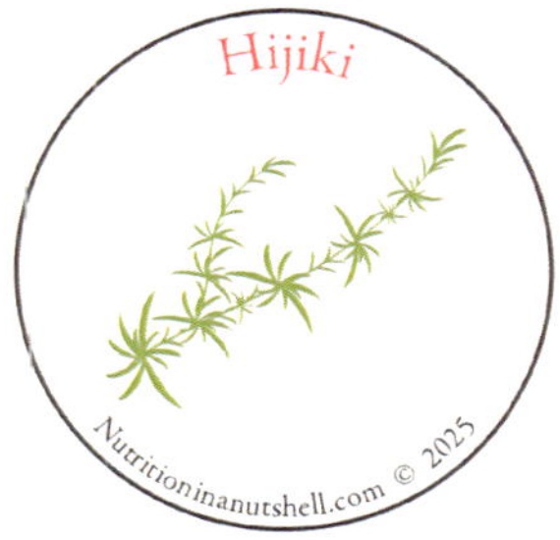

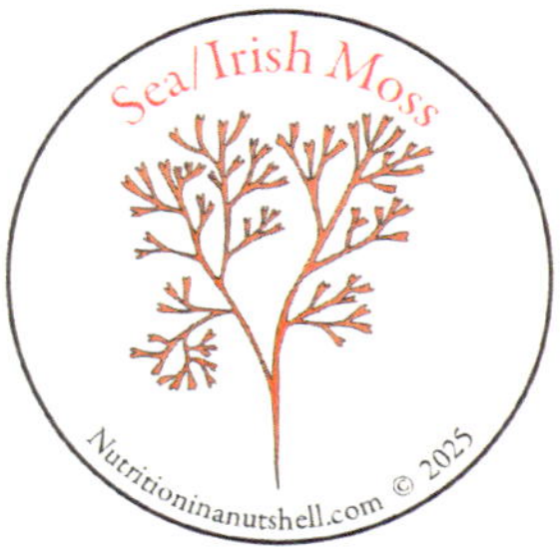

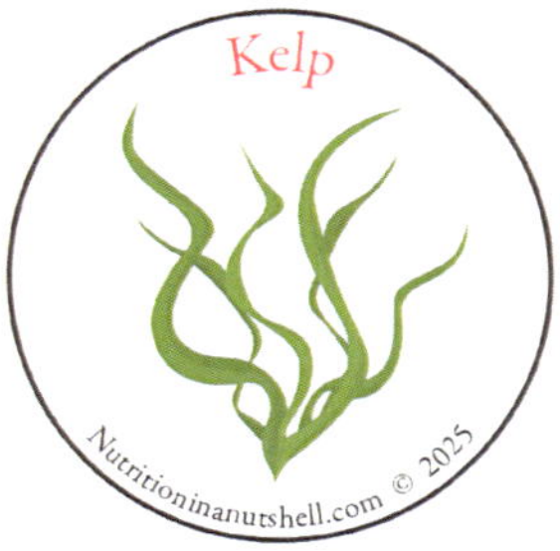

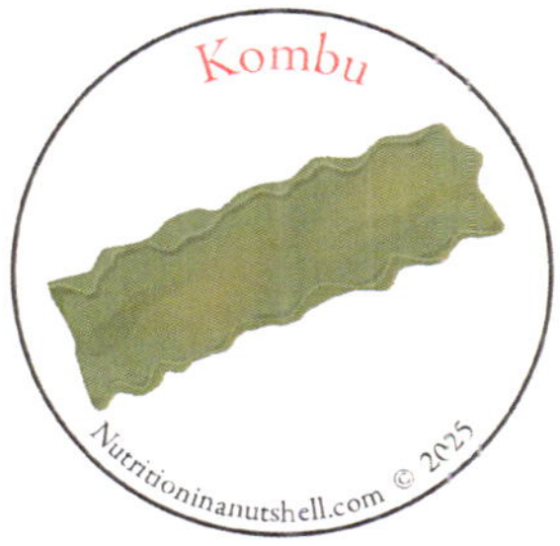

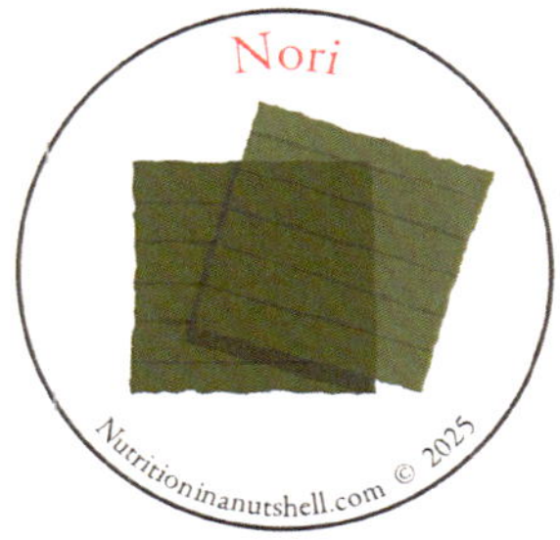

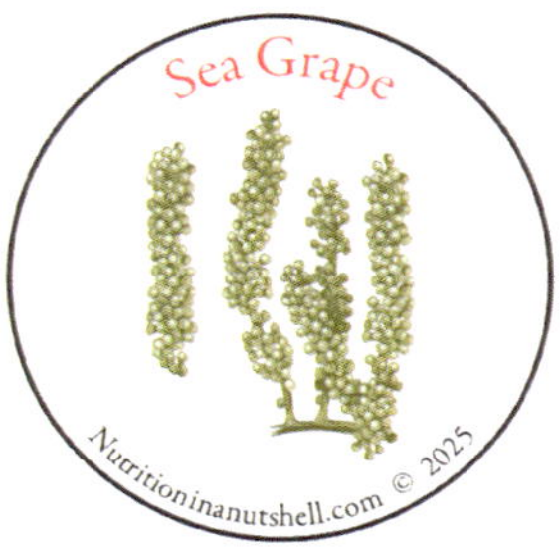

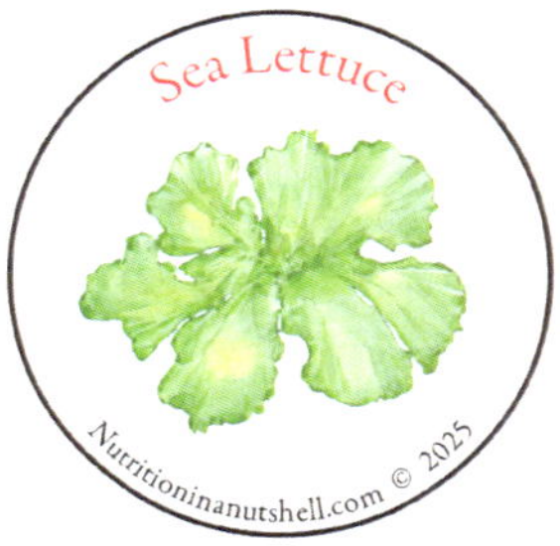

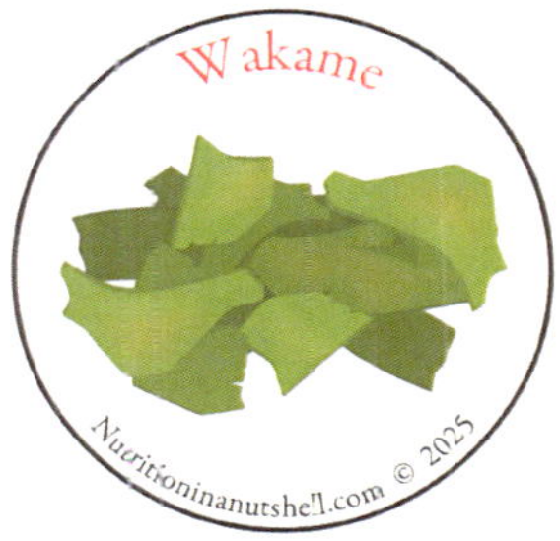

Cyanobacteria

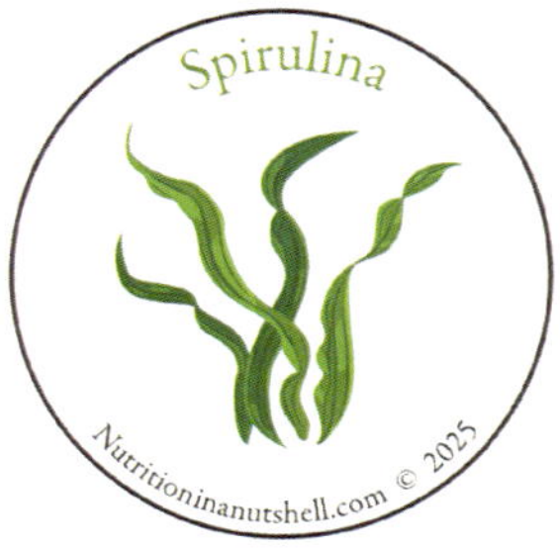

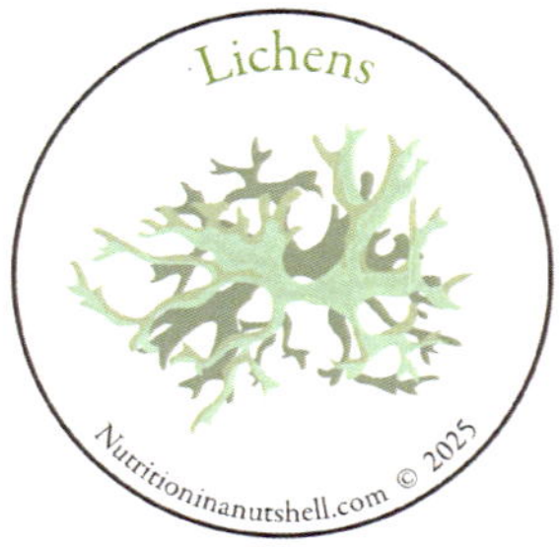

Spirulina are ancient photosynthesizing, single-celled cyanobacteria that live in colonies, inhabiting fresh and saltwater ecosystems. Although spirulina are part of the *Bacillati* Kingdom (*Bacteria* Domain), they have similar attributes to algae and are, therefore, often thought of as blue-green algae.

Lichens are colonies of green algae and/or cyanobacteria living symbiotically among filaments of multiple species of micro-fungi. They are generally used for medicinal purposes rather than as a food because they can cause indigestion. Additionally, lichens should only be harvested from pristine environments because they easily absorb pollutants.

Probiotic Ferments (Bacteria & Fungi)

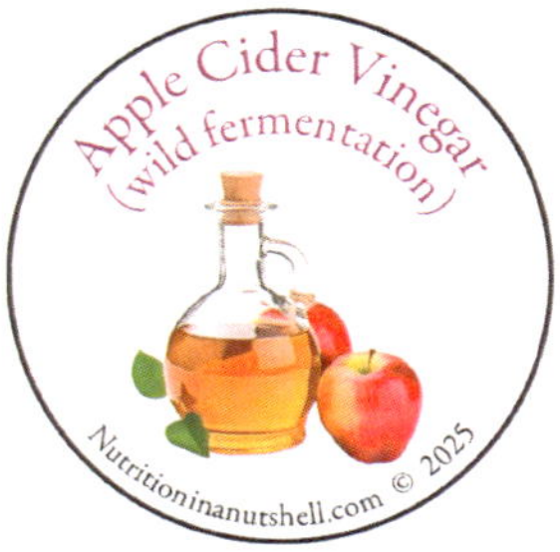

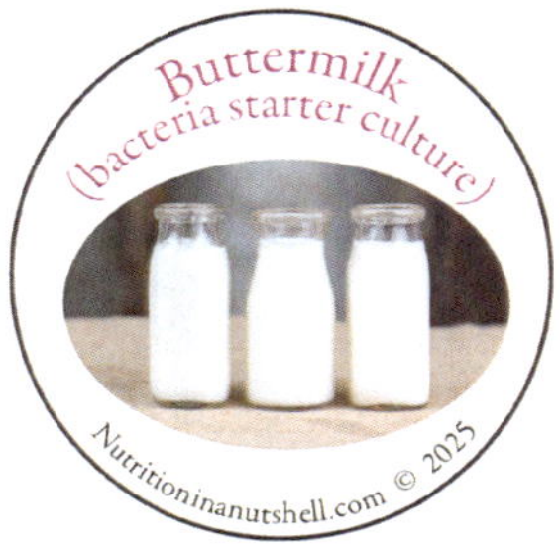

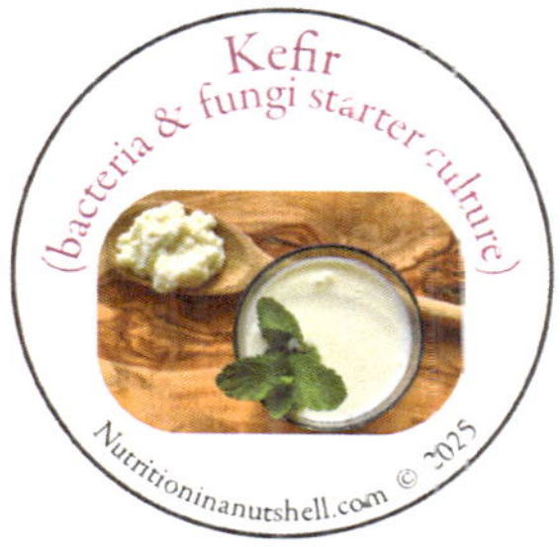

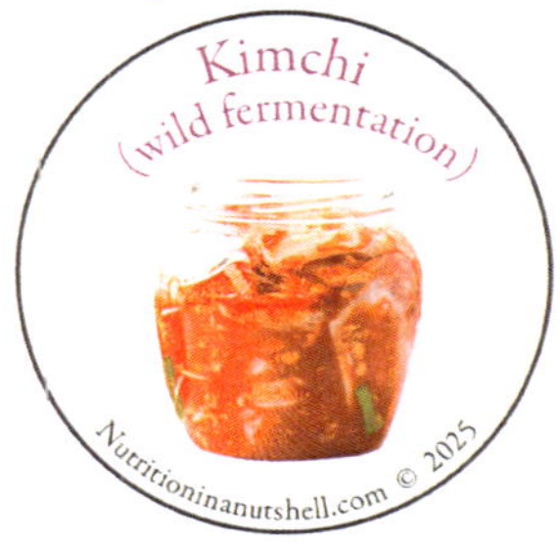

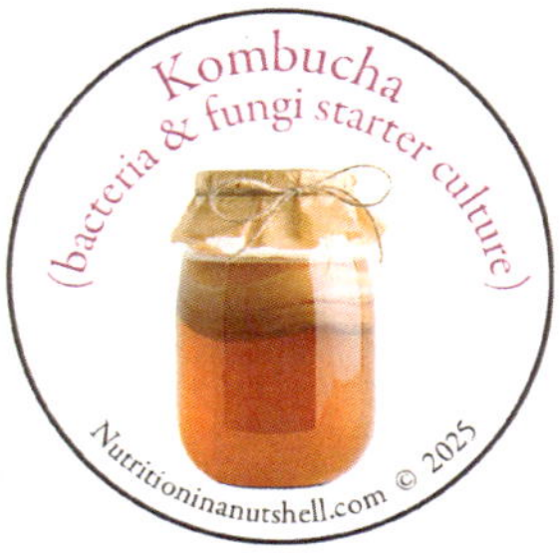

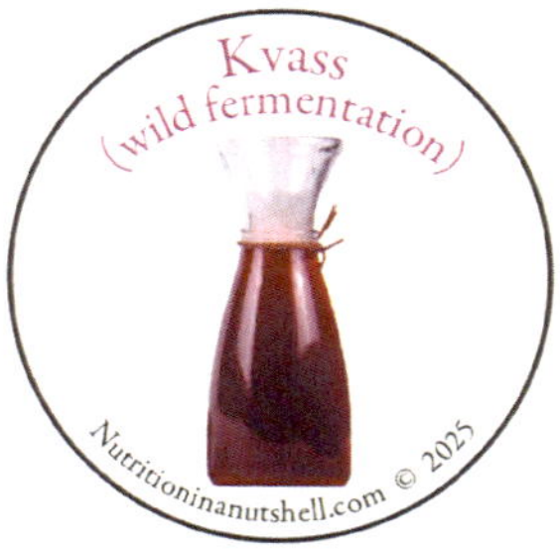

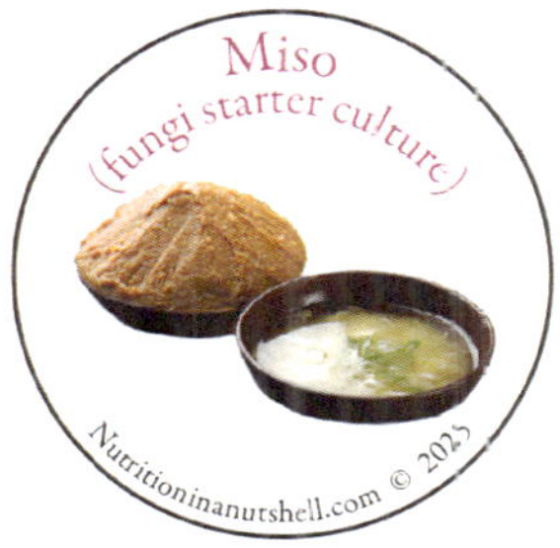

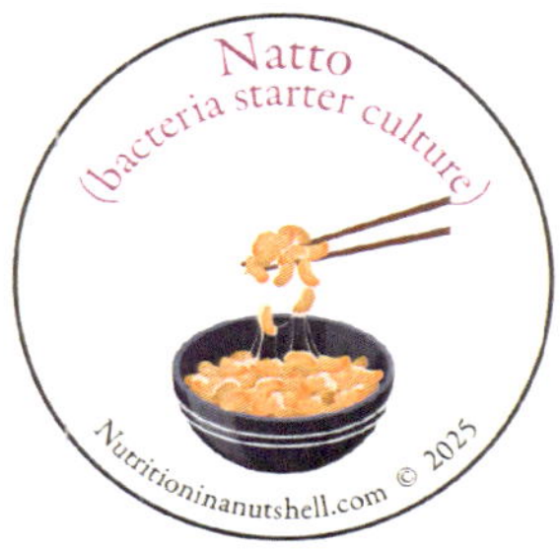

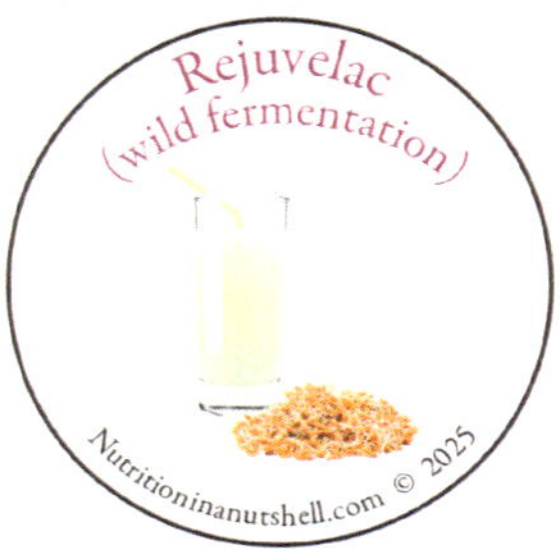

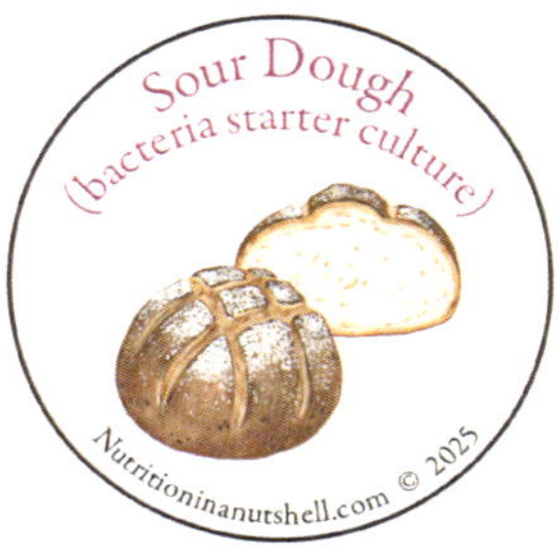

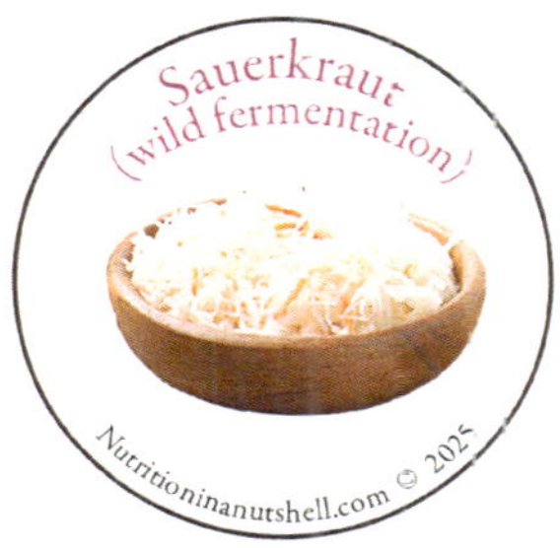

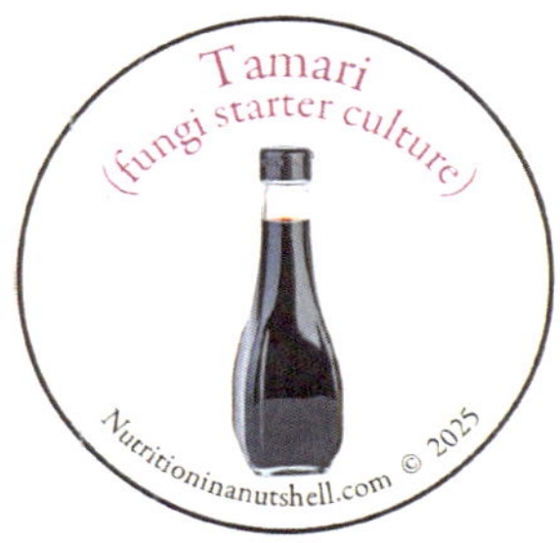

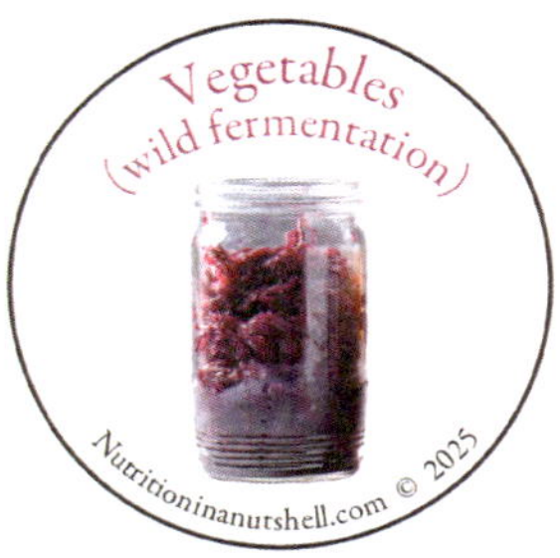

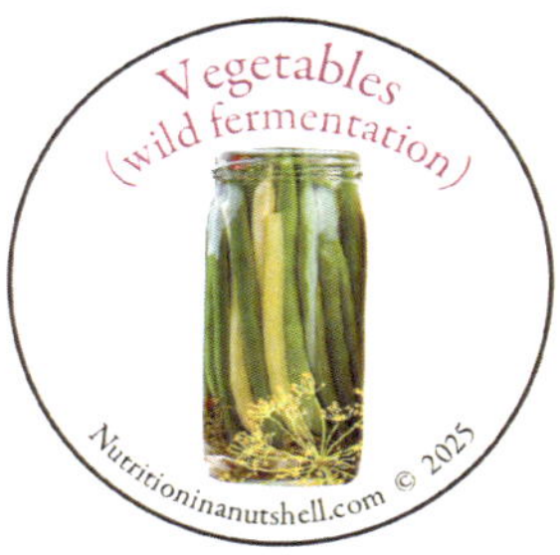

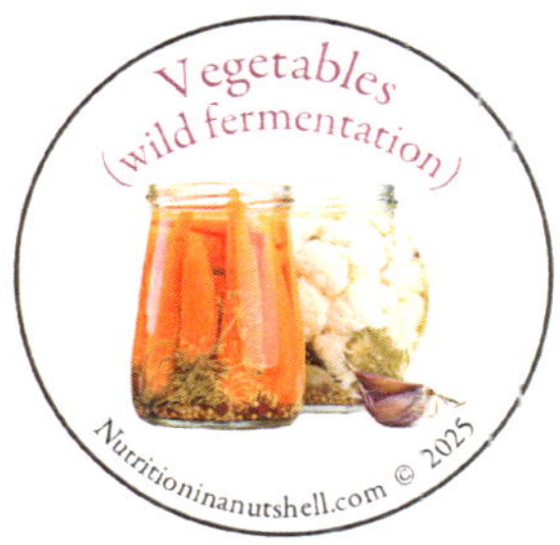

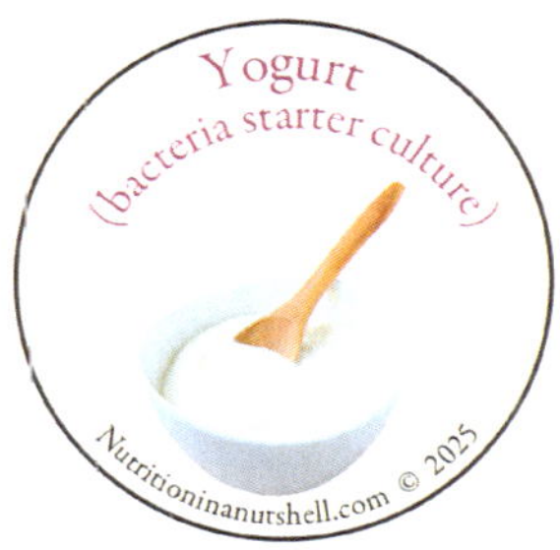

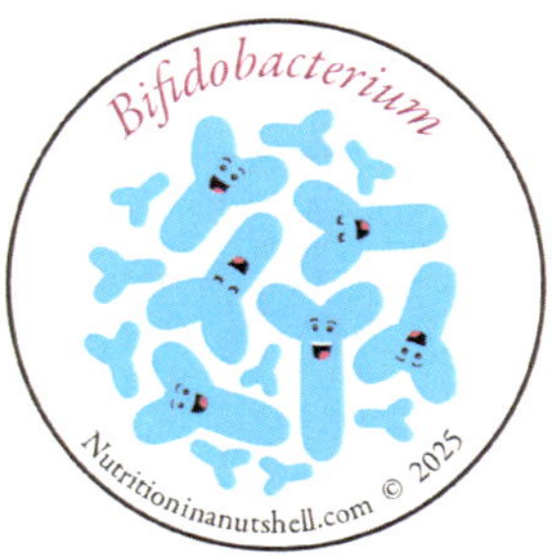

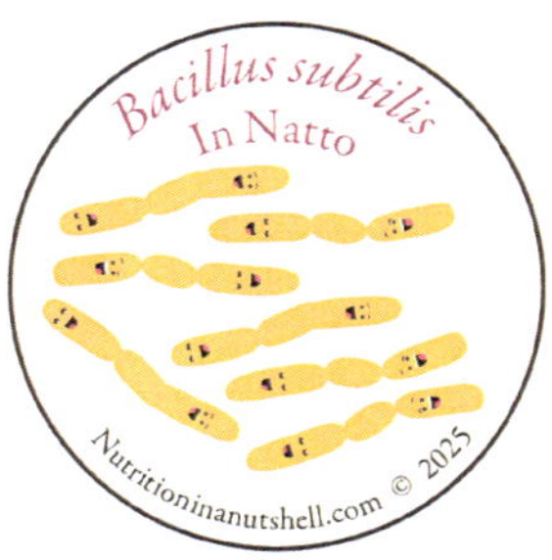

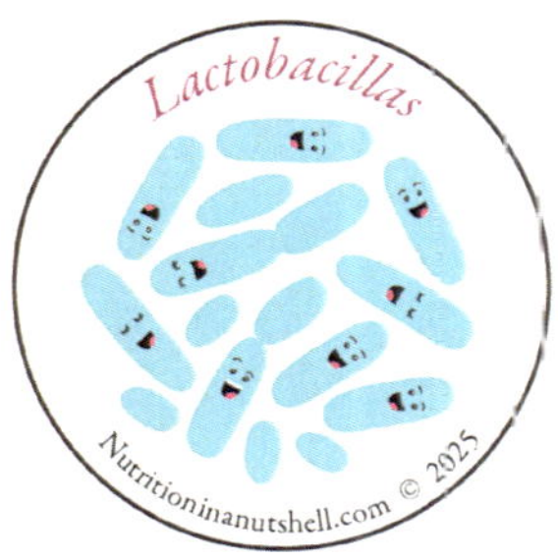

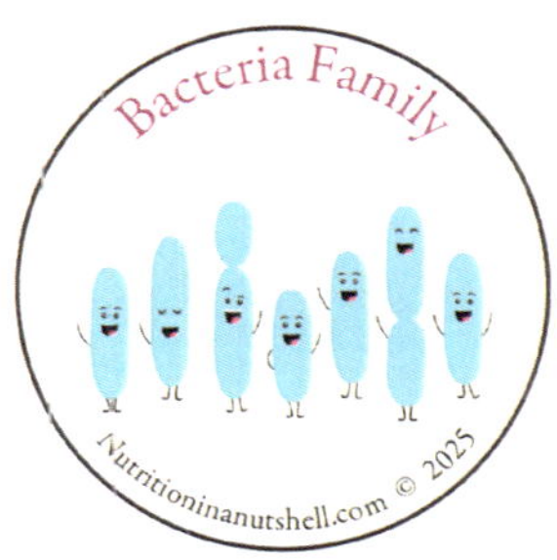

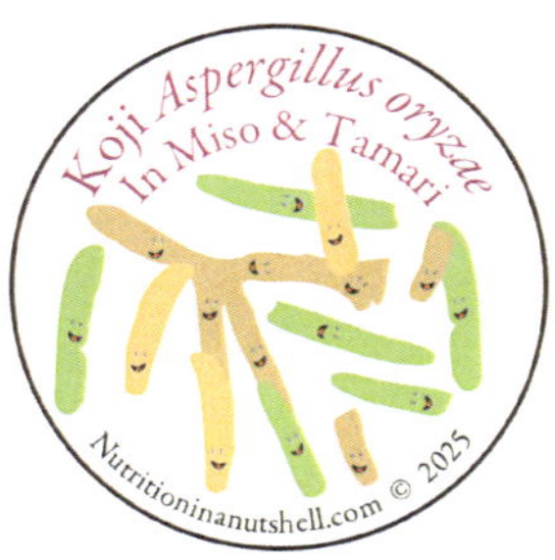

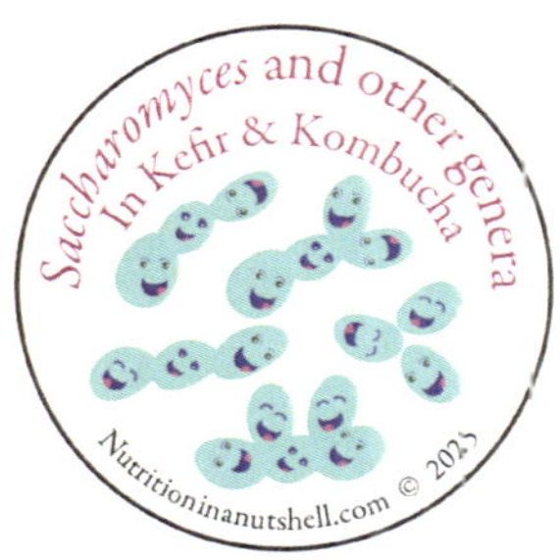

Natural Living

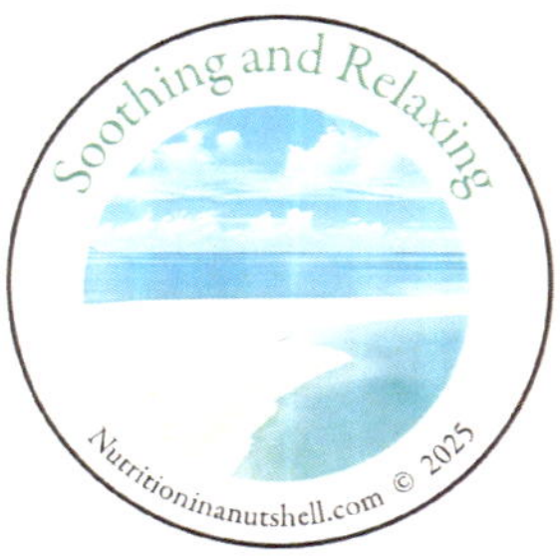

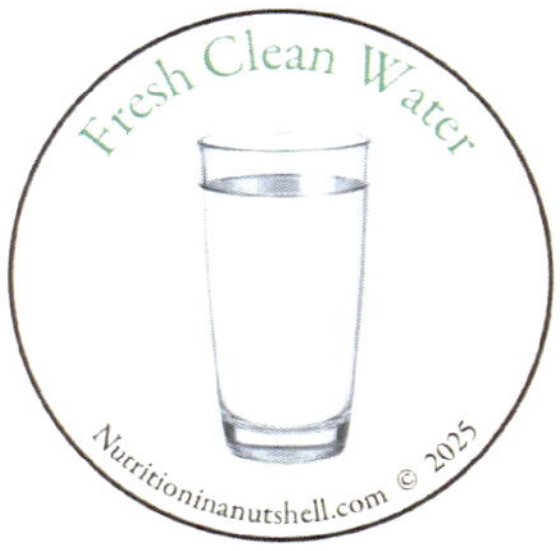

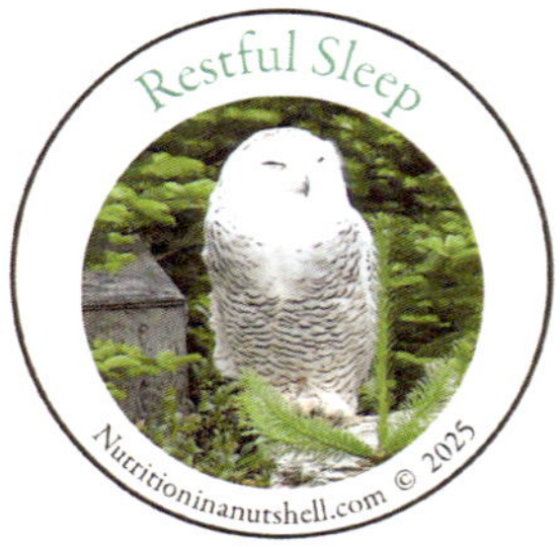

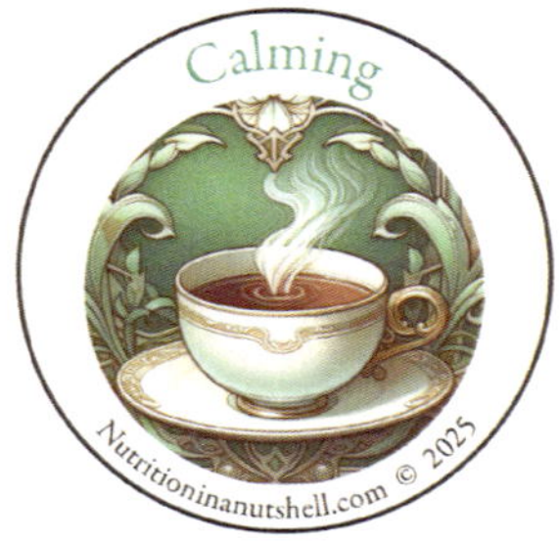

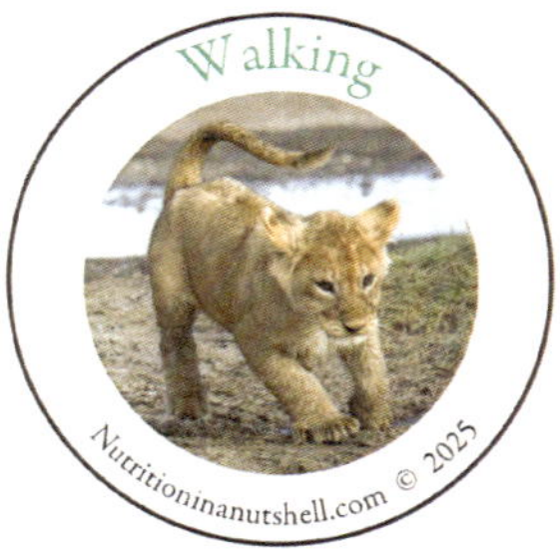

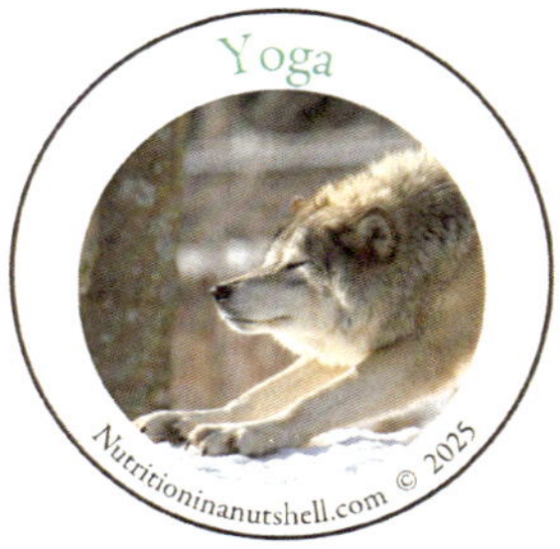

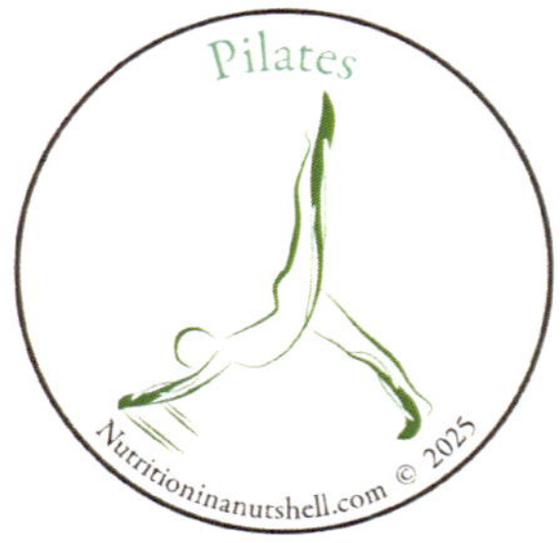

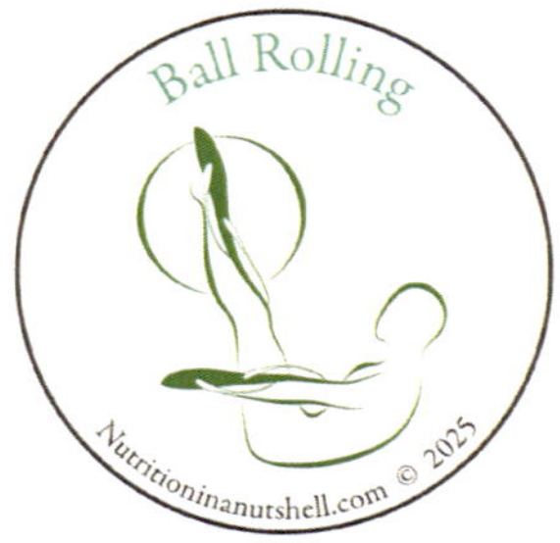

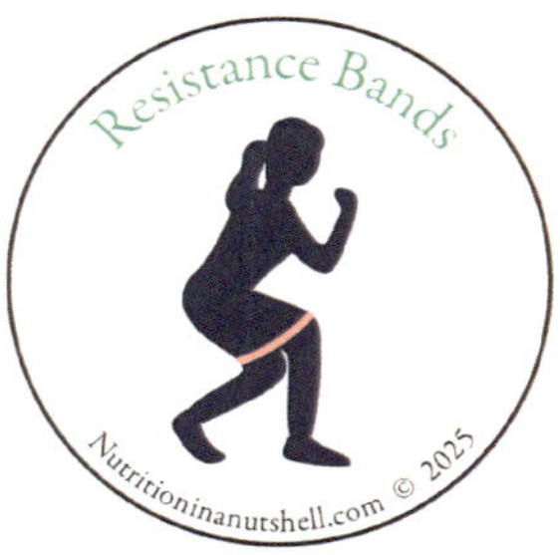

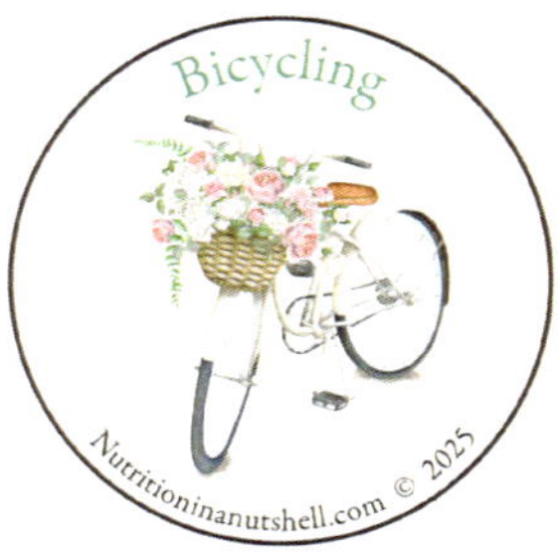

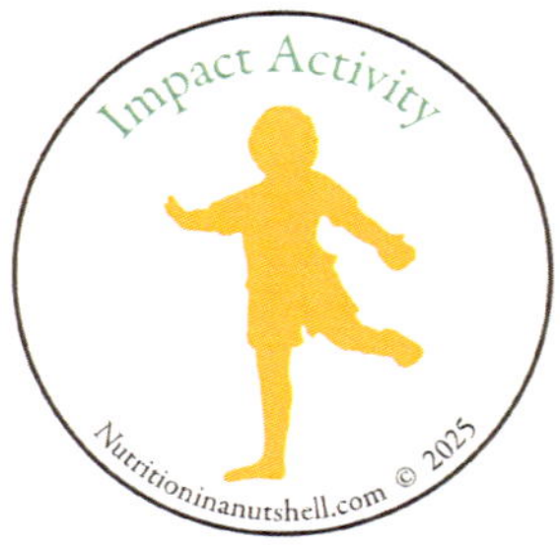

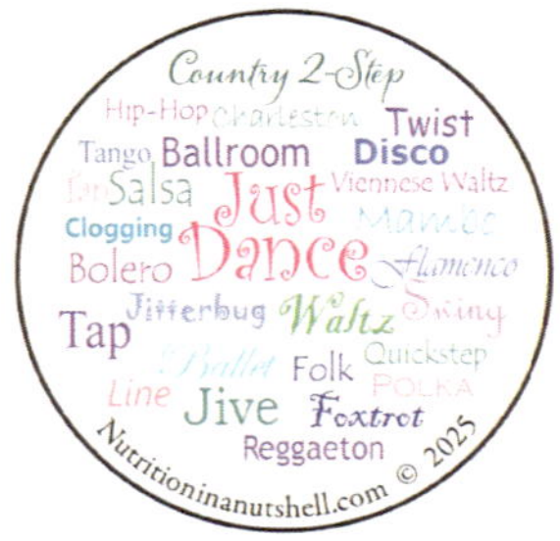

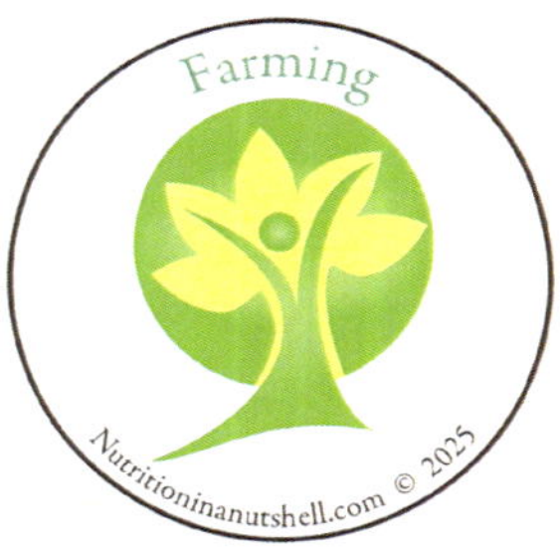

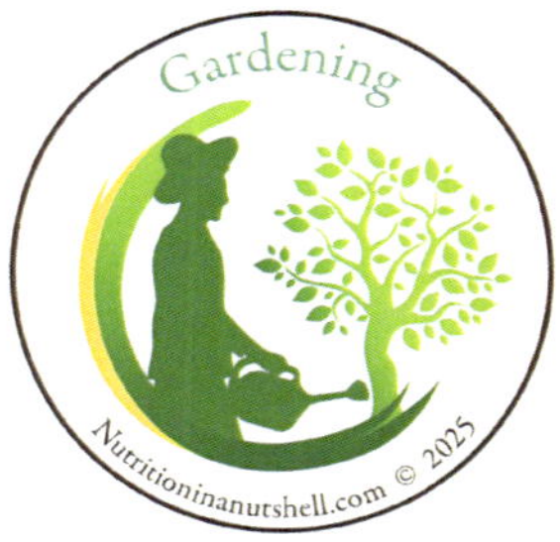

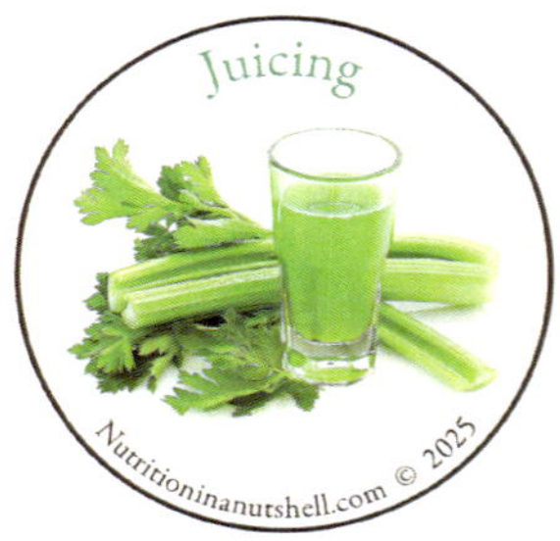

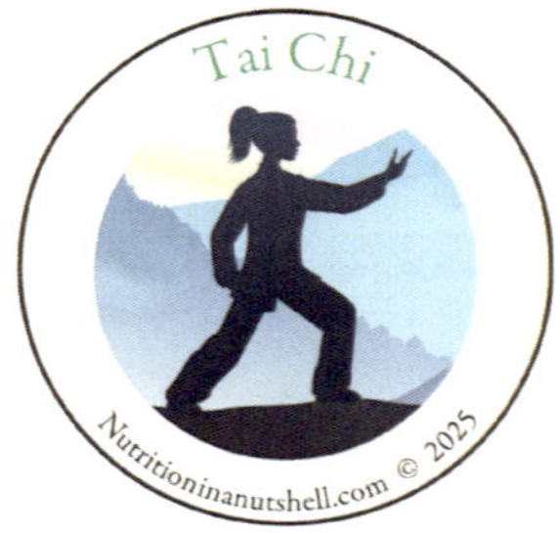

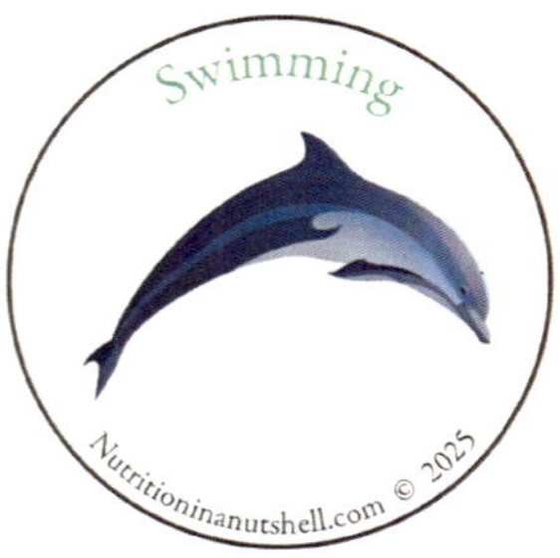

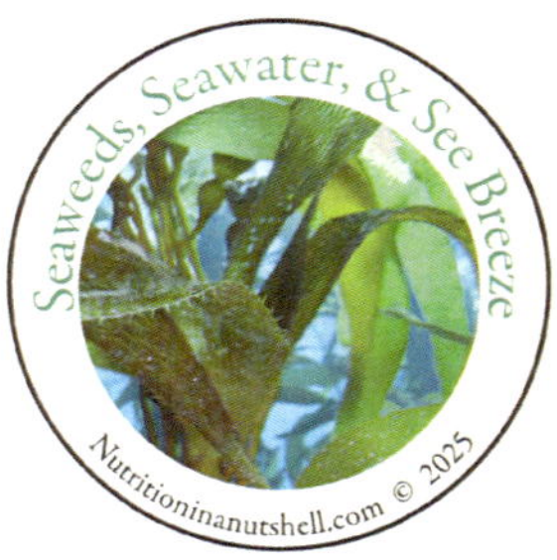

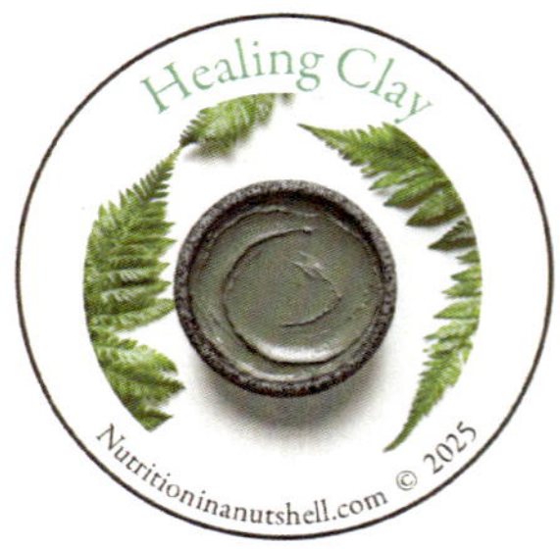

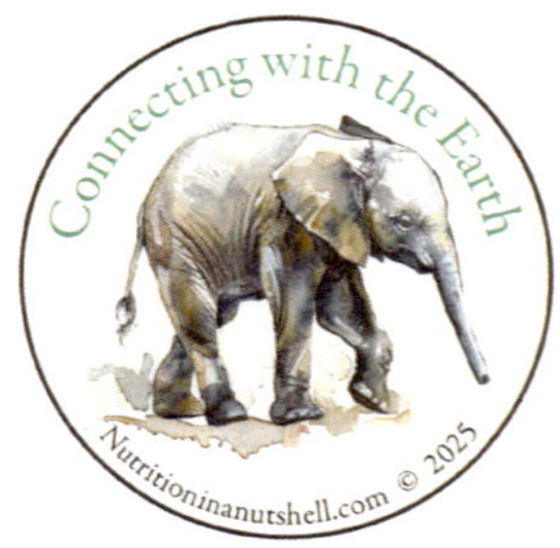

NutritioninaNutshell.com

Visit our website to find:

Natural Foods *from the* Tapestry *of* Life and companion ACTIVITY BOOK–Full Version

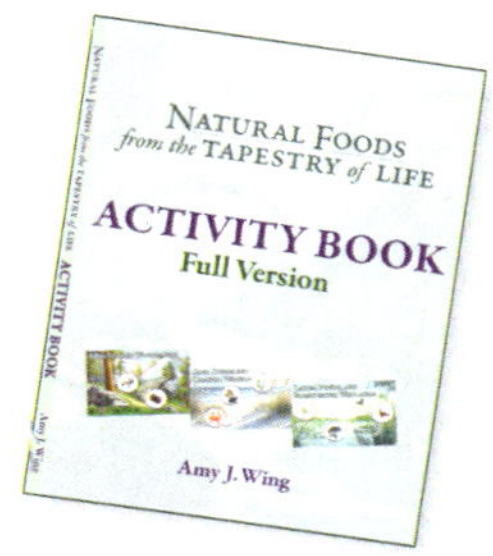

Nutrition Charts and Natural Foods Sticker Gift Package

These exquisite and detailed educational materials are designed for educators and anyone studying nature and holistic health

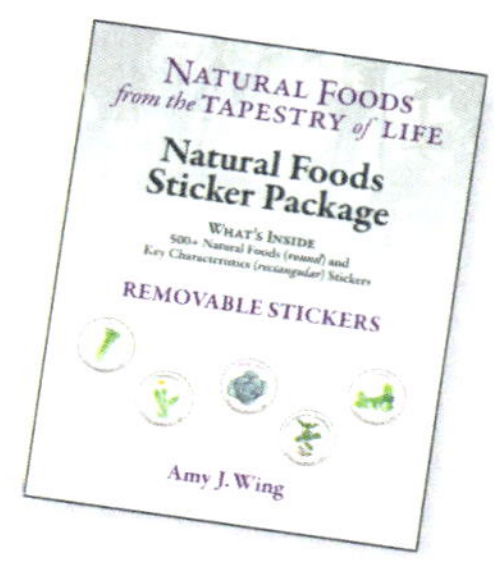

Organic, regenerative farm store links to traditional, artisan-prepared natural foods

www.ingramcontent.com/pod-product-compliance
Lightning Source LLC
LaVergne TN
LVRC080247220926
848482LV00042B/343

* 9 7 9 8 9 9 8 5 1 8 3 0 0 *